The Vanishing Black African Woman

A Compendium of the Global Skin-Lightening Practice

Volume One

Yetunde Mercy Olumide

Langaa Research & Publishing CIG
Mankon, Bamenda

Publisher:
Langaa RPCIG
Langaa Research & Publishing Common Initiative Group
P.O. Box 902 Mankon
Bamenda
North West Region
Cameroon
Langaagrp@gmail.com
www.langaa-rpcig.net

Distributed in and outside N. America by African Books Collective
orders@africanbookscollective.com
www.africanbookscollective.com

ISBN:9956-763-56-X

Dedication

The writing of this book was inspired by the Holy Spirit. He ***taught*** me, gave me ***understanding, guided*** *me* and ***directed*** me throughout the writing of the book. He ***empowered*** me and gave me the sustained ***strength*** to do the needed work, day and night, throughout the months when I had to gather my thoughts, conduct the necessary bibliographic search and write the book. With God there is no distinction between 'spiritual' /'religious' and 'secular' matters. God is omniscient. Science is the discovery of what God has created.

"Every gifted artisan in whom the LORD has put wisdom and understanding, to know how to do all manner of work for the service of the sanctuary, shall do according to all the LORD has commanded." (Exodus 36:1)

"I will instruct you and teach you in the way you should go;
I will guide you with My eye." (Ps 32:8)

To God be all the glory!

About the Book

Skin lightening is currently one of the most common forms of harmful body modification practices in the world and African women are among some of the most widely represented users of skin lightening products. The first Chapter describes the background problem, purpose and scope of the book, and the materials and methods used. There is a compilation of one or more Story Highlights at the beginning of every chapter. Since skin bleaching is an offshoot of slavery, racism, colorism and colonialism, the historical institutions that are related to skin bleaching are well characterized. Chapter 3 defines the global magnitude of the problem. Nigeria is regarded as the hot house of the skin bleaching practice, hence the chapter on Nigeria can truly be regarded as the microcosm of the skin bleaching culture in Sub-Saharan Africa. The skin bleaching stories on representative countries in West, Southern, East, Central and North Africa are also discussed. In a globalized world, cosmetic skin bleaching has no boundaries. Hence, some insight is given about skin bleaching in the Caribbean, India, South East Asia, Latin America, North America and the United Kingdom. Furthermore, skin bleaching is not only practiced by homeland Africans but also diasporic Africans. The Determinants that provide social and cultural impetus towards skin bleaching are extensively characterized, since these factors must be taken into consideration if meaningful intervention strategies are to be created and employed to counteract the trend towards skin bleaching. The chemicals, products and methods used for skin bleaching and the adverse health effects are clearly described. Finally, guideline recommendations that would help attenuate the burden and possibly eliminate the injuries related to skin bleaching are prescribed. Potential developments and future directions are discussed.

About the Author

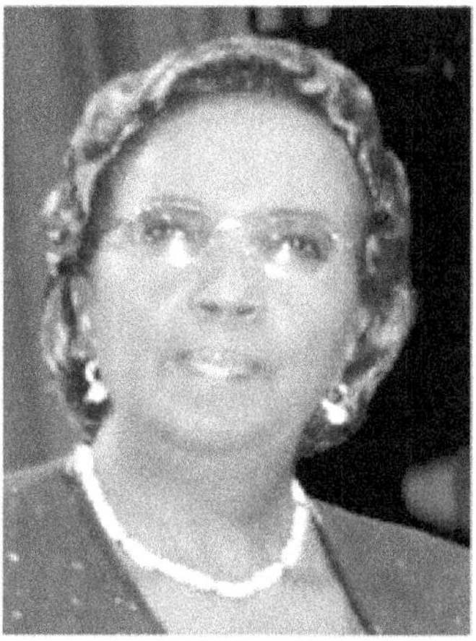

Yetunde Mercy Olumide (Née: ỌKẸGẸ) is an Emeritus Professor of Medicine of the University of Lagos, Nigeria, and a Consultant Physician, Dermatologist and Venereologist. She graduated from the Medical School of the University of Ibadan in 1968. Yetunde commenced her dermatology training in 1971 at the University Cantonal Hospital in Geneva, Switzerland, under the tutelage of Professor Paul Laugier for two years. She later pursued the University of London Postgraduate Diploma Course in Dermatology at the London Institute of Dermatology, St. John's Hospital for Diseases of the Skin, and successfully concluded the course in 1974.

In 1975, Yetunde commenced the Residency Training Programme of the National Postgraduate Medical College in Internal Medicine (Physic), and successfully concluded the Fellowship programme in 1979. She is also a Fellow of the West African College of Physicians, a Fellow of the American Academy of Dermatology, a Fellow of the Nigerian Academy of Science and a Member of the British Association of Dermatologists. As a University Lecturer in Internal Medicine and Dermatology, her special research interest was in the field of Contact and Occupational Dermatology. Her Thesis on this subject earned her a University of Ibadan Doctorate Degree in Medicine (MD) in 1990.

Yetunde has published over seventy scientific research papers in learned journals. She has authored and co-authored several relevant textbooks in her specialty. She is the sole author of all the **three** relevant textbooks for training medical students and Continuing Medical Education (CME) of family physicians in Dermatology, Venereology, and HIV/AIDS.

Yetunde is a member of a collaborative interdisciplinary and transnational research team on the skin bleaching culture in Sub-Saharan Africa. Yetunde, who is indeed the **first** and to date, the **only** female Emeritus Professor in the 54 years history of the University of Lagos, is a recipient of several awards both nationally and internationally. She was adjudged the Best Teacher in the Department of Medicine, College of Medicine of the University of Lagos; the Most Outstanding Female Medical Practitioner at the first ever Pan African Award for Women Entrepreneurs and Achievers—WEAN'07 Awards, and Life Fellowship Status of the American Academy of Dermatology for "commitment to continuing education and dedication to professional excellence."

God's mighty revelation to Yetunde Olumide on the existing prophecy of HIV/AIDS in the Holy Bible culminated in her writing a 3,500-page book (2 Vols) of Prophecy to the Church in 2002. This was followed by over 35 Christian pastoral books, papers, and ministrations at various churches, schools, and tertiary institutions, imparting Christian moral values.

Acknowledgement

I am a member of a collaborative interdisciplinary and transnational research team on the skin bleaching culture in Sub-Saharan Africa, through the kind invitation of Prof. Susan Levine, a social anthropologist and Prof Lester Davids, a molecular cell biologist–both of the University of Cape Town in South Africa. This book is a direct outcome of a Workshop held in March 2015, hosted by the University of Cape Town and funded by the Programme for the Enhancement of Research Capacity (PERC). Susan Levine asked me to prepare an original working paper on my research for discussion at the Workshop. I ended up preparing a 326-page document (within three months) for the Workshop. On sighting my document, Susan's spontaneous reaction was that I should get the document published as a book. I instantly saw this suggestion by Susan as Holy Spirit inspired, hence I developed an extraordinary interest in **all** the presentations at the Workshop, so as to be able to expand the scope of the book. Hitherto, I had perceived the problem of skin bleaching purely from the medical perspectives. The Workshop was instrumental in broadening my horizon on the subject to understand the complex issue bound up with skin colour, skin-lightening and public health discourse and to appreciate the pivotal relevance of other disciplines such as social anthropologists, sociologists, historians, psychologists and media practitioners. I received tremendous encouragement from other members of the research team which include Prof. Lynne Thomas, a professor of history at the University of Washington and Prof Ncoza Dlova, a dermatologist of the University of KwaZulu Natal. Indeed that singular workshop truly *enhanced* my research capacity. I thank them all.

Prof Ngide Okubadejo of the College of Medicine, University of Lagos, proof-read the original copy of the document for the Workshop. Evelyn Ugomma Osuagwu, Omolabake Elizabeth Adefuye and Gabriel Ogor Edigbo worked tirelessly to typeset the book. I thank them all.

My fervent prayer for all those who have been directly or indirectly involved with the preparation of this book is for the good Lord to enlarge your coasts, hear your prayers, show you His great favours and meet you all at your points of need.

Table of Contents (Volumes One & Two)

Chapter 3

Chapter 4

Chapter 5

Volume Two Contents

Chapter 1

The Vanishing Black African Woman
A Compendium Of The Global Skin-Lightening Practice

Background
Purpose and Scope
Materials and Methods

Background

Up till the early 1960s the people who inhabited the geographic space called Nigeria were homogenously **chocolate brown**-skinned (Fitzpatrick scale VI). Light skin was associated with the Fulani people of Northern Nigeria, some ethnic groups in South Eastern Nigeria, albinos and biracial people who were largely found in the coastal regions of Nigeria due to first contact with foreigners who arrived by boat to trade with Nigeria. Indeed in the South Eastern regions of Nigeria some **genetically** light skinned people are regarded as "outcast"—'Osus'—due to some ill-understood ancestral reasons. Osus were stigmatized and ostracized, and it was regarded an abomination for anyone to marry an 'Osu'. This prejudice against the Osus even still exists up to the present time. Furthermore, albinos are regrettably ostracized and stigmatized like the Osus up to the present day. Decades ago, Nigerians were very proud of their brown colour and bleaching of the skin was literally unheard of. People who were genetically light skinned were exceptional in the minority.

However, in **current** times, It may not be hyperbolic to state that the vast majority about 70% of women in Nigeria are light complexioned. One just needs to do a cursory scan of the complexion of women at any public gathering e.g parties, churches, university lecture halls, public transport, national assembly sessions featured on TV, politicians and wives of politicians, television newscasters/presenters, Nollywood film actresses, female patients at the skin clinic etc. One is likely to find that two out of every three women have various shades of light skin from light brown (caramel colour or *café-au-lait*) to pale light (Fitzpatrick II-III). (See chapter 12 on COLOUR DISCOURSE—MELANIN for Fitzpatrick classification of skin colour). In Nigeria, it is common practice to print a serial lifetime photogallery in a commemorative brochure when celebrating landmark birthdays (e.g 50, 60, 70) and in a funeral programme. It is common finding to discover, **for the first time**, that the *seemingly* light-skinned celebrant or dead woman was actually a dark-skinned school girl in childhood who has transformed over the years to the light skin tone in adulthood due to the use of skin lightening products. It is also not unusual to find these seemingly pale-skinned Nigerian women wearing blond wigs. The physical transformation achievable from the current body modification technology is phenomenal. Hence dark skinned women in Nigeria are gradually going into extinction—this observation of metamorphosis/transformation from the traditional "trade mark" of **chocolate brown** skin among Nigerian women inspired the title of this book-THE VANISHING BLACK AFRICAN WOMAN. This colour transformation is not an isolated phenomenon in Nigeria but has been observed in other African nations, hence the adjective "African" (not just 'Nigerian').

Nigeria, the largest black African country, has been described as "the world capital for skin bleaching". According to the World Health Organization (WHO), 77 percent of women in Nigeria use skin-lightening products, the world's highest percentage. Against the position of all credible data that most Nigerians survive on less than US$2 a day, most people find it hard to believe this new report from another world body.

The World Health Organization defines bleaching as the "Intentional alteration of one's natural skin colour to one relatively if not substantially, lighter in colour, through the use of chemical skin lightening agents, either manufactured, homemade or the combination of the two."

Skin-lightening involves the application of various cosmetic products to the skin with the aim of obtaining a lightened complexion by reducing its melanin content. Skin-lightening is currently one of the most common forms of potentially harmful body modification practices in the world and African women are among some of the most widely represented users of skin-lightening products. Despite government efforts to ban these products and public health campaigns to discourage their use, the desire for light skin has accelerated over the last few decades and the market for skin-lightening products has boomed in many parts of the world. Studies indicate that their use is growing fastest among young, urban literate and illiterate women in the global South where light-skin operates as a form of symbolic capital. It is believed that the racial legacy of colonialism alone is not a sufficient explanation for the recent rise in the use of skin-lighteners.

The spectrum of skin bleaching chemicals is no longer restricted to mercury, hydroquinone and corticosteroids. A product pandemic has led to a tsunami of new skin-lightening chemicals which have now flooded the global market, some in the form of injectables and pills. This product pandemic has led to a plethora of cheap, affordable over-the-counter (OTC) products touted to be the "next best thing" for lightening the skin. Even some local individuals have begun manufacturing their own brand of skin creams for the home market creating a new "background industry". More worrisome is the emergence of reports that some mothers have now resorted to bleaching the skin of their babies. Salons are now known to use corticosteroid creams on the scalp of their clients to promote faster hair growth. Studies suggest that much misinformation exists around the health consequences of skin lighteners and users rarely understand the important role of the pigment—melanin, in the skin. Such are the advances in the technology of skin lightening that surgical laser procedures have also been introduced.

Skin bleaching in Africa cuts across all sociodemographic strata. In current times, an African girl child is most likely to have mother and grandmother who are skin bleachers. When she goes to school and finds her teacher who is also a skin bleacher, and goes to the hospital and sees the doctor and nurse who are skin bleachers, she inevitably develops the impression that it is healthy to bleach and that skin bleaching is an accepted way of life and part of the culture. Such a girl child is bound to see skin bleaching products as part of the armamentarium of womanhood (just like feminine sanitary pads)! Sadly, a whole generation and indeed future generations of young girls are being proselytized to be skin bleachers! The current scenario is dire and if allowed to continue unchecked has disastrous social, economic, political and health consequences for the continent.

The psychology for social acceptance, more opportunities, and improved self-image is already an epidemic that has reached a critical mass. There are social, economic and psychological complexes—*enemy within* affecting individuals / families / organizations / communities and nations alike, which make people want to change their skin colour from dark to light.

The cosmetic practice of skin lightening, poses increasing concern to dermatologists and scientists around the world. While most medical practitioners and pharmacists tend to affiliate this harmful practice with sub-Saharan Africa and third-world countries, the phenomenon is far-reaching. Evidence of skin lightening is rife, from rural, underprivileged areas and even at the foreground of pop culture. Moreover, the range of scientifically untested products and constituents flooding the market, makes for a disastrous situation to the uninformed lay public. The increase in dermatological and systemic organ damage is increasing throughout the continent.

Although there is ample evidence that skin bleaching poses a serious health risk, there is a paucity of research on incidence and prevalence of adverse health outcomes from skin bleaching, and there is currently no tracking system to fill this gap to further understand the scope of this problem. Furthermore, health authorities do not see skin bleaching as a priority because people are not dying in masses from associated conditions, and in places with limited access to health resources, skin diseases can be a low priority. However, injury associated with current skin bleaching practices will likely decrease quality of life and contribute significantly to sickness and health costs. Further, the largely unregulated chemical content of skin bleaching products, especially in developing countries, makes the direct marketing and promotion of such practices especially dangerous.

It is regrettable that skin bleaching has been viewed largely as an individual problem and has focused largely on changing individual behavior, often portraying women who bleach as uninformed and pathological, not acknowledging the real or imagined social benefits women may gain from a lighter skin tone, or institutionalized privileges based on skin colour—colorism. Furthermore focusing on government regulation alone–policy change alone is largely ineffective in changing health-risky behaviours such as skin bleaching. In order to achieve success in addressing current harmful skin bleaching practices, both government and community-based approaches need to be considered.

The added pressure of mega-advertising campaigns for skin lightening using Hollywood and Nollywood celebrities and the global issue of idealized depictions of women and men in the media is another factor that needs to be addressed. Complexion ideals in local and Western media are a source of anxiety in women who then turn to harmful forms of body modification.

Furthermore, the monumental cost of this bleaching culture in Nigeria is unquantifiable. Most of the bleaching products used by the elite wealthy urban women cost several millions of dollars. Most of them can afford to purchase the products online from far countries like the UK, USA, Japan, China, the Philippines etc and have them delivered at their doorsteps just by the click of the mouse. They can also afford to travel out to those countries for skin lightening cosmetic surgical procedures at monumental cost. Nigeria's economy is currently reeling under the current serious tide of "medical tourism", oblivious of the impact of the subterranean practice of "cosmetic tourism".

The global cosmetic market stands at a staggering 113 billion dollar industry. Skin lightening/bleaching products form a significant part (up to 15%) of this market. The powerful economic forces at play need to be understood and confronted. The manufacturing, advertising and selling of skin-lighteners have become a major growth market for multinational corporations. These corporations play a leading role in the creation and manipulation of needs and desires often overtly supporting capitalist white supremacy.

The current situation is dire and needs attention. This calls for a drastic re-evaluation of the factors driving this devastating phenomenon. Government regulations and policies as well as public campaigns need to be based on an understanding of the motives behind the practice and of course the driving force behind this skin bleaching culture.

In the literature there have been many works on the dangers and prevalence of skin-lightening practices but few offer plausible solutions to help ameliorate the sad situation. The bleaching phenomenon has been rightly described metaphorically as a "syndrome" which means that skin bleaching should not be regarded as an isolated phenomenon, but should be rightly seen and treated as one of a group of "symptoms and signs," which, when considered together, are known or presumed to characterize a disease or lesion. There is therefore a compelling need to analyze the constellation of "symptoms or signs" with a view to determining which of them are significantly linked as probable results of the same underlying cause or causes.

Evidence presented from various studies suggest that multiple factors provide the social and cultural impetus towards skin bleaching and these factors should be taken into account if meaningful strategies are to be created and employed to counteract the trend.

In recent years, the practice of skin bleaching in Africa and among populations of Africa descent throughout the diaspora has gained international attention. Journalistic as well as scholarly coverage of the phenomenon has generally focused on two key issues—the medical problems associated with bleaching, and the psychosocial and cultural implications of the desire for lighter or white skin.

Questions have been asked about how the huge investment in skin bleaching products elsewhere differs from the multi-million dollar African American hair weave market in the US? Although many African-American women style their hair in various ways, quite a lot of women who weave their hair are motivated by the fact that longer hair, curly or straight, is viewed as more attractive. Observations have also been made that the future of campaigns that encourage Africans and Asia Pacific individuals to reject paler complexion as damaging and demeaning while embracing the quest for a lighter shade of pale looks bleak, especially if North American and European standards are anything to go by. Just as Africans and Asians undergo body altering practices such as skin bleaching, so too do white North Americans and Europeans self-inflict wounds through tanning salons and tanning creams. Whites subject themselves to self-mutilation to siphon off unwanted fat through wrinkling-reducing Botox or Liposuction procedures. Perhaps these trends reinforce a possible global truth namely, *a universal longing to be impossibly beautiful by doing what comes unnaturally to achieve the unattainable.*

Having practiced as a dermatologist for about four and half decades in Nigeria, seeing and managing skin bleachers both within and outside health facilities, probably the highest number of skin bleachers in Nigeria, it is most timely and desirable to formally document a firsthand knowledge of this bleaching phenomenon and profer plausible solutions to help ameliorate the sad situation. This book is not a theoretical discussion nor a cognitive treatise. Icons of black beauty are given appropriate 'airtime' to demonstrate a lifestyle achievable because we Africans have seen it lived out in these ladies. The book sets out to adopt a **holistic** approach to the subject.

> "The quest for fairness in skin colour through the use of skin lighteners is based on many 'unfair' problems and in the long term has very unfair and unhealthy results. The practice of skin lightening is a public health issue as well as, genetic, social, behavioral, psychological, socioeconomic and environmental determinants. The root cause being a response to a deep-seated need for individuals to cope with suffering they perceive or experience resulting from social norms. In this sense, skin lightening could be regarded as a "disease" in the broader definition of health as a "state of mental and social wellbeing." *Malangu Ntambwe.*

Purpose and Scope

The overall objective of this book is to provide up-to-date evidence-based recommendations for reducing the global burden of cosmetic skin bleaching and preventing injuries related to skin bleaching in sub-Saharan Africa and Africans in diaspora.

The book aims to:

- offer an appraisal of all relevant literature on cosmetic bleaching practices to-date, focusing on any key developments.
- identify and address important medical, public health issues as well as historical, genetic, psychosocial, cultural, behavioral, socioeconomic, political, institutional and environmental determinants.
- provide guideline recommendations that would help attenuate the burden and possibly eliminate the injuries related to skin bleaching.
- discuss potential developments and future directions.

Materials and Methods

Articles pertaining to all aspects of skin bleaching practices globally were explored from databases that publish research in biomedical, public health, and social science literatures. Scholarly literature, journalistic publications, feature articles in magazines, videos, social media e.g Twitter, Facebook, Blogs, Youtubes etc were extensively consulted and explored for this study. There is an incredibly rich repertoire of literature on the issue of complexion dissatisfaction that gave birth to skin bleaching. This repertoire of relevant literature is extensively used and some of the publications are not just cited but reproduced, with acknowledgement, so that the importance of the message conveyed is fully appreciated and not overlooked nor lost.

Since the Holy Bible and the Christian religion were the original instruments used to **invent** racism, the Holy Bible is liberally used to expose the truth of God's plan and will for mankind.

The interviews granted by different women both upwardly mobile and those at the fringes of the society are documented. Interviews granted by women from several different generations are explored to find if the views of women's varying complexions are different or has changed from one generation to the next. Comments from individuals—both men and women, bleachers and non bleachers, posted on social media are studied and documented.

Scope

The study explores and analyzes previous research concluded on the overall complexion dissatisfaction globally. Since the main focus of the book is on the skin bleaching practice in sub-Saharan Africa and Africa in diaspora, virtually no publication on the subject emanating from sub-Saharan African countries was ignored. Countries in sub-Saharan Africa may be regarded as coeval in the skin bleaching practice though the rate of progression of the practice may vary. Each of the countries in sub-Saharan Africa is featured separately because they may have different experiences on the matter and because each recommendation may not be universally applicable in different cultural and religious settings. Therefore each country is given the chance and choice to decide on culturally acceptable intervention strategies. There are no stories in this book on some of the countries in sub-Saharan Africa. This is because nothing has been documented as regards skin bleaching in such countries or that no worthwhile research findings have been identified in the literature. Furthermore, the extent of write-up on each country is commensurate to the volume and spectrum of *existing* documentation of the subject on each country. Also the choice of countries for discourse depends on regional spread to ensure that the culture of each region on the continent is represented and covered.

Nigeria is regarded as the hot house of the skin bleaching practice. Hence Nigeria is featured as the "**CASE STUDY**" in this book. Literally all locally conducted studies and feature articles on the matter in Nigeria are explored. Since the author of this book is a Nigerian with unprecedented first-hand knowledge of the skin bleaching culture in Nigeria, about four and a half decades—literally from the inception of the skin bleaching practice in Nigeria to-date, the chapter on

NIGERIA can be truly regarded as the microcosm of the skin bleaching culture in sub-Saharan Africa.

Although the primary purpose of this book is to characterize cosmetic skin bleaching practices in sub-Saharan Africa, existing literature clearly identifies skin bleaching as a **global** practice. Like communicable diseases, cosmetic skin bleaching has no boundaries because we live in a globalized world. Hence some insight is given about skin bleaching in the Caribbean—Jamaica as a case study, India, South East Asia, Latin America, North America, and the United Kingdom which has a large population of Africans, Caribbeans and Indians. Furthermore, skin lightening is not only practised by homeland Africans but also by diasporic Africans. Apart from the effect of cross border smuggling of the bleaching products, there are valuable lessons to be learnt from the motives and intervention strategies put in place by these other countries which may be helpful to the African countries.

The magnitude of the problem

The epidemiology of the skin bleaching practice globally is described because no meaningful intervention strategies can be recommended nor put in place if the magnitude of the problem, the distribution and the factors that fuel and drive the bleaching culture—are not well defined and characterized

Chemicals and Adverse health effects

The bedrock of any argument on the medical implications of the skin lightening culture is a well articulated chapter on the chemicals/procedures used and the adverse health consequences of such chemicals and procedures. Therefore, in this book a detailed description of the chemicals and toxic effects of the chemicals and clinical illustrations of the cutaneous manifestations are given the needed attention and space.

The issue of Racism

Skin bleaching is a global phenomenon driven by colorism which is an offshoot of racism. Racism is the belief that humans are subdivided into distinct groups that are different in their social behavior and innate capacities that can be ranked as superior or inferior. There are some taxonomies of race that have fabricated merely subjective built-in pejorative expressions and innuendos that can only evoke prejudice and confine the so-called "inferior" race to debasing stereotypes that negatively impact self-worth and self-esteem. The over-arching influence of race and racism cannot be over-estimated. In this book the **invention** of racism is given the needed attention hence there is a dedicated section on race, racism and its progeny colorism and apartheid.

Why do people bleach?

There are several motivations for the skin-bleaching practice, and these are primarily connected to issues of fashion, beauty, popularity, self-image and acceptability. Unequivocally, the most recurring motive globally for skin bleaching in the female gender is to enhance their chances in the marriage market. However, this marriage burden has assumed a monstrous dimension in sub-Saharan Africa which cannot be dissociated from cultural imperatives like polygamy, bigamy, absence of inheritance rights, childlessness, and lack of economic empowerment of women in Africa. The book therefore explores the literature to know more about the lives and culture of different people for choosing such drastic measures for changing their appearance.

The psychology of why skin lighteners are such a viable market in Africa requires elucidation. Therefore the psychological imperatives—paradigms—that have been theorized which gave birth to the skin bleaching culture are extensively explored and described in the book. Most articles describe the practice and participants of skin bleaching through a framework of social pathology that had a racial dimension. Skin bleaching is believed to be an offshoot of racism which emerged from the transatlantic slavery. The institutions of transatlantic slavery, racism and its sister institutions—colorism and apartheid need elucidation in order to understand the link to the genesis of skin bleaching.

While it is true that skin bleaching represents a multifaceted phenomenon, with a complexity of historical, cultural, sociopolitical, and psychological forces motivating the practice, the large majority at the very least acknowledge the institutions of colonialism and enslavement historically, and global White supremacy contemporarily, as dominant and culpable instigators of the penchant for skin bleaching. These institutions shall be well defined.

Determinants

There is a compelling need to identify the factors that provide the social and cultural impetus towards skin bleaching; the cultural factors and institutions that drive the practice. These factors should be taken into account if meaningful strategies are to be created and employed to counteract the trend towards skin bleaching.

Perspectives

Furthermore, there is need to identify and describe peoples (bleachers and non bleachers) perspectives on skin bleaching, peoples way of thinking, peoples attitude towards skin bleaching, peoples view point on skin bleaching, and the benefits, real or imaginary, that are accruable from skin bleaching. These must be clearly defined before recommendations are made so that the much needed interventions would be successfully implemented. As regards perspectives, the social media came in very useful as it provided a very broad spectrum of opinions, thoughts, view points and suggestions on perspectives

The issue of failed interventions

Virtually most African countries have "legally" banned the manufacture, importation and sale of these cosmetic skin bleaching products in their countries. Some have even gone further to put in place laudable intervention strategies to stem the tide of skin bleaching in their countries. However, it is regrettable that **no** African country has succeeded in stemming the tide of cosmetic skin bleaching practices. The reasons for this gloomy state of affairs are explored and well described in this book as a prelude to proffering the Recommendations for reducing the burden and injury from cosmetic skin bleaching practices.

The issue of Beauty

The multi-billion cosmetic industry thrives on exploiting women's insecurities and society's perceptions of what constitutes beauty. The society's influence on perception of beauty has come under criticism as it reinforces a possible global truth namely, *a universal longing to be impossibly beautiful by doing what comes unnaturally to achieve the unattainable.* The factors that have contributed to this quest to achieve the "unattainable beauty" have come under the search-light in a chapter entitled "BEAUTY, PHYSICAL ATTRACTIVENESS AND SEXUAL ATTRACTIVENESS

The issue of colonization and neo-colonization

It is believed that people who lighten their skin suffer from a colour complex issue that can be traced back to issues related to colonization. All the countries in sub-Saharan Africa were at one time colonies of foreign powers. The institutions of colonization/neo-colonization are well defined and described as to their relevance to complexion dissatisfaction among inhabitants of its former colonies.

The issue of colorism

Colorism is a form of prejudice and discrimination in which human beings are treated differently based on the social meaning attached to skin colour. Colorism disadvantages dark-skinned people, while privileging those with lighter skin. Within the United States, the legacy of slavery created a bifurcated system which affected the social and economic stratification of Blacks. However, in the majority of countries in sub-Saharan Africa like Nigeria, the people are homogenously dark skinned. What form of "colorism"—real or imaginary—exists in these African countries to justify skin bleaching? Nigeria is used as a **Case Study** for this discourse.

The issue of beauty icons

The entertainment industry has been blamed for the fact that so many young women choose to bleach. To what extent is this true? This matter is extensively laid bare in the chapter on CELEBRITY DISCOURSE.

The role of the media

Identity by nature is dual because it is elaborated internally, having been constructed externally. People internalize identity construction, which manifests itself in the appearance of social actions. The spread of the ideology that fair skin is better can be attributed in part to new media vehicles such as Facebook, Myspace, Twitter, Instagram, Blogs etc. These are social media representation women see and interact with everyday. Effort is made in this book to understand the implications of the globalization of media representation that promote skin bleaching practices and to discover any correlations between advertisements, media representation, and skin bleaching. The subject is analyzed under the heading THE MEDIA AS A MAJOR DRIVING FORCE OF SKIN BLEACHING

The cost of skin bleaching

The global production and marketing of skin bleaching products is a very lucrative industry and continues to become more popular in that these products are being requested globally. There is a perpetually evolving cosmetic products. Skin bleaching is practiced in some countries where more than half the population lives on less than US$1 a day, yet these people would rather starve to have funds to purchase skin lightening products. Skin bleaching is a multi-billion dollar industry. The question is often asked "what justifies this investment on skin bleaching products?"

Story highlights

Each chapter or section starts with 'Story highlights'. The 'Story highlights' is not a summary, not an abstract and not a conclusion. The purpose of the 'Story highlights' is to highlight some critical or noteworthy parts of the story that are related to the primary objective of the book—to reduce the burden and injury from the skin bleaching culture. Therefore, 'Story highlights' simply highlights parts of the story that should not be ignored for meaningful recommendations and intervention strategies. The design and structure of the Story highlights vary according to the message, hence not all of them are bullet pointed. Some of them exceed a page depending on the overall message the author wishes to convey that would impact the needed response and actions by (i) the government (ii) the individuals, (iii) the community and (iv) the various institutions relevant to the story of the skin bleaching practice.

Final self appraisal questions

This book is not just an academic exercise. It has addressed skin bleaching as a problem of social and public health concern which has implications for national policy, practice and theory. It is left to the Government of each country to decide on the appropriate line of action.

At the **individual** level there is need to ask ourselves some searching questions which may help us position ourselves to respond appropriately. The questions are as follows:

i. Are the health risks of skin lightening made clear enough?
ii. Is it not a woman's right to choose what she does with her body?
iii. If it were proven that lightening your skin meant you were more likely to be successful in life, would you be compelled to bleach your skin?
iv. If you had $20b to spend on helping young women improve their chances in life, how would you spend it?
v. Do you bleach? Would you consider doing it? If yes, what are your motivations?
vi. Why would you never consider bleaching your skin?
vii. To what extent is the entertainment industry to blame for the fact that so many young women choose to bleach?
viii. Should adverts for skin lightening products be banned?
ix. Should the skin bleaching products themselves be banned?

Chapter 2

The Invention Of Racism

Story highlights I

The invention of racism

- Racism, Colorism and Colonialism are legacies of the Transatlantic slavery. Skin bleaching is an offshoot of racism, colorism and Colonialism

- "Global White Supremacy" is a system that emerged with the European colonial project and has led to today's racially inflicted social, economic and political culture "structured to advantage white." In this context, skin bleaching would manifest as a seemingly most "logical" method through which to approximate the white ideal and thus empower oneself

- Manichaen view is one that not only divides the world into dualities, but sees those dualities as ***irreconcilable*** oppositions. In this way, the Manicheans conceived of darkness, or black, and things associated with it as evil; while light or white, symbolized those things that were good.

- White Supremacy was a historically based, institutionally perpetuated system of exploitation and oppression of continents, nations, and peoples classified as "non-white" by continents, nations, and peoples who, by virtue of their white (light) skin pigmentation and/or ancestral origin from Europe, classify themselves as "White".

- European Christianity has been thought and felt in distinctly white ways for most of its history due explicitly to doctrinal persistence of the Manichean dualism of white versus black.

—Ideologies were built around different skin tones to maintain control over the indigenous populations

—Anyone that was dark was considered demonic and unworthy of life; they were considered lower than dirt and they had no human rights

—Light skin was considered beautiful and almost God-like in appearance, anyone with light skin was considered closer to God and has human rights and a right to have a better standard of living

—The above ideologies were ingrained in the minds of slaves to maintain a system of racial oppression and class divisions among the different skin tones

—Colonization and racism perpetrated the idea that light skin slaves were more beautiful, smart and cooperative and they often got jobs working in the house— "house negroes"; while their darker relatives slaves in the fields — "field negroes" were considered as inferior.

—Whiteness—"godliness", "the light" moral, good—represents everything that blackness is not.

Hence darkness represents damnation, immoral and evil, wicked, depressing, gloomy, angry, sullen, morbid, and absence of light

—Manichaeism inherent to heretical/European Christianity has been instrumental in the defining of what is now referred to as "White nationalism"—an expression of European nationalism which identifies Caucasian racial characteristics with superiority and African racial characteristics with inferiority

—The [European] Christian structure of — whiteness associated with "the light," or salvation, godliness and morality versus blackness associated with darkness, or damnation, devilish and immorality led to whitening of religious imagery particularly that of Christ

—Christ, the iconic measure of perfection, was (re)interpreted, (re)imagined, and (re)presented as not just white skinned, but extremely white; so white as to illuminate. Additionally Christ is depicted with blonde hair and blue-eyes, eerily reflective of the proclaimed racial superiority of the Nordic race

—If, Christ, the son of God, is portrayed as white, the logical assumption is that God too is white

—If God made man in His image and gave him authority over all other creatures, approximation of this whiteness when embodied by "man on earth" communicated not only a greater nearness to God, but humanity itself.

—In the Manichean sense, then, **whiteness** embodied by humanity, communicates moral and physical superiority. Conversely, **blackness**, the absence of whiteness communicates inhumanity, immorality, and physical inferiority, **divinely** subjected to the dominance of God and/or His earthly counterpart —White man!

—In fact, the Christianity of the colonial order characterizes black skin not only as punishment from God via the "curse of Ham," but divine justification for the enslavement of Africans.

—Manichaeism inherent to European construct materializes as one of the ideological antecedents of hierarchical racial demarcation that not only hold whiteness as superior and inherently good, and blackness as inferior and inherently evil, but **necessitate** the domination of those who embody darkness/ blackness by those who embody whiteness. It is this Manichean Christian worldview that would not only substantiate and proliferate global White nationalism, but also further validate European colonialism and enslavement of African people.

—In this way, those Europeans who had gained power by way of their embodiment of God and acquisition of knowledge claimed to have a **divine responsibility** to choose for those who were ungodly and ignorant—Africans. Thus legitimatizing, precipitating and further maintaining the colonization of Africa by Europe and the enslavement of Africans by Europeans.

— It provided the **ideological** justification for the systematic and systemic racial subjugation that would come to be known as global White supremacy.

— **Ideology** is a "system of beliefs or theories held by an individual or a group. It is the image a society gives of itself in order to perpetuate itself. Therefore the word **"race"** as is propagated in modern times as European/White identity versus African/Black identity is a **social** construct fabricated to perpetuate an ideology of White supremacy.

Story highlights II

Biblical Christianity debunking the ideology of racial superiority

- The Manichaen European Christian ideology of White Supremacy was ***demon-inspired.***
- God doesn't judge people on the basis of race, gender, ethnic or national origin. The Holy Scriptures classically divides all humans into two classes: **godly** or **ungodly**; **natural (unspiritual)** or **spiritual**. These two classes are ***reconcilable*** by God's ***grace*** through the process of **redemption, regeneration** and **sanctification**
- **As regards lights (white) or darkness (black); In the Scriptures**

God is pictured as **light** (Ps 18:28; Ps 27:1; Isaiah 60:19-22)

Jesus is the **light** of God (Jn 1: 4, 5; Rev 21:23)

The Bible often compares goodness with light and evil with **darkness** or shadow (Jas 1:17; 1, Jn 1:5, 6)

Believers are children of **light** (Eph 5:8; Mat 5:15, 16; Prv 4:18, 19)

The Word of God —the Holy Scriptures—is **light** (Ps 119:105)

The Gospel of Christ is **light** (2 Cor 4:4,6)

If you love a Christian brother or sister you are in the **light** (1 Jn 2:10, 11)

Light makes us know the will of God (Jn 11:9, 10)

Evil people love **darkness** and hate **light** (Jn 3: 19-21)

Satan represents **darkness** (2 Cor 6:14, 15)

- **In what ways are we made in the image (likeness) of God?**

God is spirit. He is not a physical being. Moreover no one has ever seen Him. Therefore no one can describe His colour. Jesus was born a Jew. Jews are not of the Nordic race (extremely light-skinned with blond hair and blue eyes). Even at Jesus transfiguration, we are simply told that His "clothes", not His skin, became "white" (Mat 17:2; Mk 9:3). Though we are created in the "image"/"likeness" of God, God did not create us *exactly* like himself because God has no physical body. Instead, we are reflections of God's glory. God has unique attributes which human beings do not have. These attributes exclusive to God are: He is omnipresent, omniscient, omnipotent, transcendent, eternal, unchangeable, perfect and holy—completely without sin, and God is **triune** in nature.

However human beings at creation possess the **moral** attributes of God which became corrupted as a result of the Fall. The moral attributes of God are: He is good, He is love, He is merciful and gracious, He is compassionate, He is patient (longsuffering) and slow to anger, God is truth, faithful and just. Christ is the **perfect** expression of God in human form. What made his humanity unique was his freedom from sin. Jesus was born a Jew. God chose Israel not because the people merited it but in His love and mercy, He wanted a special nation on earth to represent His way of life, to teach His Word, and to be an agent of salvation to the world. All human beings of whatever race or color tone originated from one blood—that of Adam.

- Although God created human beings in His image, after the Fall, (when Adam and Eve disobeyed God), ***moral and spiritual death occurred***. Moral death consisted in the death of God's life in them and their nature became sinful; spiritual death meant that their former relationship to God in innocence was destroyed, resulting in a state of sinfulness. Since the sin of Adam and Eve, every person born comes into the world with a sinful nature and slaves to sin.
- How do human beings **regain** the moral and spiritual image of God which were corrupted as a result of the Fall ? Four critical words describe the process—**Grace, Re-creation, Redemption** and **Sanctification**. The meaning and implications of all these words are clearly elucidated in the remaining part of the chapter.

- The foremost character of God is His **holiness**. Holiness means morally perfect, pure, and set apart from all sin. Because sin cannot exist in the presence of a holy God, God chose to **re-create** sinful human beings in His likeness and empower us to remain in fellowship with Him. This process of re-creation is also called regeneration/spiritual rebirth/born again. This **initiative** of God is called **Grace.**

- In the Holy Bible ***Canaan*** (Ham's son) was cursed (Gen 9:25). Noah's curse on Ham's son however, wasn't directed toward any particular race, but rather at the Canaanite nation—a nation God knew would become wicked. The curse was fulfilled when the Israelites entered the Promised Land and drove the Canaanites out. Nowhere did the Bible tell us Canaan was black, nor the skin tone of Ham nor Canaan.

- The curse of Ham's son (Canaan) has ***no*** bearing whatsoever to any racial group nor the institution of slavery. Slavery was ***not*** ordained by God. Nowhere does the Bible condone slavery, but recognizes its existence. God's laws offered many guidelines for treating slaves properly, and there were very harsh consequences for violators of God's law as regards slavery. Paul and the early church expressed an even higher standard. Although Christians may be at different levels in earthly society, we are all equal before God. God does not play favorites; no one is more important than anyone else. Paul and the early church set forth Christian principles that removed the harshness of Roman slavery and eventually led to its banishment altogether within Christianity. Racism or Favoritism is contemptible in God's sight.

- Furthermore, when the descendants of Noah were scattered by God when they erected the tower of Babel (Gen 11: 1-9), the Bible did not tell us which group went to settle in geographical spaces called Africa, Europe etc. We are simply told ———————
[8]*"So the LORD* ***scattered*** *them abroad from there over the face of all the earth, and they ceased building the city.* [9] *Therefore its name is called Babel, because there the LORD confused the language of all the earth; and from there the LORD* ***scattered*** *them abroad over the face of all the earth* (Gen 11: 8-9).

- All human beings of whatever colour or race originated from Adam and Eve. The Holy Bible does **not** tell us about the "evolution" of man **nor** the colour of Adam and Eve. All we know today is that there is a direct correlation between the geographic distribution of Ultraviolet (UV) radiation (UVR) and the distribution of indigenous skin pigmentation around the world. Areas that receive higher amounts of UVR, generally located closer to the equator, tend to have darker-skinned populations. Areas that are far from the tropics and closer to the poles have lower intensity of UVR, which is reflected in lighter-skinned populations. Researchers have proposed various **theories** about how and when the skin of some people "became" dark over the centuries (see the chapter on THE COLOR DISCOURSE). The truth is that the Holy Bible has **not** told us **how** and **when** this occurred nor the skin color of Adam and Eve. All we know is that the **all-knowing** and **all-wise God**, the Creator of the universe—mankind, the sun and the whole earth, the tropical and temperate regions of the world, **chose** to protect those inhabiting the geographical space with high intensity of UVR by endowing us with the **melanin** pigment as a natural 'umbrella' against the harmful effects of excessive UVR

Preamble

What is the relationship between history, slavery, colonialism, global white supremacy and skin bleaching?

While it is true that skin bleaching represents a multifaceted phenomenon, with a complexity of historical, cultural, sociopolitical and psychological forces motivating the practice, the large majority of scholars who examine skin bleaching at the very least acknowledge the institutions of colonialism and enslavement historically, and global White supremacy contemporarily, as dominant and culpable instigators of the penchant for skin bleaching. As an introduction to the special comprehensive discourse on skin bleaching, it is necessary to critically examine the symbolic significance of whiteness, the history of global white supremacy, both ideologically and politically, discussing its subsequent promulgation, and further investigating its relationship to the historical and contemporary skin bleaching phenomenon. Since the ideology was promulgated from heresy emanating from *mis*interpretation of the Holy Bible, the only valid response to debunk the heresy shall be extracted from the Holy Bible.

One may ask up front, what can be the possible relationship between history, colonialism and global white supremacy and skin bleaching? Historically most people were colonized and conquered by the Europeans, Arabs and the Spaniards. Most of these imperialists have lighter skin due to their climate and geographical location. They also built ideologies around different skin tones to maintain control over the indigenous populations. Anyone that was dark was considered demonic and unworthy of life; they were considered lower than dirt and they had no human rights back then. While the light skin was considered beautiful and almost God-like in appearance, anyone with light skin was closer to God and has human rights and a right to have a better standard of living. Back then these ideologies were ingrained in the minds of slaves to maintain a system of racial oppression and class divisions among the different skin tones.[1] Colonization decisively embedded skin-tone hierarchies into indigenous society in Africa.

One may also ask—What is the relationship between slavery and skin bleaching? In Europe, during the industrial revolution, light skin was associated with high social status as those with tanned skin were the poorer classes who worked outdoors. Colonization and racism perpetrated the idea that light skin slaves were more beautiful, smart and cooperative and they often got jobs working in the house—"house negroes"—while their darker relatives slaves in the fields—"field Negroes," were considered as inferior. Lighter skin amongst blacks still retains its elevated status to the point that studies have associated blackness with low self-esteem.[2] Furthermore, in the slave-trade era, it was discovered that the slave master (Europeans) had their skin affected by long exposure to sun. The experience prompted the European slave master to adopt various methods (skin bleaching) that brought improvement to their skin! Thus, skin bleaching was practiced in the 16th century.

'Global white supremacy' is a system that emerged with the European colonial project and has led to today's racially inflicted social, economic and political culture 'structured to advantage white.'

"Skin bleaching is a widespread global phenomenon. Within the context of global white supremacy skin color communicates one's position to and within the document power structure. Given this reality, many people, namely those historically subjected to white domination, colonization, and enslavement, have internalized projected notions that the basis of their inferior condition is their skin color. In this context, skin bleaching would manifest as a seemingly most "logical" method through which to approximate the White ideal and thus empower oneself. As the political offshoot of European/White nationalism, global White supremacy continually creates an image of itself in order to perpetuate itself, and thus continues to employ and rely upon the fabrication and projection of imagery to forcibly convince the masses, particularly those oppressed under its systemic exploitation, that the White ideal is in fact the human ideal."[1]

References

1. Blay Yaba Amgborale. Skin bleaching and Global White Supremacy: By Way of introduction. *The Journal of Pan African Studies*. 2011 June; 4:4.
2. Nyabuoy Gatbel. Skin bleaching and the South Sudanese Community. (http:www.nyabuogabeldeng.com/blog/skin-bleaching-and-the-south-sudanese-community#comments)

THE INVENTION OF RACISM

Manichaeism, Dualism, and the Heresy of White Supremacy in Manichaen/European Christianity

Manichaeism

Manichaeism[1,2,3] was a major Gnostic religion that was founded by the Iranian prophet Mani in the Sasanian Empire. Manichaeism tought an elaborate dualistic cosmology describing the struggle between a good, spiritual world of light, and an evil, material world of darkness. Through an ongoing process which takes place in human history, light is gradually removed from the world of matter and returned to the world of light from whence it came. Its beliefs were based on local Mesopotamian Gnostic and religious movements.

Manichaeism was quickly successful and spread far through the Aramaic—Syriac speaking regions. It thrived between the third and seventh centuries, and at its height was one of the most widespread religions in the world. Manichaean churches and scriptures existed as far east as China and as far west as the Roman Empire. It was briefly the main rival of Christianity in the competition to replace classical paganism. Manichaeism survived longer in the East than in the West, and it appears to have finally faded away after the 14th century in southern China, contemporary to the decline in China of the church of the East. While most of Mani's original writings have been lost, numerous translation and fragmentary texts have survived.

An adherent of Manichaeism is called, especially in older sources, a **Manichee**, or more recently **Manichaean**. By extension, the term "Manichean" is widely applied (often disparagingly) as and adjective to a philosophy or attitude of moral dualism, according to which a moral course of action involves a clear (or simplistic) choice between good and evil, or as a noun to people who hold such a view.

Heretical/European Christianity, White Ideal, and the Rise of White Nationalism

Although it developed initially as a misappropriation of more ancient African religious traditions, namely Memphite theology and Gnosticism,[5] heretical/European Christianity has been thought and felt in distinctly white ways for most of its history due explicitly to doctrinal persistence of the Manichean dualism of white versus black and the subsequent whitening of religious imagery, particularly that of Christ.[6,7] In this context, particularly during the period of expansionism and colonialism, whiteness came to be projected and furthermore perceived in a manner consistent with both Manichean and Christian ideologies such that whiteness—godliness, "the light," moral, good—represents everything that blackness is not[8]. Hence darkness represents damnation, immoral and evil. Thus, the Manichaeism inherent to heretical/European Christianity has been instrumental in the defining of what is now referred to as White nationalism—"an expression of European nationalism which identifies Caucasian racial characteristics with superiority and African racial characteristics with inferiority"[9]

In his discussion of the psychology of the oppressed/colonized, Fanon[10,11] used the term "Manichean" to describe the world of the oppressed/colonized. Of or relating to Manichaeism, "a doctrine based on the ideas of the Persian philosopher Manes, which saw the world as polarized between forces of absolute good and evil, symbolized in the oppositions of light and darkness, black and white".[7] A Manichean view is one that not only divides the world into dualities, but sees those dualities as irreconcilable oppositions. In this way, the Manicheans conceived of darkness, or black, and things associated with it as evil, while light, or white, symbolized those things that were good.

White Supremacy was a historically based, institutionally perpetuated system of exploitation and oppression of continents, nations, and peoples classified as "non-white" by continents, nations, and peoples who, by virtue of their white (light) skin pigmentation and/or ancestral origin from Europe, classify themselves as "White". Although history illuminates the *fabrication*, changeability, and contingencies of Whiteness (e.g. the case of Irish and Italians once being denied entry into the White "race"), it is important to note that this global power system is structured and maintained not for the purpose of legitimizing racial categories as much as it is for the purpose of maintaining and defending a system of wealth, power, and privilege. Thus, it has been Whites who have constructed racial categories based on the economic, political, and social aspirations of Whites for the benefits of Whites.[12] In this way, Whites define who is White; a definition that has changed and will likely continue to change based upon the particular economic, political, and social conditions of the moment (e,g. the case of Egyptians now being classified as White when they were once classified as Arab, and previously as Black). It is clear then that White supremacy is based less on racial Whiteness (as evidenced by skin color) than it is on ideological Whiteness—the exclusive value assigned that involves "a series of immunities, privileges, rights, and assumptions." This value is not inherent, natural, or biologically determined. Rather it reflects artificial beliefs created by social, economic, and political conditions. Given the historical fact that White supremacy has been constructed by Whites for the benefit of Whites, White supremacy is routinely interpreted as a code word for White people.

Manichean worldview also influenced semantics,[13] "the study of the way in which language expresses meaning." While some of the literal definitions of "white" include "the achromatic color of maximum lightness, unsullied, pure, and snowy;" and "black" "without light, soiled, as from soot, dirty, evil, wicked, depressing, gloomy, angry, sullen, morbid, and absence of light."[14] these definitions are best understood in the context of their moral symbolic meanings—white dove of peace, White Christmas, white collar, and white lie as opposed to Black Death, blackball, blackmail, Black Market, and black eye.

While the impact of both Manichaeism and Christianity on European thought has been profound, the most powerful implications of this dualistic and hegemonic ordering has been on the construction if identities—that of a superior White (European) identify as well as that an inferior Black (African) identify. The [European] Christian structure of "feeling"—whiteness associated with "the light," or salvation, godliness and morality/blackness associated with darkness, or damnation, devilish and immorality—"are realized in concrete images and stories [centered] on embodiment "and **further mapped into skin color** difference.[7] **No human being has a truly (completely) white skin and no human being has a truly (completely) black skin**. Human beings possess various shades of pale (light colored) skin and Africans possess various shades of brown (dark colored) skin. Even though Christianity developed out of African/Jewish religious precursors, once it became a tool of both

European and White nationalism, Christ, the iconic measure of perfection, is (re)interpreted, (re) imagined, and (re) presented as not just white skinned, but extremely white; so white as to illuminate. Additionally, Christ is depicted with blonde hair and blue-eyes, eerily reflective of the proclaimed racial superiority of the Nordic race. "It was necessary that this man, the incarnation of God, be so far removed as possible from everything that could suggest darkness even indirectly".

If, Christ, the Son of God, is portrayed as White, the logical assumption is that God too is White. And if, as according to Christian doctrine, God made man in His image and gave him authority over all other creatures, approximation of this whiteness when embodied by "man on earth" communicates not only a greater nearness to God, but humanity itself. In the Manichean sense, then, whiteness embodied by humanity, communicates moral and physical superiority. Conversely, blackness, the absence of whiteness communicates inhumanity, immorality, and physical inferiority, **divinely** subjected to the dominance of God and/or His earthly counterpart —White man! In fact, the Christianity of the colonial order characterizes black skin not only as punishment from God via the "curse of Ham," but divine justification for the enslavement of Africans.[6,15,16] Here we witness the Manichaeism inherent to Christianity materialize as one of the ideological antecedents of hierarchical racial demarcation that not only hold whiteness as superior and inherently good, and blackness as inferior and inherently evil, but **necessitate** the domination of those who embody darkness/ blackness by those who embody whiteness. It is this Manichean Christian worldview that would not only substantiate and proliferate global White nationalism, but also further validate European colonialism and enslavement of African people.

One of the first steps in advancing the notion of European superiority in the minds of both Europeans and African was the explorer's metaphorical construction of Africa as the "Dark Continent." Described as an impenetrable and hostile environment whose balmy heat and rampant disease "invited mental prostration and physical debility."[17] Africa represented everything that the "Enlightened" West (Europe) was not. Thus, 'logically" any people able to survive in what was later termed the "White Man's grave" represented everything that Europeans were not—barbaric, unintelligent, and powerless.

The missionary, relying on the accounts of both the explorer and the soldier counterposed the Manichean/Christian doctrine metaphor of darkness as sin and ignorance with the "light" of Christian doctrine and epistemology. Because his whiteness positioned him nearer to God, the missionary considered himself the embodiment of supreme good, and because of his blackness, the missionary portrayed the African as the incarnation of evil.[18] He thus on the divinely ordained mission to "save the natives' souls"[17,19]

Each of these figures accounts of their experiences with Africa and her people constituted a type of knowledge and discourse about Africa and her people.[19] Moreover, each of these figures' knowledge and discourse constituted a type of **power over** the objects of which they were knowledgeable.[19] In this way, those who had gained power by way of their embodiment of God and acquisition of knowledge—Europeans—had a **divine responsibility** to choose for those who were ungodly and ignorant—Africans—thus legitimatizing, precipitating and further maintaining the colonization of Africa by Europe and the enslavement of Africans by Europeans. Colonization and enslavement thus served to actualize European nationalism and came to symbolize and solidify a unity in European consciousness[19] that would influence the contact and interaction of cultures (races) for countries to come.

Most important to note about the history of White nationalism is that insofar as it espoused the "natural" and **divine** superiority of Whites, and ultimately constructed a system of Black exploitation for the purpose of maintaining and defending a system of White wealth, power and privilege, it provided the **ideological** justification for the systematic and systemic racial subjugation that would come to be known as global White supremacy. In this regard then, we should neither take our definition nor conceptual understanding of the term "Ideology" for granted. Beyond a "system of beliefs or theories held by an individual or a group."[20]

"Ideology is how the existing ensemble of social relations represents itself to individuals; it is the image a society gives of itself in order to perpetuate itself. Ideology uses the fabrication of images and the processes of representation to persuade us that how things are is how they ought to be and that the place provided for us is the place we ought to have."[21]

Thus, as an ideology, global White supremacy is exceptionally potent, particularly as it attempts to create an "image of itself in order to perpetuate itself." Insofar as the superior European/White identity was constructed on Manichean grounds, Europeans/Whites would be continually dependant not only upon the "construction" of Africans/Blacks as inferior[8] but furthermore in the projection of corroborating imagery. Not only did Europeans create images to substantiate their falsified and inflated sense of self, but in form true to their capitalistically exploitative nature, they "dressed-up" commodities with these images, thus profiting from their marketing and sale —commodity racism.

At the same time that European colonialists were creating and instituting color hierarchies vis a vis Manichaeism/Christianity, they were also taking additional measures to assert the power "inherent" to whiteness. Commodities, with their ability to produce forms of knowledge, subjectivity, identity and consciousness[22] represented vehicles through which the colonial order was able to not only gain capital, but also advance both its White nationalist agenda and its "civilizing mission." Through commodities, namely soap, Europeans positioned and furthermore advertised whiteness as the color of civilization. For example a simple commodity like soap became a very symbol of whiteness—cleanliness and further became a vehicle of skin bleaching chemicals which are designed to wash off the "dirty" pigment of blackness. Soap was even advertised as being so effective as to wash black hands so clean that they became "white"! (See the section on "THE MEDIA AS A MAJOR DRIVING FORCE OF SKIN BLEACHING" (See chapter 6).
Therefore the word **"race"** as is propagated in modern times as European/White identity Vs African/Black identity is a **social** construct fabricated to perpetuate an ideology of white supremacy (See Chapter 18).

References

1.Blay YA. Skin Bleaching and Global White Supremacy: By Way of Introduction. The *Journal of Pan African Studies* June 2011; 4 (4)37
2.Manichaeism—*Wikipedia, the free encyclopedia.* http://en.wikipedia.org/wiki/Manichaeism
3.Dualism (n.d) Retrieved from http://www.artsci.wustl.edu/~philos/MindDict/dualism.html.
Fanon F. *The Wretched of the Earth* (1963) New York: Grove Press
4.Manichaeism. (n.d.) Retrieved from http:/www.catholic-forum.com/saintS/heresy03.htm.
5.Ashby MA. *African Origins of Civilization, Religion, Yoga Mystical Spirituality and Ethics Philosophy.* Miami FL: Cruzian Mystic Books/Sema Institute of Yoga. 2002
6.Akbar N. *Breaking the Chains of Psychological Slavery.* Tallahassee, FL: Mind Productions & Associates. 19967.Dyer R. *White.* New York: Routledge 1997

7. Dyer R. white. New York: Routledge 1997
8.Blay YM. Editorial: Struck by Lightening: The Transdiasporan Phenomenon of Skin Bleaching. *Jenda: A Journal of Culture and African Women Studies*, 2009a; 14:1-10
9. Ani M. *Yurugu: An African-centered Critique of European Cultural Thought and Behavior.* Trenton, NJ: Africa World Press. 1994.
10.Fanon F. *The Wretched of the Earth.* New York: Grove Press. 1963
11.Fanon F. *Black Skin White Masks.* (1967) New York: Grove Press.
12.Ross L. White Supremacy in the 1990s. Political Research Associates Public Eye. *http://www.publiceye-org/eyes/whitsup.html*
13.Harrell CJP Manichean Psychology: *Racism and the Minds of People of African Descent.* Washington. GC: Howard University Press 1999
14.The America Heritage Dictionary. New York: Bantam Dell 2001
15.Bestide B. Color, Racism, and Christianity. In J. H. Franklin (Ed) *Color and race.* Boston: Houghton Mifflin Company 1968.
16.Gomez MA. *Reversing Sail: A History of the African Diaspora.* New York: Cambridge University Press 2005
17.Jarosz L. Constructing the Dark Continent. Metaphor as Geographic Representation of Africa. *Geografiska Annales. Series B, Human Geography*, 1992; 74, 105-15
18.Bulhan HA. *Frantz Fanon and the Psychology of Oppression.* New York: Plenum Press 1985.
19.Mudimbe VY. *The Invention of Africa: Gnosis, Philosophy and the Order of knowledge.* Bloomington: Indiana University Press. 1988
20.The American Heritage Dictionary New Dictionary of Cultural Library. New York: Houghton Mifflin Company 2005
21.Nichols B. *Ideology and the Image.* Bloomington: Indiana University Press 1981
22.Burke T. *Lifebuoy Men, Lux Women: Commodification, Consumption, and Cleanliness in Modern Zimbabwe.* Durham NC: Duke university Press 1996.

BIBLICAL CHRISTIANITY DEBUNKING THE DOCTRINE OF MANICHAEISM, DUALISM AND THE HERESY OF WHITE SUPREMACY IN CHRISTIANITY

(1). WHAT IS THE CURSE OF HAM?

Read Genesis 9:18-27

"Cursed be Canaan;
A servant of servants he shall be to his brethren."
(Gen 9:25).

This verse has been wrongfully used to support racial prejudice and slavery. Noah's curse, however, wasn't directed toward any particular race, but rather at the Canaanite nation— a nation God knew would become wicked. The curse was fulfilled when the Israelites entered the Promised Land and drove the Canaanites out (see the book of

Joshua). Nowhere did the Bible tell us Canaan was black, nor the skin tone of Ham or Cannan.

Gen 9:25 "Cursed be Canaan." When Noah learned of Ham's shameful action, he pronounced a curse on Ham's son Canaan (though not on Ham himself). (1) Perhaps Canaan was in some way involved in Ham's sin or possessed the same character faults of his father. The curse indicated that Canaan's descendants (**who were not black**) would be oppressed and under the control of other nations. In contrast, Shem and Japheth's descendants would be blessed by God (vv. 26-27). (2) This prophecy of Noah was **conditional** for all concerned. Any descendants of Canaan who turned to God would also receive the blessings bestowed on Shem (Josh 6:22-25; Heb 11:31), while any descendants of Shem and Japheth who depart from God would experience the curse bestowed on Canaan (cf. Jer 18:7-10).

What does the Bible say about descendants being "Cursed"/suffering because of the sins of Parent/s?

God Judges each person individually

A classical example is that of the **sons of Korah**

Psalms 42-49, 84, 85; 87, 88 were writing by the sons of Korah. Korah was a Levite who led a rebellion against Moses (Num 16:1-35). Korah was the leader of a rebellion against Moses and Aaron while Israel was camped in the wilderness of Paran (Num 16). Korah, Dathan, and Abiram led a confederacy of 250 princes of the people against Aaron's claim to the priesthood and Moses' claim to authority in general. The rebels contended that the entire congregation was sanctified and therefore qualified to perform priestly functions. As punishment for their insubordination, God caused the earth to open and swallow the leaders and their property. A fire from the Lord consumed the 250 followers. Korah was killed, but his descendants remained faithful to God and continued to serve God in the temple. David appointed men from the clan of Korah to serve as choir leaders (1 Chr 6:31-38), and they continued to be temple musicians for hundreds of years (2 Chr 20:18, 19). Levite descended from Izhar, of the family of Korah (Exod 6:21; 1 Chr 6:22, 37). The sons of Korah and Asaph were the two most prominent groups of temple singers (cp. 2 Chron 20:19).

A False Proverb Refuted

"What do you mean when you use this proverb concerning the land of Israel, saying:
'The fathers have eaten sour grapes,
And the children's teeth are set on edge'? (Ezek 18:2)

Read Ezekiel chapter 18

The people of Judah believed they were being punished for the sins of their ancestors, not their own. They thought this way because this was the teaching of the Ten Commandment (Ex 20:5). Ezekiel taught that the destruction of Jerusalem was due to the spiritual decay in previous generations. But this belief in the corporate life of Israel led to fatalism and irresponsibility. So Ezekiel gave God's new policy for this new land because the people had misconstrued the old one. God judges each person individually. Although we often suffer from the effects of sins committed by those who came before us, God does not punish us for someone else's sins, and we can't use their mistakes as an excuse for our sins. Each person is accountable to God for his or her actions.

In addition, some people of Judah used the corporate umbrella of God's blessing as an excuse for disobeying God. They thought that because of their righteous ancestors (18:5-9) they would live. God told them that they would not; they were the evil sons of righteous parents and, as such, would die (18:10-13). If, however, anyone returned to God, he or she would live (18:14-18).

How do people suffer from the sins of parents

"Keeping mercy for thousands, forgiving iniquity and transgression and sin, by no means clearing the guilty, visiting the iniquity of the fathers upon the children and the children's children to the third and the fourth generation." (Ex 34:7)

Exodus 34:7. Why would sins affect grandchildren and great-grandchildren? This is no arbitrary punishment. Children still suffer for the sins of their parents. Consider child abuse or alcoholism, for example. While these sins are obvious, sins like selfishness and greed can be passed along as well. The dire consequences of sin are not limited to the individual family member. Be careful not to treat sin casually, but repent and turn from it. The sin may cause you little pain now, but it could sting in a most tender area of your life later—your children and grandchildren.

i).Indeed the only place where someone was described by skin color in the Bible was in Acts 13:1—*Simon,* a Christian teacher and prophet at Antioch
ii).Another place where a tanned skin was referred to is Song of Solomon

[5]*"I am dark, but lovely, O daughters of Jerusalem, like the tents of Kedar, like the curtains of Solomon.* [6]*Do not look upon me, because I am dark. Because the sun has tanned me. My mother's sons were angry with me, They made me the keeper of the vineyards, but my own vineyard I have not kept."* (Songs 1:5, 6).

1:5 *the tents of Kedar.* Tents were usually made of black goat hair. Kedar was an Arabian tribe descended from Ishmael (Gen 25:13; cf. Is 21:16-17); thus some have suggested that the bride was an Arabian princess.

1:6 The vineyard mentioned here was apparently by Solomon (because he came to visit it) and leased to the girl's step-brothers (her "mother's Sons"), who made her take care of the vineyards in the hot sun. Thus she could not take care of her own skin (my own vineyard I have not kept"). When she was brought to Jerusalem, the young girl was embarrassed about her tanned complexion because the girls in the city had the fair, delicate skin that was considered much more beautiful. But Solomon loved her dark skin.

1:6 *mine own vineyard have I not kept.* The cruel brothers of the maiden forced her to guard and care for their vineyards, something she had not done for her own. This outdoor work may be the reason her skin was so dark, a marked contrast to the sun-bonnetted beauties of Jerusalem—though hard work had not destroyed her real beauty (v. 5). In light of these verses it is hard to see how some suppose the speaker here was the daughter of Pharaoh (1 Ki 3:1). This Shulamite maiden was probably the princess Solomon first loved and married before he began to enter marriages for the sake of political alliances.

Note! Solomon loved the dark skin of his bride inspite of the fair skin of the other women who where considered much more beautiful.

(2) HOW ARE PEOPLE CLASSIFIED IN THE HOLY BIBLE

God doesn't judge people on the basis of race, gender, socioeconomic status, ethnic or national origin. He judges them on the basis of their faith in him and their response to his revealed will. There are only two

paths of life before us—God's way of obedience or the way of rebellion and destruction.
Psalm 1:1-6 has as its theme: Life two roads. The life of the faithful person is contrasted with the life of the faithless person. The Holy Scriptures typically divides all humans into two classes:

—godly or ungodly
—natural (unspiritual) or spiritual

Characteristics of the godly

The godly are characterized by righteousness, love, obedience to God's Word and separation from fellowship with the world (Ps 1:1-2). The lives of those who delight in God and His Word have a root system that draws life from God and prospers. The righteous can be distinguished by their lifestyle and associations (v1) and by the things in which they delight (v2)

Those who diligently try to obey God's will are blessed. Their happy condition is like healthy, fruit-bearing trees with strong roots (Jeremiah 17:5-8), and God promises to watch over them. God's wisdom guides their lives. No person can experience God's blessing (Lit. **'blessed is the man that"** (v1) without turning from harmful or destructive associations (v1) to become rooted and established in God's word (v2). Only then are they "like a tree planted by the rivers of water" (v3). Those who are blessed by God not only turn from evil, but also build their lives around the instruction of the Lord. They genuinely take pleasure in God and his beauty, and pattern their lives according to His Word. What motivates their actions is love for God and His Word. As they draw life from God, they live fruit bearing lives (v 3).

Characteristics of the ungodly

Psalm 1:4-6 describes the ungodly, who represent the ways and counsel of the world, who do not abide in God's Word (or counsel), who are cynical about God and mockers of that which is holy, and who consequently have no part in the assembly of God's people (vv. 4-5). The ungodly are unrepentant sinners with three awful pictures: (1) they are like "chaff" blown away by the winds of God's judgments —forces they cannot see (v4), and have no part in God's kingdom (1 Cor 6:9); (2) they will be condemned before God on the judgment day (v5); (3) they will perish for eternity

The two classes of people

"For those who live according to the flesh set their minds on the things of the flesh, but those who live according to the Spirit, the things of the Spirit." (Rom 8:5)

Read Rom 8:5-14

8:5 live according to the flesh…according the Spirit.

Paul describes two classes of people: Those who live according to the sinful nature and those who live according to the Spirit. (1) To live 'according to the flesh" is to be occupied with its desires, thoughts, emotions and physical gratification. This includes not only sexual immorality, adultery, hatred, selfish ambition, outbursts of anger, and so forth (see Gal 5:19-21), but also drug addiction, obscenity, pornographic pleasure from sex scenes in plays, books, magazines, TV, movie, video, the internet and the like

(2) To live "after the Spirit" is to seek and submit to the Holy Spirit's direction and enablement, and to focus one's attention, thoughts, energy and values on the things of God (see Gal 5:22,23). It is to live consciously at all times in the presence of God, trusting Him to give us the help and grace we need to accomplish His will in and through us.

(3) There is tremendous contradiction and tension when attempting to follow the sinful nature and the Spirit at the same time (vv. 7-8; Gal 5:17-18). Those who are (in any way) "in the flesh cannot please God" (v. 8). Paul says the outcome is clear: "If you live according to the flesh, you shall die [spiritually]: but if you through the Spirit do mortify the deeds of the body, you shall live [now and eternally]" (v.13)

Characteristics of the natural, or unspiritual, man/woman

"But the ***natural*** *man does not receive the things of the Spirit of God: for they are foolishness to him; nor can he know them, because they are* ***spiritually*** *discerned. But he who is spiritual judges all things, yet he himself is rightly judged by no one."* (1 Cor 2:14-15)

The natural, or unspiritual, man/woman (Gk *psuchikos*, 1 Cor 2:14) identifies the **unregenerate** person, i.e, one governed by mere natural instincts (2 Pet 2:12). This kind of person does not have the Holy Spirit (Rom 8:9), is under Satan's dominion (Acts 26:18), and is enslaved to the body and its passions (Eph 2:3). He or she belongs to the world, is in sympathy with it (Jas 4:4) and rejects the righteous ways of the Spirit (1 Cor 2:14). The unspiritual person is not able to understand God and His ways, but instead relies on human reasoning or emotions.

Characteristics of the spiritual man/woman

The spiritual man/woman (Gk *pneumatikos,* 1 Cor 2:15; 3:1) identifies the **regenerated** person, i.e., one who has the Holy Spirit. This person is spiritually minded, thinks the thoughts of God (1 Cor 2:11-13) and lives by the Spirit of God (Rom 8:4-17; Gal 5:16-26). Such an individual believes in Jesus Christ, strives to follow the leading of the indwelling Spirit, and resists sensual desires and sin's dominion (Rom 8:13-14).

How does one become a spiritual man/woman? When a person accepts by faith the salvation provided through Christ, he or she is regenerated; the Holy Spirit imparts to him or her a new nature by an infusion of divine life (2 Pet 1:4). He or she is born again (John 3:3, 5, 7), renewed (Rom 12:2) and made a new creation (2 Cor 5:17) and recipient of God's righteousness through faith in Christ (Phil 3:9).

(3) THE MANICHAEN EUROPEAN CHRISTIAN IDEOLOGY OF WHITE SUPREMACY WAS DEMON-INSPIRED

False Religious Teachers are demon inspired

Read 1 Timothy 4:1-5

"Now the Spirit expressly says that in latter times some will depart from the faith, giving heed to deceiving spirits and doctrines of demons. [2]speaking lies in hypocrisy, having their own conscience seared with a hot iron." (1 Tim 4:1,2)

Paul said the false teachers were hypocritical liars who encouraged people to follow "deceiving spirits and doctrines of demons." Satan deceives people by offering a clever imitation of the real thing. Such False Teachers are *not* connected to Christ (Col 2:19); they distorted the truth (2 Cor 11:4; Mt 24:23,24)

As early as the New Testament times heretics had infiltrated the Christian Church. Apostle Paul had warned the church to beware of heretics in Colossians chapter 1,2 and 3. He was fully aware that the devil will inspire heresies (1 Tim 4:1). Paul knew how dangerous and destructive heretics could be that he cursed them.

"If any man preach any other gospel unto you than that ye have received, let him be accursed." (Gal 1:8, 9). John the apostle also gave similar warnings about heretics when he enjoined Christians not to believe every spirit. John distinguished about the Spirit of Truth (know as the Spirit of God, 1 Jn 4:2) and the Spirit Error (known as the spirit of the Antichrist, 1 Jn 4:3).

It is not enough that a teacher appears to know what he is talking about, is disciplined and moral, or says that he is speaking for God. If his words contradict the Bible, his teaching is false. Like Timothy, we must guard against any teaching that causes believers to dilute or reject any aspect of their faith. Such false teaching can be very direct or extremely subtle. False teachers were and still are a threat to the church. Jesus and the apostle repeatedly warned against them (see, for example, Mark 13:21-23; Acts 20: 28-31; 2 Thess 2:1-12; 2 Pet 3:3-7). The danger that Timothy faced in Ephesus seems to have come from certain people in the church who were following some Greek philosophers. Hence the Manichaean philosophy/religion that marked the "European Christian thought" was demon inspired. The church formally denounced Manichaeism heresy because of the pegan roots. Indeed this human tendency to re-create God in our minds, to define Him into what we would wish Him to be, so that He can fit into our own mould is one of the pivotal reasons for God's 2nd Commandment to mankind.
"You shall not make for yourself a carved image—any likeness of anything that is in heaven above, or that is in the earth beneath, or that is in the water under the earth; [5]you shall not bow down to them nor serve them." (Ex 20 :4; Deut 5:8).

Over the centuries both before and after Christ arrived on earth, human beings with finite minds have disobeyed God's law and have circumvented the injunction by fashioning for themselves tangible useless objects made of wood, clay, metals etc

The people of Athens at least were honest enough to admit that God was unknown to them (Acts 17:23). However, when Paul taught them that God has revealed Himself to mankind, to the extent that He wished to be known through His son Jesus Christ, "some men joined him and believed" (Acts 17:34). It is noteworthy that the Holy Bible was not available to the men of Athens as it is to us today. Therefore, when men and women who today have access to the **truth** in the Holy Bible, deliberately distort it for selfish interest so as to mislead and exploit people through false philosophy / doctrines, such people are certainly in league with Satan and his cohorts—demons. This was why Apostle Paul affirmed that a False Teachers is not connected to Christ, but is demon inspired. "... *intruding into those things which he has not seen, vainly puffed up by his fleshly mind. [19]and not holding fast to the Head,.."* (Col 2:18, 19)

Therefore, those who have not seen God (face to face), because *God in Spirit*, but claim to know the color of His skin, are under the wrath of God. The only time when we can see Him face to face and be like Him is stated in 1 Jn 3:2

"Beloved, now we are children of God; and it has not yet been revealed what we shall be, but we know that when He is revealed, we shall be like Him; for we shall see Him as He is. [3]And everyone who has this hope in Him purifies himself, just as He is pure." (1 Jn 3:2, 3)

(4) HOW LIGHT AND DARKNESS ARE USED IN THE BIBLE

(1) God is pictured as light

"The LORD is my light and my salvation;
Whom shall I fear?
The LORD is the strength of my life; Of whom shall I be afraid?" (Ps 27:1)

Fear is a dark shadow that envelops us and ultimately imprisons us within ourselves. Each of us has been a prisoner of fear at one time or another—fear of rejection, misunderstanding uncertainty, sickness, or even death. But we can conquer fear by using the bright liberating light of the Lord who brings salvation. If we want to dispel the darkness of fear, let us remember with the psalmist that "the LORD is my light and my salvation."

Read Isaiah 60:19-22

[19]*"The sun shall no longer be your light by day, Nor for brightness shall the moon give light to you; But the LORD will be to you an everlasting light,——. For the LORD will be your everlasting light."* (Isaiah 60:19, 20)

Isaiah 60:19. This verse looks forward to the Jerusalem of the new heaven and new earth, in which God and the Lamb will be the everlasting light of His people.

See Revelation 21:23, 24 and 22:5, where this beautiful reality is also promised.

(ii) Jesus is the light of God

"In Him was life, and the life was the light of men. [5]And the light shine in the darkness, and darkness did not comprehend it." (Jn 1:4,5)

"The life was the light," *zôç; phôs.* "Life," Gk *zôç,* is a featured term in John's Gospel and epistles. Jesus is the life (14:6), the bread of life

(6:35, 48) and the living water (4:10-11; 7:38). His words are the words of eternal life (6:68). He is the giver of life (6:33; 10:10). Thus, the life revealed in Jesus is imparted to us as we abide in intimate relationship with Him by faith (1 John 1:1-3). This life is eternal life enjoyed now and is ours in its fullness through our future resurrection (5:28-29; 6:39-40, 54). "Light" (Gk *phôs*) is mentioned 23 times in John's Gospel, more than in any other NT book. Jesus is the light and through Him we become children of light (12:36) and must walk in the light and develop the fruit of light (Eph 5:9; 1 John 1:7).

"The darkness did not comprehend it" means the darkness of evil never has and never will overcome or extinguish God's light. Jesus Christ is the Creator of life, and his life brings light to mankind. In his light, we see ourselves as we really are (sinners in need of a Savior). When we follow Jesus, the true Light, we can avoid walking blindly and falling into sin. He lights the path ahead of us so we can see how to live. He removes the darkness of sin from our lives. Have you allowed the light of Christ to shine into your life? Let Christ guide your life, and you'll never need to stumble in darkness.

"That was the true Light which gives light to every man coming into the world." (Jn 1:9)
gives light to every man. Christ illumines all who hear His gospel by imparting a measure of grace and understanding in order that they may freely choose to accept or reject that message. Apart from this light of Christ, there is no other light by which we may see the truth and be saved.

"[35]Then Jesus said to them, "A little while longer the light is with you. Walk while you have the light, lest darkness overtake you; he who walks in darkness does not know where he is going. [36]While you have the light, believe in the light, that you may become sons of light.". (Jn 12:35,36)

Jesus said he would be with them in person for only a short time, and they should take advantage of his presence while they had it. Like a light shining in a dark place, he would point out the way they walk. If they walked in his light, they would become sons of light," revealing the truth and pointing people to God. As Christians, we are to be Christ's light bearers, letting his light shine through us. How brightly is your light shining? Can others see Christ in your actions?

(iii) The Bible often compares goodness with light and evil with darkness or shadow (Jas 1:7)

"Every good gift and every perfect gift is from above, and comes down from the Father of lights, with whom there is no variation or shadow of turning." (Jas 1:17)

The Bible often compares goodness with light and evil with darkness or shadow. For other passage where God is pictured as light, see Psalm 27:1, Isaiah 60:19-22, John 1:1-14.

"This is the message which we have heard from Him and declare to you, that God is light and in Him is no darkness at all. [6]If we say that we have fellowship with Him, and walk in darkness, we lie and do not practice the truth." (1 Jn 1:5,6)

Light represents what is good, pure, true, holy, and reliable. Darkness represents what is sinful and evil. The statement "God is light" means that God is perfectly holy and true and that he alone can guide us out of the darkness of sin. Light is also related to **truth** in that light exposes whatever exists, whether it is good or bad. In the dark, good and evil look alike; in the light, they can be clearly distinguished. Just as darkness cannot exist in the presence of light, sin cannot exist in the presence of a holy God. If we want to have a relationship with God, we must put aside our sinful ways of living. To claim that we belong to him but then to go out and live for ourselves is hypocrisy. Christ will expose and judge such deceit.

(iv) Believers are children of light
"For you were once darkness, but now you are light in the Lord. Walk as children of light." (Eph 5:8)
As children of light your actions should reflect your faith. You should live above reproach morally so that you will reflect goodness to others. Jesus stressed this in the Sermon on the Mount (Mathew 5:15, 16)

"But the path of the just is like the shining sun, that shines ever brighter unto the perfect day. [19]The way of the wicked is like darkness; they do not know what makes them stumble". (Prv 4:18, 19)

(v) The Word of God is light
"Your word is a lamp unto my feet, and a light unto my path." (Ps 119:105)

Thy word is… a light unto my path. God's Word contains the spiritual principles that will help us avoid many sorrows, pitfalls and tragedies brought on my wrong decisions and choices; consequently, we must treasure its wisdom and steadfastly hold on to its precepts in all life's situations (vv. 106,112).

To walk safely in the woods at night we need a light so we don't trip over tree roots or fall into holes. In this life, we walk though a dark forest of evil. But the Bible can be our light to show us the way ahead so we won't stumble as we walk. It reveals the entangling roots of false values and philosophies. Study the Bible so you will be able to see your way clear enough to stay on the right path.

"Oh, send out Your ***light*** *and Your truth!*
Let them lead me;
Let them bring me to Your holy hill
[4]*And to Your tabernacle.*
Then I will go to the altar of God,
To God my exceeding joy;
And on the harp I will praise You,
O God, my God. (Ps 43:3,4)

43:3,4 The psalmist asked God to send his light and truth to guide him to the holy hill, the temple, where he would meet God. God's truth (see 1 John 2:27) provides the right path to follow, and God's light (see 1 John 1:5) provides the clear vision to follow it. If you feel surrounded by darkness and uncertainty, follow God's light and truth. He will guide you.

(vi) The Gospel of Christ is light
"Whose minds the god of this age has blinded, who do not believe, lest the light of the gospel of preach ourselves, but Christ Jesus the Lord, should shine on them. [6]*For it is the God who commanded light to shine out of darkness, who has shone in our herts to give the light of the knowledge of the glory of God in the face of Jesus Christ."* (2 Cor 4:4,6)

4:4 ***god of this world.*** The "god of this world" refers to Satan (cf John 12:31; 14:30; 16:11; Eph 2:2; 1 John 5:19), who holds power over much of the activity of this present age. His rule is, however, temporary and conditional. He continues only by God's permissive will until the end of history (Rev 19:11-20:10). Those who do not submit themselves to Jesus Christ remain under Satan's sway. He blinds their eyes to the truth and glory of the gospel in order that they might not be saved. The solution to this situation is to bind his activity through intercession and to preach the gospel in the power of the Spirit (Acts 1:8) in order that people may hear, understand and choose to believe and be saved (vv. 5-6; see Mat 4:10)

Satan (devil). Satan (Heb, meaning "accuser" or "adversary") was a great angel created perfect and good. He was appointed to be a minister at the throne of God; yet before the world began, he rebelled and became the chief antagonist of God and humanity (Ezek 28:12-15)

(1) In his rebellion against God, Satan drew with him a multitude of lesser angels (Rev 12:4) who are probably to be identified, after their fall, with demons or evil spirits. Satan and many of these lesser angels were exiled to the earth and the atmosphere around it, and operate within this sphere under God's permissive will.

(2) Satan, also called "the serpent," caused the fall of the human race (Gen 3:1-6; see 1 Jn 5:19).

(3) Satan's kingdom (12:26) is a highly systemized empire of evil that has authority over the kingdom of the air (Eph 2:2), fallen angels (Mat 25:41; Rev 12:7), unregenerate humanity (Mat 4:8-9; John 12:31; Eph 2:2) and the world (Luke 4:5-6; 2 Cor 4:4; see 1 John 5:19). Satan is not omnipresent, omnipotent or omniscient; therefore, most of his activity is delegated to demons (Mat 8:28; Rev 16:13-14; see Job 1:12).

(4) Jesus came to earth to destroy the works of Satan (1 John 3:8), establish the kingdom of God and deliver us from Satan's dominion (Mat 12:28; Luke 4:18; 13:16; Acts 26:18). By His death and resurrection, Christ initiated the defeat of Satan and thereby ensured God's ultimate victory over him (Heb 2:14).

(5) At the end of the age Satan is to be confined to the Abyss for a thousand years (Rev 20:1-3). After his release he will make a final attempt to overthrow God; this will result in Satan's final defeat and his being thrown into the lake of fire (Rev 20:7-10).

(6) Satan presently wars against God and His people (Job 1-2; Eph 6:11-18), seeking to draw them away from loyalty to Christ (2 Cor 11:3) and into sin and bondage to this present world system (cf. 2 Cor 11:3; 1 Tim 5:15; 1 John 5:16). Believers must pray constantly for deliverance from Satan (Mat 6:13), be on the alert concerning his schemes and temptations (Eph 6:11), and resist him through spiritual warfare, while remaining firm in the faith (Eph 6:10-18, 1 Pet 5:8-9).

(vii) If you love a Christian brother or sister you are in the light

"He who loves his brother abides in the light, and there is no cause for stumbling in him. [11]But he who hates his brother is in darkness and walks in darkness, and does not know where he is going, because the darkness has blinded his eyes." (1 Jn 2:10, 11)

Does this mean that if you dislike someone you aren't a Christian? These verses are not taking about disliking a disagreeable Christian brother or sister. There will always be people we will not like as well as others. John's words focus on the attitude that causes us to ignore or despise others, to treat them as irritants, competitors, or enemies. Christian love is not a feeling but a choice. We can choose to be concerned with people's well-being and treat them with respect, whether or not we feel affection toward them. If we choose to love others, God will help us express our love.

"A new commandment I give to you, that you love one another; as I have loved you, that you also love one another. [35]*By this all will know that you are My disciples, if you have love for one another."* (Jn 13:34, 35)

13:34 ***love one another***. The Christian is commanded to love, in a greater and special way, all true Christians, whether or not they are members of one's own church or followers of one's particular theological persuasion. (1) Believers must distinguish true Christians from those whose profession is false by examining their love for and obedience to Jesus Christ and their loyalty to God's holy Word (5:24; 8:31; 10;27; Mat 7:21; Gal 1:9).

(2) Any person who possesses a living faith in Jesus Christ and remains loyal to God's inspired and inerrant Word as he or she sincerely understands it, while standing against the prevailing popular spirit of our day, is my brother or sister in Christ and one who deserves my special love and support.

(3) Loving all true Christians, including those who are not of our church, does not mean that we must compromise or accommodate our particular Biblical beliefs or doctrinal differences. Nor does it mean we must necessarily seek organizational unity.

(4) Christians must never compromise God's holiness. Love for God and His will as revealed in His word must control and direct our love for others. Love for God must always be first.

13:35 ***know that you are my disciples***. Love (Gk *agapę*) must be the distinguishing mark of Christ's followers (1 John 3:23; 4:7-21). This agape love is basically a self-giving and sacrificial love that seeks the good of another (1 John 4:9-10). Thus, the relationship among all believers must be characterized by a devoted concern that sacrificially seeks to promote the highest good of our brothers and sisters in Christ. Christians must befriend each other in trials, be careful of each other's feelings and reputation, and deny themselves in order to promote each other's welfare (cf. 1 Cor 13; Gal 6:2; 1 Thes 4:9; 2 Thes 1:3; 1 Pet 1:22; 2 Pet 1:7; 1 John 3:23).

(viii) Light makes us know the will of God

"Jesus answered, "Are there not twelve hours in the day? If anyone walks in the day, he does not stumble, because he sees the light of this world. [10]But if one walks in the night, he stumbles, because the light is not in him." (Jn 11:9,10)

Day pictures the knowledge of God's will and *night* the absence of this knowledge. When we move ahead in darkness, we will be likely to stumble.

ix) Evil people love darkness and hate light

"And this is the condemnation, that the light has come into the world, and men loved darkness rather than light, because their deeds were evil. [20]For everyone practicing evil hates the light and does not come to the light, less his deeds should be exposed. [21]But he who does the truth comes to the light, that his deeds may be clearly seen, that they have been done in God." (Jn 3:19-21)

3:19 ***loved darkness rather than light.*** A fundamental characteristic of the wicked is that they love darkness, i.e, they find their pleasure in sin and immorality (Rom 1:18-32; Phil 3:19; 2 Tim 3:2-5; 2 Pet 2:12-15). On the other hand, truly born-again persons love righteousness and hate wickedness (see Heb 1:9), and are grieved when they see the unrighteous deeds of depraved people (1 Cor 13:6). They take no pleasure in the sensual entertainment or the expression of sinful conduct shown so openly in contemporary society (Ps 97:10; Prv 8:13; Rom 12:9; see 2 Pet 2:8, Rev 2:6).

3:19-21 Many people don't want their lives exposed to God's light because they are afraid of what will be revealed. They don't want to be changed. Don't be surprised when these same people are threatened by your desire to obey God and do what is right, because they are afraid that the light in you may expose some of the darkness in their lives. Rather than giving in to discouragement, keep praying that they will come to see how much better it is to live in light than in darkness.(See 1 Pt 4:3,4).

(x) Satan represents darkness

Read 2 Cor 6:14-18

"Do not be unequally yoked together with unbelievers. For what fellowship has righteousness with lawlessness? And what communion has light with darkness? [15]And what accord has Christ with Belial? Or what part has a believer will an unbeliever?" (2 Cor 6:14, 15)

6:14 unequally yoked... with unbelievers. In God's eyes people ultimately are divided into two categories: those who are in Christ and those who are not (vv. 14-16). Believers are instructed not to be partnered or in intimate association with unbelievers. This includes partnership in business, secret orders (lodges), dating, marriage and close friendship. A Christian's association with unbelievers should be only such as is necessary for social or economic existence, or to show unbelievers the way of salvation.

6:14-18 Paul urges believers not to from binding relationships with nonbelievers, because this might weaken their Christian commitment, integrity, or standing. It would be a mismatch. Earlier, Paul had explained that this did not mean isolating oneself from nonbelievers (see 1 Corinthians 5:9, 10). Paul even tells Christians to stay with their nonbelieving spouses (1 Corinthians 7:12, 13). Paul wants believers to be active in their witness to nonbelievers, but they should not lock themselves into personal or business relationships that could cause them to compromise the faith. Believers should do everything in their power to avoid situations that could force them to divide their loyalties.

(5) SLAVES AND SLAVERY IN THE HOLY BIBLE

Some people justified slavery by saying that it existed in biblical times and was neither condemned by God nor Paul the apostle.
Let us now examine **slave** and **slavery** in the Holy Bible.

Why Joseph's brothers sold him into slavery to the Ishmaelities

Read Genesis 37. Joseph the favorite son of Jacob, is sold into slavery by his jealous brothers.

"28Then Midianites traders passed by; so the brothers pulled Joseph up and lifted him out of pit, and sold him to the Ishmaelites for twenty shekels of silver. And they took Joseph to Egypt." (Gen 37:28)

Although Joseph's brother didn't kill him outright, they wouldn't expect him to survive for long as a slave. They were quite willing to let cruel slave traders do their dirty work for them. Joseph faced a 30-day journey through the wilderness, probably chained and on foot. He would be treated like baggage, and once in Egypt, would be sold as a piece of merchandise. His brothers thought they would never see him again. But God was in control of Joseph's life.

Why Pharaoh turned Hebrews into slaves

9"And he said to his people, "Look, the people of the children of Israel are more and mightier than we; 10come, let us deal shrewdly with them, lest they multiply, and it happen, in the event of war, that they also join our enemies and fight against us, and so go up out of the land." (Exo 1:9,10)

Pharaoh was afraid the Israelites were becoming so numerous that they would organize and threaten his kingdom so he made them slaves and oppressed them to kill their spirit and stop their growth. Slavery was an ancient practice used by almost all nations to employ conquered people and other captives. Most likely, the great pyramids of Egypt were built with slave labor. Although Israel was not a conquered nation, the people were foreigners and thus lacked the rights of native Egyptians.

The law concerning slavery

Read Leviticus 25:39-55; Ex 21:2-11; Deut 15:12-18

44 "And as for your male and female slaves whom you may have—from the nations that are around you, from them you may buy male and female slaves." (Lev 25:44)

Why did God allow the Israelites to purchase slaves? Under Hebrew laws, slaves were treated differently from slaves in other nations. They were seen as human beings with dignity, and not as animals. Hebrew slaves, for example, took part in the religious festivals and rested on the Sabbath. Nowhere does the Bible condone slavery, but recognizes its existence. God's laws offered many guidelines for treating slaves properly.

Slavery was a fact of life in Biblical days. That God allowed Israel to buy slaves from the pagan nations around them was a blessing for the slaves purchased, for God required His people to treat their slaves with much more dignity than they would have received in their own country (cf. Ex 20:10).
Read Exodus 21:2-11

2"If you buy a Hebrew servant, he shall serve six years; and in the seventh he shall go out free and pay nothing." (Ex 21:2)

The Hebrews, though freed from slavery, had slaves (or servants) themselves. A person could become a slave because of poverty, debt, or even crime. But Hebrew slaves were treated as humans, not property, and were allowed to work their way to freedom. The Bible acknowledges the existence of slavery but never encourages it.

Although God did not immediately abolish such evils as slavery or polygamy in Israel, He did regulate them in order to make them more humane (cf. Lev 25:39-40; Deut 15:12-18). On the one hand, these practices were not God's ideal. On the other hand, He permitted them for a time because of the hardness of human hearts (cf. Mat 19:8; see Gen 29:28). Furthermore, God's laws concerning slavery were much more humane than the customs of the nations surrounding them. In the NT, however, God expressed an even higher standard (see John 13:34; Col 3:22-25).

Read Deut 15:12-18. The Law Concerning Bondservants

"And when you send him away free from you, thou shall not let him go away empty handed." (Deut 15:13)

not let him go away empty handed. The Israelites were not allowed to send their slaves away without adequate provision (cf. v. 12). Love for others (cf. lev 19:18) demanded that sufficient food and supplies be given to them so that they began to earn a living. Similarly, the principle of love and justice under the new covenant requires that we treat our employees with compassion, fairness and justice.

Deut 15:12-15. The Israelites were to release their slaves after six years, sending them away with enough food so that they would be amply supplied until their needs could be met by some other means. This humanitarian act recognized that God created each person with dignity and worth. It also reminded the Israelites that they, too, had been slaves in Egypt, and that their present freedom was a gift from God, we do not have slaves such as these today, but God's instructions still apply to us. We must still be sure to treat our employees with respect and economic fairness.

Consequences for violators of God's law for slavery – treacherous treatment of slaves

Read Jeremiah 34:8-22

"But afterward they changed their minds and made the male and female slaves return, whom they had set free, and brought them into subjection as male and female slaves (Jer 34:11)

brought them into subjection. When the Babylonian siege of Jerusalem was temporarily interrupted by an Egyptian challenge to the

Babylonia army (cf. vv. 21-22), the Jews forced their slaves back into bondage. This action showed that the previous freeing of the slaves (v.8) had not been motivated by a concern for justice and God's law, but rather by selfishness. About these flagrant violators of His law, God states: *"Their dead bodies shall be for meat unto the fowls of the heaven"* (v.20).

Paul's instructions for master-servant relationship
Read Ephesians 6:5-9
"And you, masters, do the same things to them, giving up threatening, knowing that your own Master also is in heaven, and there is no partiality with Him." (Eph 6:9)

Although Christians may be at different levels in earthly society, we are all equal before God. He does not play favorites; no one is more important than anyone else. Paul's letter to Philemon stresses the same point. Philemon, the master, and Onesimus, his slave, were brothers in Christ.
Read Col 3:22-25

"Servants, obey in all things your masters according to the flesh; not with eyeservice, as menpleasers; but in singleness of heart, fearing God:" (Col 3:22)
Servants… masters. Paul instructs slaves how to live in a Christian way even within their undesirable situation. He never indicates that the slave-master relationship is ordained by God or should be perpetuated. Rather he sows the seeds for its abolition in Philem 10, 12, 14-17, 21, and in the meantime seeks to regulate it to the benefit of both masters and slaves (Eph 6:5-9; 1 Tim 6:1-2; Tit 2:9-10; cf. 1 Pet 2:18-19).

The Epistle of Paul to Philemon
Background
First, Philemon was a slaveowner (v.16) and church member at Colosse (compare vv. 1-2 with Col 4:17), and probably was a convert of Paul (v.19). Second, Onesimus was Philemon's slave who had run away to Rome for freedom. While in Rome Onesimus came into contact with Paul, who led him to Christ. A strong bond of friendship developed between Paul, the spiritual father, and Onesimus, his son in the Lord (vv.9-13). Paul now reluctantly sends onesimus back to Philemon but with this powerful letter of appeal.

Purpose
Paul wrote Philemon to deal with the specific problem of his runaway slave Onesimus. According to Roman law, a runaway slave could be

punished by death. Paul intercedes on Onesimus's behalf with Philemon and appeals for him to graciously receive Onesimus back as a fellow believer and as Paul's companion, with the same love with which he could receive Paul himself.

Survey

Paul's appeal to Philemon goes as follows: (1) He appeals to Philemon as a Christian brother (vv. 8-9, 20-21) to receive Onesimus back, not as a slave but as a brother in Christ (vv. 15-16). (2) In a wordplay Paul observes that Onesimus (whose name means "useful") was formerly "un-profitable," but now is "profitable," or useful, to both Paul and Philemon (vv. 10-12). (3) Paul wishes Onesimus could remain with him in Rome to serve him in his practical needs while in chains, but he feels constrained instead to send him back to his lawful master {vv. 13-14). (4) Paul offers himself as a substitute for Onesimus's debt and reminds Philemon of his indebtedness to Paul (vv. 17-19). The letter concludes with greetings from some of Paul's co-workers in Rome (vv. 23-24) and with a benediction (v.25).

Special features

More than any other NT portion, it illustrates how Paul and the early church dealt with the problem of Roman slavery. Rather than attacking it directly and thereby stirring up armed rebellion in the Roman Empire, Paul set forth Christian principles that removed the harshness of Roman slavery and eventually led to its banishment altogether within Christianity. (3) It provides unique insight into Paul's inner life, for he identifies himself with a slave so closely that he calls Onesimus "mine own bowels" (v.12).

The spiritual meaning of slavery

Slavery to sin

"Jesus answered them. "Most assuredly, I say to you, whoever commits sin is ***slave*** *of sin.* [35]*And a* ***slave*** *does not abide in the house forever, but a son abides forever."* (Jn 8:34, 35)

8:34 Whoever commits sin. The NT clearly teachers that the Lord Jesus Christ Himself breaks the power and dominion of sin in the lives of those who are His true followers (vv.31-32,36). Individuals who habitually sin are still slaves to sin and unrighteousness and therefore are the children of the devil (cf. 1 John 3:6-10). The union of sincere believers with Christ in His death and resurrection will result in freedom from sin's power and dominion (see 8:36, cf. Rom 6)

The spiritual meaning of freedom

"Then Jesus said to those Jews who believed Him, "If you abide in My word, you are My disciples indeed. [32]And you shall know the truth, and the truth shall make you free." (Jn 8:31,32)

8:32 the truth shall make you free. In the context of human knowledge, many things are true. Yet there is only one truth that will set people free from sin, destruction and Satan's dominion, i.e., Jesus Himself and His revelation of truth in Scripture. Three important observations about truth are as follows: (1) Scripture, especially the original revelation of Christ and the NT apostles, testifies to the truth that frees one from sin, the world and the demonic (see Eph 2:20). (2) Further revelation of "truth" is not needed to complete or make more adequate the gospel of Christ. (3) Saving truth is revealed only from God "by his Spirit" (1 Cor 2:10) and does not originate from any person or humanistic wisdom (1 Cor 2:12-13).

"Therefore if the Son makes you free, you shall be free indeed." (Jn 8:36)
8:36 ye shall be free indeed. Unsaved persons are slaves to sin, impurity and Satan (v. 34; Rom 6:17-20). They live according to the cravings of the sinful nature and the ways of Satan (Eph 2:1-3). (1) As true believers, we possess salvation in Christ with the accompanying grace of the indwelling Holy Spirit and are set free from the power of sin and immorality (Rom 6:17-22; 8:1-17). When we face temptation to sin, we now have the power to act according to the will of God. We are free to be enslaved to God and righteousness (Rom 6:18,22).

(2) Freedom from sin's bondage is one sure criterion by which we may test whether we have eternal life with its regenerating and sanctifying grace living in us. Anyone presently in bondage to immorality either has never experienced spiritual rebirth by the Holy Spirit or, having experienced spiritual regeneration, has yielded to sin and once more entered into the spiritual death that brings slavery to sin (Rom 6:16,21,23;8:12-13; see 1 John 3:15)

(3) This is not to say, however, that we as believers are free from spiritual warfare against sin. Throughout our lives, we will have to constantly fight against the pressures of the world, the sinful nature and the devil (see Gal 5:17, Eph 6:11-12). Full freedom from temptation and the pull of sin will come only with complete redemption at death or at Christ's return for His faithful. What Christ offers us now is the sanctifying power of His life, whereby we who follow the Spirit are set free from the desires of the sinful nature (Gal 5:16-24), and enabled to live holy and blameless lives before Him in love (Eph 1:4).

"For you, brethren, have been called to liberty; only do not use liberty as an opportunity for the flesh, but through love serve one another" (Gal 5:13)
"Now the Lord is that Spirit; and where the Spirit of the Lord is there is liberty." (2 Cor 3:17)

3:17 the Spirit… there is liberty. The freedom that comes through Christ (Gal 5:1) is, first and foremost, liberation from the condemnation and slavery of sin (vv.7-9; Rom 6:6, 14; 8:2; Eph 4:22-24; Col 3:9-10) and the whole dominion of Satan (Acts 26:18; Col 1:13; 1 Pet 5:8). (1) True liberation begins with the believer's union with Christ (Acts 4:12; Eph 1:7) and his or her receiving the Holy Spirit. Liberation from spiritual bondage is maintained through the Spirit's continued indwelling and through obedience to His direction (Rom 8:1ff, Gal 5:18 cf. John 15:1-11).

(2) Freedom provided by Christ is not a freedom for believers to do what they want (1 Cor 10:23-24) but to do what they should (Rom 6:18-23). Spiritual freedom must never be used as a cover up for evil or as a justification for conflict (Jas 4:1-2; 1 Pet 2:16-23). **Christian liberation frees believers for service to God** (1 Thes 1:9) **and other people** (1 Cor 9:19) **in the way of righteousness** (Rom 6:18ff). We are now Christ's slaves (Rom 1:1; 1 Cor 7:22; Phil 1:1), living to God by grace (Rom 5:21; 6:10-13).

"While they promise them liberty, they themselves are salves of corruption; for by whom a person is overcome, by him also he is brought into bondage" (2 Pt 2:19)

2:19 A person is a slave to whatever controls him or her. Many believe that freedom means doing anything we want. But no one is ever completely free in that sense. If we refuse to follow God, we will follow our own sinful desires and become enslaved to what our bodies want. If we submit our lives to Christ, he will free us from slavery to sin, Christ frees us to serve him, a freedom that results in our ultimate good.
"But he who looks into the perfect law of liberty and continues in it, and is not a forgetful hearer but a doer of the work, this one will be blessed in what he does." (James 1:25)

1:25 "The perfect law of liberty" could also be called "the perfect law that gives freedom." It seems paradoxical that a law could give us freedom, but God's law points out sin in us and gives us the opportunity to ask for God's forgiveness (see Romans 7:7, 8). As Christians, we are saved by God's grace, and salvation frees us from sin's control. As believers, we are free to live as God created us to

live. Of course, this does not mean that we are free to do as we please (see 1 Pt 2:16). We are now free to obey God.
1:25 **Law of liberty.** This law (cf. 2:12) is the will of God internalized in our hearts by the indwelling Holy Spirit (cf. Ezek 11:9-20). Through faith in Christ we receive not only mercy and forgiveness (2:12-13), but also the power and freedom to obey the moral law of God (Rom 3:31; see Rom 8:4). **It is called the "law of liberty" because the believer desires to do the will of God: "I will walk at liberty: for I seek out thy precepts"** (Ps 119:45). Freedom is not permission to violate the commandments of Christ and God's moral precepts in Scripture, but rather is the **freedom and power to obey them and be what we were created for.**

What true freedom is in the Holy Bible
"For you, brethren, have been called to liberty; only do not use liberty as an opportunity for the flesh, but through love serve one another." (Gal 5:13)
5:13 Paul distinguishes between freedom to sin and freedom to serve. Freedom or liberty to sin is no freedom at all, because it enslaves you to Satan, others, or your own sinful nature. Christian, by contrast, should not be slaves to sin, because they are free to do right and to glorify God through loving service to others.

"Christ has redeemed us from the curse of the law, having become a curse for us (for it is written, "Cursed is everyone who hangs on a tree" (Gal 3:13)

Redemption refers to Christ setting sinners free from slavery to sin. In Old Testament times, a person's depts could result in his being sold as a slave. The next of skin could redeem him—buy his freedom. Christ purchased our freedom and the price was His life.
Salvation by grace through the activity of faith in Jesus Christ includes not only being **saved *from* condemnation, but also being saved *for* initimate and holy fellowship with God and a life of good** works (as the fruit of faith) (Eph 2:10). **The present stage of salvation saves us from the bondage, power and dominion of sin, and brings us into the fellowship of the Holy Spirit.**

(6) WHAT IS THE COLOR OF THE SKIN OF GOD?

(i). What made Jesus' humanity unique?
(ii). Was Jesus of the Nordic race—extremely light skinned, with blond hair and blue eyes?
(iii). Is God a Jew? Why did God choose Israel as His nation?
(iv). Is the origin of light-skinned people different from dark-skinned people e.g Africans?

What is the color of the skin of God?

Nobody knows the colour of God. Nobody has God face to face!
"You cannot see My face; for no man shall see Me, and live." (Ex 33:20)
"God is Spirit" (Jn 4:23)

"God is Spirit" means He is not a physical being limited to one place. He is present everywhere at the same time. God is **omnipresent** (Ps 139:7-12; cf, Jer 23:23-24; Acts 17:27, 28)
"No one has seen God at any time"
The only begotten Son, who is in the bosom of the Father, He has declared Him." (Jn 1:18)

God communicated through various people in the Old Testament, usually prophets who were told to give specific messages. But no one ever *saw* God. "The only begotten Son, who is in the bosom of the Father" is a title showing that Jesus is both God and the Father's unique Son. In Christ, God revealed his nature and essence in a way that could be seen and touched. In Christ, God became a man who lived on earth.

Only those in heaven shall see God's face.

"---Those who are saved ----they shall see his face." (Rev 21:24; 22:4)
"Blessed are the pure in heart; for they shall see God" (Mat 5:8)

Was Jesus of the Nordic race—extremely white, with blond hair and blue eye?

Jesus was born a Jew. Jews are not of the nordic race. His genealogy is given in Mathew. 1:1-17; and His earthly parents—Mary and Joseph subjected Him to the Jewish ceremonies when He was born. Read Luke 2:21-24.

Jesus was God's Son, but his family carried out these ceremonies according to God's law. Jesus was not born above the law; instead, he fulfilled it perfectly.

Is God a Jew? Why did God choose Israel as his nation

"Now therefore, if you will indeed obey My voice and keep My covenant, then you shall be a special treasure to Me above all people; for all the earth is Mine." (Exo 19:5)

Why did God choose Israel as his nation? God knew that no nation on earth was good enough to deserve to be called his people, his "special treasure." He chose Israel, not because of anything they had done, but in his love and mercy he chose Israel in spite of the wrong

the nation had done and would do. Why did he want to have a special nation on earth? To represent his way of life, to teach his Word, and to be an agent of salvation to the world. "All the nations of the earth" would be blessed through Abraham's descendants (Genesis 18:18). Gentiles and kings would come to the Lord through Israel, predicted Isaiah (Isaiah 60:3). Through the nation of Israel, the Messiah, God's chosen Son, would be born. God chose one nation and put it through a rigorous training program, so that one day it could be a channel for his blessings to the whole world.
Jesus was born a Jew. Jews are **not** extremely white, with blonde hair and blue eyes like the Nordic race.

Is the origin of light-skinned people different from dark-skinned people e.g Africans?
All human beings of all races and all colours originated from Adam and Eve. Adam and Eve, our first ancestors, were the highlight of God's creation. Genesis 2:4-25, 4:1, 2.

"And He has made ***from one blood every nation of men to dwell on all the face of the earth****, and has determined their reappointed times and the boundaries of their dwellings."* (Act 17:26)

"And Adam called his wife's name Eve, because ***she was the mother of all living****.*" (Gen 3:20)

"Therefore, just as through **one man** *sin entered the world, and death through sin, and thus death spread to all men, because all sinned—"* (Rom 3:12)

Christ is the perfect expression of God in human form (Jn 1:14; Col 2:9; 1 Tim 3:16; Heb 1:3)
"And the Word became flesh and dwelt among, and we beheld His glory, the glory as of the only begotten of the Father, full of grace and truth." (Jn 1:14)

When Christ was born, God became a man. He was not part man and part God; he was completely human and completely divine (**Colossians 2:9, Heb 1:3).** Before Christ came, people could know God partially. After Christ came, people could know God fully because he became visible and tangible in Christ. Christ is the perfect expression of God in human form. The two most common errors people make about Jesus are to minimize his humanity or to minimize his divinity. Jesus is both God and man.

What made Jesus' humanity unique

"Let this mind be in you which was also in Christ Jesus,[6] who, being in the form of God, did not consider it robbery to be equal with God,[7] but made Himself of no reputation, taking the form of a bondservant, and coming in the likeness of men." (Phil 2:5-7)

2:5-7 The Incarnation was the act of the preexistent Son of God voluntarily assuming a human body and human nature. Without ceasing to be God, he became a human being, the man called Jesus. He did not give up his deity to become human, but he set aside the right to his glory and power. In submission to the Father's will, Christ limited his power and knowledge. Jesus of Nazareth was subject to place, time, and many other human limitations. *What made his humanity unique was his freedom from sin.* (Jn 8:46; 2 Cor 5:21; 1Pt 2:22, His sinlessness was also demonstrated at His temptation Mat 4:1ff). In his full humanity, Jesus showed us everything about God's character that can be conveyed in human terms. The incarnation is explained further in these passages: John 1:1-14; Romans 1:2-5; 2 Corinthians 8:9; 1 Timothy 3:16; Hebrews 2:14; and 1 John 1:1-3.

Racism/Favoritism/Partiality are contemptible in God's sight God is not a respecter of persons, He shows no partiality nor favoritism

"Ye shall not respect persons in judgment: but you shall hear the small as well as the great; you shall not be afraid of the face of man; for the judgment is God's and the cause that is too hard for you, bring unto me, and I will hear it." (Deut 1:17)

"You shall not oppress a hired servant who is poor and needy, whether one of your brethren or one of the aliens who is in your land within your gates. 15 Each day you shall give him his wages, and not let the sun go down on it, for he is poor and had set his heart on it; lest he cry out against you to the Lord, and it be sin to you." (Deut 24:14,15)

poor and needy. God often warned Israel not to take advantage of the poor but to treat them with compassion and respect. Believers who fail to treat the poor and needy fairly will bring God's condemnation upon themselves (v. 15; cf. Jas 5:1-6)

"For there is no distinctions between Jew and Greek, for the same Lord over all is rich to all who call upon Him." (Rom 10:12)

"Greek," Here the word for Greek is *hellçnos,* meaning "a person of Greek language and culture." In the KJV "Greek" is often used in a generic sense to refer to all Gentiles. It is also used of the pagan world under the Romans who were dominated by Greek culture. This broader sense was used of Gentiles in contrast to Jews.

"There is neither Jew nor Greek, there is neither slave nor free, there is neither male nor, female; for you are all one in Christ Jesus." (Gal 3:28)

3:28 neither male nor female. Paul removes all ethnic, national, socioeconomic and gender barriers with regard to one's spiritual relationship with Jesus Christ. All who are "in Christ" are equal heirs of "the grace of life" (1 Pet 3:7), the promised Spirit (v.14; 4:6) and renewal in God's image (Col 3:10-11). On the other hand, within the context of spiritual equality men remain men and women remain women (Gen 1:27). Their God-assigned roles in marriage, childbearing, family and society remain unchanged (1 Pet 3:1-4; see Eph 5:22-23, 1 Tim 2:13, 15).
Some Jewish males greeted each new day by praying "Lord, I thank you that I am not a Gentile, a slave, or a woman." The role of women was enhanced by Christianity. Faith in Christ transcends these differences and makes all believers one in Christ. Make sure you do not impose distinctions that Christ has removed. Because all believers are his heirs, no one is more privileged than or superior to anyone else.

It's our natural inclination to feel uncomfortable around people who are different from us and to gravitate toward those who are similar to us. But when we allow our differences to separate us from our fellow believers, we are disregarding clear biblical teaching. Make a point to seek out and appreciate people who are not just like you and your friends. You may find that you have a lot in common with them.
"For by one Spirit we were all baptized into one body—whether Jews or Greeks, whether slaves or free—and have all been made to drink into one Spirit." (1 Cor 12:13)

"Where there is neither Greek nor Jew, circumcised nor uncircumcised, barbarian, Scythian, slave nor free, but Christ is all and in all." (Col 3:11)

3:11 The Christian church should have no barriers of nationality, race, education level, social standing, wealth, gender, religion, or power. Christ breaks down all barriers and accepts all people who come to him. Nothing should keep us from telling others about Christ or accepting into our fellowship any and all believers (Eph 2:14,15). Christians should be building bridges, not walls.

Table 2.1 Racism/Favoritism/Partiality are contemptible in God's sight
==

Read James 2:2-4

Why it is wrong to show favoritism.	1. It is inconsistent with Christ's teachings.
	2. It results from evil thoughts.
	3. It insults people made in God's image.
	4. It is a by-product of selfish motives.
	5. It goes against the biblical definition of love.
	6. It shows a lack of mercy to those less fortunate.
	7.It is hypocritical.

8. It is sin.

---

(7) IN WHAT WAYS ARE WE MADE IN THE IMAGE (LIKENESS) OF GOD?

"Then God said, "Let Us make man in Our image, according to Our likeness; let them have dominion over the fish of the sea, over the birds of the air, and over the cattle, over all the earth and over every creeping thing that creeps on the earth." (Gen 1:26)

In what ways are we made in God's image? God obviously did not create us exactly like himself because God has no physical body. Instead, we are reflections of God's glory. Some feel that our reason, creativity, speech, or self-determination is the image of God. More likely, it is our entire self that reflects the image of God. We will never be totally like God because he is our supreme Creator. But we do have the ability to reflect his character in our love, patience, forgiveness, kindness, and faithfulness.

Knowing that we are made in God's image and thus share many of his characteristics provides a solid basis for self-worth. Human worth is not based on possessions, achievement, physical attractiveness, or public acclaim. Instead it is based on being in God's image. Because we bear God's image, we can feel positive about ourselves. Criticizing or downgrading ourselves is criticizing what God has made and the abilities he has given us. Knowing that you are a person of worth helps you love God, know him personally, and make a valuable contribution to those around you.

1:26 **let us make man.** In Gen 1:26-28 we read about the creation of human beings; Gen 2:4-25 gives more specific details about their creation and environment. These two accounts are complementary and teach several things. (1) Both man and woman were a special creation of God, not a product of evolution (v.27; Mat 19:4; Mark 10:6).

(2) Man and woman were both created in the "image" and likeness" of God. On the basis of this image, they could respond to and have fellowship with God and uniquely reflect His love, glory and holiness. They were to do so by knowing God and obeying him (2:15-17). (a) They possessed a moral likeness to God, for they ***were*** sinless and holy, possessing wisdom, a heart of love and the will to do right (cf. Eph 4:24). They lived in a personal fellowship with God that involved moral obedience (2:16-17) and intimate communion. When

Adam and Eve sinned, their moral likeness to God was corrupted (6:5). *In redemption believers must be renewed to the original moral likeness (*Eph 4:22-24; Col 3:10). (b) Adam and Eve possessed a natural likeness to God. They were created personal beings with spirit, mind, emotions, self-consciousness and power of choice (2:19-20; 3:6-7; 9:6). (c) In some sense man and woman's physical makeup is in God's image in a way not true of animals. God gave to human beings the image in which He was to appear visibly to them (18:1-2) and the form that His Son would one day assume (Luke 1:35; Phil 2:7; Heb 10:5).

(3) That human beings were made in the image of God does not mean they are divine. They have been created on a lower order and are dependent on God (Ps 8:5).

(4) All human life is derived initially from Adam and Eve (Gen 3:20; Rom 5:12; Acts 17:26).

It is critical for human beings to know that although we are "created in God's image". There are *unique* attributes of God which human beings do not have.

Unique attributes of God

1.God is omnipresent " ie, He is present everywhere at the same time. (Ps 139:7-12; cf. Jer 23:23-24; Acts 17:27-28).

2.God is omniscient – ie. He knows everything (Ps 139:1-6; 147:5).

3.God is omnipotent – ie. He is all-powerful and has ultimate authority over all things and all creatures (Ps 147:13-18; Jer 32:17; Mat 19:26; Luke 1:37.

4.God is transcendent – ie, He is different and independent from His creation (see Ex 24:9-18; Is 6:1-3; 40:12-26; 55:8-9).

5.God is eternal— ie, He is from everlasting to everlasting (Ps 90:1-2; 102:12; Is 57:15).

6.God is unchangeable – ie, there is no change in God's attributes, in His perfections or in His purpose for humankind (Num 23:19; Ps 102:26-28; Is 41:4; Mal 3:6; Heb 1:11-12; Jas 1:17).

7.God is perfect and holy– ie, He is completely without sin and absolutely righteous (Lev 11:44-45; Ps 85:13; 145:17; Mat 5:46)

8.God is triune – ie, He is one God (Deut 6:4; Is 45:21; 1 Cor 8:5-6; Eph 4:6; 1 Tim 2:5), who has manifested Himself in three divine persons. Father, Son and Holy Spirit (e.g, Mat 28:19; 2 Cor 13:14; 1 Pet 1:2). Each person is fully divine, equal with the other two, yet they are not three Gods, but one)

It is also critical for human beings to know the ***moral*** attributes of God which bear similarities to human qualities and are related to our being created in God's image. The presence of His grace (His Holy Spirit) in our lives enables us to reflect these moral attributes.

Many characteristics of the one true God, particularly His moral attributes, bear similarity to human qualities; however, His attributes all exist to a degree incomparably greater than they do in us. For example, even though both God and humans possess the ability to love, no human is able to love to the degree and intensity that God does. Moreover, it must be stressed that our ability to exercise these characteristics is related to our being created in God's image (Gen 1:26-27) and to the presence of His grace in our lives. In other words, we are like Him, not He like us.

Moral attributes of God

These are reflected in human beings also as a result of their being created in God's image.

1. **God is good** (Ps 25:8; 106:1; Mark 10:18)
2. **God is love** (1 John 4:8) His love is a selfless love that embraces the entire world of sinful humankind (John 3:16; Rom 5:8)
3. **God is merciful and gracious** (Ex 34:6; Deut 4:31; 2 Chr 30:9; Ps 103:8; 145:8; Joel 2:13; He does not cut off and destroy humanity as our sins deserve (Ps 103:10), but offers forgiveness as a free gift to be received through faith in Jesus Christ (Ps 103:11-12; Rom 6:23; 1 Cor 1:3-4; Eph 2:8-9; Tit 2:11; 3:4-5)
4. **God is compassionate (**2 Kg 13:23; Ps 86:15; 111:4). To be compassionate means to feel sorrow for someone else's suffering, with a desire to help.
5. **God is patient (longsuffering) and slow to anger** (Ex 34:6; Num 14:18; Rom 2:4; 1 Tim 1:16).
6. **God is truth** (Deut 32:4; Ps 31:5; Is 65:16; John 3:13).
7. **God is faithful** (Ex 34:6; Deut 7:9; Is 49:7; Lam 3:23; Heb 10:23).
8. **God is just** (Deut 32:4; 1 John 1:9).

8) THE CONSEQUENCES OF THE FALL

"And when the woman saw that the tree was good for food, and that it was pleasant to the eyes, and a tree to be desired to make one wise, she took of the fruit thereof, and did eat, and gave also unto her husband with her; and he did eat." (Gen 3:6)

The woman…did eat, and …her husband with her. When Adam and Eve sinned, moral and spiritual death came immediately (cf. 2:17), while physical death came later (5:5). (1) God had said, "In the day thou eatest thereof thou shall surly die" (2:17). Thus spiritual and moral death occurred at once when they sinned (cf. John 17:3). Moral death consisted in the death of God's life in them and their nature becoming sinful; spiritual death meant that their former relationship to God in innocence was destroyed, resulting in a state of sinfulness. Since the sin of Adam and Eve, every person born comes into the world with a sinful nature ("in/after the flesh"; "carnally minded") (Rom 8: 5-8). This corruption of human nature involves the innate desire to go one's own selfish way without concern for God or others, and it is passed on to all human beings (5: 3; 6:5; 8:21; see Rom 3:10-18, Eph 2:3)

(2) Note, however, that nowhere does Scripture teach that all sinned when Adam sinned or that his guilt was imputed to the whole human race (see Rom 5:12). The Bible does teach that Adam introduced the law of sin and death to all humanity (cf. Rom 5:12; 8:2; 1 Cor 15:21-22).

"Therefore, just as through one man sin entered the world, and death through sin, and thus death spread to all men, because all sinned" (Romans 5:12)

5:12 **through one man sin entered.** In the fall of Adam, sin as an active principle or power gained entrance into the human race (vv. 17,19; Gen 3; 1 Cor 15:21-22. (1) Two results followed: (a) Sin and corruption entered into Adam's heart and life-stream of the human race corrupting all people thereafter. All humans are now born into the world with an impulse towards sin and evil (v. 19; 1:21; 7:24; Gen 6:5, 12; 8;21; Ps 14:1-3; Jer 17:9; Mark 7:21-22; 1 Cor 2:14; Gal 5:19-21; Eph 2:1-3; Col 1;21; 1 John 5:19).

(2) Paul does not explain how Adam's sin is transmitted to his descendants. Nor does he say that all people were present in Adam and participated in his sin, and therefore inherit Adam's guilt. Nowhere does Paul say that Adam was the federal head of his descendants and that his sin was imputed to them. All are guilty before God because of their own personal sin, "because all sinned." The only doctrine that finds Biblical support is that men and women inherit a moral corruption and an impulse toward sin and evil.

(3) Death entered the world through sin, and now all people are subject to death, "for that all have sinned" (vv 12, 14; cf. 3:23; Gen 2:17; 3:19)

Table 2.2

WHAT WE HAVE	*What we have as Adam's children*	*What we have as God's children*
AS CHILDREN	Ruin 5:9	Rescue 5:8
Romans	Sin 5:12, 15, 21	Righteousness 5:18
Chapter 5	Death 5:12, 16, 21	Eternal life 5:17, 21
	Separation from God 5:18	Relationship with God 5:11, 19
	Disobedience 5:12, 19	Obedience 5:19
	Judgment 5:18	Deliverance 5:10, 11
	Law 5:20	Grace 5:20

(9) HOW DO WE REGAIN OUR RELATIONSHIP WITH GOD AND BECOME GODLY/SPIRITUAL

Four critical words describe God's **initiative** to restore His relationship with the Fallen (separated sinful) mankind. These are:

(i) Grace
(ii) Redemption
(iii) Regeneration (Re-creation, Spiritual rebirth, Born again)
(iv) Sanctification

What is grace?

Salvation is purely by the grace of God

"For all have sinned, and come short of the glory of God; Being justified freely by his ***grace*** *through the* ***redemption*** *that is in Christ Jesus."* (Rom 3:23, 24) Grace is God's initiative, love and favor that make possible our salvation in Christ as we receive Him. Salvation does not come by our efforts to keep the law, but by the Holy Spirit and Christ's grace coming into our lives to regenerate our spirits and to re-create us in Christ's image.

"For by ***grace*** *are ye saved through faith; and that not of yourselves: it is the gift of God:* ***Not of works****, lest anyone should boast."* (Eph 2:8, 9)

Not of works. One cannot be saved by works, good deeds of love or strenuous efforts to keep God's commandments. One must be saved by the grace of God. The reasons for this are the following: (1) All the unsaved are spiritually dead (v.1), under Satan's dominion (v.2), enslaved to sin (v.3) and under God's condemnation (v.3).

(2) In order to be saved one must receive God's provision of salvation (vv. 4-5), be forgiven of sin (Rom 4:7-8), be made spiritually alive (Col 1:13), be delivered from the power of Satan and sin (Col 1:13), be made a new creation (v.10; 2 Cor 5:17) and receive the Holy

Spirit (John 7:37-39; 20:22). No amount of self-effort can accomplish the above.

(3) What brings salvation is the grace of God through faith (vv.5, 8). God's gift of grace includes the following: (a) First comes the call to repentance and faith (Acts 2:38). With this call comes the work of the Holy Spirit within a person, giving him or her the power and ability to respond to God. (b) Those who respond in faith and repentance and accept Christ as Lord and Savior receive additional grace to be regenerated or born again by the Spirit and to be filled with the Spirit (Acts 1:8; 2:38; Eph 5:18). (c) Those who become new creatures in Christ receive continuing grace to live the Christian life, resist sin and serve God (Rom 8:13-14; 2 Cor 9:8). Believers strive to live for God by His grace that works within them (1 Cor 15:10). The grace of God operates within committed believers both to will and to act according to God's good purpose (Phil 2:12-13). From beginning to end, salvation is by the grace of God. See GLOSSARY for description of "Election and Predestination."

What is Redemption?

The root meaning of "redemption" (Gk *apolutrçsis*) is ransom by the payment of a price. The expression denotes the means by which salvation is procured, namely, by the payment of a ransom. **After the Fall we had to be redeemed from what we have as Adam's children** (see Table 2:2).

"Knowing that you were not redeemed with corruptible things, like silver or gold, from your aimless conduct received by tradition from your fathers, [19]*but* ***with the precious blood of Christ,*** *as of a lamb without blemish and without spot."* (1 Pt 1:18, 19)

A slave was "redeemed" when someone paid money to buy his or her freedom. God redeemed us from the tyranny of sin, not with money, but with the precious blood of his own Son. (Rom 6:6, 7; 1 Cor 6:20; Col 2:13, 14; Heb 9:12). We cannot escape from sin on our own; only the life of God's Son can free us.

Why shed blood?

"And according to the law almost all things are purified with blood, ***and without shedding of blood there is no remission."*** (Heb 9:22)

Why does forgiveness (remission of sin) require the shedding of blood? This is no arbitrary decree on the part of a bloodthirsty God, as some have suggested. There is no greater symbol of like than blood; blood keeps us alive. Jesus shed his blood—gave his life—for our sins so that we wouldn't have to experience spiritual death, eternal separation from God. Jesus is the source of life, not death. He gave his own life to pay our penalty for us so that we might live. After shedding his blood for us, Christ rose from the grave and proclaimed victory over sin and death.

Why not animal blood as in the Old Testament?
Read Heb 9:13, 14, 15; 10:4

When the people sacrificed animals, God considered the people's faith and obedience, cleansed them from sin, and made them **ceremonially** acceptable according to Old Testament law. But Christ's sacrifice transforms our lives and hearts and makes us clean on the inside. His sacrifice is infinitely more effective than animal sacrifices. No barrier of sin or weakness on our part can stifle his forgiveness.

People in Old Testament times were saved through Christ's sacrifice, although that sacrifice had not yet happened. In offering unblemished animal sacrifices, they were anticipating Christ's coming and his death for sin. There is no point in returning to the sacrificial system now that Christ had come and had become the **final,** perfect sacrifice.

"For it is not possible that the blood of bulls and of goats should take away sins." (Heb 10:4)

10:4 **the blood of bulls.** The blood of animals was only a temporary provision or atonement for the sins of the people, ultimately, a human was needed to serve as a substitute for humanity. Thus Christ came to earth and was born as a human so that he might offer Himself in our place. (see Heb 2:9,14). Furthermore, only a human who was free from sin could take our punishment for sin (2:14-18; 4:15) and thus adequately and perfectly satisfy the demands of God's holiness and justice (cf. Rom 3:25-26).

[14]how much more shall the blood of Christ, who through the eternal Spirit offered Himself without spot to God, clense your conscience from dead works to serve the living God?" (Heb 9:14)

9:14 **the blood of Christ**. The blood of Jesus Christ is central to the NT concept of redemption (1 Cor 10:16; 11:27; Eph 2:13; 1 Pet 1:2; Rev 7:14; 12:11). On the cross Christ shed His innocent blood in order to remove our sins and to reconcile us with God (5:8; Rom 5:19; Phil 2:8; cf. Lev 16).

By His blood Christ accomplished the following (1) His blood forgives the sins of all who repent and believe (Mat 26:28). (2) His blood ransoms all believers from the power of Satan and evil powers (Acts 20:28; Eph 1:7; 1 Pet 1:18-19; Rev 5:9; 12:11). (3) His blood justifies all who believe in Him (Rom 3:24-25). (4) His blood cleanses believers' conscience that they might serve God without guilt in full assurance of faith (9:14; 10:22; 13:18). (5) His blood sanctifies the people of God (13:12; 1 John 1:7-10). (6) His blood opens the way for believers to come directly before God through Him in order to find grace, mercy, help and salvation (7:25; 10:19; Eph 2:13, 18). (7) His blood is a guarantee of all the promises of the new covenant (10:29; 13:20; Mat 26:28; 1 Cor 11:25). (8) The saving, reconciling and purifying power of the blood of Christ is continually appropriated to believers as they come to God through Him (7:25; 10:22; 1 John 1:7). Because those whom Jesus came to redeem are flesh and blood humanity, Jesus also had to become a human being. For only as a true human being could He qualify to redeem the human race from sin and Satan's power (Heb 2:14).

Table 2.3 Summary

WHY DID JESUS HAVE TO DIE TO MAKE US GODLY?

==================================

The Problem	We have all done things that are wrong, and we have failed to obey God's laws. Because of this, we have been separated from God our Creator. Separation from God is death; but, by ourselves, we can do nothing to become united with God.
Why Jesus Could Help	Jesus was not only a man; he was God's unique Son. Because Jesus never disobeyed God and never sinned, only he can bridge the gap between the sinless God and sinful mankind.
The Solution	Jesus freely offered his life for us, dying on the cross in our place, taking all our wrong doing upon himself, and saving us from the consequences of sin— including God's judgment and death.
The Results	Jesus took our past, present, and future sins upon himself so that we could have new life. Because all our wrongdoing is forgiven, we are reconciled to God. Furthermore, Jesus' resurrection from the dead is the proof that his substitutionary sacrifice on the cross was acceptable to God, and his resurrection has become the source of new

> life for whoever believes that Jesus is the Son of God. All who believe in him may have this new life and live it in union with him.

Regeneration (Re-creation; Spiritual rebirth; Born again; new birth)

Jesus confirmed the importance of Re-creation

"Jesus answered and said to him, "Most assuredly, I say to you, unless one is born again, he cannot see the kingdom of God." (Jn 3:3)

In John 3:1-8, Jesus discusses a foundational doctrine of the Christian faith: spiritual birth, or regeneration. Without the new birth one cannot see the kingdom of God, and receive eternal life and salvation through Jesus Christ. The following are important facts concerning the New birth.

What is the meaning of 're-creation' or 're-generation'?
"Therefore, if anyone is in Christ, he is a new creation; old things have passed away; behold, all things have become new". (2 Cor 5:17)

Christians are brand-new people on the inside. The Holy Spirit gives them new life, and they are not the same anymore. We are not reformed, rehabilitated, or reeducated—we are re-created (new creations), living in vital union with Christ (Colossians 2:6, 7). At conversion we are not merely turning over a new leaf; we are beginning a new life under a new Master.

he is a new creation. Through the creative command of God (2 Cor 4:6), those who accept Jesus Christ by faith are made a new creation that belongs to God's totally new world in which the Spirit rules (Rom 8:14; Gal 5:25; Eph 2:10). The believer becomes a new person (Gal 6:15; Eph 2:10, 15; 4:24; Col 3:10), renewed after the image of God (2 Cor 4:16, 1 Cor 15:49; Eph 4:24; Col 3:10), sharing His glory (3;18) with a renewed knowledge (Col 3:10) and understanding (Rom 12:2), and living a life of holiness (Eph 4:24).

This newly created person is *"in Christ Jesus"* (Rom 8:1) enjoys a spiritual life, freedom from condemnation, victory over sin and fellowship with God come through union with Christ by the indwelling Holy Spirit. By receiving and following the Spirit, we are delivered from sin's power and are led onward to final glorification in

Christ. This experience is the normal Christian life under the full provision of the gospel of Christ. The "law of the Spirit of life" (Rom 8:2) is the regulating, activating power and life of the Holy Spirit operating in the hearts of believers. The Holy Spirit comes into sinners and frees them from the power of sin (cf Rom 7:23). The law of the Spirit comes into full operation as believers commit themselves to obey the Spirit (Rom 8:4-5, 13-14). They find a new power operating within, a power that allows them to overcome sin. "The law of sin and death" (Rom 8:2) is the controlling power of sin, which places people in bondage (Rom 7:14) and reduces them to wretchedness (Rom 7:24). Anyone that does not have the Spirit of Christ (The Holy Spirit) does **not** belong to Christ (Rom 8:9) hence, that person is **not** re-created and cannot please God (Rom 8:8). Essentially, a re-created person has "the Spirit of life in Christ Jesus" by whom he/she is "freed from the law of sin and death" (Rom 8:2).

The indwelling Holy Spirit empowers believers to live righteous lives by obeying the "moral law"
"I will put My Spirit within you and cause you to walk in My statutes, and you will keep My judgements and do them." (Ezek 36:27).

"For it is God who works in you both to will and to do for his good pleasure" (Phil 2:13)

"That the righteous requirement of the law might be fulfilled in us who do not walk according to the flesh but according to the spirit." (Rom 8:4.)

'The law might be fulfilled in us'. The Holy Spirit working within believers allows them to live lives of righteousness, which is seen as the fulfillment of God's "moral" law. Thus, the operation of grace and obedience to the law of God are not in conflict (cf 2:13; 3;31; 6:15; 7:12,14) they both point to righteousness and holiness.

A Christian is anyone who has the Spirit of God living in him or her
"But you are not in the flesh but in the Spirit, if indeed the Spirit of God dwells in you. Now if anyone does not have the Spirit of Christ, he is not His." (Rom 8:9)

If...the Spirit of God dwells in you. All believers from the moment of their spiritual birth and faith in Jesus Christ have the Holy Spirit living in them (cf. 1 Cor 3;16; 6:19-20; Eph 1:13-14). Have you ever worried about whether or not you really are a Christian? A Christian is anyone who has the Spirit of God living in him or her. If you have sincerely trusted Christ for your salvation and acknowledged him as

Lord, then the Holy Spirit has come into your life, and you are a Christian. You won't know that the Holy Spirit has come if you are waiting for a certain feeling; you will know he has come because Jesus promised he would (Jn 14:17, 18, 23). When the Holy Spirit is working within you, you will believe that Jesus Christ is God's Son and that eternal life comes through him (1 John 5:5); you will begin to act as Christ directs (Romans 8:5; Galatians 5:22, 23); you will find help in your daily problems and in your praying (Rom 8:26, 27); you will be empowered to serve God and do his will (Acts 1:8; Romans 12:6ff); and you will become part of God's plan to build up his church (Ephesians 4:12, 13)

The Holy Spirit is "the Spirit of life" even to our "mortal bodies"

[10]"And if Christ is in you, the body is dead because of sin, but the Spirit is life because of righteousness. [11]But if the Spirit of Him who raised Jesus from the dead dwells in you, He who raised Christ from the dead will also give life to your mortal bodies through His Spirit who dwells in you." (Rom 8:10-11)

8:10 The body is dead because of sin. Because of sin and its ravaging effects, the body in the natural state is under the process and sentence of death, even for the believer. Our bodies ultimately will be redeemed by resurrection or transformation at Christ's second coming (cf. 1 Cor 15:50-54; 1 Thes 4:13-17). But because Jesus came to give us life here and now (cf. John 10:10), the Holy Spirit who raised Jesus from the dead desires to impart life even to our "mortal bodies" as we embrace His life within us. The Holy Spirit is "the Spirit of life" (cf 8:2).

A believer must *consciously* decide to *surrender* sinful desires of the "flesh"

'For if you live according to the flesh you will die; but if by the Spirit you put to death the deeds of the body, you will live." (Rom 8:13) NKJV

'For if ye live after the flesh, ye shall die: but if ye through the Spirit do mortify the deeds of the body, ye shall live" (Rom 8:13) KJV

8:13 mortify the deeds of the body. Paul emphasizes the necessity for continual warfare against all that would limit God's work in our lives (cf. 6:11-19), for sin is always striving to regain control over us. (1) This spiritual conflict, although directed against Satan and evil spiritual force (Eph 6:12), is primarily against the passions and desires of the "flesh" (Gal 5:16-21; Jas 4:1; 1 Pet 2:11). We as believers must continually decide whether we will surrender to sinful desires or to the demands of the divine nature in which we participate (Gal 5:16, 18; 2 Pet 1:4).

(2) The result of failing to put to death the misdeeds of the body is spiritual death (vv. 6, 13) and the loss of inheritance in God's kingdom (Gal 5:19-21). The words "ye shall die" mean that a Christian can pass from spiritual life back into spiritual death. Thus, the life of God that we receive at our new birth (John 3:3-6) can be extinguished in the soul of a believer who refuses to put to death by the Spirit the misdeeds of the body.

▪ Why is regeneration pivotal to our relationship with God and seeing the kingdom of God?

In other to understand our relationship with God and His requirements from us, it is critical to know God's **innate** character as regards His **holiness.**

Holiness is the foremost character of God

God is perfect and holy—i.e., He is completely without sin and absolutely righteous (Lev 11:44-45; Ps 85:13; 145:17; Mat 5:48). Adam and Eve were created without sin (cf Gen 1:31) but with the capability of sinning. God, on the other hand, cannot sin (Num 23:19; 2 Tim 2:13; Titus 1:2; Heb 6:18). His holiness also includes His dedication to carrying out His purposes and plan.

What is holiness?

Rev 4:8. ***"Holy, holy, holy".*** The Greek word *hagios* means primarily "separate, holy" Holiness means morally perfect, pure, and set apart from all sin. God is completely separate from all creation and all evil and is absolute in purity and holiness. God's holiness is His first and foremost quality that is repeatedly emphasized and praised in this the first of many hyms/songs in Revelation. This is God's nature and character that is encountered most immediately when in His awesome presence.

Isaiah 6:3 ***Holy. holy, holy.*** The foremost characteristic of God revealed to Isaiah is His holiness, signifying His purity of character, separation from sin and opposition to all that is evil.

Isaiah 1:4 ***"The Holy One of Israel."*** The expression as a title for God occurs 26 times in Isaiah, five additional times God is referred to simply as "the Holy One." By using this name for God, undoubtedly derived in part from Isaiah's powerful encounter with God and His holiness (ch 6), the prophet not only emphasized God's distinctively holy character, but also that God's people must be holy if they are to continue in a covenant relationship with Him.

▪ **Without holiness no one can see God**

Sin cannot exist in the presence of a holy God.

"Pursue peace with all men, and holiness, without which no one will see the Lord" (Heb 12:14)

Pursue peace with all men, and holiness. Holiness is being separated from sin and being set apart for God; it is to be close to God, to be like Him, and to seek His presence, righteousness and fellowship with all our hearts. Above all things, holiness is God's priority for His followers (Eph 4:21-24).

(1) Holiness was God's purpose for His people when he planned their salvation in Christ (Eph 1:4)

(2) Holiness was Christ's purpose for His people when He came to this earth (Mat 1:21; 1 Cor 1:2,30). (3)Holiness was Christ's purpose for His people when He gave Himself up for them on the cross (Eph 5:25-27)

(4) Holiness is God's purpose in making us a new creation and in giving us the Holy Spirit (Rom 8:2-15; Gal 5:16-25; Eph 2:10).

(6) Without holiness there is no nearness to or fellowship with God (Ps 15:1-2)

(7) Without holiness no one will see the Lord (Heb12:14; Mat 5:8)

When do we *see* God?

Read Rev 22:1-5

"And they shall see His face, and His name shall be on their foreheads." (Rev 22:4)

They shall see His face. This is the ultimate goal of redemptive history: God living among His faithful people on an earth purged from all evil. On this new earth the saints will see and live with Jesus, the Lamb of God, who through love redeemed them by His death on the cross. Their greatest happiness will be: 'Blessed are the pure in heart: for they shall see God" (Mat 5:8; cf. Ex 33: 20, 23; Is 33:17; John 14:9;1 John 3:2).

▪ **Why is Regeneration necessary?**

Regeneration is necessary because all people, prior to turning to Christ, are in their inherent natures, sinners who are spiritually dead, and who are incapable of obeying and pleasing God (Ps 51:5; Jer 17:9; Rom 8:7-8; 1 Cor 2:14; Eph 2:3).

- **How do we receive Regeneration?**

Regeneration comes to those who repent of sin, turn to God (Mat 3:2), and put their faith in the Lord Jesus Christ alone for salvation (See John 1:12)

Read the parable of the prodigal son in Luke 15:11-24. The father of the prodigal son in that parable represents God the Father. The prodigal son represents sinful mankind separated from God (Isaiah 53:6). The prodigal son **humbled** himself, recognized his lost state and helplessness to save himself and consciously chose to return to his father in contrition and repentance. This was made possible through the grace to God—the work of the Holy Spirit who convicts our hearts of sin (Jn 16:8) and is gently knocking on the door of our hearts to let Him in (Rev 3:20). God loves every one of His creation but He does not gatecrash the soul. He comes in only as we give our consent. God has gone to the utmost lengths to save us through the atoning blood of His Son Jesus Christ. When we allow the Holy Spirit to tabernacle in our hearts, God then works His divine alchemy in our lives by progressively transforming us into His likeness (Rom 8:29) to be all He wants us to be in holiness—**Sanctification.**

- **How do we know if we are still connected to Christ, that is, *"in Christ"*?**

The Holy Spirit gives Assurance of salvation

Read Rom 8:12-17

"For if you live after the flesh, you shall die: but if you through the Spirit do mortify the deeds of the body, you shall live. 14For as many as are ***led by the Spirit of God,*** *they are the sons of God."* (Rom 8:13, 14)

8:14 **led by the Spirit of God.** The Holy Spirit lives within the child of God in order to lead him or her to think, speak and act according to God's Word. (1) He leads primarily by **promptings** that (a) are inward urgings to do God's will and to put to death the misdeeds of the body (v. 13; Phil 2:13; Tit 2:11-12); (b) are always in harmony with Scripture (1 Cor 2:12-13; cf. 2 Pet 1:20-21); (c) are intended to give direction in life (Luke 4:1; Acts 10:19-20; 16:6-7); (d) are opposed to sinful desires (Gal 5:17-18; 1 Pet 2:11); (e) are concerned with the guilt of sin, Christ's standard of righteousness and God's judgment against evil (John 16:8-11); (f) exhort believers to persevere in the faith and warn them concerning falling away from personal faith in Christ (v. 13; Heb 3:7-14); (g) become weaker the longer believers resist obeying the Spirit's prompting (1:28; Eph 4:17-19, 30-31; 1 Thes 5:19); (h) result in spiritual death when rejected (vv. 6, 13); (i) result in spiritual life and peace when obeyed (vv.6, 10-11,13; Gal 5:22-23).

(2) The Spirit's prompting comes by (a) reading God's Word (John 14:26; 15:7,26; 16:13; 2 Tim 3:16-17); (b) praying and fasting (Rom 8:26; Acts13:2-3); (c) listening to godly preaching and teaching (2 Tim 4:1-2; Heb 13:7,17); (d) earnestly desiring and valuing the manifestations of the Spirit (see 1 Cor 12:7-10; 14:6); and (e) heeding the counsel of Christian parents and trustworthy spiritual leaders (Eph 6:1; Col 3:20).

Rom 8:14 **they are the sons of God.** Paul gives the basis for the assurance of salvation here. If we are consistently putting to death the misdeeds of the body, then the Spirit is leading us. Those led by the Spirit are the children of God.

- **What are the rewards for regeneration and remaining a true child of God?**

You may wish to ask "what is in there for me"?

The future stage of salvation (Rom 13:11-12; 1 Thes 5:8-9; 1 Pet 1:5) includes: (i) our deliverance from God's coming wrath (Rom 5:9; 1 Cor 3:15; 5:5; 1 Thes 1:10; 5:9); (ii) our sharing in Christ's glory (Rom 8:29; 1 Cor 15:49) and receiving a resurrected or transformed body (1 Cor 15:52); and (iii) our receiving rewards as faithful overcomers (see Rev 2:7). This future salvation is the goal toward which all Christians strive (1 Cor 9:24-27; Phil 3:8-14). All present warnings, discipline and punishment have as their purpose that believers should not forfeit this future salvation (1 Cor 5:1-13; 9:24-27; Phil 2:12, 16; 2 Pet 1:5-11; see Heb 12:1).

As children of God we inherit God Himself *"And if children, then heirs— heirs of God, and joint-heirs with Christ; if indeed we suffer with Him, that we may also be glorified together"* (Rom 8:17)

What is Sanctification?

Sanctification (Gk *hagiasmos*) means to make holy, to consecrate, to separate from the world, and to be set apart from sin so that we may have intimate fellowship with God and serve Him gladly. ***Holiness is the goal and purpose of our election in Christ*** (Eph 1:4); It means being like God and being dedicated to Him (i.e., living to please Him). Sanctification describes the operation of the Holy Spirit through salvation in Christ by which He delivers us from sin's bondage and power (Rom 6:1-11), separates us from the sinful practices of this present world, renews our nature according to the image of Christ, produces in us the fruit of the Spirit, and enable us to live holy and victorious lives of dedication to God (John 17:15-19,23; Rom 6:5, 13, 16, 19; 12:1; Gal 5:16-22-23). Through the Holy Spirit we are able not to sin (1 Jn 2:1; 3:6), even though we never come to the place where we are free from temptation and possibility of sin.

Sanctification is the process of being made holy. God's goal is to bring "many sons into glory" (Heb 2:10); the glory spoken of here is God's people transformed into God's likeness (2 Cor 3: 18; Rom 8:29). "Sanctification is glory begun, and glory is sanctification completed." Jesus is the One who sanctifies (Heb 2:11; 13:12). The reason Jesus suffered rejection and death outside the city of Jerusalem as an outcast was to sanctify His people, so that we would be presented to God and could share in His glory (see Heb 2:11)

Sanctification was God's will for the Israelites in the OT; they were to live holy or sanctified lives, separated from the lifestyles of the nations around them (see Ex 19:6; Lev 11:44; 19:2; 2 Chro 29:5). Likewise sanctification is a requirement for believers in Christ. (1 Pet 1:15, 16). Scripture teaches that ***"without [holiness] no man shall see the Lord"*** (Heb 12:14). Sanctification is both a work of God and a work of His people (Phil 2:12-13).

We are made holy by the sanctifying work of the Holy Spirit (1 Pt 1:2), by the power of the cross in delivering us from sin (Rom 6), by being renewed in the image of Christ, and by an infusion of grace to obey God according to His Word (cf Gal 5:16, 22-23, 25; Col 3:10; Tit 3:5; 2 Pet 1:9).
In order to accomplish God's will in sanctification, believers must participate in the Spirit's sanctifying work by ceasing to do evil (Rom 6:1-2) , purifying themselves from all filthiness of the flesh and spirit, perfecting holiness in the fear of God" (2 Cor 7:10, and keeping themselves from being polluted by the world (2 Cor 6:17-18; 1 Jn 2:15-16; Jas 1:27; 4:8).

True sanctification requires that believers maintain intimate communion with Christ (see John 15:4), engage in fellowship with believers (Eph 4:15-16), devote themselves to prayer (Mat 6:5-13; Col 4:2) obey God's Word (John 17:17), be sensitive to God's presence and care (Mat 6:25-34), love righteousness and hate wickedness (Rom 12:9; Heb 1:9), put sin to death (Rom 6), submit to God's discipline (Heb 12:5-11), continue to obey, and be filled with the Holy Spirit (Rom 8:14; Eph 5:18).

In the NT, sanctification is not pictured as a slow process of forsaking sin little by little. Rather, it is presented as a definitive act by which the believer by grace is set free from Satan's bondage and makes a clear break with sin in order to live for God (Rom 6:18; 2 Cor 5:17; Eph 2:4-6; Col 3:1-3). At the same time, however, sanctification is described as a lifelong process by which we continue to put to death the misdeeds of the body (Rom 8:1-17), are progressively transformed into Christ's likeness (2 Cor 3:18), grow in grace (2 Pet 3:18), and exercise a greater love for God and others (Mat 22:37-39; 1 John 4:7-8,11,20-21).

GLOSSARY OF SOME BIBLICAL WORDS/CONCEPTS

- Definitions of some crucial words used in the Scriptures as regards God's acts of salvation

==

ELECTION..............God's choice of an individual or group for a specific
Romans 9:10-13 purpose or destiny
JUSTIFICATION.........God's act of declaring us "not guilty" for our sins.
Romans 4:25; 5:18
PROPITIATION.........The removal of God' punishment for sin through the
Romans 3:25 perfect sacrifice of Jesus Christ
REDEMPTION......... Jesus Christ has paid the price so we can go free.
Romans 3:24; 8:23 The price of sin is death; Jesus paid the price.
SANCTIFICATION....Becoming more and more like Jesus Christ through
Romans 5:2; 15:16 the work of the Holy Spirit.
GLORIFICATION.... The ultimate state of the believer after death when he or
Romans 8:18, 19, 3 she becomes like Christ (1 John 3:2).

■ Election and Predestination

"Just as He chose us in Him before the foundation of the world, that we should be holy and without blame before Him in love, 5having predestined us to adoption as sons byJesus Christ to Himself, according to the good pleasure of His will"
(Eph 1:4,5)

Election. God's choice of those who believe in Christ is an important teaching of the apostle Paul (see Rom 8:29-33; 9:6-26; 11:5,7,28; Col 3:12; 1 Thes 1:4; 2 Thes 2:13; Tit 1:1). Election (Gk *eklegó*) refers to God choosing in Christ a people whom He destines to be holy and blameless in His sight (cf. 2 Thes 2:13). Paul sees this election as expressing God's initiative as theGod of infinite love in giving us as

His finite creation every spiritual blessing through the redemptive work of His Son (Eph 1:3-5).

Predestination. Predestination (Gk *proorizç*) means "to decide beforehand" and applies to God's purposes comprehended in election. Election is God's choice "in Christ" of a people (the true church) for Himself. Predestination comprehends what will happen to God's people (all genuine believers in Christ).
(1) God predestines His elect to be: (a) called (Rom 8:30); (b) justified (Rom 3:24; 8:30); (c) glorified (Rom 8:30); (d) conformed to the likeness of His Son (Rom 8:29); (e) holy and blameless (Eph 1:4); (f) adopted as God's children (Eph 1:5); (g) redeemed (Eph 1:7); (h) recipients of an inheritance (Eph 1:14); (i) for the praise of His glory (Eph 1:12; 1 Pet 2:9); (j) recipients of the Holy Spirit (Eph 1:13; Gal 3:14); and (k) created to do good works (Eph 2:10).
(2) Predestination, like election, refers to the corporate body of Christ (i.e., the true spiritual church), and comprehends individuals only in association with that body through a living faith in Jesus Christ (Eph 1:5,7,13; cf. Acts 2:38-41; 16:31).

Summary. Concerning election and predestination, we might use the analogy of a great ship on its way to heaven. The ship (the church) is chosen by God to be His very own vessel. Christ is the Captain and Pilot of this ship. All who desire to be a part of this elect ship and its Captain can do so through a living faith in Christ, by which they come on board the ship. As long as they are on the ship, in company with the ship's Captain, they are among the elect. If they choose to abandon the ship and Captain, they cease to be part of the elect. Election is always only in union with the Captain and His ship. Predestination tells us about the ship's destination and what God has prepared for those remaining on it. God invites everyone to come aboard the elect ship through faith in Jesus Christ. Therefore, the whole purpose of God's grace is to bring us safely home to our Father's mansion.

- **Salvation**

"For I am not ashamed of the gospel of Christ, for it is the power of God to salvation to every- one that believes; for the Jew first, and also for the Greek." (Rom 1:16)

Salvation (Gk *sçtêria*) means "deliverance," "bringing safely through," keeping from harm"; already in the OT God revealed Himself as the One who saves His people (Ps 27:1, 88:1; see Deut 26:8; Ps 62:1; Is

25:6; 53:5). It is described in the NT as "the way" or road that leads through life to eternal fellowship with God in heaven (Mat 7:14; Mark 12:14; John 14:16; Acts 16:17; 2 Pet 2:2, 21; cf Acts 9:2; 22:4; Heb 10:20). This road of salvation must be walked to the very end. (Rev 2:7). See the ***Summary*** of **Election and Predestination** above.

- **What is Eternal life?**

"And this is eternal life, that they may know You, the true God, and Jesus Christ whom You have given Me to do." **(John 17:3)**

"Eternal life" also called "Everlasting life" (Jn 3:16) is the gift God bestows upon us when we are born again. "Everlasting" not only expresses perpetuity but also quality of life—a divine type of life, a life that frees us from the power of sin and Satan and removes us from what is merely earthly in order to know God (cf Jn 8:34-36)

Eternal life is more than endless existence. It is a special quality of life that we as believers receive when we partake of the essential life of God through Christ; this allows us to know God in an ever-growing knowledge and fellowship with the Father, Son and Holy Spirit. In the NT eternal life is described as:

(1)A *present* reality (John 5:24; 10:27-28). The present possession of eternal life requires a living faith. Eternal life is not secured and maintained merely by an act of repentance and faith occurring in the past (see 5:24, notes). It involves also a present living union and fellowship with Christ (1 John 5:12); there is no eternal life apart from Him (John 10:27f; 11:25f; 1John 5:11-13).

(2)A *future* hope. Eternal life is associated with the coming of Christ for His faithful (see John 14:3, note; cf. Mark 10:30; 2 Tim 1:1, 10; Tit 1:2; 3:7) and is contingent upon living by faith and by the Spirit (Rom 8:12-17; Gal 6:8).

- **What is Faith?**

"The just shall live by his faith". (Hab 2:4; Rom 1:17)

Two words describe faith: confidence and certainty. These two qualities need a secure beginning and ending point. The beginning point of faith is believing in God's character—he is who he says. The end point is believing in God's promises—he will do what he says, When we believe that God will fulfill his promises even though we don't see those promises materializing yet, we demonstrate true faith (see John 20:24-31).

Throughout the Scriptures faith is the trustful human response to God's self-revelation via His words and His actions.

"So Jesus said to them...if you have faith as a mustard seed, you will say to this mountain, 'Move from here to there, 'and it will move; and nothing will be impossible for you." (Mat 17:20)

faith... nothing shall be impossible. Jesus frequently comments on the nature of true faith. He speaks of a faith that can move mountains, cause miracles and healing, and accomplish great things for God. Just what is this faith that Jesus speaks of? (1) Faith produces results: "it shall remove" mountains.

(2) Faith is not a belief in "faith" as a force or power, but it is a "faith in God" (Mk 11:22).

(3) Faith is a work of God within the hearts of Christians (Mk 9:24; Phil 2:13). It involves an awareness divinely imparted to our hearts that our prayers are answered (Mark 11:23). The Holy Spirit creates it within us; we cannot produce it in our own minds (Rom 12:3, 1 Cor 12:9

(4)Since faith is a gift imparted to us by Christ, it is important to draw near to Christ and His Word and to deepen our commitment to, and confidence in, him (Rom 10:17; Phil 3:8-15). We are dependent on him for everything; "for without me ye can do nothing" (John 15:5; see also John 3:27; Heb 4:16; 7:25). In order words, we must seek Christ as the author and finisher of our faith (Heb 12:2). His presence and our obedience to His Word are the source and the secret of faith (9:21: John 15:7).

(5) Faith is under God's control. It is given on the basis of His love, wisdom, grace and kingdom purpose. It is given to accomplish His will and to express His love for us. It is not to be used for our own selfish interests (Jas 4:3).

▪ Who is Jesus?

"And Thomas answered and said unto him, my Lord and my God." (John 20:28)

My Lord and my God. The Scriptures declare that Jesus is God. This is the foundation of the Christian faith and is of utmost importance for our salvation. Without Christ being divine, He could not have made atonement for the sins of the world. The deity of Jesus Christ is shown by the following:

(1) Divine names are given to Him in Scripture:

(a) God (Jn 20:28; Is 9:6; Rom 9:5; Tit 2:13; Heb 1:8); (b) the Son of God (Jn 5:25; Mat 16:16-17; 8;29; 27:40,43; Mark 14:61-62; Luke 22:70); (c) the first and the last (Rev 1:17; 2:8; 22:13); (d) the Alpha and the Omega (Rev 1:8; 22:13); (e) the beginning and the end (Rev 22:13; (f) the Holy One (Hos 11:9, Acts 3:14); (g) the Lord (Luke

2:11; Acts 4:33; 9:17; 16:31; (h) Lord of all and Lord of glory (Ps 24:8-10; Acts 10:36; 1 Cor 2:8).

(2) Divine worship is given to Christ (John 5:23; 13:13; 20;28; Mat 14:33; Luke 5:8), and prayers are addressed to Him (Acts 7:59; 1Cor 1:2; 2Cor 12:8-9).

(3) Divine offices are assigned to Christ: (a) creator of the universe (John 1:3; Col 1:16; Heb 1:8,10; Rev 3:14); (b) sustainer of all things (Col 1;17; Heb 1:3); (c) forgiver of sins (Mark 2:5, 10; Luke 7:48-50); (d) bestower of resurrection life (John 5:28-29; 6:39-46; Acts 17:31; 2 Tim 4:1); (f) giver of salvation (John 5:24-26; 6:47; 10:28; 17:2)

(4) The NT sees Christ in OT statements about the Lord. Compare Ps 23:1 with John 10:11; Ps 102:24-27 with Heb 1:10-12; Is 8;13-14 with 1 Pet 2;7-8; Jer 17:10 with Rev 2:23; Ezek 34:11-12 with Luke 19:10.

(5) The name of Jesus Christ is associated with that of God the Father (Jn 14;1, 23; Mat 28: 19; Rom 1:7; 2 Cor 13:14; Col 2:2; 1 Thes 3:11; Jas 1:1; Rev 5:13; 7:10).

(6) Christ's sinlessness and holiness testify to His deity (Luke 1:35; 2Cor 5:21; Heb 4;15).

(7) Christ was declared to be the Son of God by His resurrection (Rom 1:4).

These conclusive proofs of Christ's deity mean that believers must act toward Christ in exactly the same manner as they act toward God the Father. They must believe in Him, pray to Him, serve Him and love Him (see also John 1:1, and Mark 1:11).

▪ Who is the Holy Spirit?

God is three persons in one—the Father, the Son, and the Holy Spirit. God became a man in Jesus so that Jesus could die for our sins. Jesus rose from the dead to offer salvation to all people through spiritual renewal and rebirth. When Jesus ascended into heaven, his physical presence left the earth, but he promised to send the Holy Spirit so that his spiritual presence would still be among mankind (see Luke 24:49). When Jesus said: "I will not leave you orphans, I will come to you," (John 14:18) he meant it. Although Jesus ascended to heaven, he sent the Holy Spirit to live in believers, and to have the the Holy Spirit is to have Jesus himself. The Holy Spirit first became available to all believers at Pentecost (Acts 2). Whereas in Old Testament days the Holy Spirit empowered specific individuals for specific purpose, now all believers have the power of the Holy Spirit available to them. For more on the Holy Spirit, read 14:16-28; Romans 8:9; 1 Cor 12:13 and 2 Cor 1:22.

The Holy Spirit is also called "the Spirit of God" (Rom 8:9); "the Spirit of Christ" (Rom 8:9); "the Spirit of holiness" (Rom 1:4), the Spirit of adoption (Rom 8:15); and "the Spirit of truth" (Jn 14:17). Jesus referred to the Holy Spirit as "another Helper/Comforter" (Jn 14:16; 16:26). The Holy Spirit is imparted to us through the **breath** of Jesus Christ (John 20:22). "God is Spirit "(John 4:24); The Holy Spirit is the "breath/Spirit" of God that gives life. (cf Gen 2:7; Ps 33;6, Ezek 37: 1-14). It is through the Holy Spirit that God acts, reveals His will, empowers individuals and discloses His personal presence.

The most important thing about the Holy Spirit is that **He is Holy**. His holy character, along with the manifestation of that holy character in the lives of believers, is what matters most (cf. Rom 1:4; Gal 5:22-26).

Helper/Comforter. The Holy Spirit is called the 'Helper' because, among other functions, He helps (empowers) us to obey God's laws (Ezek 36:27; Phil 2:13) so that we become all that God wants us to be. The Spirit will be by the disciples'/believers' side to help and strengthen them (cf. Mat 14:30-31), to teach the true course for their lives (v.26), to comfort in difficult situations (v.18), to intercede in prayer for them (Rom 8:26-27; cf 8:34), to be a friend to further their best interest (v.17) and to remain with them forever.As the "Spirit of adoption," at regeneration, the Holy Spirit gives us the right to become the children of God. (John 1:12, 13; Gal 4:5-7).
"The Spirit of truth, whom the world cannot receive, because it neither sees Him nor knows Him; but you know Him, for he dwells with you and will be in you" (Jn 14:17)

The Spirit of truth. The Holy Spirit is called "the Spirit of truth" (15:26; 16:13; cf. 1 John 4:6; 5:6), because He is the Spirit of Jesus, who is the truth. As such, He testifies to the truth (18:37), enlightens concerning the truth , exposes untruth (16:8) and guides the believer into all truth (16:13). Those who are willing to sacrifice truth for the sake of unity, love or any other reason deny the Spirit of truth, whom they claim lives in them. The church that abandons the truth abandons its Lord. The Holy Spirit will not be the Counselor of those who are indifferent to the faith or halfhearted in their commitment to the truth. He comes only to those who worship the Lord "in spirit and in Truth" (4:24)

What is the law?

Read Matthew 5:17-20

"Do not think that I came to destroy the Law or the Prophets. I did not come to destroy but to fulfill" (Mat 5:17)

5:17 God's moral and ceremonial laws were given to help people love God with all their hearts and minds. Throughout Israel's history, however, these laws had been often misquoted and misapplied. By Jesus' time, religious leaders had turned the laws into a confusing mass of rules. When Jesus talked about a new way to understand God's law, he was actually trying to bring people back to its *original* purpose. Jesus did not speak against the law itself, but against the abuses and excesses to which it had been subjected. (See John 1:17).

5:17-20 If Jesus did not come to destroy the law, does that mean all the Old Testament laws still apply to us today? In the Old Testament, there were three categories of law: ceremonial, civil, and moral.

(1) The *ceremonial law* related specifically to Israel's worship (see Leviticus 1:2, 3, for example). Its primary purpose was to point forward to Jesus' death and resurrection. While we are no longer bound by ceremonial laws, the principles behind them—to worship and love a holy God—still apply. Jesus was often accused by the Pharisees of violating ceremonial law.

(2) The *Civil law* applied to daily living in Israel (see Deuteronomy 24:10, 11, for example). Because modern society and culture are so radically different from that time and setting, all of these guidelines cannot be followed specifically. But the principles behind the commands are timeless and should guide our conduct. Jesus demonstrated these principles by example.

(3) The *moral law* (such as the Ten Commandments) is the direct command of God, and it requires strict obedience (see Exodus 20:13, for example). The moral law reveals the nature and will of God, and it still applies today. Jesus obeyed the moral law completely.

The purpose of the Law

Note that the law was given in connection with the covenant that God made with His people; it set forth the covenant stipulations they were expected to obey in loyalty to the Lord God to whom they belonged. The Israelites formally accepted these covenant obligations (Ex 24:1-8).

Israel's obedience to the law was to be grounded in God's mercy and in His deliverance of the people (Ex 19:4). Note that the law was given *after* they had been saved by the blood of the Passover lamb and redeemed from slavery (Ex 20:2), and while they were living as pilgrims on the earth by God's grace (Ex 19:4).

The Old Testament (OT) law and covenant were not complete, nor were they intended to be permanent. The law acted as a temporary guardian for God's people until Christ came (Gal 3:22-26). The old covenant has now been replaced by the new covenant, in which God has disclosed fully His plan of salvation through Jesus Christ (Rom 3:24-26; see Gal 3:19). (1) The law was given by God "because of transgressions" (Gal 3:19), i.e, in order to show sin as the violation of God's will and to awaken humanity's sense of need for God's mercy, grace and salvation in Christ (Gal 3;24; cf Rom 5:20; 8:2)
(2) Although the OT law was holy, good and righteous (Rom 7:12), it was inadequate in that it could not impart spiritual life or moral strength (Gal 3:21; Rom 8:3; Heb 7:18-19).
(3) The Law acted as a temporary tutor for God's people until salvation through faith in Christ came (Gal 3: 22-26).
(4) The Law was given "to lead us to Christ that we might be justified by faith (Gal 3;24).

References

1. Life Application Bible. New King James Version. (NKJV) TYNDALE
2. Life in the Spirit Study Bible. ZONDERVAN
3.The World of Llife Study Bible NKJV. NELSON
4.Selwyn Hughes. **Every Day with Jesus**. *Alive.* Jan/Feb 2016 and *The Presence of God.* May/June 2016.

Chapter 3

The Epidemiology Of Skin Bleaching Practices

Story highlights

- Body modification practices is a global phenomenon; skin bleaching is one of the body modification practices.

- The preference for fair skin in the majority of the Global South is manifested in a variety of ways: the most tangible of which is the widespread use of skin bleaching products. Skin bleaching employs dermatological, cosmetic, or homemade depigmentation products that inhibit the production of melanin and/or remove the top layer of the epidermis

- This bleaching industry has spawned a new language with terms either being derogatory or flattering e.g. **'Whitening,' 'lightening,' 'bleaching,' 'toning,' 'bukes/beauxing,' 'browning,' 'cake soap,'** '***tetrasaiklini,'*** **'Yellow fever,' "Fanta face, Cocoa cola body"** ***"na nso eben,"*** **"Otupa palor,"** ***"Mafuta,"*** **"FBI,"** ***Xessal, "tcha-tcho", "kwitukuza", "ambi"*** and "***maquillage".***

- According to estimated values, skin bleaching is practiced, at least occasionally, by two out of three inhabitants of Brazzaville, Congo, (and one out of four men); seven out of ten patients in two hospitals in Pretoria, South Africa practiced skin bleaching; in Cote d'voire, it is estimated that "eight out of every ten seemingly fair-complexioned women use skin—lightening products on a regular basis; among Zambian women aged 30-39, as many as 60% reportedly use skin bleaching agents; in East Africa about 30% of the women bleach. It seems that in many parts of the continent, skin bleaching is nothing less than a way of life.

- Prevalence from studies in specific countries in Africa are Mali 53%, Nigeria 77%, Senegal 67.2%, Togo 60%, Ghana 39.2%, East Africa 30%, Rwanda 35%, South Africa 35%, Republic of Benin 36.6%, Saudi Arabia 38.95, Jordan 60.7%.
- Men also bleach their skin in several countries including Nigeria, Ivory Coast, Rwanda, Congo, Zambia and Jamaica. Male skin bleaching is institutionalized in India.

- Skin lightening products are manufactured in many countries including UK, Italy, China, the Dominican Republic, Lebanon, Mexico, India, Pakistan, the Philippines, Thailand, Indonesia and the USA. The products can also be purchased online.

- Skin whitening products have remained prominent over time, often due to historical beliefs and perceptions about fair skin. Sales of skin whitening products across the world grew from $40 billion to $43 billion in 2008. Corporations have created product lines in a wide range of price categories, such that whiteners are financially accessible.

- Light skin tone can be transformed into social capital (social networks), symbolic capital (esteem or status), or even economic capital (high-paying job or promotion). The motives for current skin bleaching in Africa can be grouped under the following headings; aesthetics and beauty; social domination, attraction and seduction, fashion, strengthening of self, success, compliance, pleasure and sensuality and medical reasons.

- Unquestionably, right across the continent of Africa (except perhaps South Africa, Sudan and Liberia where there is institutional colorism), the primary motive why women lighten their skin is to attract the opposite gender and improve their chances in the marriage market.

- The production and marketing of skin-lightening products offering the promise of lighter, and whiter skin has become a multi-billion dollar international industry. Skin lightening has been incorporated into transnational flows of capital and culture and is implicated in both the formal global economy and various informal, often underground economies. Multinational corporations have jumped on the bandwagon and are spending large sums of money on research and development of both mass and specialised skin-lightening markets.

- The rise of skin bleaching around the globe can also be attributed to the constant, current mass-marketing of contemporary images of white beauty. Wealthy nations like the United States, Japan, and many European nations create many of the global images of white (or light) beauty. In turn, these same nations are also home to the cosmetics companies that produce some of the top-selling skin-bleaching creams, including L'Oreal, Unilever, Schiseido, Vaseline, Emami, Revlon and others.
- Supporting women in altering their natural phenotypes to conform to a Eurocentric beauty standard only validates the racism and colorism behind the beauty standard itself. Moreover, not only is skin bleaching ideologically problematic, it presents a myriad of health risks.

- Dangerous homemade concoctions containing caustic and toxic chemicals are fabricated by poor women in Africa for bleaching because they cannot afford the expensive high-end products

- With the high rates of migration, the prevalence and complications of skin lightening cosmetics can no longer be seen as a health issue in African countries alone, but a global health challenge.

- The practice of skin bleaching has also been reported in Africans and Afro-Caribbeans living in European countries, including the United Kingdom and France. 16% to 28% of adult African women seeking dermatological treatment in Paris are regular users of skin bleaching agents.

- In the United Kingdom, Asians, Africans and Afro-Caribbeans make up 14 percent of the country's 86 million people. They make up part of a cosmetics market in Europe alone worth, at least, US $200 million. Ethnic consumers of skin bleaching in UK account for around one in 10 people. The motives for skin bleaching in UK are similar to the motives back in their home countries—largely viz for aesthetic reasons and improve their chances in the marriage market. The products used contain very potent corticosteroids, hydroquinone and mercury. Corticosteroids are not legally over-the-counter drugs in the UK as they are prescription drugs.

Hydroquinone has been banned decades ago in cosmetics in the UK because of its toxicity. Mercury is banned both in cosmetics and medicinal because it is a very toxic chemical.

However, the law in UK allows manufacturers to make products banned in UK as long as they are for export. These products find their way back to Europe among immigrant communities who use them. Toxic mercury-containing bleaching creams and soaps made in UK have been found in dozens of countries in Africa. Extensive research, funded by the Danish Council for development research, carried out in Tanzania and Kenya on the use of these mercury containing products, have found high levels of mercury in hair samples and very high prevalence of nephrotic syndrome (kidney damage) among women who use the products as bleaching agents and also toxic environmental pollution with methylmercury from effluent of bath soaps and creams containing mercury. This is expected to inevitably, lead to consumption of toxic fish containing mercury in such communities.

- **Jamaica** is an island of 2.6 million people, a plural society in which groups mix, but they do not combine. There are three separate and unique cultural sections: white, brown and Black with their distinctive institutions. 80% are Afro-Caribbeans. The three sections reflect and are guided by their racial and cultural ancestry. Jamaica is a colorized society.

There is no study to define the exact prevalence of skin bleaching in Jamaica, although dermatologists in Jamaica say about 20% of their patients present with complications of the skin bleaching chemicals. Poorer women in Jamaica slums are still the primary consumers of black market commodities often creating concoctions from household products to strengthen the potency of these creams and probably make the cost affordable. The women have become so desperate to the extent of debasing themselves by swallowing "fowl pill," an anti-infection drug approved only for veterinary use in Jamaica for chickens and other fowls. This product is labeled "poison…not for human use" but the women simply call it "fowl pill."

Successive governments in Jamaica have put in interventions based on increased awareness of the health hazards—they have all failed. The responses from the women have been that of **indifference,**

defiance, **resentment** and a **feeling of inequity in the society due to colorism.**

- In **India**, pale skin is considered more attractive, while dark skin is associated with a lower class status, creating a massive market for skin whitening creams. Fairer skin tones also correlate to higher caste status in the Hindu social order. 60 to 65 percent of the women in India use skin lightening products on a daily basis. Skin lightening in India is a US $400 million business with customers across the socio-economic spectrum. The fairness cream sector is growing at 25% per year compared with 15% for the cosmetic industry as a whole. Nearly 61% of skin care products in India contains bleaching agents. In India issues such as employment and matrimonial matters often rest on skin tone. In professions such as aviation, films and modeling, white skin is a prerequisite. Indian men both urban and rural are obsessed with white skin. Perhaps no other country in the world is there a perpetually evolving skin lightening products which include whitening creams, soaps, lightening after-shaves, fairness wipes, armpits whitener, genital whitener, fairness baby oil etc.

- **In South and East Asian countries,** light skin has traditionally been seen as more attractive, and a preference for lighter skin remains prevalent and skin whitening cosmetic products are popular. Four out of ten women surveyed in Hong Kong, Malaysia, the Philippines and South Korea use a skin whitening cream, and more than 60 companies globally compete for Asia's estimated US$18 billion market. Philippino women are the highest users with 50% using whitening products. Some two thirds of men surveyed in Hong Kong said they prefer lighter skinned women and almost half of young Asia adults have admitted to use skin whiteners in attempts to achieve lighter complexion. Asian colorism is not "racism" but an issue of "class/status" because dark skin is associated with peasantry—outdoor work. Asian colorism isn't about preserving racial purity and killing off dark-skinned people. The *product* of Asian colorism, however, isn't much different from the products of American racism. Both systems instill in darker skinned people a sense of low worth.
- In parts of **Latin America**, light skin is seen as more attractive. In Mexico and in Brazil, light skin represents power. Skin color is such an obsession in some countries that specific words describe distinct skin tones from "*jincha*," Puerto Rican slang for "glass of milk" to "*morena*," literally "brown". Colorism is highly prevalent in

Brazil which has the largest population of African descendants in the world as a result of the transatlantic slave trade. The use of skin lightening products is heavily practised in Brazil. Indeed there is an aphorism "In Brazil money bleaches!" In Latin American countries, there are families who constantly want their children to ***'mejorar la raza'*** (improve the race) by marrying lighter skinned or if they are lucky, white people.

- In the **United States** (USA) skin-bleaching has been as much a part of USA national history as the organized system of slavery and legalized racial segregation. In 1990, $ 44 million of over-the-counter skin-bleaching products were purchased. Skin lightening in the USA is a tragic but reasonable response to the narrow American representation of beauty, power, and womanhood. Based on historical and current ideas in American society, skin-lightening products allow entry into a more accepted, respected, and desired sect of society. No formal studies have assessed the prevalence of skin lightening in the USA. However, the tide shifted after the Civil rights and Black Pride movements began and took root, and there is evidence that the sale of skin-bleaching products actually came down. In current times, skin lightening creams also exist but they differ in the fact that they are used to **even out** skin tones than to lighten the skin. A 'beauty cream' manufactured in Mexico but imported into the US was found to contain very high levels of mercury. This product caused signs of mercury toxicity among Hispanic women and household members in the border communities of Arizona, California, New mexico and Texas. Recently, toxicity associated with mercury-containing soap has been reported from OTC products purchased in Chicago stores and some online products. Currently in the USA there is a black market for creams with prescription strengths hydroquinone, strong corticosteroids and mercury. They are available in local salons, ethnic food stores, eBays, flea market, herb shops, local beauty stores and bodeja market. Many of these products are produced in Africa, India, Mexico, the Philippines but imported and sold in the US illegally. This is of particular importance given the fact that the demographics of the USA is changing with a higher proportion of the US population predicted to be of African and Hispanic decent in the future. Doctors in the US have reported seeing cases with complications of these products especially among people from West Africa and the Caribbean Ancestry. Both the FDA and Health officials have warned that skin lightening creams from outside US can be hazardous.

THE EPIDEMIOLOGY OF SKIN BLEACHING PRACTICES

Skin bleaching: a global problem

Skin bleaching is the use of home-made products, cosmetic creams, and dermatological creams to reduce the melanin in the skin. This chemical alteration of the physicality is a global phenomenon. Several studies have documented the occurrence of skin bleaching in Latin America,[1] North America,[2,3,4] Europe,[5,6] Asia,[7,8,9] the Caribbean,[10,11,12,13] Africa,[14,15] and the Middle East.[14,15]

The worldwide awareness of the cultural practice of skin bleaching originates from the work of Findlay *et al*,[17] who in 1975 first reported on the occurrences of exogenous ochronosis in South African women. These women had used high concentrations (3.5-7%) of hydroquinone-containing agents over the course of many years for bleaching their skin. Skin bleaching remained a problem in South Africa and by 1986 the total sales volume of skin lighteners was an estimated 30 million pounds. The first report from West Africa about skin bleaching was by Marchand *et at*, in 1975,[18] in a study in Senegal, other reports soon followed. Currently, skin bleaching continues to have an impact on dermatological practice in many sub-Sahara African communities.

References

1. Winders J, Jones JP III & Higgins MJ. Making gueras: Selling white identities on late-night Mexican television. *Gender, Place and Culture*. 2005; 12:71–93.

2 . Hall RE. The "bleaching syndrome": Implications of light skin for Hispanic American assimilation.Hispanic Journal of Behavioral Sciences. 1994; 16: 307–14.

3.Hall RE. The bleaching syndrome: African Americans' response to cultural domination vis-a'-vis skin color. *Journal of Black Studies*. 1995a; 26:172-84.

4.Hall RE. The color complex: The bleaching syndrome. *Race, Gender & Class*. 1995b; 2:99–110.

5. Mire A. Pigmentation and empire: The emerging skin whitening industry. *Counter Punch*. 28 July, 2005. http://www.counterpunch.org/mire07282005.html.

6. Petit A, Cohen-Ludmann C, Clevenbergh P, Bergmann JF, & Dubertret L. Skin lightening and its complications among African people living in Paris. *Journal of American Academy of Dermatology*. 2006; 55: 873-8

7. Ashikari M. Cultivating Japanese whiteness—The whitening cosmetics boom and the Japanese identity. *Journal of Material Culture*. 2005; 10: 73–9.

8. Easton A. Women have deadly desire for paler skin in the Philippines. *Lancet*. 1998; 352:1–2.

9. Karan K. Obsessions with fair skin: Color discourses in Indian advertising. *Advertising Society & Review*. 2008; 9:1–13.
10. Charles CAD. Skin bleaching, self-hate and Black identity in Jamaica. *Journal of Black Studies*. 2003a; 33:711–28.
11.Charles CAD. Skin bleaching and the deconstruction of Blackness. *Ideaz*. 2003b; 1: 78–105.
12. Hope DP. Fashion ova style: Contemporary notions of skin bleaching in Jamaican dance hall culture. *Jenda: A Journal of Culture and African Women Studies*. 2009; 14:101–26.
13. Menke J. Skin bleaching in multi-ethnic and multicolored societies: *The case of Suriname*. Paper presented at the Caribbean Studies Association Conference, Nassau, Bahamas. 2002, May 27–June 1.
14. Blay YA. Yellow fever: Skin bleaching and the politics of skin color in Ghana. Ph.D. Dissertation. Temple University. 2007.
15. de Souza MM. The concept of skin bleaching in Africa and its devastating health implications. *Clinics in Dermatology*. 2008; 26:27–29.
16. Al-Saleh I & Al-Doush I. Mercury content in skin lightening creams and potential hazards to the health of Saudi Women. *Journal of Toxicology and Environmental Health*. 1997; 51:123–30.
17. Findlay GH, Morrison JGL, and Simson IW. *Brit J Derm*. 1975; 93:613.
18. Marchand JP, N'daiye B, Arnold J, Sarrat H. Les accidents des pratiques dépigmentants cutanés cosmétiquechez la femme africaine. *Bull Soc Med Afr Noire Lque Frse*. 1976; 21:190-9.

Understanding Skin Bleaching in the Global South[1]

The preference for fair skin in the majority of the Global South is manifested in a variety of ways, the most tangible of which is the widespread use of skin bleaching products. Skin bleaching employs dermatological, cosmetic, or homemade depigmentation products that inhibit the production of melanin and/or remove the top layer of the epidermis. Skin lightening has long been practiced in societies around the world.[2] Dating back at least a century, it has not been uncommon for women to produce homemade bleaching products or to buy lightening creams and soaps from small vendors.[3] These products were typically either ineffective or contained hazardous agents such as mercury or lead that effectively bleached the skin while presenting serious health consequences. Today, skin lightening has mushroomed into a multi-billion-dollar industry, which is currently dominated by three large multinational corporations: France's L'Oreal, Japan's Shiseido, and the U.K.'s Unilever.[3] These corporations and others have perfected the art of marketing and distributing bleaching products that appeal to women aged 18-35 around the world.

Interestingly, in much of the developing world, skin-lightening practices span class levels, though the use of such products is concentrated in urban areas. Corporations have created product lines in a wide range of price categories, such that whiteners are financially accessible for both rural villagers and white-collar urban professionals.[3] In some cases, such as the Shona women of Zimbabwe, the consumption of skin lightening products is actually most concentrated in working class communities.[3,4] Such pitches for whitening creams for men have been particularly successful in villages, in India where personal care companies sell credit-card-size plastic sachets of lotions for as little as 6 rupees (about a dime). Rural markets contribute significantly to volume sales "and are an important factor for driving growth", Emami said in a statement. "People in the cities have more options and are better educated," says Naveen Vyas, an analyst at Microsec Capital in Kolkata. "It's the rural market that is most important for fairness creams. It's a very big market that nobody can afford to ignore." (See the section below on MEN ALSO BLEACH). In Ghana, and in much of West Africa, middle and upper class women use more expensive imported bleaching products, such as Vantex Skin Bleaching Creme from the African-American company Fashion Fair Cosmetic.[5] Poor and working-class women more often use homemade concoctions that are more likely to include mercury and other ingredients that make creams more physically dangerous than high-end products.[6,7,8]

Skin bleach companies often market their products as rejuvenating one's "natural" fairness that the consumer had as an infant before the skin was "damaged" by the sun and the wear of everyday life. Many products make rhetorical appeals through the fact that they were produced in "scientific laboratories" in the U.S. and Western Europe to build a sense of validity for customers in the developing world.[9] Interestingly, many who ideologically support the manufacturing and use of skin lightening products consider them a path towards female empowerment. Light skin tone can be transformed into social capital (social networks), symbolic capital (esteem or status), or even economic capital (high-paying job or promotion). Blay found that women in Ghana who used bleaching products were trying to attain beauty vis a vis light skin. She argues that light skin and beauty were the vehicles through which women attempted to gain social capital.[10] In the 19th century, before the birth of the modern cosmetic industry, "Beauty may have been considered the birthright of only wealthy or fortunate women."[11] Today, many skin bleach proponents and industry leaders argue that cosmetic companies have made beauty easily attainable, even for "'working women unable to afford the time and money leisured women spent on beauty culture.'"[11] Cosmetic advertisers have long used this selling point of democratizing beauty.

"Beauty's first requisite since time immemorial has been a fair complexion. Formerly it was nature which decided on face-appeal of different people but now fortunately science steps in and a pearly-white skin may be easily attained by any-one who uses PEARLEX."[12]

The directors of Fair & Lovely, India's largest skin bleach brand, claim that their products are fulfilling a social need for women in the developing world. Like an education, they argue, fair skin is regarded as "a social and economic step up."[13] However, the moral defense of the skin lightening industry breaks down under scrutiny. Supporting women in altering their natural phenotypes to conform to a Eurocentric beauty standard only validates the racism and colorism behind the beauty standard itself. Moreover, not only is skin bleaching ideologically problematic, it presents a myriad of health risks.

References

1. Imani Franklin. Living in a Barbie World: Skin Bleaching and the preference for fair skin in India, Nigeria and Thailand.Senior Honors thesis. Center for Democracy, Development, and the Rule of Law. (CDDRL) Stanford University. May 14, 2013.

2. Dicker Ron. "Plastic Surgery Spending is Up, As Number of Chin Augmentations Surges." Huffington Post. April 18, 2012. http://www.huffingtonpost.com/2012/04/18/plastic-surgery-spending-up-2011_n_1435512.html.

3. Glenn Evelyn Nakano. *Shades of Difference: Why Skin Color Matters*. Stanford CA: Stanford University Press. 2009; 65

4. Gwaravanda Ephraim Taurai. "Shona Proverbial Implications on Skin Bleaching: Some Philosophical Insights." *The Jounal of Pan African Studies*, Vol. 4, no.1. no. 4, June 2011:201.

5. Pierre, Jemima. 'I Like Your Colour!' Skin Bleaching and Geographies of Race in Urban Ghana." Feminist Review, 2008: 15. http://www.palgravejournals.com/fr/journal/v90/n1/pdf/fr200836a.pdf

6. Olumide YM, Akinkugbe AO, Altraide Dan, Mohammed T, Ahamefule N, Ayanlowo S, Onyekonwu C, Essen N. Complications of chronic use of skin lightening cosmetics. *International Journal Dermatol.* 2008; 47: 344-53.

7.Delle Edmond. In: Dying To Be White: by Sylvia Arthur. http://www.clutchmagonline.com/2008/01/dying-to-be-white.

8. Lewis KM, Harris S, Camp C, KAlala W *et al.* The historical and cultural influence of skin bleaching in Tanzania. In: The Melanin Millennium: Skin Color as 21st Century International Discourse. Publisher Springer Netherlands 2013; pp 19-38.

9. Amina Mire. The Scientification of Skin whitening and the Entrepreuneurial University—Linked Corporate Scientific Office. *Canadian Journal of Science, Mathematics and Technology Education.* 2012; 12 (3): 272-91.

10. Blay YA. Yellow Fever: Skin bleaching and the politics of skin-colour in Ghana. PhD Dissertation: Temple University. 2007.

11. Glenn Evelyn Nakano via Kathy Peiss. Shades of Difference: Why Skin Color Matters. Stanford, CA: Stanford University Press, 2009, 78.

12. Thomas Lynn. Interview by Imani Franklin. Phone interview. March 15, 2013.
13. Karnani Aneel. "Doing Well by Doing Good – Case Study: 'Fair & Lovely' Whitening Cream." *Strategic Management Journal*, 2007: 1352.http://onlinelibrary.wiley.com.ezproxy.stanford.edu/doi/10.1002/smj.645/pdf

The Terminologies

This bleaching industry has spawned a new language with terms either being derogatory or flattering. Skin **whitening** and **lightening** seems more politically correct while **bleaching** is more critical. The self deceptive word **"toning"** appears to be more acceptable globally among skin bleachers. In Zambia "**bukes/beauxing**" refers to bleaching. In Jamaica, "**browning**"— light skinned female, "**cake soap**"— skin lightening products. Jamaica even has a rich repetoir of terminologies‾derogatory expressions to describe the habit of bleachers or the appearance of skin bleachers (See the chapter on Jamaica). In Tanzania, **tetrasaiklini**, is used to describe a woman whose skin has become speckled because of the use of bleaching cream. In Ghana and Nigeria "**fanta face, cocoa cola body"** is used to describe a woman who has bleached her face alone but whose extremities remain dark in colour. The terms **"Yellow fever," "Fanta face, Cocoa cola body"** were coined by Fela for skin bleachers in Nigeria. Also in Ghana the term **"na nso eben"** ('it serves you right') is used to describe the disfiguring ochronotic skin that develops as a side effect of skin bleaching practice. In Mali and Senegal, the terms "**tcha-tcho**" and "**xessal**" are, respectively, used to describe this practice. In Zambia, "**FBI**" (formally black individual) is used to describe skin bleachers; and in Nigeria "**Otupa palor"** (in Yoruba language= lamp for the parlour) is used. **'Mafuta'** is the name for skin bleaching products in Kenya; **"ambi"** in Gabon, **"kwitukuza"** in Rwanda. The practice has become so widespread that it has been nicknamed ***'maquillage'*** by the French speaking communities.[1] All the other relevant references have been cited under the country specific chapters.

Reference

1. Odongo J. Noir ou blanc? Le vécudu double dans la pratique du 'maguillage' chez les Noirs. *Nouvelle Revue d'Ethnopsychiatrie.* 1984; 2:37-65. (For the other references— see the section on each country).

Skin Lightening products marketed globally

Some of the skin whitening products marketed globally include Porcelana Skin-lightening Cream, Cosmetic Surgeon in a Jar, Illuminator Brightening Complexion, Darphin Clear White! Brightening and Soothing Serum, Sekkisci White Powder Wash, Fair and White so White! Skin Perfector Brightening Cream, Clinique DermaWhite, Shisheido White Lucent, Loreal White Perfect, Ambi Fade Cream. Indians best-selling Fair & Lovely (for women) and Fair & Handsome (for men), with varied prices.

Reference

Hunter LM. Buying racial capital: skin-bleaching and cosmetic surgery in a globalized world. *J Pan Afr Stud* 2011; 4:143-64.

Prevalence of the use of skin lightening in Africa

Limitations of study designs

Skin lightening is the use of home-made products, cosmetic creams, and dermatological creams, pills, injectables and surgical methods to reduce the melanin pigment in the skin. This chemical/surgical alteration of the physicality is a global phenomenon used by a large proportion of the population of men and women globally in people of colour, primarily women and young girls in Africa, Asia, Latin America, and even in Europe, Canada, North America either among coloured indigenes or immigrant population. Skin bleaching is the practice by which depigmenting agents are used typically by people with skin phototypes IV to VI on a cosmetic basis, primarily to lighten normally dark skin. With the high rates of migration, the prevalence and complications of skin lightening cosmetics can no longer be seen as a health issue in African countries alone, but a global health challenge.

Obtaining prevalence rates on skin bleaching practices is challenging but researchers have made progress in estimating rates in different parts of the world. The papers were subject to bias both across studies and based on the bias inherent in each individual study design. Across studies the selection criteria used may bias results; only articles written in English, published and accessible in select databases were included. This reduced the scope and diversity of information that was reviewed regarding the safety of skin bleaching products. Further, individual articles were subject to bias based on sampling procedures. For example, many of the articles used non-random sampling that may not accurately represent the overall population of interest (e.g epidemiological methods). In some studies, participants were recruited at hospitals and clinics and many of the studies included small sample sizes. These selection biases may limit generalizability of findings. Another consideration is that true experimental design is not feasible with the topic of skin bleaching since it would constitute harm to participants, limiting the ability to state directly causal links between skin bleaching and injury/disease in many cases. Further, many studies relied on participants self-report which may have skewed findings toward more socially desirable answers. Also, because of the limited attention to skin bleaching in the scholarly literature some of the articles reviewed were published in non-peer reviewed studies or were more descriptive in nature. Furthermore, injury caused by these practices is not tracked. However, a simple google search shows that the global phenomenon of skin bleaching remains prevalent worldwide. The serious public health risks that these practices pose cannot be ignored and incorporating efforts to prevent skin bleaching under the umbrella of global injury prevention may give this understudied topic a necessary boost.

Since most of the studies are based on interviews and/or questionnaires, the study subjects may have given inaccurate histories about their cosmetic use of cutaneous depigmenting agents. Also, studies in hospital-based settings may overestimate the prevalence of skin bleaching, as individuals attending dermatology clinics are more likely to have primary dermatological problems for which they would have sought out cutaneous depigmenting agents.

As regards the frequency of complications from the use of skin-lightening products, the figures given in various hospital studies are grossly inaccurate for the following reasons:

i. Only a fraction of such cases seek hospital intervention, Adebajo's[6] study on skin lightening was a community study (not hospital based). When the respondents were asked how they react when they developed complications, only **7.5%** said they go to the hospital. 35.6% said they simply discontinue use; 11.5% visit the herbalist for treatment, and 45.4% ignored the complications.
ii. Skin bleachers for various reasons, very often deny the use of the products. (See the section on FURTHER NOTES ON PREVALENCE IN NIGERIA—Chapter 4). The danger from denial is that many of the symptoms and signs of the complications of skin lightening chemicals are not specific to the skin lightening chemicals. The unpleasant sequelae of denial often leads to failure in making prompt diagnosis of the adverse health consequences, and delays in appropriating effective medical interventions and management.
iii. Adverse health consequences are often reported in terms of skin complications e.g acne, striae and exogenous ochronosis. **Systemic** complications like cancers, nephropathies, neuropathies, fetal

toxicity, other public health complications, and infections from injectables (e.g HIV/AIDS, Tetanus and hepatitis) are hardly linked to possible complications from the use of skin bleaching agents because the cause and effect relationship are not easy to prove nor investigated. Hence such systemic complications are hardly documented.

In 2012, Indians reportedly consumed an estimated 233 tones of bleaching products, and in terms of sheer numbers, Indians make up to the largest skin bleaching market. A synovate market survey in 2004 showed that 50% of respondents in the Philippines reported using skin lighteners. In places like Japan, China, Taiwan, and Korea, global surveys report that 20-50% of the respondents had used skin bleaches and that 20-50% would use more if they are available. In parts of Latin America, and in the US, women of all races, including Europeans and whites, have long legacies of skin whitening or lightening. And these indicators probably underestimate the practice of skin bleaching around the globe.

Finally, skin bleaching is a highly stigmatized practice in most countries in Africa which people are unwilling to discuss and often keep to themselves as a secret. Unless they have problems they are not likely to reveal the habit and even when complications compel them to seek, medical help, they tend to deny the use of skin bleaching agents but would rather divert the attention of the dermatologist/health care provider to an imaginary causal "allergy" from diet. Some studies have also shown that some analphabetic women genuinely do not know that the cosmetic product they are using contain skin lightening chemicals. It is therefore not sufficient to base studies solely on questionnaires; the products used should also be analyzed for the active ingredients when possible. In countries with highly repressive laws on skin bleaching (like the Gambia), the patient will never admit the use of bleaching agents. (see further details in the country specific chapters).

References

1. Glenn EN. Yearning for lightness transnational circuits in the marketing and consumption of skin lighteners. *Gender & Society*. 2008; 22 (3): 284-95.

2. Jalika C Street, Karie Gaska, Kelly M Lewis, Michael L Wilson. Skin bleaching: A neglected form of injury and threat to global skin. *African Safety Promotional Journal*. 2014; 12 (1): 52-71

3. Daizie OE, Petit A. Skin bleaching: highlighting the misuse of cutaneous depigmenting agents. Prepare in June 2009, *EADV online CME*.

4. Olumide YM, Akinkugbe AO, Altraide Dan, Mohammed T, Ahamefule N, Ayanlowo S, Onyekowu C, Essen N. Complications of chronic use of skin lightening cosmetics. *International Journal Dermatol.* 2008; 47: 344-53.
5. Ofondu EO. Cosmetic use of bleaching cream in Enugu. [*Nigerian FMCP Dissertation*] National Postgraduate Medical College, Nigeria 2003.
6. Adebajo SB. An epidemiologic survey of the use of skin lightening cosmetics among traders in Lagos, Nigeria. *West Afri J Med* 2002; 21: 51-5.

Estimated Prevalence in Africa

Beyond impacting communicates "of color," in general, the skin bleaching phenomenon has long affected African communities in particular.[1] Paradoxically situated within the first wave of the African independence movements, skin bleaching surfaced as an increasingly popular cosmetic practice as early as the late 1950s and is currently widespread.[2,3] Surveys conducted from 1986 to present days show that skin bleaching is practiced, (a) at least occasionally, by two out of three inhabitants of Brazzaville, Congo, (b) by one out of four women living in Bamako, Mali, (c) by one out of two women living in Dakar, Senegal (and one out of four men), by about three out of four women and men living in Lagos, Nigeria. This phenomenon is not limited to West Africa. A study conducted twenty five years ago showed that seven out of ten patients in two hospitals in Pretoria, South Africa practiced skin bleaching.[4] In Cote d'voire, it is estimated that "eight out of every ten seemingly fair-complexioned women use skin—lightening products on a regular basis.[5] Among Zambian women aged 30-39, as many as 60% reportedly use skin bleaching agents.[6] In East Africa about 30% of the women bleach.[7] In Ghana, dermatologists estimate that upwards of 30% of the population, primarily women, use bleaching creams regularly.[8,9] It seems that in many parts of the continent, skin bleaching is nothing less than a way of life.

References

1. Blay YA. Editorial: Struck by lightening: The Transdiasporan Phenomenon of skin bleaching. *Jenda: A Journal of Culture and African Women Studies*. 2009a; 14:1-10.
2. Blay YA. Ahoofe Kasa!": Skin bleaching and the function of beauty among Ghanaian women. *Jenda: A Journal of Culture and Africa Women Studies.* 2009b; 14:1-10.
3. da Souza MM, The concept of skin bleaching in Africa and its devastating health implications. *Clinics in Dermatology* 2008; 26:27-29.
4. Hardwick N, Van Gelder LW, Van der Merwe CA, & Van der Merwe MP. Exogenous ochronosis: an epidemiological study.*Br J Dermatol.* 1989; 120: 229-38.
5. Gender Bulletin: Cote d'Ivoire-Skin Bleaching Health authorities Decry skin Bleaching. (1998, September 24). [Electronic Version] Africa News service. Retrieved 2003 from http://www.highbeam.com
6. Pitché P, Kombaté K & Tchangai-Walla K cosmetic use of skin-bleaching products and associated complications. *Int J Dermatol.* 2005; 44:39-40.

7. Lewis KM, Harris S, Camp C, KAlala W et al. The historical and cultural influence of skin bleaching in Tanzania. In: the Melanin Millennium: Skin Color as 21st Century International Discourse. Publisher Springer Netherlands 2013; pp 19-38.
8. Delle Edmund. In Dying to be white by Sylvia Arthur. http://www.cluthmagonline.com/2008/01/dying-to-be-white.
9. Mckinley C. Yellow Fever. *Honey Magazine.* May 2001; 96-9

Prevalence from studies in specific countries in Africa

Mali 53%,[1] Nigeria 77%,[2] Senegal 67.2%,[3] Togo 60%,[4] Ghana 39.2%,[5] East Africa 30%,[6] Rwanda 35%,[7] South Africa 35%,[8] Republic of Benin 36.6%,[9] Saudi Arabia 38.95,[10] Jordan 60.7%.[11]

Further notes on the epidemiology of the skin bleaching practices in Africa are elaborated under specific countries.

References

1. Mahé A, Blanc L, Halna JM, Kéita S, Sanogo T, Bobin P. an epidemiologic survey on the cosmetic use of bleaching agents by the women of Bamako (Mali) *An Dermatol Venereol* 1993; 120 (12):870-3.
2. Adebajo SB. An epidemiologic survey of the use of cosmetic skin lightening cosmetics among traders in Lagos, Nigeria. *West Afr J Med.* 2002; 21 (1): 51-5.
3. ne I, Tat-Dia A, Diallo OF, Badian M. *et al.* Prevalence of the use of skin bleaching cosmetics in two areas in Dakar. (Sénégal). *Dakar Med.* 2000; 45 (2): 157-7.
4. Pitche P, Afanou A *et a.l* Prevalence of skin disorders associated with the use of bleaching cosmetics by Lome women. *Sante.* May-Jun 1997; 7 (3): 161-4 http://www.ncbi.nlm.nih.gov/pubmed/9296805
5. Kuffour RA, Dartey E, Owusu W, and Dabuoh PM. Level of awareness of effects of the use of cosmetic bleaching products among women. A Case Study of Bolgatanga municipality in Ghana. Research on Humanities and Social sciences. 2014; 4 (11): 57-62.
6. Lewis KM, Harris S, Camp C, Kalala W *et al.* The historical and cultural influences of skin bleaching in Tanzania. In: The melanin Millennium: Skin Color as 21st century International Discourse. *Springer Netherlands.* 2013 pp 19-38.
7. Léocadie Kamagaju, Renato Morandini, Françoise Gahongayire *et al.* Survey on skin-lightening practices and cosmetics in Kigali, Rwanda. *International Journal of Dermatology.* 2015; 1-7.
8. Malangu Ntambwe. Mirror mirror on the wall, who is the FAIREST of them all?" *Science in Africa*: Africa's first On-line Science Magazine. March 2004. http://www.scienceinafrica.com/old/index.php?q=2004/march/skin/i...
9. Atadokpédé F, Adégbidi H, Koudoukpo C, Téclessou J, Aholoukpé C, Dedboé B, do Ango-padonou F, and Yedomon H. Epidemiological and clinical aspects of skin bleaching in Secondary schools in Bohicon , Benin. *Journal of cosmetics, Dermatological Sciences and Applications.* 2015; 5:1-6.

10. AlGhamdi KM. The use of topical bleaching agents among women: a cross-sectional study of knowledge, attitude and practices. *Journal of the European Academy of Dermatology and Venereology JEADY*. 2010. DOI:10.IIII/j.1468-3082.2010.03629.x
11. Hamed Saja H, Tayyem Reem Reema, Nimer Nisreen, and AlKhatib Hatim S. Skin-lightening practice among women living in Jordan: prevalence, determinants, and user's awareness. *The International Society of Dermatology*. 2010; 49:414-20.

Cross-sectional study

Karl Peltzer *et al*[1] in 2015 carried out a cross-sectional study with a network of collaborators in 26 participating countries globally: 5 countries in the Caribbean and South America, 7 countries in Sub-Saharan Africa; 5 countries in North Africa, Near East and Central Asia; 4 countries in South Asia and China; and 5 countries in Southeast Asia. Using the World Bank, New Country Classification[2] the countries were classified as Low, Lower middle income, Upper middle income and High income countries. The aim of the study was to investigate the use of skin lighteners as its social correlates in university students. Using anonymous questionnaires, data were collected from 19,624 undergraduate university students (mean age 20.8, SD 2.8) from 27 universities in 26 countries. Multivariate logistic regression analysis was used to identify associations between sociodemographic, social, health risk, mental health and abuse, and the use of skin lighteners.

Overall, the prevalence of previous 12-month skin lightener use was 24.5; 16.7% in male and 30.0% in female students. The prevalence rate by country ranged from 0% in Turkey to 83.8% in Thailand, a country which also has a high prevalence of use of highly hazardous mercury-containing skin bleaching products. In multivariate logistic regression analysis among both men and women, social variables (highly-organized religious activity and lack of personal mastery) and health variables (inconsistent condom use) were associated with skin lightening use. In addition, male students from a lower income country, having a lack of social support, and a history of childhood sexual abuse were more likely to use skin lighteners, and women aged 20-21 years old, residing on the university campus, being a student of health and welfare, and having a lack of personal control, inadequate physical activity, and depressive symptoms were more likely users of skin-lightening products.

The researchers concluded that at-risk groups point to a picture of individuals who have low self-esteem, depression, and trauma. Knowledge of this vulnerable population needs to be given careful consideration particularly concerning planning of interventions, which should target these underlying issues

References

1.Karl Peltzer, Supa Pengpid, and Caryl James. The globalization of whitening: prevalence of skin lighteners (or bleachers) use and its social correlates among university students in 26 countries. *Int J dermatol* 2016; 55: 165-72.

2.World Bank, New country Classifications, 2013. Available at. *http://data.worldbank.org/news/new-country-classifications.* [Assessed April 10, 2014]

Prevalence of skin lightening in Europe

The practice of skin bleaching has been reported in Africans and Afro-Caribbeans living in European countries, including the United Kingdom and France.[1,2,3] Although hydroquinone in cosmetics has been banned in Europe, over-the-counter use of hydroquinone and various other depigmenting agents remain available illegally in many markets in Europe.[4] In a multicentre study conducted in the Paris region, it has been estimated that 16% to 28% of adult African women seeking dermatological treatment in Paris are regular users of skin bleaching agents.[2] Furthermore, in a recent study by Petit *et al*[3] on 46 subjects from various African countries attending a dermatology clinic in Paris for side-effects of skin lighteners, 31% had begun their practice of skin bleaching in France. See also the chapter on UNITED KINGDOM—Chapter 15.

References

1. Bongiorno MR, Aricò M. Exogenous ochronosis and striae atrophicae following the use of bleaching creams. *Int J dermatol* 2005; 44: 112-5.

2. Arsouze A, Fitoussi C, Cabotin P-P *et al.* Presenting skin disorders in black Afro-Caribbean patients: a multicentre study conducted in the Paris region. *Ann Dermatol Venereol* 2008; 135:177-82 (in French).

3. Petit A, Cohen-Ludman Clevenberge P, Bergmann J-F, Dubertret L. Skin lightening and its complications among African people living in Paris. *J Am Acad Dermatol* 2006; 55: 873-8.

4. Keane FM, Munn SE, Taylor NF, du Vivier AW. Unregulated use of clobetasol propionate. *Br J Dermatol* 2001; 144:1095-6.

Prevalence of skin lightening in North America

See the chapter on NORTH AMERICA for a detailed discussion on the prevalence of skin lightening practices in the USA—Chapter 15.

Prevalence of skin lightening in India

In 2012 there 240 brands of lightening creams available in India alone and according to Didier Villanueva, a manager for L'Oréal India, 60 to 65 percent of the women use the products on a daily basis. Skin lightening in India is a $400 million business with customers across the economic spectrum. Although the practice is rampant in Africa, the industry's popularity extends far beyond the continent. Nearly 61% of skin care products in India contain bleaching agent, and 40 percent of women in China, Malasia, the Philippines, and the Republic of Korea admit to bleaching. One does not need smooth skin to navigate life. It is desirable because, for women especially, men find smooth skin attractive. The India matrimonial site Shaadi.com conducted a poll of nearly 12,000 people and skin tone was the most important criteria for choosing a partner in three northern Indian states[1]. Fair skin is generally associated with beauty, greater affluence and increased employability. Bollywood frequently sings of goro mukhdas (a fair complexion) and white skin. Until a few ago, fairness creams were marketed mainly to women.

The quest for whiter skin runs deep in India. MidasCare Pharmaceuticals in 2012 began selling its Clean and Dry intimate wash that promises women a "fair" look for their vaginas. And on shaadi.com and bharatmatrimony.com, the nation's two biggest matchmaking website, users can screen by complexion—dark, fair, wheatish, and very fair. "We definitely see a large segment where complexion matters" for both brides and grooms, says Gourav Raksit, chief operating officer of shaadi.com. Skin-care sales in India grew about 20 percent in 2013, to $1.2 billion, according to analysts surveyed by Bloomberg, with whiteners comprising about a quarter of that market. Emami introduced its Fair and Handsome cream in 2005; Unilever's men's line followed in 2006, and L'Oréal's (OR:FP) Garnier unit launched its PowerLight men's products in 2009. Analysts say men now account for 10 percent of fairness cream sales. See also the chapter on INDIA—Chapter 16.

References

1. Ronda Racha Penrice. Skin lightening is serious business in India. *The Grio*. July 19, 2010 Http://thegrio.com/2010/07/19/skin-lightening-is-serious-business-in-i...
2. Dan Morrison of National Geographic Voices. Has India's Skin-Lightening. Obsession Reached the Final Frontier? April 12, 2012. http://voices.nationalgeographic.com/2012/04/12/has-indias-skin-lig..

Prevalence of skin lightening in Asia

In Asia a preference for lighter skin remains prevalent and skin whitening cosmetic products are popular.[1, 2] Ashikari[3] when writing on the Japanese culture, states that since the late 1980s, consumption of skin 'whitening' cosmetics has remained at consistently high levels and a white complexion has been considered trendy and desirable in

Japan, being a symbolic physical characteristic for identifying Japanese people. In June 2004 synovate, a global market research company, conducted a survey on skin whitening products use in Hong Kong, Malaysia, South Korea, Taiwan and the Philippines. The survey found that Filipino women were the highest users with 50% using whitening products. Four out of ten women surveyed in Hong Kong, Malaysia, the Philippines and South Korea used a skin whitening cream, and more than 60 companies globally compete for Asia's estimated $18 billion market.[2,4] Indeed despite the world-wide economic downturn, the multibillion dollar whitening cosmetics industries of Europe, Japan, India and elsewhere are robust, and show no sign of shrinking, according to an Asian-wide group, the ASEAN Cosmetic Association. Global skincare companies have tapped into this booming business. In the late 1980s and early1990s, only local companies were providing consumers with whitening products, according to Tina Arceo-Dumlao of Change Agent, a marketing research magazine. By the mid 1990s, global companies like Nivea and l'oreal found their way in. Tang *et al*[5] reported the case of a woman who developed minimal change nephropathy as a complication of the use of mercury containing skin-lightening cream. Furthermore, following an index case of mercury poisoning, a survey was conducted in Hong Kong to describe the demographic characteristics, patterns of use and other laboratory parameters in people who had used the same skin whitening cream. Among 314 cream users, 27% were using it as a skin whitening agents.[6] Health concerns of skin whitening in 2002, Marianne Bray of CNN reported that 1,262 people contacted a Hong kong health department hotline that was set up after reports that Rosedew and La Rose Blanche, two popular skin whitening products, had levels of mercury 9,000 to 65,000 times higher than recommended.[7] Mercury can cause liver demage, kidney failure, demage to the central nervous system and fatel seizures. Corticosteroid and hydroquinone are other ingredients sometimes added to whitening products.

Skin whitening in Asia has a long history and stems back to Ancient China and Japan. To these cultures to be light in an environment where the sun is harsh, meant that one was upper class and rich enough to stay indoors and leave the outdoor work to servants.[4] In many Asian cultures colorism is taught to children in the form of fairy tales, just like the Grimm fairy tales with the light skinned white princess or maiden, Asian mythological protagonists are typically fair and depict virtue, purity, and goodness. Lightness is equated with feminine beauty, racial superiority, and power and has strong influences on marital prospects, employment, status, and income.[8]

With globalization, the obsession with whiteness has become even more prevalent in Asia's newfound hypercommercialism and consumer culture. In metropolises such as Hong Kong light skinned Asian models cover billboards, magazine covers and counter spaces at department stores. **Some two thirds of men surveyed in Hong Kong said they prefer lighter skinned women and almost half of young Asian adults have admitted to use skin whiteners in attempts to achieve a lighter complexion**. (See also the chapter on ASIA—Chapter 16)

References

1.Discrimination based on skin color.
http://en.wikipedia.org/wiki/Discrimination_based_on_skin_color#cite_note_22
2. "Skin whitening big business in Asia." Public Radio International. 30 March 2009.
3. Ashikari M. Cultivating Japanese whiteness: the 'whitening' cosmetics boom and the Japanese identity. J Mat Cult. 2005; 10:73-91.
4. Rosana San Vicente. Skin Whitening and dark beauty in the Philippines Suit 101.com. from the bundle Beauty Min Thesis Resources.
http://bundlr.com/chips510bd398aaa6b10002000c4e
5. Tang HL, Chu KH, Mak YF et al. Minimal change disease following exposure to mercury-containg skin lightening cream. Hong Kong Med J. 2006; 12: 316-8.
6. Sin KW, Tsang HF. Large-scale mercury exposure due to a cream cosmetic: community-wide case series. Hong Kong Med J. 2003; 9: 329-43.
7. "Skin Deep: Dying to be White" CNN. 2002-05-15. Retrieved 09-08-2010.
8. Verma Harsh. "Skin 'fairness'–Culturally Embeded Meaning and Branding Implications" Global Business Review 2011; 12 (2): 193-211.
Doi:10.1111/097215091101200202.

Men also bleach their skin

One of the most controversial celebrity endorsement came in 2007 when mega-successful Bollywood actor, Shah Rukh Khan endorsed the skin-lightening product, "Fair and Handsome." Created by the British company, Unilever, and marketed as the masculine companion product to best-selling Fair and Lovely, Fair and Handsome became the first major skin-lightening product and mass-marketed exclusively to men. Khan's endorsement was read by the Indian public as an endorsement of skin-bleaching itself and as an endorsement of a strongly color-based system of privilege in India.[1]

Similarly, USA baseball star Sammy Sosa, originally of the Dominican Republic, recently attracted international media attention when he appeared at the Latin Grammy Awards with notably lighter skin than he had during his career in Major League Baseball.[2] Sosa has suggested that he was negotiating an endorsement deal with the cosmetic company that manufactured his skin-lightening cream. His *de facto* celebrity endorsement of skin-bleaching elicited significant feedback including a televised ridiculing from former NBA basketball star, Charles Barkley. Despite the media furor, Sosa's actions reinforce the idea that skin bleaching is a mainstream route to building racial capital.

Nigeria

An African lady who works in a Beauty supply store in Lagos has this to say:

"I deal with these customers first hand. It means a lot to me as I am myself an African and was shocked about how naturally they use that stuff. The skin won't revert to its normal state and becomes thinner till it is like paper. I was invited to a Congolese wedding one day and everyone was bleached except me, my boyfriend (Caribbean) and his best friend (Cameroon). We were so shocked about these orange faces we were speechless. That was the first time when I realized that lighter skin is also desired by the men which was strange to me."[3]

A study of market traders in Lagos, Nigeria, reported a prevalence of 77.3% comprising **27.6% males** and 72.4% females.[4] Another study among students of a tertiary institution in Enugu, Nigeria, report as prevalence of 71.9% in women and **53.3% in men.**[5] Another tertiary institution in Benin Nigeria,[6] reported a prevalence rate of 70.7% among female students and **52.2% among male** student

Many high profile ***men*** e.g a former head of state, state governors, traditional rulers, a deputy speaker of the House of Assembly and some clergy men have bleached their skin.[21] Some male Television News casters have also bleached their skin.

When some of the male bleachers were asked in the skin clinic why they found it necessary to bleach, invariably they usually responded with a guilty grin of embarrassment on their faces and say:

"I use whatever my wife uses on her skin because she buys the cosmetics"

"I sell the beauty products in my shop in the market and I need to advertise them on my body."

"I don't deliberately bleach. I have some skin rash all over my body and I want to remove them with the cream"

Some of the male skin bleachers are homosexuals. They never admit this when asked because homosexuality still remains a grievous crime in Nigeria, but there are some stigmatas which may be helpful in identifying them—atimes the perianal area is bleached; the anal orifice is more patulous and the perianal region may be studded with lesions of verruca vulgaris—viral warts. Some of them are HIV positive. Some of them bleach the phallus.

Ivory Coast

"While the craze is most widespread among women, some men use the creams too." Ekra said[7]

Rwanda and Congo

"Men are increasingly becoming culprits of bleaching with the Congolese men leading the pack. Koffi Olomide, Madilu System and General Dafao are the list of Congolese men who are known to have bleached themselves."[8]

Skin-lightening is not just a fascination and obsession of women. Congolese hair stylist Jackson Marcelle says he has been using special injections to bleach his skin for the past 10 years. Each injection lasts for six months.[9] "I pray every day and I ask God, 'God why did you make me black?' I don't like being black. I don't like black skin," Marcelle said. Mr Marcelle[9]—known in this busy community as Africa's Michael Jackson—says his mother used to apply creams on him when he was young in order to make him appear "less black". "I like white people. Black people are seen as dangerous; that's why I don't like being black. People treat me better now because I look like I'm white," he adds.

Entrenched in the minds of many Africans from a young age is the adage "if it's white, it's all right", a belief that has chipped away at the self-esteem of millions.

Zambian men with bleached skins: new trend[10]

"BLACK is beautiful, so goes the saying. But not for some people, so it seems. A colleague told me how one day, while he was in a beauty supply shop, he saw the shelf stockpiled with Deprosone, Betazole, Dermo Gel, Amira C, Top Lemon, Lemonvate, Extra Claire, Bio Claire, Carolite, Maxlight, Bu-tone *et cetera.* He was having a conversation with the owner of the shop, a dark-skinned woman, when a man, thought to be in his late 20s, came-in and picked an assortment of skin bleaching products from the shelf. The guy did not look embarrassed at all, but he could notice a little of discomfort from the shop owner as the man downloaded the bleaching stuff on the counter ready to purchase. After he had left, she explained to my friend that **make-up and bleaching creams are increasingly becoming popular among men**. And she can't be mistaken; it is easy nowadays to come across Zambian men with make-up as well as those using bleaching skins in the name of keeping with trendy world of fashion. This is unlike in the past when men were associated with moderate, comfortable and conservative outlooks. **In fact, in the past**, and please no offence intended, any **man with a bleached skin was thought to be from Congo, specifically, a Kasai**. The easiest way to identify a Kasai was through their skin appearance".

"Now, with all these risks, it is difficult to understand why Zambian men, would embrace skin bleaching. A bit of make-up for purposes of photo shots or television camera is understandable, but skin bleaching is certainly out of our system as black Zambian men. The argument of going with the fashion trends does not even hold water. If anything the argument or discussion about dark skin and light skin is actually dumb. A lot of people do not like dark skinned people because they think they are ugly while mistakenly thinking that light-skinned people are prettier. I strongly think that it does not matter what colour your skin is, as long as you feel confident in the one you have."[10]

Jamaica[12,13]

Jamaica dancehall artist Vybz Kartel has bleached his skin and also released a range of skin lightening products.

Along with fear of ridicule or harassment, men in particular, hide because of the stigma attached to men bleaching their skin. Another societal view of bleaching is that it is a female practice and men who bleach their skin are homosexual. Since the bleaching practice is viewed as being cosmetic in nature, and therefore, the prerogative of women, men who bleach are at risk of being labeled homosexual, and disgustingly effeminate, worthless, without personal ambition.

Most of the men interviewed in the group mentioned the positive effect their bleaching or toning was having on their social life, particularly as it related to dating women. Some went as far to say that the reason for bleaching or toning was to get women. The term 'browning' is a popular nickname for individuals who are considered light-skinned (especially women.)

A male skin bleacher said:
"You get a lot of girls! You get popular because people just take notice of you. Those who did not notice before, start to see you now. Those who did not talk to you, start talking to you now, and those who were not your friends, want to become your friends because you start to become popular." "It is so important to me because it makes me feel good when I am looking good and it makes other people look at me and admire me when I am looking good."

Rice Bag, a man who has been using skin lightening products, explained that the main reason he started using the products was to remove spots and bumps from his face. The added benefit to a blemish-free complexion is the extra attention from women.

While females insist that men should not bleach their skin, the males boast that they are considered more attractive because they bleach and ultimately get more girls.

Both bleachers and toners report the intermittent, time-consuming, laborious, costly, yet addictive nature of the bleaching phenomenon in Jamaica. Their responses indicate that bleaching/toning requires commitment on various levels—financial, time and effort.

According to Kayja, (a retailer of the products) she analyzed the market and found that bleaching products would prove to be a wise investment as skin bleaching was a popular and fashionable trend. Her motivations are obviously to capitalize on the popularity of the bleaching trend and to earn money from it, despite the illegal nature of the business. As a retailer of the products, she explained that while she may not be in full support of people bleaching their skins, she would keep selling the products as she had bills that needed to be paid. Further, she clarified that she has in the past discouraged people from bleaching, if she noticed that they were overdoing it and causing severe problems to the skin, but soon admitted that she would not be insistent as she needed the business.

India

As regards male bleaching in India, see the section on INDIA—Chapter 16.

References

1. Parameswaran R, & Cardoza K. Melanin on the margins. Advertising and the cultural politics of fair/light/white beauty in India. *Journalism & Communication Monographs.* 2009; 11 (3): 213-74.

2. Mitchell F. Sosa says he's preparing to endorse skin product. *Huffington Post.* Retrieved from *http://www.chicagobreakingsports.com/2009/11/sosa-says-hes-preparing-to-endorse-skin-product.html*
3. Britni Danielle. Nigerian Singer Release 'whitenicious' Skin Lightening Cream and it's sold out. Jan 20, 2014. *http://www.xojane.com/issues/nigerian-singer-releases-whitenicious.*
4. Adebajo SB. An epidemiologic survey of the use of skin lightening cosmetics among traders in Lagos, Nigeria. *West Afr J Med* 2002; 21:51-5.
5. Ofondu EO. Cosmetic use of bleaching cream in Enugu. *Nigeria FMCP Dissertation.* National Postgraduate Medical College, Nigeria, 2003.
6. Ofili AN, Eze EU, Onunu AN. Prevalence of use of Skin lightening agents amongst University of Benin undergraduates in Benin City, Nigeria. *Nigeria Medical Practitioner.* 2006; 49:24-7.
7. Standard Digital News%Kenya; Ivory Coast bans skin whitening creams. http://www.standardmedia.co.ke/article/2000161357/ivory-coast-bans-...
8. Léocadie Kamagaju, Renato Morandini, Francoise Gahongayire et al. survey on skin-lightening practices and cosmetics in Kigali, Rwanda. International Journal of Dermatology 2015; 1-7 doi:10.êêêê/ijd.12833
9. Pumza Fihlani. Africa: Where black is not really beautiful. *BBC NEWS, Johannesburg.* / January 2013. http://www.bbc.com/news/world-africa-2044789.
10. Daimone Siulapwa. Zambia men bleach skins: new trends? December 23rd, 2010 http://ukzambians.co.uk/home/2010/10/31/zambian-men-b;eached-skins-trends/
11. Ina Skosana. When lightening strikes, it brings pale ailments. *Mail & Guardian. http://mg.co.za/2014-10-31-00-when-lightening-strikes-it-bring...* 31 Oct 2014. p2.
12. Robinson Petra Alaine. Skin bleaching in Jamaica: A colonial legacy. *A Dissertation* submitted to the Office of Graduate Studies of Texas A&M University in partial fulfillment of the requirements for the degree of DOCTOR OF PHILOSOPHY May 2011.
13. Charles C. skin Bleaching and the Deconstruction of Blackness. *IDEAZ* 2003; 2 (1): 43-54

Where are the products manufactured?

Skin lightening products are manufactured in many countries; for example, consumer protection agencies in the European Union[1-6] and the United States of America (USA)[7,8] have identified mercury-containing products made in China,[1,4,7,8] the Dominican Republic,[7,9] Lebanon,[1,9] Mexico,[7,11] Pakistan,[1,2] the Philippines,[1,3] Thailand,[1,5,12] and the USA.[1,6]

Skin-lightening or bleaching, has reached pandemic levels in scores of nations around the globe and especially in many African nations. Although both men and women engage in skin-whitening practices of various sorts, women generally have higher rates of skin-whitening than men, and women also sometimes apply skin-whitening products on their children.[13]

A 2011 survey funded by the German Federal Ministry for the Environment, Nature Conservation and Nuclear Safety noted that individuals from Brazil, Kyrgyzstan, Mexico and the Russian Federation believe that mercury-containing skin lightening products are easy to obtain.[14,15]
Some manufacturers are no longer using mercury as a preservative in mascara and eye makeup cleansing products as a result of consumer pressure. However, most jurisdictions still allow the sale of makeup products containing mercury compounds.[16]

So lucrative is the skin bleaching cosmetic market in Nigeria, that in January, 2015, one "Pastor" of a church in Nigeria brought a consignment of cosmetics including skin bleaching products made in **Spain** for me to prescribe them for my patients in the clinic. I simply told him that I prescribe drugs not cosmetics. He promised to go round the Spas in Lagos to introduce the products for use on clients. This type of casual dealers and importers of bleaching products is not uncommon. Anyone may just decide to try out his potentials in the Nigerian market. Hence a variety of products are imported from hitherto unknown manufacturers globally for sale and distribution to Spas around the country. As regards skin bleaching products in general, in **addition** to the above countries, products on sale in Nigeria have come from France, Italy, Nigeria. Some products come with user instructions that are written in mostly strange Chinese or Arabic languages.[17,18]

Skin lightening cosmetics have no borders because they are available in any country where there are users, through the following routes.

1. The individual immigrant users transport the products from their home country either for personal use or for sale to friends/compatriots in foreign lands. This is often done as a ready source of foreign exchange for the immigrant.
2. The products are shipped from Nigeria and some other African countries, with ethnic foodstuffs to foreign lands where there are immigrants e.g Europe, Canada, USA. The products are then made available to immigrants at the ethnic food shops in those countries[21]
3. Many of these products are homemade or mixed and manufactured in cottage industries locally in Nigeria and other African countries (see Online Marketing Strategy below)

Africa has become the dumping ground for the world's banned products; goods that were prohibited in Europe years ago but are still manufactured solely for export to Africa. Some companies manufacturing exclusively for the continent produce creams with dangerously high levels of the bleaching agents hydroquinone and mercury.

References

1. UNEP *Mercury in products and wastes.* Geneva, United Nations Environment Programme, Division of Technology, Industry and Economics,Chemicals Branch. 2008.(http://www.unep.org/chemicalsandwaste/Portals/9/Mercury/AwarenessPack/Englih/UNEP_Mod1_UK_Web.pdf).
2. Ladizinski B, Mistry N, Kundu RV. Widespread use of toxic skin lightening compounds: medical and psychosocial aspects. *Dermatologic Clinics*, 2011; 29:111–123.
3. RAPEX . *The Rapid Alert System for Non-Food Products* 2011 (http://ec.europa.eu/consumers/dyna/rapex/rapex_archives_en.cfm; enter "mercury" in the search box).
4. RAPEX. *The Rapid Alert System for Non-Food Products.* 2011 week 31, No. 33, Reference 0461/11 (http://ec.europa.eu/consumers/dyna/rapex/create_rapex.cfm?rx_id=385).
5. RAPEX. *The Rapid Alert System for Non-Food Products.* 2007 week 29, No. 22, Reference 0732/07 (http://ec.europa.eu/consumers/dyna/rapex/create_rapex.cfm?rx_id=142).
6. RAPEX. The Rapid Alert System for Non-Food Products, 2009 week 49, No. 8, Reference 1625/09 (http://ec.europa.eu/consumers/dyna/rapex/create_rapex.cfm?rx_id=268)
7. RAPEX. *The Rapid Alert System for Non-Food Products.* 2009 week 28, No. 3, Reference 0954/09 (http://ec.europa.eu/consumers/dyna/rapex/create_rapex.cfm?rx_id=245).
8. RAPEX. The Rapid Alert System for Non-Food Products, 2006 week 31, No. 13, Reference 0491/06 (http://ec.europa.eu/consumers/dyna/rapex/create_rapex.cfm?rx_id=91)
9. USFDA. *Import alert: Detention without physical examination of skin whitening creams containing mercury.* Silver Spring, MD, United States Department of Health and Human Services, Food and Drug Administration (Import Alert No. 53-18; http://www.accessdata.fda.gov/cms_ia/importalert_137.html).
10. USFDA. *Import alert: Detention without physical examination of unapproved new drugs promoted in the U.S.* Silver Spring, MD, United States Department of Health and Human Services, Food and Drug Administration (Import Alert No. 66-41; http://www.accessdata.fda.gov/cms_ia/importalert_190.html).
11. RAPEX (2006). *The Rapid Alert System for Non-Food Products*, 2006 week 24, No. 16, Reference 0356/06 (http://ec.europa.eu/consumers/dyna/rapex/create_rapex.cfm?rx_id=83)
12. Peregrino CP, Moreno MV, Miranda SV, Rubio AD, Leal LO.Mercury levels in locally manufactured Mexican skin-lightening creams. *International Journal of Environmental Research and Public Health*, 2011; 8(6):2516–2523.
13. Anonymous. FDA bans skin whitening products due to mercury content. The Manila Paper, 6 August 2011 (http://manila-paper.net/fda-bans-skin-whitening-products-due-to-mercury content/8021).

14. Uram E, Bischofer BP, Hagemann S. *Market analysis of some mercury-containing products and their mercury-free alternatives in selected regions*. Gesellschaft für Anlagenund Reaktorsicherheit (GRS) mbH, March 2010 (GRS-253; http://www.ipen.org/ipenweb/documents/ipen%20documents/grs253.pdf)
15. Weinberg J. *An NGO introduction to mercury pollution.* International POPs Elimination Network. 2010 (http://www.ipen.org/ipenweb/documents/book/ipen%20mercury%20booklet_s.pdf).
16. Counter SA and Buchanan LH. Mercury exposure in children: A review. *Toxicology and Applied Pharmacolopy* 2004; 198 (2): 209-30.
17. Olumide YM Editorial. BMT 2010; 341: c6102
18. Olumide Y.M. Akinkugbe AO, Altraide D et al. Complications of Chronic use of skin lightening cosmetics. *Int J Dermatol* 2008: 47: 344-53.
19. Mistry N, Shapero J, Kundu RV, Shapero H: Toxic effects of skin-lightening products in Canadian immigrants. *J Cutan Med Surg.* 2011 Sept-Oct; 15 (5): 254-8.
20. Rosen HN, Alseddeeqi E, Rivera J. Cosmetic agents causing endocrinopathy in an African immigrant *Canadian Family Physician* February 2012; 58 (2): 169-171.
21.Markey AC, Kobza Black A, Rycroft RJG, Confetti-like depigmentation from hydroquinone. Contact Derm 1989; 20:148-9.

Where can these products be purchased?

Recent observations suggest that bleaching practices exist among the African population in Europe, West Indies and Asia. Markey *et al*[1] have noted that large quantities of skin lightening creams are sold in Britain to Afro-Caribbeans and Asians. In Europe, most products can be found without any control in specialized African shops and sold as "innocent" cosmetic creams. These creams are also readily available in Europe, USA and Canada to immigrants who either bring them from their home country or purchase them in stores where ethnic foodstuff is sold (See chapter 15 on UNITED KINGDOM).

Ethical concerns

As the global industry grows and more consumers are affected by its devastating consequences, ethical questions abound. Studies report the dumping of substandard products in the global south by overseas industries. Often these products were not passed for human use in their country of origin.[1] Many of the mercury soaps used by Africans are manufactured in the European Union (EU), where they are allowed to be manufactured as long as the product is exported. EU manufactured soaps are reportedly smuggled back into EU where they are sold to African immigrant communities.[2] A number of third-world countries are believed to be used as off-shore production and distribution sites for western-based pharmaceutical companies.[3] The Nigeria, South African, Zimbabweans, Gambian and Kenyan governments have banned the import and sale of mercury and hydroquinone products. However, these bans are often poorly enforced and difficult to control due to the fact that they are smuggled in from other African or European nations.

References

1. Alphonso Van Marsh. UK's skin bleaching trade exposed. UK's Skin Bleaching trade exposed-CNN.com Nov 26, 2007. http://edition.cnn.com/2007/HEALTH/11/26vanmarsh.skinbleaching/i...
2. Antony Barnett and Zoe Smith. Toxic creams for sale as thousand seek whiter skin. The guardian UK. Sunday 16 Octerber 2005. http://www.theguardian.com/uk/2005/oct/16/health. healthandwellbeing.
3. Glahder Christian M. Appel Peter Will and Asmund Gert. Mercury in Soap in Tanzania. NERT Technical Report NO 306. 1999. http://www2.dmu.dk/Lviden/2_publikationer?3_fagrapporter/rapporter/fr306.pdf
.

The location of Online manufacturers, marketers and suppliers in Nigeria

Mercury-containing skin lightening products are available for sale over the Internet. A cursory search on any Internet search engine reveals hundreds of skin lightening websites that provide information for would-be consumers about the "best" skin-lightening products and strategies. Lighter skin.org, whiterskin.com, skinwhitening.org, skin-whitening-product.com, and skinwhitening experts. com—all purport to share with readers the newest information on, and reviews of, skinlightening products.

Manufacturers, Marketers and suppliers spread through all the length and breath of Nigeria:

Agege, Gwarinpa, Ikeja, Ikorodu, Isolo, Lagos Island West, Lagos Mainland, Lekki, Port Harcourt, Surulere, Aba North, Agbado/Oke-Odo, Amuwo Odofin, Asokoro, Central Business District, Aba, Ibadan Central, Ibadan North, Ifako Ijaiye, Igando/Ikotun, Ijebu Ode, Ikoyi-Obalende, Ojodu, Onitsha North, Oredo/Benin-City, Oshimili South/Asaba, Oshodi, Owerri – Municipal, Wuse, Yaba and more!

The location of retail marketers

In most cities in Nigeria, the products are universally available. A visit to the cosmetic department of some pharmacy shops, departmental stores or supermarkets that sell cosmetics and toiletries will reveal this. The sections devoted to cosmetics are heavily adorned with a broad spectrum of skin lightening cosmetics and toiletries, elegantly and attractively packaged and imported from across the globe. A departmental store in high brow Lekki Phase 1 in Lagos, devoted five shelves in the cosmetic department to skin lightening products alone. Each shelf contained **13 different** products. Hence, there were 65 (sixty-five) **different** products on sale in that single store alone. One level of the shelves had products whose names and instructions were inscribed in the French language alone.

Roadside vendors sell tubes and plastic bags of powders and ointments from cardboard boxes stacked alongside walks in market districts. Most of such products are unlabelled. Moreover most of those who patronize these roadside vendors are not literate and even cannot read nor understand the few labeled tubes which are mislabeled, misbranded or counterfeit. In most markets in Nigeria, business is booming for shops selling skin-lightening products. Both local and imported products line the shelves of such shops. Ijeoma Eze who works at God First Cosmetic shop, said, "bleaching creams sell these days and we have varieties almost everyday. I'm not an expert on cream but by the time people come here, especially ladies, to ask for a particular cream or soap, often I know it's to bleach and so, I recommend it for others too who come looking for bleaching cream or soap and they say, it works". Ijeoma said, "most of these soaps and creams are not costly, "anyone can easily buy them".

Over the last few years this 'product pandemic' has led to a flood of cheap and affordable over the counter (OTC) products touted to be the "next best thing" for lightening the skin.The products are available everywhere, from big shops in the elite areas of Victoria Island, Ikoyi and Allen Avenue, to the local markets in the neighbourhoods of Mushin, Oshodi, Agege, Oyingbo, Ajegunle, among others. Street hawkers also peddle them, as well as the various types of medicated soaps and similar items which have come within easy reach of residents in the metropolis. With the advent of online marketing, the products can be ordered and delivered, same day, at your door steps just by the click of the mouse! The impact of online marketing is so serious that it is discussed under a special heading below.

Products are also available in a variety of price ranges from a few cents per ounce to over one hundred U.S. dollars per ounce. In addition to these more expensive products created by multinational cosmetics companies, many small mom-and-pop vendors offer local products in informal markets throughout the Global South and in smaller markets catering to immigrant communities in the West.

These products, often created and sold outside of formal regulatory channels, frequently contain active ingredients illegal in many nations, or legal chemicals in illegal doses[5].

Sylvia Arthur[8,9] said "someone in Ghana wanting to buy an ordinary body cream or lotion would be hard pressed to find one that doesn't contain a bleaching agent among the hundreds that do; and even those believed to be non-bleaching are not always so". (See chapter 7 on GHANA)

In Nairobi, Kenya,[10] bleaching products are sold on Nairobi's River Road – a hotbed for black market transactions. (See chapter 9 on KENYA).

In Sudan,[11] the bleaching products are available in make-up and skin care stores with the exception of steroid and hydroquinone–containing creams having a pharmaceutical presentation which can be obtained only from pharmacy. However, all brands regardless of their composition can be obtained without any medical prescription from pharmacies. (See chapter 9 on SUDAN).

Online manufacturers and marketers

Online market

Skin lightening or whitening is probably the most searched term on the internet when we talk about beauty. Searches related to skin lightening products in Nigeria include:
Skin lightening products for **black people**
Skin lightening products **for dark skin**
Skin lightening products **without hydroquinone**
Skin lightening products **with kojic acid**
Skin lightening products **for African Americans**
Skin lightening products **used by celebrities**
Skin lightening products **boots**

Natural skin lightening products.
Skin cream suppliers
African skin creams
Suppliers skin bleaching
Cream suppliers

People from all walks of life, from Africa, Asia to America, men and women, all want to know how they can significantly whiten their skin without burning holes in their pockets. Indeed, tons of the so-called best skin whitening products are out on the market all of which promise a fairer, age defying, more radiant skin tone.

Most of these products are also priced incredibly expensive but there are some priced affordably. Nigerians at home or in diaspora can purchase African foods and hard-to-find African products; all shipped right to your doorstep with the click of a mouse. Indeed Nigerians now consult beauty therapists and purchase customized **"mix"** without stepping out of their homes. In Europe, Canada, USA and elsewhere it is likely that these skin-lightening products are shipped with food items as the products are clearly displayed and sold where ethnic foods are sold e.g African, Indian, Caribbean food stores.[1,2,3]

Some examples of online adverts read thus:
"If you desire to have a flawless glowing skin, we definitely have products for you. Natural skin lightening products that 'll give you even tone, blemish free skin. Even your friends will wonder what your secret is."
"Place your order now and we'll deliver right at your doorstep.

Call: Name—phone number—Company
You can also join our membership club and enjoy more benefits: http://... and beauty.com/membership-club/"

Consultations are made Online; responses are sent Online. You are given the name and number to call for details, and the product is delivered at your doorstep—same day.

The following details give an insight into this pernicious subterranean market in Nigeria.

Some of the locations of the Online manufacturers/suppliers in Nigeria
Marketers and suppliers spread through all the length and breath of Nigeria (See page 135).

Some of the promotional claims on the product include:
- To make you flawless and confident
*[1] Anti aging soap, slimming soap etc
- Flawless and spots soap
- Maximum impact and satisfaction for your desired whitening looks
- Professional that deals with issues of light skin, dark skin, chocolate skin

- Glowing cream that repair with combined effect of radiance
- Get the whiten flawless ageless look like the celebs . . . .

-* **Learn how to mix cream and start making money**

- Sunburn removal, soft dark knuckles
- halfcast cream, stretch mark, darkspot, knuckles, scar …

*2 1 week empowerment programme, training on,
Base cream production, mixing of toning, glowing, and whitening cream, medicated soap production, essential oil extract

- Whitening liquid Bath Wash
- Whitening bath gel
- Whitening cleansing oil
- Whitening and exfoliating bath scrub
- Extra whitening multi action cream, the powerful anti-oxidant glutathione, green-tea, olive …

*3 Instant whitening body lotion, moisturizes, even tone boosts, uv protection

*3 Extra whitening visible result in 3 days

- Whiten skin fast with triple strength formula
- Visible whiten skin in 10 days; proven 24 hours moisturization, leaving skin silky smooth

*3 Instant smothering whitening

- Mild whitening milk
- Age Defying Whitening Body lotion, brings moisture back by helping the skin recover from sun uv
- Cosmetics for your pimples eradicators, stretch mark cream, black knuckles clean up, body polish cream/soap – ultra glow, Night body oil
- Clear and radiant skin, with no side effects … our product is biochemically tested
- Flawless face and body cream plus whitening papaya soap

*4 L Glutathione 700mg capsules – whitens skin, antioxidant, clears the skin

- It's all about flawless ageless skin
- Whitening body polish

*5 Teeth whitening strips, Light, Pen, Stick, Gel Pen

*5 Teeth Peeling Stick

- Rejuvenating, lightening and mild exfoliation

*5- Whiter teeth for under $50US – Simple, Quick, and Effective

*6- China wholesale Online – buy Direct from China Factories, Free shipping & Buyer Protection

Note!

(1) *[1] Anti aging soap, **slimming soap** etc are available online
(2) *[2] Online schools are available for training in **mixing** ingredients for bleaching
(3) *[3] Skin whitening can be achieved "instantly", in "3 days", in "10 days"!
(4) *[4] Bleaching capsules are available
(5) *[5] **Teeth Whitening** is a common practice
(6) *[6] Products can be shipped directly from China factory online and "buyer Protection" is guaranteed at no extra cost. (The method of protection is unknown).
(7) Note the polyvalent (multipurpose) nature of most of the products

References

1. Markey AC, Kobza Black A,Rycroft RJG. Confetti-like depigmentation from hydroquinone, *Contact Derm* 1989; 20:148-9
2. Olumide YM Editorial. *BMJ* 2010; 341:c6102
3. Olumide Y.M. Akinkugbe AO, Altraide D et al. Complications of Chronic use of skin lightening cosmetics. *Int J Der*matol 2008:47: 344-53.
4. Mistry N, Shapero J, Kundu RV, Shapero H: Toxic effects of skin-lightening products in Canadian immigrants. *J Cutan Med Surg.* 2011 Sept-Oct; 15 (5): 254-8.
5. Rosen HN, Alseddeeqi E, Rivera J. Cosmetic agents causing endocrinopathy in an African immigrant *Canadian Family Physician* February 2012; 58 (2): 169-171.
6. Centres for Disease Control and Prevention (CDC): Mercury exposure among household users and nonusers of skin-lightening creams produced in Mexico-California and Virginia, 2010, M M M R Morb Wkly Rep; 2012
7. Gabler E, and Roe S. Some skin whitening creams contain toxic mercury, testing finds. *Chicago Tribune*, May 18, 2010.http://articles.chicagotribune.com/2010-15-18/.health/ct-met-mercury-skin-creams-20100518/skin-lightening-creams-mercury-testing.
8. Sylvia Arthur for TBWT. Ghana Web. General News of Thursday, 7 March 2002 http://www.ghanaweb.com/GhanaHomePage/NewsArchive/artikel.php?ID=22240.
9.Sylvia Arthur Dying to be White http://www.clutchmagonline.com/2008/01/dying-to-be-white/
10. Annabel Fenwick Elliott http://www.dailymail.co.uk/femail/article-2650766/Kenya-men-like-women-whiter-skin-The-rise-wealthy-Nairobi-women-illegally-INJECTING-skin-lightening-creams.html.
11. Hamed S H, Tayyem R, Nimer N, and Alkhatib HS. Skin-lightening practice among women living in Jordan: prevalence, determinants, and user's awareness. *International Journal of Dermatology* 2010; 49:414-20.

Chapter 4

NIGERIA

Story highlights I

- The WHO adjudged Nigeria as the country with the highest prevalence of skin bleaching in the world with a prevalence rate of 77%.

The prevalence of skin bleaching in Nigeria from various studies in different study populations are **consistently** high 77.3%, 62.4%, 40%, and 64.9%.

- Both men and women bleach the skin in Nigeria; it is just that the prevalence is higher among women.

- Skin bleachers come from all socio-demographic variables and professional groups which regrettably, include doctors, nurses, pharmacists and school teachers.

- The story of skin bleaching practices in Nigeria is a microcosm of the global problem.

- Although there is a history of pre-colonial light skin colour preference in Africa, the aetiopathogenesis is completely different from the **current** rage of post-colonial skin bleaching phenomenon. Africans used shared culture, language and traditions, rather than skin tone as a means of identification, whereas the idea of "biology ***determines*** destiny" is what undergirds modern Western racism.

- Although skin bleaching practices started sometime in the 1940s the ***current rage*** of skin bleaching commenced in Nigeria in the early 1960s as a 'copycat-mentality' or 'bandwagon syndrome' following African-Americans and South Africans who bleached out of expediency in a milieu of pernicious racism and colorism.

- Popular dancehall music of Victor Olaiya was one of the factors that fueled the skin bleaching culture among the Yorubas.

- Another popular musician, Fela Ransome-Kuti, denounced the practice and coined the pejorative terms "Yellow fever" and "Fanta face/Cola Cola legs."

- The motives for bleaching in Nigeria can be classified under the following headings: attraction and seduction, enhancement of marriage prospects, fashion, strenthening the self, social domination, success, compliance, pleasure and sensuality, skin 'cleansing'.

- Skin bleaching in Nigeria should be seen as a ***'cry for help'*** that is, seeking for attention, because the single most important motive for skin bleaching **is to *marry and remain happily married,*** which in the context of the Nigerian culture, translates to three words **'security,' 'self-worth'** and **'significance.'**

- The Federal Government of Nigeria's intervention culminated in the UK Department of Trade and Industry (DTI) prohibiting the exporting or supplying of toxic mercury containing cosmetics and toiletries to Nigeria in 1988. The campaigns by a London TV station BANDUNG (Channel 4) and AB's Luncy Hannan's investigative journalism helped to ***positively*** influence a crack down on the trade.

- In Nigerian, the electronic media—specifically Television, has not been forthcoming in the campaign against skin bleaching, possibly because the manufacturers of the skin-lightening products are sponsors of TV programmes and many TV newscasters and presenters engage in skin bleaching.

- The Nigeria Government published a ban on the manufacture, importation and sale of skin bleaching products in Nigeria in 1995, but the ban was ineffective due to smuggling and trading corruption at high level in Nigeria.

- Several scholarly and journalistic publications and feature articles have emerged in Nigeria on the subject.

- All the various skin bleaching products and methods are available on the market for use by Nigerians including systemic skin bleaching pills and injections and surgical techniques. There is as yet unquantifiable ***cost of cosmetic tourism*** on the burden from the skin bleaching culture in Nigeria.

- Injury associated with current skin bleaching practices decreases quality of life and contributes significantly to sickness and health costs.

- Bootleg versions of skin-bleaching products abound in the market. The product labels on the packages have no bearing on the chemical composition because analyzed products were found to contain **mixtures** of high concentrations of hydroquinone **and** mercury which were not reflected on the product labels. Misbranded, adulterated and counterfeit products abound.

- Several laboratory studies done by scientists in Nigeria show that the cosmetic products on sale in a broad spectrum of geographic locations contain unexpected high concentrations of heavy metals as **contaminants**. This shows that Good Manufacturing Practices (GMP) were not used in the process to ensure the quality and safety of the products.

- Apart from locally made cosmetics, the cosmetics in the Nigerian market were found to have been manufactured in Ivory coast in particular, Europe (Italy, UK and Germany); others were manufactured in India, Indonesia, Philippines and USA.

- The significant increase in the levels of serum renal indices among skin bleachers in Nigeria shows that these agents might be nephrotoxic after prolonged usage; while increase in copper level with accompanying renal dysfunction may be an indication that copper mediates in oxidative-induced renal dysfunction.

- Laboratory investigations also show that some common skin lightening creams available in Nigeria caused mutations in bacteria and were possibly carcinogenic.

- The researchers found that expensive cosmetics are not necessarily "safe" in terms of the toxic metals content. The researchers recommend that there was a need for more stringent control of cosmetics in the market by the regulatory bodies, appointed by the government, to check the quality of cosmetics in the market.

Story highlights II

Unanswered questions for further research in Nigeria

Extensive laboratory studies in Nigeria by scientists have shown that the chemical ingredients in the cosmetics and toiletries, as reflected on package labeling, have no bearing on the **actual** chemicals in the products which were found to contain very high levels of mercury and other heavy metals well above WHO permissible levels. The scientists have also found that even the expensive products are not "safe"!

- Mercury in skin-lightening cosmetics have been found through experimental studies to be absorbed through the skin into the blood stream. Apart from the already establish toxicity on the kidneys and nervous system, mercury has been found to accumulate in the ovaries of mice and is a potential cause of infertility and birth defects (reminiscent of thalidomide story).

  There is need to conduct studies comparing the infertility rates (reproductive risk potential) between chronic skin bleachers and non-bleachers, and the prevalence of congenital abnormalities (genotoxic risk potential) between the babies born to mothers who bleach and non-bleachers.

- The global issue of skin bleaching or lightening has become a public health crisis of epic proportions. Many people of color purchase and use skin bleaching products that later cause serious health problems both to the users and non-users. For example, household members of users of high concentrations of mercury containing bleaching creams have been found to be exposed to toxic levels of mercury vapour. Also mercury in soaps and creams eventually enters waste water and then enters the food chain as highly toxic methyl mercury. Pregnant women who consume fish containing methyl-mercury transfer the mercury to their fetuses that can later result in neurological deficits in children. There is need to explore the evidence on the human health effects of low-level methylmercury exposure.

- Babies of mothers who use mercury containing cosmetics are at risk both *before* birth because methylmercury is transmissible through the placenta and *after* birth by ingesting mercury through the breast milk and sucking the nipple skin coated with mercury containing creams, and inhaling mercury vapour from the skin of the mother. Mercury toxicity manifests in babies as *micro*cephaly (reminiscent of the Zika virus effect), severe neurological and intellectual deficits which may manifest years after exposure e.g epilepsy, unsteady gait, visual or hearing impairment and poor intellectual performance. All these may manifest in a child even in the absence of clinical evidence of mercury toxicity in the mother. There is need to study the effects of mercury in cosmetic skin lightening products on the newborn and follow-up studies on neurological and intellectual deficits.

- Measurable toxic levels of mercury vapours have been identified in the homes of users of mercury-containing cosmetics and toiletries. Hence close family members, including spouses, are vulnerable to inhalation of the toxic vapours. Mercury is a notable cause of Young's syndrome in men. Male infertility is one of the manifestations of Young's syndrome because mercury causes hyperviscosity of the semen and impaired motility of sperm cells. Gynaecologists and Urologists have identified rising prevalence of male infertility and that the current male:female ratio of infertility among spouses in Nigeria is 1:1. Could mercury in skin-lightening creams be the occult contributory factor in the current high prevalence of infertility in Nigeria which Gynaecologists have now given as one in every four married couples? There is need for further research.

- The international Agency for Research on Cancer (IARC) has released alarming world cancer statistics. The most recent statistics in 2013 show that in Nigeria, a woman is diagnosed of breast cancer every 20 minutes and 40 (forty) women die every day from the disease.

1,4 Dioxane is a known **breast** carcinogen. It is not indicated on ingredient labels because 1,4 dioxane is a contaminant created when common ingredients form the compound are **mixed** together. Most of the skin-lightening products in Nigeria are products **mixed** for individuals and beauty spas. Indeed there are online schools where the art of "**mixing ingredients**" are taught. Dioxane is not a skin bleaching ingredient but a veritable contaminant during the **mixing** process. Research shows that 1,4-dioxane readily penetrates the skin.

Is the alarming rise in breast cancer in Nigeria related to 1,4 Dioxane in skin lightening cosmetics? There is need for research to answer the question.

NIGERIA

History of skin bleaching in Nigeria

Some facts about Nigeria

Nigeria, officially called the Federal Republic of Nigeria, is a country located in the West coast of Africa. The capital of Nigeria is Abuja. Built in the 1980s, Abuja is one of the most well planned cities in the country. It became the capital of Nigeria on December 12, 1991, replacing Lagos. Nigeria has a population of 173.6 million (2013) World Bank. The currency is Nigeria naira. Official languages are English, Hausa, Yoruba and Igbo. English is the **main** official language in Nigeria and is extensively used for education, business transactions and for official purposes. Nigeria is bordered by the Republic of Benin on the west, Chad and Cameroon on the east, and by Niger on the north. On the south it borders the Gulf of Guinea. Nigeria is a country covering a total area of 356,667 square miles. Nigeria is a country comprising thirty-six states and one Federal Capital Territory. The states are further divided into 774 Local Government Areas (LGAs). Nigeria is Africa's most populous country and is the seventh most populous country in the world. Nigeria is composed of more than 250 ethnic groups; the following are the most populous and politically influential: Hausa and Fulani 29%, Yoruba 21%, Igbo (Ibo) 18%, Ijaw 10%, Kanuri 4%, Ibibio 3.5%, Tiv 2.5%. As regards religion Muslim 50%, Christian 40%, indigenous belief 10%. Also there are minority groups of British, American, East Indian, Chinese, white Zimbabwean, Japanese, Greek, Syrian and Lebanese immigrants in Nigeria. Lagos is the largest city in Nigeria covering an area of 385.9 square miles. It is the third-most populous city in Africa with an estimated population of 7,937,932. As of now, it is the second-fastest growing city in Africa. It was once the capital of the country, and is the economic and financial capital of the country at present. The national day in Nigeria is celebrated on October 1 every year. The day is celebrated to commemorate the independence of Nigeria from the United Kingdom on this day in 1960. The country was declared a Republic on October 1, 1963.[1]

Skin colours of Nigerians

The geographic space called Nigeria today is inhabited largely by homogenously ***dark skinned indigenous*** African people. In the South there is an imperceptible sprinkling of biracial light skinned people from two different historical events: (i) products of miscegenation in the coastal regions of Nigeria's trade routes and (ii) descendants of Nigerians who travelled to Europe to study. With this exposure, some of them returned home with Caucasian wives and, of course, the resultant biracial offsprings. These biracial people ('half-casts' or 'mulattoes' as they are usually called) constitute less than 1% of the Nigerian population. Interestingly, there is a high prevalence of inbreeding among them, probably a strategy to preserve or improve on whatever level of 'whiteness' they already have rather than 'risk' the dilutional effect of mating with a 100% dark skinned Nigerian. Furthermore, now that skin bleaching is in vogue, some of these biracial women have now joined the league of skin bleachers so that they now have a lighter level of pale skin than the characteristic *café au lait* colour of biracial people. When asked in the skin clinic why they found it necessary to bleach their skin further, they have consistently claimed it was to erase the darkening effect of the sun. One then wonders the psychology behind mulattoes wanting to consciously erase any vestiges of darkness on their skin while the Caucasians consciously torment themselves under the sun to acquire the tan.

In the northern part of Nigeria there are light skinned Fulani (Fula) people, an ethnic group of people spread over many countries, predominantly in West Africa, but found also in Central Africa and The Sudan of east Africa. The Fulas are not a majority in every country they live, but in Guinea they represent a plurality of the population (largest single group). The Fulanis constitute only 9% of the Nigeria population. The Fulanis are traditionally a nomadic, pastoralist, trading people, herding cattle, goats and sheep across the vast dry hinterlands of their domain, keeping somewhat separate from the local agricultural population.

The early origin of Fulani People is most fascinating and deepened in mystery with widely divergent opinions. Many scholars believe that they are of Judaeo-Syrian origin. However, it is generally recognized that Fulani descended from nomads from both North Africa and from sub-Saharan Africa. They came from the Middle-east and North Africa and settled into Central and West Africa from the Senegal regions they created the Tekruur Empire which was contemporary to the Ghana Empire. Then, they spread in all the countries in West Africa, continuing to lead their nomadic life style. The history of the Fulani seems to begin with the Berbers of North Africa around the 8th or 11th century AD. The Fulani themselves believe they are related to the Tuaregs and Arabs.[2,3]

Morphological analyses of the Fulani have been interpreted to suggest a Middle Eastern origin. The identifiable physical qualities of a Fulani are a light colour, slight bone structure, straight hair, thin lips, and above all, a long narrow nose. These are obviously 'Caucasoid' characteristics, and the natural explanation is that the Fulani have a partly Caucasian ancestry, either from East Africa (e.g Ethiopean) or more likely from the North (e.g Tuareg). From early times explorers and anthropologists have been intrigued by the appearance of the Fulani, which differs from that of the Negroid people around them. The Fulani are not basically of Negro stock, although it is clear that through the centuries Fulani populations have interbred in various degrees with the Negro populations among whom they are dispersed, retain non-Negroid physical characteristics to the greatest extent, and speak the purest Fulfulde. Interestingly **'Whiteness' among this ethnic group is less about skin colour, and more about "genealogical connection to important people in the historical and religious pantheon of Arab Islam. Blackness, by contrast, was defined most fundamentally by the lack of such connections.**[3]

Pre-colonial skin colour preference in Nigeria

Even in the pre-colonial past, there were African people who prized light-skin. Amadioha, the Igbo deity of thunder and lightning, is said to be the patron of light-skinned Igbos,[4] and some scholars have argued that Igbo people admired whiteness before they encountered Europeans. Yet Igbo people do not have a tradition of skin-bleaching, at least not that I know of. Peter frost extensively reviewed the literature on studies done as regards skin color preference in sub-Saharan Africa.[5] There is ample evidence that this aesthetic preference for light skin is native to Africa. Ardener found it to be widespread among the Igbos of Nigeria, including generations born before the colonial period.[6] Peter frost featured several extracts from ethnographic literature to corroborate this cross cultural preference for lighter skin in women. Among the Igbos of Nigeria, in the choice of a wife, 'yellow-skinned' girls are regarded as beauties, and other things being equal, they command higher bride prices. (See the section on SKIN-COLOR PREFERENCE IN SUB-SAHARAN AFRICA—Chapter 11). There are parents who would compliment their light-skinned kids on their "beautiful light skin", unaware of the potential psychological damage their comments might be causing. Suddenly the kid is made conscious of something he/she needs to maintain in order to be liked. Meanwhile, any dark-skinned kids overhearing the compliment start to have a complex about their skin tone and grow up with particular ideas about standards of beauty. Light skinned children are often fondly given the moniker—'Oyinbo' (the white man) while the dark-skinned child is called 'blackie.' We hear such compliments today, parents complimenting kids, men complimenting women based on skin colour, and women commenting on other women's skin tone.[7]

A colleague of mine, a dermatologist in Nigeria, once told me she has a set of dizygotic (fraternal) twin sons—one light-skinned and the other is dark-skinned. She noticed that whenever friends or relations came to visit them at home, the visitors **spontaneously** polarized towards the light complexioned one (of the twins), played with him and ignored the dark-complexioned twin brother. The mother of the twins, is understandably disturbed about this unsolicited preferential affinity for only one of her twin sons because the dark-complexioned son is already developing a complex and getting withdrawn, feeling unloved and may end up bleaching his skin later in life to attract attention and feel loved. Traditionally, adulation of the beauty of brides on their wedding day is often described in terms of their fair skin colour.

> "It has never been a secret that Nigerian men prefer their wives, light, bright, and voluptuous. Anytime a man picks his future wife, there is high praise if she happens to be lighter than him. I remember attending several weddings as a kid, and hearing the grown-ups relentlessly discuss how gorgeous the bride was with emphasis placed on her light skin. A bride with a darker complexion never gets the same amount of attention." **Ezinne Ukoha[8]**

Paradoxically, there is a clan in the South Eastern part of Nigeria, with genetically light skinned people called OSUs. For some ill-understood ancestral reasons, the OSUs are regarded as outcasts and, till date, it is regarded an abomination to marry an 'Osu'. Albinos too are light-skinned and regrettably, there still exists great prejudice against Albinos.

> Among the Yorubas in the West the traditional beauty standard is full bosoms, wide hips, dark skin like ebony to contrast with the brightness of white eyes[9] enhanced with the traditional cosmetic eyeliner 'tiro' (in Yoruba), 'kwali' (in Hausa) and 'otanjele' (in Igbo).

The beginning of Skin bleaching in Nigeria

Nigeria is **not** a multiracial country where one race could dominate the other. Unlike the USA, South Africa and Liberia where racially

black populations are often only a subset of larger populations, Nigeria boasts of a racially homogenous population and we are all predominantly of chocolate brown dark skin, stratified only by socio-economic factors **not** color. In addition, independent Nigeria, at least, has never had official discourses and practices denigrating blackness and elevating lighter skin color. Nigerians **copied** the bleaching culture from the African-Americans and South Africans **but for a different motive**. Indeed at the inception of the bleaching culture only one or. two brands of bleaching creams were available on the market—notable among them were Ambi, and Artra. Indeed, if a Yoruba son or daughter wanted to marry a Caucasian, it was often met with stiff resistance from the Yoruba family; and that prejudice against marrying a Caucasian still exists even in current times.
Education researcher Irene Durasaro, cites the 1940s as the beginning of the formal use of skin lightening products in Nigeria.[10] On a regional level, sub-Saharan Africa (SSA) experienced an escalation in the use of skin bleach products throughout the second half of the 20th century. South Africa's Drum magazine expanded throughout much of SSA, including Nigeria, and, by the 1950s, became the most influential vehicle for marketing skin lightening products to African women.[11] By the 1970s, "skin lighteners were common commodities in most of southern Africa" and the industry was effectively in motion on the content.[11]

It is actually difficult to personally recall with exact precision when the **current rage** of skin bleaching culture gained root in Nigeria as it crept in imperceptibly.

The role of legendary Victor Olaiya

Sometime in the early 1960s, the most popular Nigerian highlife musician, Victor Olaiya, released an album in Yoruba with the lyrics – "Omo pupa lemin fe" which literally means – "I love light-skinned women" or "I love to marry a light-skinned woman!"[12] That song literally controlled the music air waves and dancehall at that time as it was very popular at parties, radio, the homes etc. It was a common sight to see men and women dancing ecstatically to that song. Apparently that musician was simply echoing the minds of Nigerian men like him and the song helped to cultivate and mould the minds of even more Nigerian men to develop a special affinity or taste for light-skinned women. The bleaching culture gained momentum and further acceptance among some men and women, and reinforced the craze to bleach the skin. That singular music was one of the factors that fueled the epidemic of skin bleaching, because, culturally, in

Nigeria, the **ultimate goal** for a woman is to secure a husband once she has reached the marriageable age in her twenties; and any woman without strength of character, will succumb to societal pressure, and do whatever it takes to secure a husband. See the section on MOTIVES FOR SKIN BLEACHING IN NIGERIA and THE MARRIAGE PRESSURE below.

It is tempting to play down the importance of the lyrics of Victor Olaiya's "Omo pupa lemin fe" as a driving force in skin bleaching in Nigeria. **His high profile and celebrity status** in the music industry needs some focus.[12,13] Victor Olaiya was born 31 December 1930 and is still alive at 85 years and still **continues** to play music from his rich repertoire of discography as he gets invited often to perform with new generation artists like Michael Odiong, Project Manager of the Premier Records. He still features with other celebrities, like 2 face Idibia, Nollywood's finest, Director Kunle Afolayan of "The Figurine" fame, veteran producer/director Mr Kunle Kelani, and Navio from Namibia.

In 1954 Olaiya formed his own band, the Cool Cats, playing popular highlife Music largely on love life in the Yoruba language. His band was chosen to play at the state ball when Queen Elizabeth II of the United Kingdom visited Nigeria in 1956, and later to play at the state balls when Nigeria became independent in 1960 and when Nigeria became a republic in 1963. On the latter occasion, Olaiya shared the stage with the American jazz musician Louis Armstrong. During the Nigerian Civil War of 1967-70, Olaiya was given the rank of a lieutenant colonel (honorary) in the Nigerian army and his band played for the troops at various locations. The Cool Cats later travelled to the Congo to perform for the United Nations troops. Olaiya is known as the "godfather" and "The Evil Genius of Highlife." Olaiya renamed his band to All Stars Band when they played at the 1963 International Jazz Festival in Czechoslovakia. In 1990, Olaiya received a fellowship of the Institute of Administrative Management of Nigeria. For a period, he was also president of the Nigeria Union of Musicians.
Michael Odiong, Project Manager of the Premier Records has this to say:

> *"It is pertinent that we bring back to the music industry what made Dr Victor Olaiya internationally known. His lyrics are still very relevant today and he has so many tracks that have an impact on people everywhere, and his classic love songs like "Omo pupa" "Fami Mora O" will withstand the test of*

> *time any day. We want to encourage younger stars to take advantage of these classic songs and do something new with them."*

The legendary stature of Victor Olaiya explains the impact of his music "Omo pupa leminfe" which is akin to celebrity endorsement of the bleaching culture.

Response to skin bleaching by another legendary musician–Fela Kuti (Anikulapo-Kuti, Ransome-Kuti) 1938-1997

Fela Kuti was a highly talented Nigerian multi-instrumentalist, musician, composer, pioneer of the Afrobeat music genre, human rights activist, and political marverick.

The bleaching culture truly gained full acceptance in Nigeria in the sixties. At the time James Brown released the album- "Say it loud – I'm black and I'm proud" in 1968, bleaching was already on course though not yet so prevalent in Nigeria as at present. However at the time the Afro Beat musician, Fela Anikulapo-Kuti, a social crusader, released his "Yellow Fever" song in 1971, bleaching of the face had gained some grounds. Using pidgin English as a medium of communication, Fela identified the different types of fevers—malaria, jaundice, hay, influenza, inflation, freedom and yellow—and bifurcated yellow fever into original and artificial. Fela then chronicled the different symptoms of the original and metaphorically equated skin bleaching as artificial "yellow fever". He also described the signs of artificial "yellow fever" as well as the damaging effects on the skin. He called bleaching "stupid thing, yeye thing, ugly thing, foolish thing". Indeed haters of the bleaching culture ridiculed such people and called them "yellow pawpaw," "Fanta face and Coca Cola legs"[9] (Fig 4:1). However the art and science of bleaching have been so "perfected" in current times through the availability of Spas, bleaching injections and capsules, that the disparity in the colour of the face and legs (which existed some decades ago) has been largely eliminated.

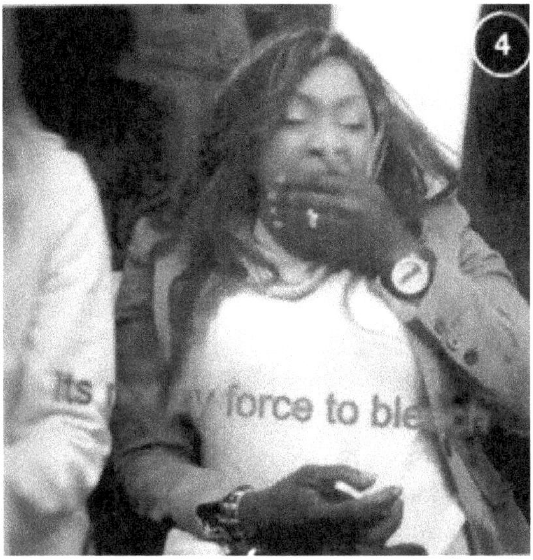

Fig 4:1 "Yellow fever" "Fanta face/coca cola body"

How relevant is the history of colonialism to this body modification practice manifested by altering the skin colour?

David EJR and Sumie Okazaki define ***colonial mentality*** as internalized oppression.[15] This oppression is driven by perceptions of ethnic and cultural inferiority created from centuries of colonial rule. Though historical indications of colorism existed before the onset of colonialism in Nigeria and some other African nations, racial hierarchies that were loosely forming beforehand were cemented during the British rule. Postcolonial African countries could be regarded as coeval in the skin bleaching practice though the rate of progression may differ.

The colonialism hypothesis for colorism essentially argues that the success in marketing and selling skin lightening agents today is "predicated upon European (colonial) promotion of idealized whiteness. It is colonization, this theory asserts, that decisively embedded skin-tone hierarchies into indigenous society in Africa. Regardless of class level, black Nigerians were residentially segregated from white colonizers, were denied quality jobs, and were regularly supervised by less-qualified whites. Nigerian elite indirectly helped cement a racial and cultural hierarchy that valorized the British. For example they could afford to send their children for quality education in England. Some of the original crop of the privileged elite who schooled in England returned home with Caucasian wives and/or biracial offsprings with *café au lait* skins (mulattoes). Now that light-complexioned skin is in vogue, some of the biracial women are now proud to wear their skin tone like a collar and have joined the league of skin bleachers. Furthermore, they belong to the upwardly mobile that can afford the highend bleaching products and some of them are now looking even light skinned like the white Britons.

On the most basic level, this colonial phenomenon equated whiteness with power and desirability. The material payoff of being or appearing white became omnipresent in everyday Nigerian life. If this race/culture-based power gradation were not enough to embed a bias towards fair skin into Nigerian society, the British also promoted white supremacist ideology and intangible assigned morality to different skin colors. Colonialism and Westernization can be understood as intersecting rather than as distinct, unrelated phenomena. In its aftermath, colonialism left a region vulnerable to Western influences, including media images that portrayed lighter-skinned individuals as valuable and more powerful. Western media images reinforced the earlier racial hierarchies that were in place. Regardless of the impetus for colorism in Nigeria, the real propeller of the preference for lighter skin is the "global association of light skin with power. Is the booming skin whitening industry a result of this inferior mentality of Nigerians? The recent rise in the use of skin lighteners cannot be seen as simply a legacy of colonialism but rather a **consequence** of the penetration of multinational capital and Western consumer culture, cultural migration and feminism. Nigerians are just doing their own thing because they want to do it—possibly a **copycat mentality/the bandwagon syndrome** following African-Americans and South Africans who bleached out of expediency from pernicious racism and colorism. Once initiated into the bleaching culture Nigerians want to claim membership in a transnational, cosmopolitan culture. In current times skin bleaching in Nigeria cuts across all demographic characteristics and people from all ethnic groups in Nigeria engage in the practice. Several other determinants came in to propel the skin bleaching practice in Nigeria. (See the sections on MOTIVES in NIGERIA below and the chapters on DETERMINANTS—Chapters 5,6).

However, the fact that Nigeria and several other African countries had pre-colonial light skin colour preferences does ***not*** absolve Europeans of their responsibility for indoctrinating non-European populations with harmful racial ideologies because

(i) Africans used shared culture, language and traditions, rather than skin tone, as a means of identifications.

(ii) Pre-European skin colour preferences (PESCP) is fundamentally different from modern western racism or colorism. The language is different. The word 'race' is a modern social construct by the Europeans who fabricated spurious "scientific evidence" to support the dichotomy, thereby providing an ideological justification for colonialism. In racism, race is defined not as a biological fact but on the processes—the institutions, ideologies and practices —that work to make race an organized principle for social relationship. Racism is the belief that humans are subdivided into distinct groups that are different in their social behavior and innate capacities and that be ranked as superior or inferior. (See the chapters on (i) THE INVENTION OF RACISM; (ii) RACE; (iii) THE LEGACIES OF SLAVERY (iv) THE LEGACIES OF COLONIALISM—Chapters 2,18.

(iii) PESCP was constructed on *benign* physical indigenous personal choices/preferences based on life-style and tradition **not** the **poisonous** ideologies of Western white supremacy. Post-colonial racism is based on one's genotype, and by extension, its phenotypic expression determines one's circumstances in life, i.e. "if you are white, you will have certain privileges as a result of your biologic heritage." The idea of "biology **determines** destiny" is what undergirds modern Western racism.[16] Hence all people with dark skin were confined within defined negative stereotypes constructed by the whites themselves.

(iv) The rise of skin bleaching around the globe can also be attributed to the constant, current mass-marketing of contemporary images of white beauty. Wealthy nations like the United States, Japan, and many European nations create many of the global images of white (or light) beauty. In turn, these same nations are also home to the cosmetics companies that produce some of the top-selling skin-bleaching creams, including L'Oreal, Unilever, Schiseido, Vaseline, Emami, Revlon and others. Supporting women in altering their natural phenotypes to conform to a Eurocentric beauty standard only validates the racism and colorism behind the beauty standard itself. Moreover, not only is skin bleaching ideologically problematic, it presents a myriad of health risks.

(v) The production and marketing of skin-lightening products offering the promise of lighter, and whiter skin has become a multi-billion dollar international industry.[17] Skin lightening has been incorporated into transnational flows of capital and culture and is implicated in both the formal global economy and various informal, often underground economies. Multinational corporations have jumped on the bandwagon and are spending large sums of money on research and development of both mass and specialised skin-lightening markets.[18] (See SCIENTIFICATION OF SKIN LIGHTENING PRODUCTS—Chapter 6).

(vi) The global beauty industry has re-invented itself in recent years in the image of multiculturalism. Many cosmetics companies that once exclusively featured white women have added **light skinned women of color** to their advertisements as spokespersons for their products. Hunter calls this maneuver the "illusion of inclusion".[19] The Illusion of inclusion is a seductive marketing strategy to draw in women of color who might otherwise feel alienated from products marketed exclusively with images of white beauty. By including a few light-skinned, Anglo-looking women of color, cosmetics distributing companies appear to be inclusive of people of color, without their message that white bodies are beautiful. The inclusion of fair-skinned women of color like Halle Berry of the US (Revlon), Aishwarya Rai of India (L'Oreal), Genevieve Nnaji of Nigeria (Lux soap), or Terry Pheto of South Africa (L'Oreal) is designed to lull women of color consumers into buying these products and believing that their bodies and beauty are being valued.[20] Ironically as the marketing strategies have added a veneer of inclusion, there has simultaneously been a boom of products offered that all claim to lighten, brighten, or whiten the skin.

As this industry grows and more consumers are affected by its devastating consequences, ethical questions abound. Studies report the dumping of substandard products in the global south by overseas industries. Often these products were not passed for human use in their country of origin.[21] Many of the mercury soaps used by Africans are manufactured in the European Union (EU), where they are allowed to be manufactured as long as the product is exported. EU manufactured soaps are reportedly smuggled back into the EU where they are sold to African and Caribbean immigrant communities.[22] A number of third-world countries are believed to be used as off-shore production and distribution sites for Western-based pharmaceutical companies.[23] (See Chapters 5,6 on DETERMINANTS).

References

1. Facts about Nigeria. www.mapsofworld.com/nigeria/facts.html
2. Tarig Anter. Special Report: Who are the Fulani people and their origins? Pointblanknews.com. June 8. 2013. Pointblanknews.com/pbn/exclusive/special-report-who-are-the-fulani-people-and-their-origins/
3. Hall Bruce. *A History of Race in Muslim West Africa*, 1600-1960. Cambridge University Press,
2011:57http://ebooks.cainbridge.org/ebook.jsf?bid=CB09780511976766
4. Why are women playing down skin-bleaching? *Cosmic Yoruba.* July 31, 2014 http://thisisafrica.me/skin-bleaching-post-tramatic-colonial-syndrome/
5. Frost Peter. Skin-color preference in Sub-Saharan Africa. The Unz Review: *An Alternative Media Selection.* December 21, 2006. http://www.unz.com/pfrost/skin-color-preference-in-sub-saharan/
6. Ardener EW. Some Ibo attitudes to skin pigmentation, Man 1954; 54:71-3.
7. Siji Jabbar. "Who taught you to hate your [dark] skin?" This is Africa. http://thisisafrica.me/who-taught-you-tohate-your-dark-skin/
8. Ezinne Ukoha. This is Forty: I bleach My Skin. Jan 21, 2014. https://thsppl.com/this-is-forty-i-bleach-my-skin-52baf76f1479.
9. Lawal Qudus. Interview by Imani Franklin. In-person interview. Stanford, CA, April 2013.
10. Durasaro AI *et al.* Perceptions of Skin Bleaching Among Female Secondary School Students in Ibadan Metropolis, Nigeria. *Journal of Education and Practice.* 2012; 3 (7):43 http://www.iiste.org/Journals/index.php/JEP/article/viewFile/1847/1802
11. Thomas Lynn. Cited in Glenn, Shades of Difference: Why Skin Color Matters. Stanford CA: Stanford University Press, 2009, 201.
12.Victor Olaiya - Wikipedia, the free encyclopedia
http://en.wikipedia.org/wiki/Victor_Olaiya
13.Vanguard July 17, 2013, Comments
http://www.vanguardngr.com/2013/07/2face-victor-olaiya-come-toge...
14.Fela Kuti. From Wikipedia, the free encyclopedia
http://en.wikipedia.org/wiki/Fela_Kuti
15.David EJR and Okazaki S. "Colonial Mentality: A Review and Recommendation for Filipino American Psychology". *Cultural Diversity & Ethnic Minority Psychology.* 2006; 12 (1):1-6.
16. Pre-European Contact Colorism and post-colonial Racism in Asia and North Africa.http:/www.colorg.orgarticle.aspx?d=2002&x=colorism
17."Pell Research" *https//www.pellresearch.com/cosmetics-and-Beauty-Products-Manufacturing.htm.* Cosmetics Manufacturing Report.
18. http://frontiersnews.com/index.php/news/3636-exclusive-bleaching...
19.Hunter M. 'If you're light you're alright: Light skin color as social capital for women of color. *Gender & Society.* 2002; 16 (2): 175-93.
20. Osuri G. Ash-colored whiteness: The transfiguration of Aishwarya Rai. *South Asian Popular Culture* 2008; 6 (2): 109-23. Consultancy Africa Intelligence (Pty) Ltd 2013.
21.Alphonso Van Marsh. UK's skin bleaching trade exposed. *UK's Skin Bleaching trade exposed-CNN.com* Nov 26,
2007.http://edition.cnn.com/2007/HEALTH/11/26/vanmarsh.skinbleaching/i.

22. Antony Barnett and Zoe Smith. Toxic creams for sale as thousands seek whiter skin. *The guardian UK*. Sunday 16 October 2005. http://www.theguardian.com/uk/2005/oct/16/health. healthandwellbeing.
23.Glahder Christian M. Appel Peter Will and Asmund Gert. Mercury in Soap in Tanzania. *NERI Technical Report* No 306. 1999. http://www2.dmu.dk/Lviden/2_publikationer/3_fagrapporter/rapporter/fr306.pdf.

Past response in Nigeria by the Nigerian Government

Several research publications on the adverse health effects of Bleaching of the skin have been published by Medical practitioners in Nigeria (see Appendix 1). The regulatory body for monitoring Cosmetics and Drugs in Nigeria was the Food and Drugs Administration of Nigeria (FDA) until 26th February, 1993, when the change in Nomenclature to National Agency for Food and Drug Administration Control (NAFDAC) was gazetted (Appendix 2). Olumide was a member of the Governing Council of the FDA when the attention of the Hon. Minister of Health, Prof. Olukoye Ransome-Kuti, was drawn to the dangerous adverse effects of the chemicals in skin lightening products. The Federal Ministry of Health in 1987 then prohibited the use of mercury as an ingredient in all cosmetic products and limited the concentration of hydroquinone to 2% in all cosmetic products manufactured in Nigeria.

However, cosmetic skin lightening products containing mercury and high levels of hydroquinone manufactured outside Nigeria continued to flood the market in Nigeria to the extent that they overshadowed the local industries, because Nigerians preferred the imported products as they were found to be more effective in lightening the skin than the locally manufactured products with lower concentration (2%) of hydroquinone. The then Hon Minister of health, through an Administrative Order in 1991 **completely** banned the manufacture and importation of cosmetic bleaching products containing mercury and hydroquinone at any concentration (Appendix 3).This was published in the legal document through an Extraordinary Gazette on the 29th December, 1995. (See Appendix 4)

The Regulation provides thus:

"No person shall offer for sale, import or manufacture any cosmetic products which are adulterated or which contains any skin bleaching agents, steroids, hydroquinone, mercuric compound and so on."

Shortly after that, officers from the Federal Ministry of Health and Law enforcement agents, in the bid to enforce the law, raided the market and shops in Balogun West in Lagos that was regarded as the "headquarters" for the importation and distribution of the products in Nigeria because rows of streets in this geographical area were found to sell in retail and wholesale assorted skin lightening products imported into Nigeria. Some of the products on the market at that time were Symba medicated cream, Mililo, Tura, Crusader, Neco, Hg1, Amber, Asepso, Jaribu, Concorde among a host of others. The exercise of raiding the shops to forcefully confiscate the illegal products for destruction was a complete failure as it only led to panic and looting and the products that were confiscated by the law enforcement agents found their way back on the market stalls. Hence the market for the product continued to boom unabated.

Sometime in April, 1991, an Importer took legal actions against the Federal Govt, Customs and Excise Revenue Division, for impounding some cosmetic products at the port of entry. The FDA Research/ Customs Laboratory analysed one of the products and found it to contain 4.3%ww hydroquinone. Olumide was invited to court to help defend the case in favour of the Federal Government. Olumide had to enquire from the FDA what the true legal position of the Federal Govt. was as regards the importation of skin lightening products – as at April 1991. A hand written reply from the FDA – Federal Ministry of Health Drug Control Division revealed that both mercury and hydroquinone had been completely banned in Cosmetics in Nigeria (see Appendix 3). The Federal Government Customs Department won the legal case against the importer and the illegal products remained impounded and eventually destroyed.

London TV Documentary on the Skin Bleaching Industry in Nigeria

In June 1988, Olumide was invited to London by a Television Station BANDUNG Channel 4 (Figure 4.2) for the recording of a documentary, titled "A Whiter Shade of Black", on the sale of both legal and illegal dangerous skin-lightening cosmetics to black people. The bitter irony was that the products were not permitted for sale in Europe but were permitted for export. Several companies that were household names engaged in the business and some even received grants, from the EEC. At that time, some of the manufacturers of the skin lightening products were Reckitt and Colman, W & E Products, Shakespeare Soaps of Manchester International Generics of Hove in Sussex, and Martal Cosmetics of London. Indeed over 20 factories within the EEC were producing mercuric soaps. (Appendix 5 shows African Business (AB) report on the skin whitening trade).

As at that time, European safeguards had outlawed the sale of certain hazardous cosmetics such as mercury soap and skin lighteners in European markets. But African Business (AB) investigations discovered that a number of European companies continued to manufacture these harmful products specifically for sale to African markets. AB's Lucy Hannan carried out on-the-spot inspections to see what was still on offer in the African marketplace and where it came from. During the January 1988 survey the petty traders of Lagos were evidently unaware that their goods were illegal and they unreservedly showed receipts that identified the suppliers. The source proved to be Balogun West, a major market on Lagos Island, where whole streets were devoted to an exclusive stock of all available brands of mercury soaps and skin-lightening creams.
While AB was unable to determine who the actual importers were, the thriving success of the trade at Balogun West was evident. **It was also evident that the operation was not on a small scale, as new stock constantly arrived in vans carrying "Government Licensed Imports" labels – suggesting that the smuggling and trading involved corruption at a high level**.

The above observation by Lucy Hannan in 1988 corroborates **today's scenario**
"Unethical practices among many local manufacturers and dubious practices by the businessmen who import from overseas, substandard and proscribed items into the country, have contributed in no small measure to the menace."

Tunde Alao—Staff Reporter. (See Appendix 8).
"Skin-toning is a huge money-maker that I'm sure has lined the pockets of enough politicians to allow it to keep being sold despite international outcry" Kingsley'Rukus'Okafor—Nigerian-Americanrapper.

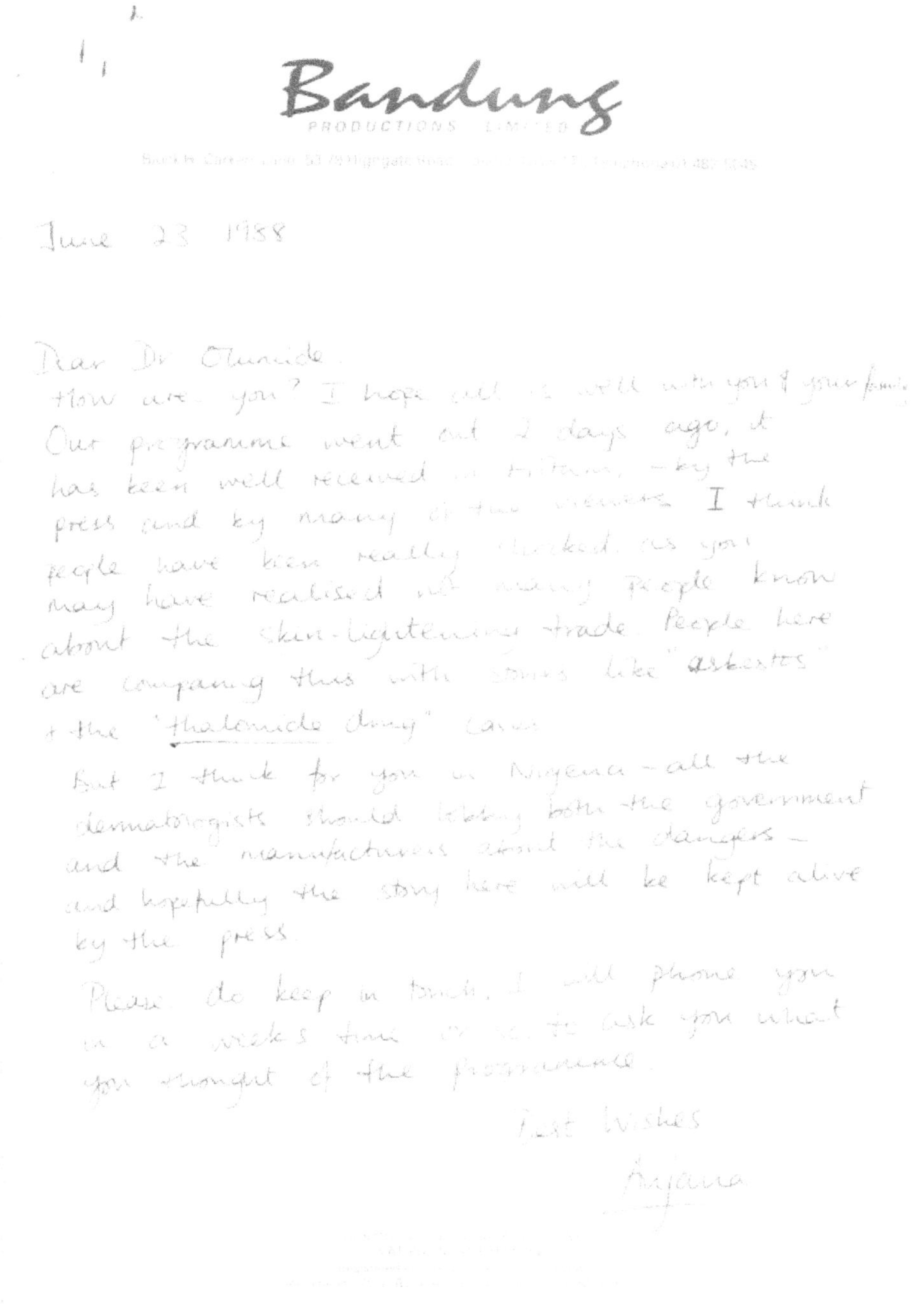

Bandung

PRODUCTIONS LIMITED

June 23 1988

Dear Dr Olumide

How are you? I hope all is well with you & your family.

Our programme went out 2 days ago, it has been well received in Britain – by the press and by many of the viewers. I think people have been really shocked, as you may have realised not many people know about the skin-lightening trade. People here are comparing this with stories like "asbestos" & the "thalomide drug" cases.

But I think for you in Nigeria – all the dermatologists should lobby both the government and the manufacturers about the dangers – and hopefully the story here will be kept alive by the press.

Please do keep in touch. I will phone you in a weeks time or so to ask you what you thought of the programme.

Best Wishes

Anjana

Figure 4.2 Letter from BANDUNG TV Channel 4 after featuring the documentary

Lucy Hannan further noted that a market flooded by foreign goods in this way encouraged a consumer preference for imported products and has the additional effect of undermining the nascent domestic industries. Some entrepreneurs circumvented consumer demand by

producing "Made in England" fakes, but the end result was a severely disadvantaged domestic market. For all these reasons, Lucy Hannan of AB investigators further noted that many African government officials contended that EEC must recognize the necessity of stopping **production** of any dangerous products at source, rather than leaving it to the importing countries to attempt to clear their markets through legislation.
The thrust of Olumide's message during the documentary by BANDUNG was that:

"The preservation of human health is the collective responsibility of all nations. If the manufacturers in Britain cannot do anything to better the health of people in Africa, at least they should not do anything to worsen the plight of Africans. It is totally immoral, totally unjustifiable to export these chemicals which have been banned in your countries to my people."

This generated some controversy.
When the Irish Development Authority (IDA) provided a £750,000 sterling ($1.4m) grant to expand W & E Products' mercury – soap operation in County Wicklow, it defended the decision by claiming that **"IDA is not in the business of making moral decisions for other countries"**

Michael Tattersall, Financial Director of the main British factory of W & E Products, continued to insist, despite a public and parliamentary campaign to stop the trade, that the soaps were actually completely harmless – whether used according to the instructions on the packet (which carry a mandatory "poison" warning) or as a skin-lightener. According to Tattersall, mercury soaps have been available in Africa for over 50 years, and *"if there were any problems with it, they would have come to light by now"*.

UK Euro MP Michael Hindley, in whose constituency W & E Products operated, dismissed any excuse from the manufacturers for a trade which he says was evidently dangerous. Hindley claims, *"Given the number of countries that have found it necessary to ban the soap, there is* ***ipso facto*** *enough evidence; even South Africa bans skin-lighteners, and South Africa is hardly known for protecting the interests of its black citizens."*

Hindley pointed out that the economic and political situation in many of the African markets facilitated sales despite any appropriate legislation – and he had, in fact, produced samples of the soap found in British and Belgian markets. It was observed that some of the products were openly on sale in Britain and that 16 different brands could be bought in Brixton alone!

Olumide dismissed Tattersall's claims. She charged that manufacturers were simply sheltering behind the difficulties all developing countries face when it comes to producing corroborative statistical and laboratory evidence.

Olumide described herself as being "propelled into research … by the number of people who flooded the clinic with hopelessly damaged skin" It is only the tip of the iceberg, she added as many people did not come to the clinic until the symptoms were for advanced. Moreover the systemic manifestations of adverse effects to these chemicals may take several years to manifest and many symptoms and signs of mercury poisoning, for example, mimic other diseases, so it may not be possible to statistically or forensically link them to skin lightening cosmetics when such patients present in other clinics e.g, Renal, Ear/Nose/Throat (ENT), Paediatric or Gynaecological clinics.

Olumide contended that "Banning the importation was not the panacea. Stopping the production from the source was manifestly the solution. In one year the Nigerians got through £20m (twenty million Pounds Sterling) worth of the stuff and that's not counting the dozens of other African countries where it was sold!

The UK Department of Trade & Industry (DTI), which had justified the policy of ***laisser-faire*** as being "based on the principle that all countries were responsible for the health and safety of their own consumers" responded to pressure by asking the manufacturers to substantiate their defence that the products were completely harmless. Sales of these products, which contained mercury and hydroquinone, were banned in Europe although their manufacture for export was not, despite evidence to suggest that workers making them could suffer miscarriages and their children suffer kidney failures.

Although DTI acknowledged that it had been receiving many complaints from African governments, the main political leverage against the factories appeared to be domestic pressure concerning the effects of mercuric poisoning on the work force. A female worker who gave birth to a baby suffering from muscular spasms, stiffness and high muscle tone – all symptoms of heavy mercuric poisoning – took legal action. The baby was found to have 10 times more mercury in his body than the amount tolerable for an adult. Another woman working at W & E Products in UK gave birth to a baby with no

kidneys, who died at three months. Both the BBC and The Observer of London drew attention to the controversy growing around mercury-soap production, which along with the pressure from Hindley, forced the DTI to reconsider its position.
Then in February 1988, as a result of the January survey in Lagos, Nigerian Health Minister, Olikoye Ransome–Kuti announced a ban of 34 brands of British-manufactured mercuric soap and skin lighteners and called on the exporting countries to "inform their industries that it was an offence to import into Nigeria any cosmetic products that contained mercury." On 18 February 1988, the DTI wrote to the factories and told them to "stop exporting or supplying the products for exporting, or a prohibition notice will be served". However, that was not the end of the trade. W & E Products simply moved its production to their Irish branch in County Wicklow and would in all probability profit from the closure of the other British factories.

According to Tattersall, over 20 other factories within the EEC were producing mercuric soaps, and many other countries were eager to get a share of the profitable market – estimated by those familiar with it to be worth of £20m ($37m) a year for the Nigerian trade alone. He claimed that many of the brands were produced in the Far East and named Korea as one country that was eager to join the market. In Lagos, the effect of the Health Minister's new crack down paradoxically only fuelled a dramatic upward surge in demand. Vendors of the banned products were reportedly buying up stock in the markets to sell later at inflated prices, and some have removed them from the shelves to make more profitable under-the-counter deals.

Martal Cosmetics of London, which produced a range of skin-lightening creams called Symba, had been on the market for over 16years and sold its products in the EEC as well as in Africa. Its content of hydroquinone was legitimate, at only 2%. Their packaging clearly states: "This product complies with the Federal Government of Nigeria Health Directives 1987". Many legitimate manufacturers and distributors pointed out that the illegal 5% preparations on the market seriously undermined sales of products bearing the correct percentage because the users identified the difference in effectiveness and potency, abandoned the legitimate 2% hydroquinone products and patronized the illegal 5% preparations.

Lucy Hannan's survey also revealed that preventing these illegal soaps from coming into the country had proved impossible for Nigeria.

Many of the brands found their way in through cross-border smuggling, which could not be curbed without massive resources to mount a counter-policing operation and which some British distributors openly exploit to sell their products. For example, Philip Winner & Co of London, which distributed a 3% mercuric soap called Sukisa Bango, were delighted to hear that their soap had found its way into Nigeria and, in response to an enquiry about supplies to Lagos, proposed a regular transaction through the Republic of Benin.

Some comments by viewers in London on the Bandung TV documentary

Appendix 6 shows some of the newspaper cuttings reacting to the London BANDUNG TV documentary in 1988.

"Some of these products are openly on sale in Britain where the black population is being sucked into the US and South African mentality of thinking "lighter is better" Ronnie Smith Morning star

"Several decades after blacks declared themselves beautiful, there is a nagging feeling that beige is better. The most horrifying aspect is that it is blacks themselves who feel this and whites, surprise, are more than willing to exploit that feeling. It is a sobering thought that although we can intellectually dismiss all the shit about whiter being nicer, emotionally some of us still want lighter skins. The cost is not paid in cash alone, nor is it restricted to the silent shame that at some subliminal level we too feel that white skin is superior. The penalty is paid physically as well as in moral and financial terms". Alkarim Jivani

"Not the least of the ironies of the modern world is that while millions of white people lie out under the sun to make their skins darker, large numbers of dark-skinned people smother themselves in preparations they believe will make them lighter. Horrific film from Nigeria showed the disfiguring rashes caused by chemicals in the skin lightening creams and compounds, while the mercury in the soaps can cause kidney failure, miscarriages and brain damage". Peter Patterson Daily Mail 22 June 1988.

"Bandung Files (C4) looked at the cynical way in which British companies illegally exploit the absence of consumer protection in Africa by selling toxic skin lighteners which can cause permanent, irreversible skin damage and which, in the case of soaps containing mercury, are linked with foetal malformation, abortion and kidney damage. Nor is the trade confined to Africa. In Brixton the team found 16 different kinds of illegal soaps on sale.

The tragedy here is less the vast profits being made by the companies concerned, more the discontent and inferiority felt by millions of black women and men who

long to have lighter skin. Colour prejudice is felt among blacks as well as between blacks and whites. Black magazines go for lighter skinned models. Blacks with lighter skins find it easier to get jobs. Here were uncomfortable issues well aired, and an excellent justification for minority programming."

Lesley Garner Daily Times 22 June 1988

"Bandung File (Channel 4). An insidious and profitable spin-off from – racist attitudes is the huge market for skin-lightening products for black people. For many who use them, particularly in South Africa, skin-lighteners are used for pragmatic, not cosmetic reasons. The market raises moral issues¯but on top of that there is an alarming medical aspect. Tonight's report presents evidence that skin-lightening soaps and creams are causing irreversible skin damage to thousands, increasing susceptibility to cancers; that they are responsible for kidney failure, brain damage and miscarriages, and that 40 percent of black South African women are suffering from their effects. Many of these products, although banned by the EEC for sale in Europe, are being made in Britain for export to Africa¯by companies which are household names here"

(Photo of Michael Jackson shown here)

A lighter skin can lead to a better life – for some. But at what risk to health?"

Sandy Smithies 21 June 1988

"Bandung File (C4)'s magazine programme, aimed at ethnic groups, often boasts some of the most professional and comprehensive journalism on television. Tonight's programme contains a report on the horrifying effects of the skin-lightening creams and soaps which are used by those people who don't have the bank balance of Michael Jackson." ST June 1988.

Response to *Bandung TV* Documentary in Nigeria

Bandung TV gave Olumide two copies of the cassettes containing the documentary used by television houses, to give the Nigerian TV Stations for Nigerian viewers so that they would be aware of the hazards and the concern in foreign lands about their health. A copy of the cassette was given to the then Hon Minister of Health and the second copy to – the main national TV station in Lagos at that time. That same year, the Toiletries and Cosmetics Manufacturers Group (of the Manufacturers Association of Nigeria), organized the 1st National Awareness Seminar with the theme: "Nigeria's Health and Body-Care under siege". It was held at the Lagos Sheraton Hotel, Ikeja on Wednesday 23rd November, 1988 and Olumide was invited to present a one hour Paper at the Seminar. The title of Olumide's presentation was "Some Observations On The Cosmetic Culture of Nigerians – Problems and Solution". On arrival at the venue on the day of the Seminar, to my utter dismay, the official printed Programme for the day had a **full page**, advert on the full range of cosmetics under the brand name Venus de Milo—showing, among other cosmetic products a **"Complexion Cream"** with the picture of a black African on the left transforming to a milky white Caucasian on the right, with by-lines which read: *"So many ways to make a woman look and feel beautiful"* ***"Beauty is clear,*** *radiant skin enticing lips... gleaming nails... an air of freshness and fragrance. Venus de Milo cosmetics make the dream come true, for the woman who wants to look and feel good in every way. Choose venue de Milo... and make the most of your charm and attractiveness... so quickly ... so easily... every day".* Appendices 7a & 7b show the cover pages of the programme and the advert.

Worse still, at the seminar several members of the group, at different times, boasted to Olumide **"that documentary on "the whiter shade of black" that was beamed on London Channel 4 TV "will never see the light of day in Nigeria"**! At first Olumide thought it was a joke and simply replied that the main Television Station in Lagos already had a copy of the cassette which *BANDUNG* told her was suitable for TV Projectors, and another cassette was also given to the Honourable Minister of Health. When the boasts persisted, Olumide asked one of the members whose Company had nothing to do with the manufacture of skin-lightening products why they thought the documentary would not be shown in Nigeria – he replied "no TV station will show any programme which is not in the interest of its sponsors; and a major transnational company, indicted in the documentary was a major sponsor, of the TV Programmes". After waiting for several months and the documentary was never aired, Olumide went to see the senior officer of the TV station who collected the cassette from her and asked for the reason for not airing the documentary; he said it was because the **"cassette was not suitable for their projectors"**, and he immediately returned the cassette to Olumide!.

NAFDAC later **endorsed** a new cosmetic product – Venus Skin Toning Cream, manufactured by a major transnational Company – PZ industries. NAFDAC not only licensed the product and gave it a NAFDAC registration number, but also helped to market it. A very senior member of staff of NAFDAC boldly and approvingly stood in front of the glittering cameras to launch **Venus Skin Toning products**, at a special event hosted by PZ industries during the botched Miss World Beauty Pageant in 2002 in Abuja. Abuja is the capital and administrative headquarters of Nigeria! Olumide gathered that PZ action was "legal" because the new skin lightening product did not contain any of the prohibited chemicals in the Federal Government Gazette and that the product was a "toning" product and not a "bleaching" product as stated in the Federal Government Gazette!

Some other actions taken in response to the menace posed by the use of bleaching products in Nigeria

1. The Medical women's Association of Nigeria (MWAN) has mounted several programmes over several years to create awareness and sensitize people about the dangerous effects of the use of skin lightening products at different fora – market place, schools, women's conferences etc. The subject was also the main theme of a symposium on Wed 25th Feb 1987. MWAN also published a 37 page book titled **"BLEACHING OF THE SKIN: What Everyone should know"** in 1988.

2. The Nigerian Association of Dermatologists (NAD) has been in the forefront of the campaign against the use of Skin Lightening products. Indeed at its annual conferences in Ibadan 2012 and Lagos 2014, NAD carried its awareness campaign rallies, tagged 'I'm proud and black", to the grassroots in the market places.

At the 2014 annual Conference of NAD, the Director General (DG) of NAFDAC was invited as the special guest of honour so that he could personally listen to the scientific presentations on the subject and sensitize NAFDAC on the need to take stricter measures to stop the manufacture importation and sale of the products in Nigeria.

3. The African Association of Dermatologists (AFRAD), at every conference had addressed the issue and deliberated on how best to control the manufacture and sale of the products. It was consistently a component of the Recommendations/Communiqué issued at the end of each conference.

4. The Print and Electronic Media have worked tirelessly on this subject. Hardly any month expires without a publication in one of the daily Newspapers addressing the issue in the form of an editorial or feature article. (See Appendix 8)

5. In April 1999, NAFDAC organized a Workshop for Cosmetic Dealers. Olumide was Guest Lecturer at the event and provided

posters with clinical photographs on the complications of the use of skin lightening products.

In 2002 NAFDAC organized another Workshop on the Subject. Olumide was also invited to present a Paper at the Workshop and she presented a paper on "Cosmetic Habits and Legislative needs in Nigeria".

6. Relevant specialist doctors and Scientists in Nigeria have published numerous research papers on the subject. Some of these publications are listed in Appendix 1.

The theme of the 5th International Conference of Drug Regulating Authorities (ICDRA) was Misuse and Control of Hazardous Cosmetics. The Conference was organized by the German Foundation for International Development (DSE) Berlin (West). Oct 1989. Olumide presented a paper as a Guest Lecturer at the event.

References

1.Ronnie Smith. Soaps danger exposed. *Morning Star* 17 June 1988
2. Alkarim Jivani. Bandung File *Television Previews.*
3. Peter Paterson's Television Review: TV Mail *Daily Mail* 22 June 1988.
4. Lesley Garner. Misdirected passion *Television Daily Times* 22 June 1988.
5. Sandy Smithies. Bandung File (Channel 4) Watching Brief. A lighter skin can lead to a better life – for some. But at what risk to health? (legend under photo of Michael Jackson) 21 June 1988.
6. Lucy Hannan. Companies still make hazardous cosmetics for Africa. Feature: Hazardous Cosmetics *African Business* May 1988.

(2) Some Studies done in Nigeria

2 (i) Olumide *et al*

Olumide and a team of researchers at the Lagos University Teaching Hospital in Nigeria have studied extensively the skin bleach culture in Nigeria and published several scientific papers in peer reviewed journals.[1-10] A most comprehensive publication on the subject was published in 2008.[8]

Olumide *et al* characterized in details the complications of chronic use of skin lightening cosmetics. The active ingredients in these cosmetic products are hydroquinone, mercury and corticosteroids. Several additives (conconctions) are used to enhance the bleaching effect. Since these products are used for long duration, on a large body surface area, and under hot humid conditions, percutaneous absorption is enhanced. The complications of these products are very serious and are sometimes fatal. Some of these complications are exogenous ochronosis, impaired wound healing and wound dehiscence, the fish odor syndrome, nephropathy, steroid addiction syndrome, predisposition to infections, a broad spectrum of cutaneous and endocrinologic complications of corticosteroids, including suppression of hypothalamic-pituitary-adrenal axis. In this era of easy travels and migration, African patients with these complications can present to physicians anywhere in the world. It is therefore critical for every practicing physician to be aware of these complications. Details of the complications are discussed in chapters 13 and 14.

References

1. Olumide YM. Cosmetic hazards and Legislative needs in Nigeria. *Nigeria Medical Practitioner.* 1985; 9:7-12.
2. Olumide YM. Abuse of topical corticosteroids in Nigeria. *Nigeria Medical Practitioner.* 1986; 11:7-13.
3. Olumide YM, Elesha SO. Hydroquinone based skin lightening creams. *Nigeria Medical Practitioner.* 1986; 11:103-6.
4. Olumide YM. Photodermatoses in Lagos. *International Journal of Dermatology.* 1987; 26:295-5.
5. Olumide YM. Contact Leucoderma. *Nigeria Quart J Hosp Med.* 1989; 4:53-62.
6. Olumide YM, Odunowo BD, Odiase AO. Regional dermatoses in the African. Part 1 Facial hypermelanosis. *International Journal of Dermatology.* 1991: 30 (3):186-9.
7. Olumide YM. A pictorial self-instructional manual on common skin diseases. (Where there is no dermatologist) 1993; Heinemann Educational Books (Nigeria) Plc.
8.Olumide YM, Akinkugbe AO. Altraide Dan, Mohammed T, *et al.* Complications of chronic use of skin lightening cosmetics. *International Journal of Dermatology.* 2008; 47:344-53.
9. Olumide YM. Editorial: Use of skin lightening creams. Lack of recognition and regulation is having serious medical consequences. *British Medical Journal (BMJ).* 2010; 341: c6102 (Published 23 November 2010). Doi:10.1136/bmj.c6102.
10. Ayanlowo OO, Olumide YM, Akinkugbe AO, Ahamneze N. Photodamage on the background of chronic use of skin lightening cosmetics. *Household and Personal Care Today.* Health Issues—Skin Lightening (Peer reviewed article) n2/2012. pp 22-4.

2 (ii) Adebajo 2002. Market traders in Lagos

Adebajo studied 450 traders selected from three major and popular markets in the Lagos metropolis between May and July 1998 using stratified sampling method. Information on their socio-demographic characteristics, knowledge, attitudes to, and the patterns of use of skin lightening cosmetics were elicited from the respondents with the assistance of a team of experienced interviewers using well-structured administered questionnaires.

The prevalence of use of skin lightening cosmetics was 77.3% comprising ninety-six males (27.6%) and two hundred and fifty two females (72.4%). The trend cuts across all socioeconomic strata, age, sex and marital status. Hydroquinone based products were the most used, although corticosteroids and mercury-base products were also widely used.

Many of the respondents (45.7%) who admitted using the cosmetics spent between N250-N500 per month on the cosmetics whilst some (12.4%) spent between N500-N1000 (at that time 100 Naira (N) was equivalent US $1.00). Over half of the respondents claimed that they discovered the skin lightening cosmetics by themselves whilst, one hundred and twenty-three (35.3%) were influenced by their friends. Other sources of influence included health workers (2.3%), pharmacies (5.5%), parents (1.4%) and the media (1.4%). Reasons for the use of skin lightening products were: makes one more attractive (30.2%); a fashionable trend (13.7%); treat skin blemishes (31.3%); cleanse/tone the face and body (21.0%); satisfy the desires of the opposite sex (4.0%).
As regards user satisfaction, 64.1% felt they were more attractive hence, they were more confident about their new look. Only 13.2% claimed they were relieved of their skin blemishes while 9.5% claimed they were better appreciated by their spouses.

Fifty percent of the three hundred and forty eight respondents developed side effects. These side effects were exogenous ochronosis, skin rash, striae, hypertrichosis, Cushionoid swelling of the face, and pedal oedema, thinning of the skin, easy bruising of the skin, worsening of existing skin condition, haematuria, weight gain and body odour. As regards how respondents reacted to the side effects 35.6% stopped using the products; 7.5% sought medical advice; 45.4% ignored the side effects; and 11.5% used local herbs to treat the complications.

From the above study it becomes clear that the pharmacy shops constitute a veritable source of the supply of skin lightening products. Furthermore, the prevalence of adverse effects recorded in the hospitals is grossly inaccurate and a tip of the iceberg, because the vast majority simply stopped using the products, ignored the adverse effects or used local herbs to treat themselves. More importantly, *no systemic* complications were sought for by the researcher.

Adebajo recommended urgent need for the Nigerian government to enact laws banning the continuous importation and local manufacture of skin lightening products. Adebayo observed that enforcing controls on the sale of skin lightening cosmetics in Nigeria may be an uphill task. Firstly, these products are to a large extent manufactured in developed countries, purely for export purposes to Africa and without regulations, they are freely sold to a predominantly ignorant population by retailers in market places, and roadside drug stores or chemists. Prosecuting these retail traders will only drive the trade under the counter. Secondly, the formulations of these cosmetics are not standardized and at the same time, manufacturers in Nigeria have not cultivated the culture of labelling and listing the ingredients used in the preparation of their products. Besides, where labels are available, the low adult literacy level (male/female) of 54/31[2], makes it difficult for a large segment of the population to appreciate the importance of the inherent dangers associated with the use of skin lightening creams.

It therefore, becomes imperative that to address this widespread problem in Nigeria, there is an urgent need for concerted efforts by the Nigerian government to enact laws banning the continuous importation and local manufacture of these cosmetics. This should be enforced at least until proper clinical trials are conducted to ascertain the safety levels acceptable for the Nigerian skin types and climate. There is also a need for mass education of the public on the short and long term dangers, which accompany the use of these drugs. At the same time, the public should be made to understand that by simply maintaining good personal hygiene and living healthy lifestyles, it is possible that everyone can stay young and radiant. Prescription habits of practicing health workers, traditional birth attendants and healers can be improved immensely by mounting refresher courses to correct wrong prescription habits and to provide current information on the principles of corticosteroid therapy.

References

1. Adebajo SB. An epidemiological survey of the use of cosmetic skin lightening cosmetics among traders in Lagos, Nigeria. *West Afr J Med.* 2002 Jan-Mar; 21 (1): 51-5.

2. FMOH/UNICEF. Children and women in Nigeria. A situation analysis. 1990; Johnmof.

2 (iii) Ofondu 2003—University Students in Enugu

Study at the Enugu State University of Science and Technology (ESUT) between February and October 2001.

298 patients were studied; 146 female (49%): 152 males (51%). Age range 16-48 years; 186 (62.4%) were skin bleachers —105 (71.9%) females, 81 (53.3%) males; 69 (23.15%) *unintentionally* were using the products; 203 (98.12%) claimed ignorance about the adverse health effects of the products.

Table 4.1 Reasons for using the products

	Total		Female	Male
For smoother skin	—	60 (20.13%)	29	31
For lighter skin	—	53 (17.78%)	30	23
Fashionable/treat blemishes	—	27 (9.03%)	16	11
Other reasons	—	118 (39.60%)	44	74

Table 4.2 Responses of subjects studied following education on bleaching cream abuse

	Total	Female	Male
No effect	82	54	28
Intend to stop	94	43	51
Non committal	122	49	73
Total	298	146	152

Table 4.3 Top 10 skin complications after use (order of frequency)

1. Periorbital pigmentation
2. Patches of lighter skin
3. Stretch marks
4. Acne
5. Skin rashes (e.g Tinea incognito)
6. Poor wound healing
7. Hypertrichosis
8. Hyperpigmented patches (Exogenous ochronosis)
9. Changes in nail colour
10. Easy bruising

Table 4.4 Top 10 skin lightening products used with Mercury and hydroquinone content in urine analysis

	Hydroquinone mg%	Mercury content (μg/L)
1. RUKA, SWISS COLLADEN	0.09	57.80
2. BETNOVATE N	30.8	47.60
3. A1, A3, LOOKING GOOD	13.62	45.50
4. MIC	29.09	28.00
5. PEAUCLAIRE	2.79	18.00
6. SIVOCLAIRE	16.25	18.00
7. TURA, LOOKING GOOD	18.61	16.00
8. VENUS	16.03	9.73
9. IKB	10.52	5.52
10. MOVATE	14.62	14.20

21 (Twenty one) manufacturers of cosmetic beauty products were found registered with NAFDAC and produce skin beauty creams.

From the above study it becomes clear that (i) the level of education did not positively influence the prevalence of skin bleaching. (ii) Men also frequently engage in skin bleaching. (iii) About a quarter of the skin bleachers claimed they were not aware that the cosmetics they used contained skin bleaching chemicals (iv) Even after educating the people about the adverse effects of skin bleaching, the majority were not prepared to stop the practice. (v) No systemic complications were sought for although high levels of concentration of hydroquinone and mercury were found in the urine of the skin bleachers.

Reference

Ofondu Eugenia Ogugua. Cosmetic use of bleaching creams in Enugu. *National Postgraduate Medical College of Nigeria Dissertation* 2003.

---

2 (iv) Ajose 2005—Skin Clinic in Lagos State University Teaching Hospital (LASUTH)

Frances Ajose described the consequences of skin bleaching in Nigerian men and women. In the survey, 92% of female patients and 5% of male patients over the age of 16 years who attended the skin clinic reported having used skin bleaching products. However 40% of the female patients and 2% of the male patients were currently using the products at the time of study (Feb-Oct 2004). None of the current users and only 3% of the long-term users (>10years) understood the protective function of skin pigment. Eighty (80%) percent of users were aware of the effect of sun exposure on their skin but only 2% took specific sun protection measures.

The depigmented agents used included hydroquinone, topical steroid, mercurials, phenolics, caustics and other unknown chemicals and plant derivatives as creams, lotions, milks and soaps. The agents were often used in combinations of two or more products. The duration of use ranged from 6 months to over 20years. The motives for use included (a) a desire to even out the skin tone (b) a desire to lighten the complexion, (c) a desire to improve the appearance of the skin prior to an event, and (d) dependence, that is inability to withdraw the use because of worsening of the skin complications – a form of addiction.

Dermatological complications reported include disease modification e.g atypical scabies, Tinea incognito and disseminated viral warts. Other cutaneous complications which have been described by Olumide *et al*[2] were also observed by Ajose. Serious systemic complications including Cushing's syndrome, renal damage which required haemodialysis, and evidence of immune suppression manifested by tuberculosis and widespread vulval warts were also documented by Ajose in her study. There were also serious psycho-social complications which have been discussed under PSYCHO-SOCIAL COMPLICATIONS OF SKIN LIGHTENING—Chapter 14.

References

1. Ajose Frances OA. Consequences of skin bleaching in Nigerian men and women. *International Journal of Dermatology*. 2005; 44 (Suppl.1), 41-3

2. Olumide YM, Akinkugbe AO *et al.* Complications of chronic use of skin lightening cosmetics. *International Journal of Dermatol.* 2008:47; 344-53.

2 (v) Nnoruka 2006. Skin clinic in Enugu

Study at the skin clinic of University of Nigeria Hospital Enugu.

Consecutive new patients who were using depigmenting agents between June – Dec 2004.

The depigmenting agents utilized were ascertained by asking the patients to come with the packets or containers of used products from which well-known active skin lightening substances were obtained.

931 consecutive new patients (skin bleachers)—75.0% Female; 25% males; aged 18-69 yrs.

Duration of use 3 months to 30 years.

Table 4.5 Products used

57.2%— Corticosteroids
43.7% — hydroquinone
6.8% — Mercurials
2.1% — Kojic acid
1.6% — alphahydroxy acids/glycolic acids
5.7% — unknown products
61.3% used the above products in combination with steroids

Adverse health disorders reported were steroid induced acne (45.3%); Facial Hyperpigmentation (37.2%); mycosis (40.4%); striae (28.3%); telangiectasis (21.3%); hypertrichosis (13.9%); and diabetes mellitus (2.1%).

Reference

Nnoruka Edith, Okoye Obiefuna. Topical steroid abuse: Its use as a depigmenting agent. *Journal of the National Medical Association* June 2006; 98 (6): 934-9.

---

2 (vi) Ofili *et al* 2006. University Students – in Benin

In this study in Benin City, a cross-sectional study was carried out among 385 undergraduate students. A multi-stage sampling method was used to select the students. Data was collected using predesigned questionnaire. One hundred and thirty four (134) were males; while two hundred and fifty one (251) were females. **64.9% of the respondents were using bleaching agents in their soaps or creams. 70.7% of the women bleached while 52.2% of men bleached.**

It is noteworthy that in this study, the respondents were asked to **show** the jars/tubes containing the cosmetic cream they used and the wrapper/cartons of the bath soap they used. When the simple question in the Questionnaire was asked ***"Do you tone?,"*** the response is given in Table 4.6.

Table 4.6 Responses of respondents to the question "Do you tone?"

Responses	Percentage %
No	79.1
Yes	16.4
Not Sure	4.2
No Response	0.3
Total	**100.0**

Table 4.6 implies that if the study depended only on asking questions, the prevalence of bleachers in that study would have been 16.4%; as opposed to physically sighting the cosmetic product 64.9%. It becomes clear that either the respondents **deliberately** deny that they bleach or they are not aware that the products they use contain bleaching agents. The former is more likely to be true because these are university undergraduates (not illiterates) who can read what is written on the products and they can **see** the effect of the products on their skin tone.

2 (vii) NOI Polls 2014 General public in Abuja

In another study in Abuja, the capital city of Nigeria, a study was conducted among the general public using NOI Polls. NOI Polls is the No 1 for country-specific polling services in the West African region, in technical partnership with Gallup (USA) to develop opinion research in Nigeria. NOI Polls is named after its creator, Ngozi Okonjo-Iweala (NOI), former Nigerian vice precident of the World Bank.

According to NOI Polls in Abuja, Nigeria, skin bleaching was reported as being mostly predominant among Nigerians within the age group of 18-25 years (48 percent) and 26-40 years (43 percent). According to NOI Polls, People of all religious groups, single or married, rich or poor, literate and illiterate, low, middle and upper class use the products. It is noteworthy that not only young ladies bleach their skin, older women and indeed boys and men do bleach. The only difference is that the preponderance is more among young ladies.

Reference

NOI Polls. Jide Ojo. Nigeria as the world capital of skin bleaching March 26, 2014 http://www.punchng.com/opinion/nigeria-as-the-world-capita-of-skin.

2 (viii) Further notes on types of chemicals and products used in lightening the skin and frequency of adverse effects on the skin in Nigeria

The products used for skin bleaching

A survey of the products displayed for sale on the shelves in supermarkets and pharmacy shops[1] shows that the active ingredients, as reflected on the packages, could contain any of the following chemicals—corticosteroids, hydroquinone, Kojic acid, arbutin, azelaic acid, niacinamide, Bearberry, Kamana Egyptian milk, glutathione, retinoids, alphahydroxy acids Vitamin C derivaties e.g magnesium-ascorbyl-phosphate (MAP) and ascorbyl-6-palmitate. (See the chapter on COSMECEUTICALS). However the studies done both in the community[2] and in the hospital clinics showed that the products used contained corticosteroids, hydroquinone and mercurials,[3] Kojic acid and alphahydroxy acids. Indeed the study done by Ofondu[4] which involved analysis of ten products showed that **all the ten** products were **mixtures** of Hydroquinone and mercury in **very high** concentrations. This showed that ingredients labeling had no bearing whatsoever on the **actual** ingredients in the products. It is noteworthy that **none** of the products listed 'mercury' on the product package. Cost of the products on display in the shops range from $ 2 or less for a jar/tube of hydroquinone or mercury based products to $ 400 US dollars for a 500ml 0.6 kg of Kanama Egyptian milk.[5] (See further notes in chapter 3 on EPIDEMIOLOGY).

Table 4:7 shows the types of chemicals used among traders in Lagos[2], Table 4.8 shows the types of chemicals used by University undergraduates in Benin City, Nigeria[6]

Table 4.7 Bleaching agents used by traders in Lagos[2]

Types of chemical based cosmetics used

	Male	Female
Corticosteroids	(39.2%)	(53.1%)
Hydroquinone	(62.3%)	(65.6%)
Mercury	(43.8%)	(48.4%)
Locally concocted Soaps/creams	(17.7%)	(19.7%)

Table 4.8 Bleaching agents present in cosmetics used by respondents[6]

Agents Present	No. of Respondents N=385	Percentage %
Body cream		
No bleaching agent present	191	49.6
Hydroquinone	170	44.2
Mercury	21	5.4
Corticosteroids	3	0.8
**Multiple responses present*		
Bathing Soap		
No bleaching agent present	274	71.2
Mercury	82	21.3
Hydroquinone	23	6.0
Corticosteroids	6	1.6
**Multiple responses present*		
Facial Cream		
No bleaching agent present	333	86.5
Hydroquinone	29	10.1
Corticosteroids	8	2.1
Mercury	5	1.3
**Multiple responses present*		
Content added to body cream		
No bleaching agent present	359	93.2
Corticosteroids	13	3.4
Hydroquinone	10	2.6
Mercury	2	0.5
Alpha hydroxyl acids	1	0.3

Misleading labeling of products

The users of skin lightening products know the agent as brand names and most of the skin lightening cosmetics and toiletries do not have the ingredients labeled on them and some of the ones that carry ingredient labels have been found to be falsely branded both in chemical content and concentration when analysed.[3,4] Bootleg versions abound in the market and shops in Nigeria.

Table 4:9 shows a list of some of the bleaching creams used by patients in Nigeria and ingredients as labeled; and Table 4:10 shows the actual contents of some of the creams analysed. The ingredients labeling on MOVATE was Betamethasone dipropionate, but when it was analysed it was found to contain 5.10mg% of Hydroquinone and 0.20mg/kg of mercury.[3,4]

Table 4.9. A list of some of the bleaching creams used by patients in Nigeria and ingredients as labeled[4]

Cream	Ingredients
Movate	Betamethasone dipropionate
Crusader Vitamed	B3 toner 2%, Escalol UV 507, Vit E Allantoin
Looking Good	2% hydroquinone, Allantoin, Sunscreen, Vit E
Peauclair	Hydroquinone, clobetasol propionate
Mic	Hydroquinone, Dimethicone, D-methyl-PABA
Tura	Octyl-Dimethyl PABA, Dimethicone, Aqua glyceryl, propylene glycol mubbery
A3	A-hydroxyl acids, methyl p-ben
Ultra	Vitamed B3 toner 2%, Escalol UV 507, Vit E Allantoin
Venus	Benzophone 3-Dimethicone, Cyclomethicone
Swiss collagen	Triethanolamine, arbomer, Dimethicone
Fashion Fair	Betamethasone dipropionate
IKB	Triethanolamine
Shirley	Natural Essences from botany
Ambi	2% hydroquinone padimate
Skin Success	2% hydroquinone Octisalate
Sivoclaire	2% hydroquinone, Vit E 1.0
Fashion Fair	Clobetasol propionate 0.05
Tony Montana	Stearic Acid, MPG, Sorbitol Jelly, Fragrance

Table 4:10. Contents of some creams analyzed[3]

Cream	Hydroquinone (mg%)	Mercury (mg/kg)
Looking Good	1.36	0.17
Movate	5.10	0.20
Crusader	3.45	0.26
Sivoclaire	0.06	0.22
Peauclaire	0.06	0.21
Mercury	1.68	0.82
Mic	0.06	0.22
Tura	1.45	0.23
A3	0.42	0.18

Frequency of adverse effects on the skin

As regards the study on the traders[2], Tables 4. 11-13 show the relevant data, the adverse effects and what the respondents did on noticing the adverse effects. As regards the study on the University of Benin undergraduates[6], Table 4.14 shows the cutaneous adverse effects.

Table 4.11: Respondents who had side effects from the use of bleaching cosmetics (n = 348)[2]

	Percentage of side effects Yes (%) (n = 174)	No (%) (n = 174)
Sex		
Male	(45.8%)	(54.2%)
Female	(51.6%)	(48.4%)
Duration of use of (months)		
<6	(31.1%)	(68.9%)
6 – 12	(52.4%)	(47.6%)
12 – 36	(56.5%)	(43.5%)
36 – 60	(46.7%)	(53.3%)
>60 months	(31.8%)	(69.2%)

Table 4.12 Side effects experienced by the respondents (n=348)[2]

Common side effects	**Frequency** **Male** (n=96)	**Female** (n=252)
Yellow brown Discoloration of skin	(26.0%)	(23.0%)
Skin rash	(17.7%)	(22.6%)
Multiple stretch marks	(4.2%)	(20.6%)
Excessive hair on the Body (hypertrichosis)	(6.3%)	(2.0%)
Swelling of the face and Limbs (oedema)	(4.2%)	(3.2%)
Thinning of the skin	(8.3%)	(9.1%)
Easy bruising of the skin	(6.3%)	(6.3%)
Worsening of existing skin Condition	(4.2%)	(21.0%)
Passage of blood in the urine	0	(3.6%)
Weight gain	(1.0%)	(2.8%)
Body odour	(8.3%)	(4.4%)

Table 4.13 What respondents did on noticing the side effects (n=348)[2]

Action taken	Frequency	
	Male	**Female**
Stopped using the cosmetics	(34.1%)	(36.1%)
Sought medical advice	(6.8%)	(7.7%)
Ignored side effects	(45.4%)	(35.4%)
Used local herbs	(13.6%)	(10.8%)

Table 4.14 Skin disorders observed among University of Benin students in Nigeria[6]

Skin disorders	Number	Proportion (%)
Dyschromia	42	32.3
Stretch marks	26	20.0
Acne	24	18.5
Superficial mycosis	17	13.1
Skin atrophy	17	13.1
Contact dermatitis	04	3.0
Total	**130**	**100**

Brand names of the products[7,8,9]

The brand names of some of the products on the market in 1988 are listed in Table 4.15. The lists do not represent the total number of products available on the Nigerian market. Each list is collated over a period from the names of products used by each patient who consulted at the skin clinic of the Lagos University Teaching Hospital.

Table 4.15 List of skin lightening products – 1988[4] (13 products)

Symba	Concorde
Milolo	Asepso
Tura	MIC
Crusader	Hg 1
Amber	Safe guard
Ikb	Neco
Jaribu	

The brand names of some of the products on the market in 1999 are listed in table 4.16.

Table 4.16. List of skin lightening products on the market in 1999 (36 Products)

Skin Beauty 5 Ways	Hypogel	Crusader
Venus	Merico	Looking Good
Dermovate	Fair & White	Peauclair
Body C	Skin Success	Mic
Nuclear	Tura	A3
Baycuten	Body Clear	Ultra
Beauty Fair	Sivu Clear	Swiss collagen
Movate Gel	Cotonou cream	Fashion Fair
Clearliss	Maxitone	IKB
Clear Essence	Visible Difference	Shirley
Beautiful lotion	Caroline	Ambi
New Age	Super – Maxitone	Tony Montana

Table 4.17. The brand names of some of the products on the market in 2014.[10] (Total 82 products)

Biocoten		
Maxiton complexion clarifying	Neomedrol	Betasol
Skin lightening serum	Mercy ointment	Premier dame
Qualiphar pomade	Fashion fair	Caike
Endix-G cream	Gmcin	Dr snow
Skineal	Carotone	Mr Mojumama
Fungicide	Marcderm	Vovi
Menoclear	B G cream	Skin white
Silver rose	Neoskin	Dr Aladin
Vista plus tripple action	HD cream	Epiderm
T3 mycin	Viodurula	HT-26 exclusive skin whitner
Ketazol	Diprosalic pomade	Toner astringent
Curaderm	Quadriderm cream	Lightening lotion
Amor white	Super medicated cream	Eskinol classic
Neurotone	Janet (clobetasol + papaya	Olay lightening cream
Daktacort	Combi uniscreen	Ojanye
Dermocream	ABF – 3 cream	Body white
Ytacan	Beneks	Look good
Maxi light	Vecuten	Hypprogel
Eye soothner	Acne away cream	Platinum skin beautifying milk
Dermovate	White field ointment	Herbal spice
Vecuten	Tenovate gel	Bioclaire
Elona –G	7 nights	Citro clear
Mycoten	Beycuten	Grace
Betasol	Candidern	DHF gold whitnizer
Agah moju	Kenacomb	Palmer skin success
Acne control cream	Esapharma	Eventon fade milk

Makari cream	QEI plu	Methaderm

Number of products on display in one Departmental Store in Lekki – an upper class residential area in Lagos in 2014

5(five) levels of shelves were devoted exclusively to skin lightening agents. Each shelf contains 13 **different** imported skin lightening products. Therefore, that store **alone** markets 65(sixty five) skin lightening products (creams, gels and serums), exclusive of another subsection which contains skin lightening soaps. One shelf was devoted exclusively to products labeled in the French Language alone. Most of the products on the shelves were labeled as either made in France / Italy / USA. Some products have the main instructions written in strange Chinese or Arabic languages. Many products have no name of manufacturer nor country of origin. The **Economist** reported in September 2012 that in Nigeria's capital Abuja, a store's cosmetics section had two aisles devoted exclusively to **different** skin bleaching products!

From all the above findings, it becomes clear that in Nigeria alone, there are probably over 200 (two hundred) skin-lightening products on sale in 2014—an exponential increase from the 1988 list when Nigeria requested Great Britain to stop the manufacture and export of skin lightening products to Nigeria. (See the Section on NIGERIA—HISTORY above.

References

1. Olumide YM. Unpublished data.

2. Adebajo SB. An epidemiological survey of the use of cosmetic skin lightening cosmetics among traders in Lagos. *West Afr J Med.* 2002 Jan-Mar; 21 (1): 51-5.

3. Nnroka Edith, Okoye Obiefuna. Topical steroid abuse: Its use as a depigmenting agent. *Journal of the National Medical Association.* June 2006; 98 (6): 934-9.

4. Ofondu Eugenia Ogugua. Cosmetic use of bleaching creams in Enugu. *National Postgraduate Medical College of Nigeria Dissertation* 2003.

5. Kamana Egyptian milk Review. April 8, 2014. *http://nigerian-reviews-evergoodproductions.com/kamana-egyptians-m...*

6. Ofili AN, Eze EU, Onunu AN. Prevalence of use of Skin Lightening agents amongst University of Benin undergraduates in Benin City, Nigeria. *The Nigerian Medical Practitioner*, 2006; 49(1/2): 24-7.

7. Olumide YM and Elesha SO. Hydroquinone induced exogenous ochronosis. *Nig Med Pract.* 1986; 11:103-4.

8. Olumide YM, A pictorial self-instructional manual on common skin diseases (where there is no dermatologist) 1st ed., *Heinemann Educational Books* (Nigeria) Plc, Ibadan, 1993; 150-72.

9. Olumide YM. Akinkugbe AO et al. Complications of chronic use of skin lightening cosmetics. *International Journal of Dermatology* 2008; 47:344-53.
10. Ayanlowo OO, Olumide YM, Akinkugbe AO, *et al* – Unpublished data.

2 (ix) Some Studies done on the chemical constituents of cosmetics emulsions in Nigeria

Toxic metals in cosmetics

Trace amounts of potentially toxic metals can be either intentionally added to cosmetics or present as impurities in the raw materials. Some potentially toxic metal exposures from skin care products have been identified apart from mercury and hydroquinone. Some of these metals are cadmium, cobalt, copper, nickel and lead. Contact with these metals can occur at occupational and environmental sources. Nickel is a notable cause of allergic contact dermatitis with a prevalence of 20% in females and 1% in males,[1] and its main source is from Jewelries, coins, and clothing accessories e.g bottons, zippers and cosmetic personal care products. Cadmium, lead, mercury, arsenic, copper, zinc, and chromium are metals of considerable health environmental concern. At low concentrations, some of these elements cause internal body organ damage in animals and in humans. Various forms of mammalian cancers, respiratory diseases, organ failures and retardation of the intellect have been traced to metal poisoning.[2] Zinc has been reported to cause the same signs of illness as does lead, and can easily be mistakenly diagnosed as lead poisoning. Although individual metals exhibit specific signs of their toxicity, the following have been reported as general signs associated with cadmium, copper and zinc poisoning: gastrointestinal disorders, diarrhoea, stomatitis, tremors, ataxia, paralysis, vomiting, convulsion, depression, and pneumonia when vapours and fumes are inhaled.[3]

In view of the above, Onwordi et al[4] carried out a study intended to determine the levels of potentially toxic metals (cadmium, cobalt, copper, nickel and lead) from body creams¯ moisturizers and skin-lightening (toning/bleaching) creams. 15 (fifteen) samples of commonly used body creams were purchased from some local stores in Lagos Nigeria. 5 (five) creams were marketed as "moisturizers;" 5 (five) marketed as "bleaching" creams; and five as "toning" creams. All the body cream products in the study were found to contain substantial levels of copper, nickel and one of the moisturizers contain cobalt and cadmium. The study shows that the use of various classes of body creams can expose users to significant levels of potentially toxic metals apart from Hydroquinone and Mercury.

In a study done by Oyedeji *et al*,[5] a broad spectrum of eighty cosmetic emulsions were purchased from a whole sale supermarket in Ibadan, Nigeria, with the aim of finding out if the creams contained hydroquinone and heavy metals at levels which were harmful to the populace. 41.25% of these emulsions were manufactured in Africa, 30.% in Europe, 1.25% in Asia and 27.50% in USA. About 51.25% of the emulsions contained hydroquinone having concentrations ranging from 9.50-50.35mg g^{-1} Iron levels of the emulsions were in the range 0.05-1.830mg L^{-1}, and lead from 0.01-0.9 mg g^{-1}. Chromium level from 0.002-0.097 mg L^{-1} and aluminum 0.320-1.002 mg L^{-1}. There were notable differences between the cosmetics manufactured in Nigerian, other African countries, Europe and USA.

All the emulsions manufactured in Nigeria contained hydroquinone with the exception of the petroleum jellies. The hydroquinone content of the emulsions ranged from 9.50-53.30mg g^{-1}. Heavy metals like Iron (Fe), Chromium (Ch), Lead (Pb) and Aluminium (Al) were present in the range 0.335-1.580, ND-0.087, 0/01-0.39 and ND-0.989 respectively. Some of them contained quaternary ammonium bases at low levels believed to be useful for skin softening and also as surface active agent, thereby reducing the surface tension of water and allowing permeability of substantive components into the skin. (ND=Not Detected)

The majority of the emulsions from Africa contained hydroquinone some of which might have been used as antioxidant rather than for skin lightening. The percentage content of hydroquinone in cosmetic emulsions from Africa ranged from 0.78-5.35% with the exception of petroleum jelly.
The percentage content of hydroquinone in cosmetic emulsions from Europe ranged from 1.20-4.70%. Only one of these emulsions had a value higher than 3.0%. The hydroquinone may have been included in most cases as an antioxidant rather than for skin lightening.

The percentage content of hydroquinone in cosmetic emulsions from USA ranged from 1.02-5.20%. The hydroquinone might have been used as antioxidant and toner. Only two emulsions have values higher than 3.0mg g^{-1}.

Another study was done in Awka, South Eastern Nigeria by Ekpunobi *et al*[6]. Thirty cosmetic skin lightening emulsions were randomly purchased from an open market in Awka and Enugu, cities of South Eastern Nigeria, with the aim of finding out if the creams contained hydroquinone and mercury at levels which were harmful to the users. Mercury was detected in two samples at concentrations of 100 and 200µg/g whereas the WHO limit is 1µg/g. None of the manufacturers indicated in the products that they contained mercury.

6 (Six) of the products were manufactured in Nigeria; 12 (twelve) of the products were manufactured in Ivory Coast; 3 (three) of the products were manufactured in India; 3 (three) of the products were manufactured in Italy; 1 (one) products was manufactured in Indonesia.1 (one) product was manufactured in United Kingdom; 1 (one) product was manufactured in Germany; 1 (one) product was manufactured in the Philippines; 1 (one) product was manufactured in the USA; 1 (one) product was manufactured in the Republic of Congo; 19 of the products were manufactured in Africa; 5 products were manufactured in Europe; 1 product was manufactured in USA; 2 from India, 1 from the Philippines and 1 from Indonesia.

All the samples, except one, contained hydroquinone. The concentration of HQ ranged from 0.010%-2.350%. The researchers recommended that there was a need for more stringent control by the regulatory bodies, appointed by the government, to check the quality of cosmetics in the market.

Ayenimo *et al*[7] in a study titled "Heavy metal exposure from personal care products" in Ile-Ife, analyzed 74 samples of 5 different classes of personal care products commonly used in Nigeria, using atomic absorption spectrophotometry. Significant levels of Cd, Cr, Cu and Zn were found in all the products. The highest values of Cd (0.553 ppm) and Cu (0.783 ppm) were observed in hair cream, while medicated cream was mostly implicated for Cr (0.383 ppm) and Zn (0.793 ppm). According to the researchers, since no limit relating to cosmetic products is available, it is difficult to ascertain if the values of metals obtained in this study are too high or low; but Cd and Cr are prohibited in any amount in cosmetics. Prolonged use of soaps and creams containing these elements may pose threat to human health and the environment.

Faruruwa and Bartholomew[8] studied heavy metals content in facial cosmetics. The cosmetics were purchased from superstores and open markets across Kaduna metropolis, Nigeria, and were analyzed to determine and compare their heavy metals composition using flame Atomic Absorption Spectroscopy (AAS). Chromium, nickel, zinc and iron were found in varying concentrations in all samples, 85% of the samples also contain Cd while 18 of the 40 samples have Pb above detection limit (0.20-31.70 mg kg-^{1}). The levels of Pb and Cd in superstores and open markets were lower in comparision to other metals under consideration, while the concentration of Fe was generally high (72.90-75.60 mg kg-^{1}) with one of the powders having the highest value of 75.60 mg kg-^{1}. The lowest value 72.90 mg kg-^{1} was found in face cleanser. Most facial cosmetics of the open market showed higher metals content in comparision to those obtained from superstore; foundation samples showed exception to the trend. The cosmetics analyzed were observed to contain heavy metals that are toxic to human health and continuous use of these cosmetics could result in increase of the metals level in human body beyond acceptable limits. The result also showed that the expensive facial cosmetics are not necessarily "safe" in terms of the metals content.

Orisakwe and Otaraku[9] in Port Harcourt analyzed metal concentrations in cosmetics commonly used in Nigeria. The levels of lead, cadmium, nickel, chromium, and mercury were assessed in 28 body creams and lotions, 10 powders, 3 soaps, 5 eye make-ups, and 4 lipsticks widely available on Nigerian markets. The increases over suggested or mandated levels of lead in these creams and lotions ranged from 6.1 to 45.9 and from 1.2 to 9.2 mg kg"^{1} when compared with Cosmetic Ingredients Review Expert Panel 2007 and German safe maximum permissible limit of lead in cosmetics, respectively. About 61% of the body cosmetics, the lotions, and the creams contained detectable levels of nickel ranging from 1.1 to 6.4–9.2 mg kg"^{1}. Chromium and mercury were undetected in 100% of the cosmetic products. Taken together, lead and cadmium were high in creams and lotions. Most of the imported creams and creamy white coloured cosmetics contained higher levels of metal contaminants than the other colours. The researcher concluded that Regulatory Agencies in developing nations should take appropriate action for cosmetics that contain lead and cadmium beyond the reference limits.

Several facial cosmetics available in Nigeria were analyzed for their contents of the heavy metals: lead, cadmium, chromium, nickel, zinc and Iron by Nnorom *at el.*[10] The levels of chromium, Iron and zinc were much higher in the samples than those of the non-essential toxic metals: lead, cadmium and nickel. The range of the geometric average for the various cosmetics is: Fe, 97-256 μg/; Ni, 8-13 μg/g; Pb, 87-123 μg/g; and Zn, 88-101 μg/g. The geometric mean values obtained for Cr and Cd were generally below 40 μg/g and about 1 μg/g, respectively. According to the researchers, the result indicates that these cosmetics are relatively safer to use when compare to the lead-based kwali eye make-up commonly available in Nigeria. These data indicate that the continuous use of these cosmetics could result in an increase in the trace metal levels in the ocular system and the human body beyond acceptable limits. The application of these cosmetics needs to be considered as a source of lead in evaluating patients with symptoms of lead intoxication in regions where this practice is common

Iyanda *et al*[11] conducted a study to determine the concentrations of trace elements in serum samples of women who are chronic users of skin-whitening agents, as well as the hepatic and renal effects of these agents on these women. The study was conducted among 23 skin-whitening users, while 25 women served as the controls. The serum concentrations of Zn, Mn, and Mg were not significantly changed in these women compared with controls ($p > 0.05$), but Cu was significantly increased in skin-whitening agent users compared with controls ($p < 0.05$). Serum urea and creatinine were significantly increased compared with the controls ($p<0.05$). Moreover, Alanine transaminase (ALT), Aspartate transaminase (AST), albumin, total protein, and bilirubin were not significantly changed ($p > 0.05$). The significant increase in the levels of renal indices shows that these agents might be nephrotoxic after prolonged usage while increase in copper level with accompanying renal dysfunction may be an indication that copper mediates in oxidative-induced renal dysfunction.

Akortha *et al*[12] tested some common skin lightening creams available in Nigeria. Their investigations showed that they caused mutations in bacteria and were possibly carcinogenic

References

1. Josefson A, Farm G, Stymne B, Meding B. Nickel allergy and hand eczema a 20-year follow up. *Contact Dermatitis.* 2006; 55:286–290.

2. Hall AH. Chronic arsenic poisoning. *Toxicol Lett* 2002; 128(1– 3):69–72

3. McCluggage D. Heavy metal poisoning. *NCS magazine*, published by the bird hospital, CO, USA. 1991 (www.cockaties.org/articles/diseases/metals.html)

4. Onwordi CT, Onebune OC, Dorcas WA, Ajani OI. Potentially Toxic Metals Exposure From Body Creams Sold in Lagos, Nigeria. *Researcher* 2011; 3(1):30-37. http://www.sciencepub.net/reseracher

5. Oyedeji FO, Hassan GO, and Adeleke BB. Hydroquinone and Heavy Metals Levels in Cosmetics Marketed in Nigeria. *Trends in Applied Sciences Research.* 2011; 6: 622-639.

6. Ekpunobi UE, Okonkwo EO, Udeh CV, Ogbuagu AS, and Duru CB. Determination of hydroquinone and mercury concentrations in some skin lightening lotions and creams sold in Southeastern Nigeria. *International Journal of Biotechnology Research.* March 2014; 2 (1):011-016.
7. Ayenimo JG, Yusuf AM, Adekunle AS, Makinde OW. Heavy metal Exposure from Personal care Products. *Bull Environ Contam Toxicol.* 2010; 84:8-14.
8. Muhammed D Faruwa, Stephen P Bartholomew. Study of Heavy Metals Contents in Facial Cosmetics Obtained from Open markets and Superstores within Kaduna Metropolis, Nigeria. *American Journal of Chemistry and Application.* 2014; 1(2) :27-33.
9. Orisakwe Orish Ebere and Otaraku Jonathan Oye. Metal concentrations in cosmetics commonly used inNigeria. *The Scientific World Journal.* 2013; Article ID 959637, 7 page http://dx.doi.org/10.1155/2013/959637.
10. Nnorom IC, Igwe JC, Oji-Nnorom CG. Trace metal contents of facial (make-up) cosmetics commonly used in Nigeria. *Afr. J Biotechnol.* 2005; 4(10):1133-38.
11.Iyanda AA, Anetor J, Adeniyi Francis AA. Altered copper level and renal dys function in Nigeria women using skin-whitening agents. Biological trace element research Dec 2011; 143 (3):1264-70. http://www.researchgate.net/profile/John_Anetor2
12.Akortha EE, Niemogha MT, Edobor O. Mutagenic and genotoxic screening of eight commonly used skin whitening creams in Nigeria. *Bayero Journal of Pure and Applied Sciences.* 1 June 2012; 5 (1): 5-10.

Home made concoctions for skin blaching

In Nigeria, a backyard industry for manufacturing skin lightening products has emerged. Various additives are used to "enhance" the bleaching effect of over-the-counter products and possibly, make them affordable. Some of the additives for the concoctions are African black soap, lemon or lime juice, sulfur powder, potash, potassium alum, tooth paste, liquid milk, pulverized naphthalene (camphor balls)—a moth proofing agents, Vitamin C tablets, hair relaxers, detergents, shampoo, laundry bleach, battery_acid, mercury containing antiseptic soaps, Cam wood, papaya, honey, ‾indeed the list is endless. All these are made into a paste, in varied and assorted combinations, applied on the skin and left overnight, before being washed off the following morning to prepare for the day's work. Furthermore, it is customary to mix several creams containing steroids, mercury and hydroquinone for use. Indeed some salons now apply corticosteroids creams on the scalp to grow the hair!

Cam Wood—Osun, in Yoruba, Majigi in Hausa, Uhie in Igbo is a reddish/orange paste obtained from *Baphia nitida* plant. Cam Wood is also know as African Sandalwood.[2-4]

The African black soap is made from plantain skin which is dried and then roasted in the clay oven along with cocoa pods (shell of the cocoa fruit). The longer the skin is cooked, the darker it becomes. Essential oils such as Shea Butter and Palm kernel are added to the roasted skin to from soap[4]

References

1. Olumide YM. Akinkugbe AO et al. Complications of chronic use of skin lightening cosmetics. *International Journal of Dermatology*. 2008; 47:344-53.
2. Mrskincare. Positive effect of Cam Wood (osun) on the skin *Nairaland Forum*. Feb 28, 2013. http://www.nairaland.com/1210657/positive-efffect-cam-wood-osun.
3. Brighten Your Skin With Camwood. *The Neni* http://www.theneni.com/2013/04/brighten-your-skin-with-camwood.html Wednesday, 17 April 2013.
4. naturalbeauty. Making a bathing soap with black soap powder & Camwood/Red Sandalwood powder (osun). http://emergingnaturalbeauty.com/making-a-bathing-soap-with-black-soap-powder-camwoodred-sandalwood-powder-osun-2

Method of application of the cosmetic product "Body Works" / "Exfoliation"

It is critical to study not only the chemicals used but also the method of application – the procedures – because this is also relevant to toxicity of the chemicals.

Exfoliants / Exfoliation as used for *facials* alone

Exfoliants are products that help slough off dry, dead skin cells to improve the skin's appearance. This is achieved either by using acids or other chemicals to loosen old skin cells, or abrasive substances to physically scrub them off. Exfoliation can even out patches of rough skin, improve circulation to the skin, clear blocked pores to discourage acne and improve the appearance and healing of scars. Exfoliants should be applied to wet, cleansed skin, avoiding the eye area; abrasive exfoliants or scrubs should then be rubbed into the skin in a circular motion for at least 30 seconds. Dry skin should only be exfoliated in spots with severe flaking, and no more than once per week; oily skins may be able to tolerate twice weekly exfoliation. Signs of over-exfoliation include sore, dry and irritated or reddened skin and excessive dryness or oiliness.

Chemical exfoliants may include citric acid (from citrus fruits), acetic acid (from vinegar), malic acid (from various fruits), glycolic acid, lactic acid or salicylic acid. They may be liquids or gels, and may or may not contain an abrasive to remove old skin cells afterwards. Abrasive exfoliants include gels, creams or lotions, as well as physical object. Loofahs, microfiber cloths, natural sponges or brushes may be used to exfoliate skin, simply by rubbing them over the face in a circular motion. Gels, creams or lotions may contain an acid to encourage dead skin cells to loosen, and an abrasive such as beads, sea salt, sugar, groundnut shells, rice bran or ground apricot kernels to scrub the dead cells off the skin. Salt and sugar scrubs tend to be the harshest, while scrubs containing beads or rice bran are typically very gentle.

"Body Works" / Exfoliation used for total body surface as used for bleaching products

The expression "Body works" is used for exfoliation by practitioners of the Skin Lightening Products in Spas in Nigeria.
Different chemicals and different procedures are used depending on the client's pocket.

For the wealthy[1,2]

The 'body works' which is also called 'exfoliation' is the initiation procedure. This is always done in 'Spas' which is well equipped with all the armamentarium for efficient and accelerated transformation of the skin. The total body is first steamed for some 30-45 minutes "to loosing out the scales of the skin, open up the pores and make the skin soft and supple like that of a baby"; The whole body is then massaged and scrubbed with brush or some specifically designed abrasive instrument and bleaching soap to totally remove the scales-"dead cells" – exfoliation. The chemicals used during the process of exfoliation are salicylic acid, hydroquinone, tretinoin and some "penetration enhancers" is then liberally applied all over the body including the private genital area for uniform and even effect. Hydroquinone is sometimes combined with hudroxyacids that exfoliate the skin to quicken the skin lightening process. Different chemicals are used depending on **how fast** the client wants the transformation process and how white she wants the end result – lighter shade of brown, "half cast" whiteness, or milky white skin like that of a Caucasian. The client is then given a tube or several tubes of the customized cream for maintenance of the bleaching process at home until the client returns for another sessions of "body works" after about four weeks or up to 3 months depending on the client's desire.

The cost of the above procedures in the Spas varies, depending on the geographical location of the Spas. In high brow areas of Lagos like Ikoyi, Victoria Island and Lekki – the consultation fee varies from about 50,000 naira or more; the cost of 'body works' also varies and may cost some hundred thousand naira or more; while the cost of the cream is usually over a thousand naira – several thousand naira. The "consultation fee" is paid just to register for the procedures and see the 'specialist practitioner' who may simply ask for your skin type and explain the procedure – to 'simulate' some professionalism. A special appointment is then given for the day of the actual "body works". Hence, one session of exfoliation in a Spa may cost up to two hundred and fifty thousand naira or more.

It is worth noting that the above procedure in the Spas is a well guarded secrete by the practitioners. One may have to pose as a client and pay the consultation fee before one is allowed to gain access to the Spa cubicle and given any information about the procedure. The client also needs to pay in advance to order for the "custom made" bleaching cream. When I insisted that I needed to know the ingredients in the cream, I was given a cut-out from the empty package where the list of ingredients was written. One of them had this written: "GLOBAL BEAUTY Moisturizing Toner. Methanol, IPA, Tumeric powder, Collagen." When I asked for the meaning of 'IPA', the 'Specialist practitioner' replied' "I don't know, I'm not a doctor". The paper was immediately retrieved from me as I was not allowed to take away even the cut out paper!

It is also important to know the credentials – level of education – of the girls that carry out the body works – they are usually school dropouts. Setting up a Spa is capital intensive and the proprietor or 'Madam' is anyone male or female who is rich enough to set up the place as a business and a money making venture. The proprietor, who may never be seen by the clients, simply hires one or two young girls, who may be school drop outs (for cheap labor) and hurriedly trained in the administration of the 'body works' on clients.

Body works /Exfoliation for the poor

For the poor who cannot afford the cost of Spas, the body works may be self-administered at home with some concoction which may contain assorted mixtures like lemon juice, cement water, potash, tooth paste, liquid milk, pulverized naphthalene (camphor) balls – a mothproofing agent, Vitamin C, peroxides and chlorates used in hair dyes, detergent and bleaching soaps, glass window cleaner, car battery water. Indeed the list is endless and not standardized.[2]

In Ghana, Delle[3] has this to say about the method of body works used by the poor living in rural communities:

"What is more disturbing is the fact that people living in rural communities, struggling to exist below the poverty line, are also bleaching in earnest and are initiating dangerous techniques to participate in the trend. Unable to afford the sophisticated creams and soaps, they create their own home-made preparations, mixing everything from toothpaste, shampoo and milk to household bleach, cement and brake fluid. In short, anything that has a corrosive effect on the skin. Some women have even devised a new procedure involving the smearing of hair relaxer all over the body and wearing up to three layers of clothing, including socks, gloves and long-sleeved tops, to protect themselves from the sun's penetrating darkening rays."

In East Africa[4], ***mkorongo*** is a potent mix of Jik, (laundry bleach), talcum powder, hair relaxer, mashed raw potatoes (for the starch) and battery acid. This is mixed with over-the-counter products like Clear Tone or Ambi, which women them smear all over their naked bodies.

Rashida Lawal[5], a cosmetic shop owner in one of the markets in Lagos, has this to say:

"About 90 percent of my clients come asking for skin whitening products," she told Al Jazeera. "I sell it to them and give advice on what product is best for them and how to use them." She says most of her customers are in great haste to lighten their skin. "Taking the color of your skin to a different colour has to be gradual. It's not something you decide one day that "I want to be fair. I want to be like Michael Jackson and you become Michael Jackson all of a sudden." That is why we have to advise them first before selling it to them," said Rashida. Rashida and her staff also **mix** different ointments and creams for customers "depending on the desired level of lightness."

It has also been found that there are subterranean & unlicensed online schools where people study the art of **mixing** customized chemicals for clients on request. The ingredients in these customized products are unknown and are usually heavily guarded trade secrets by the manufacturers. Some of the factors that dictate the nature of the chemicals and the strength are (a) how quickly the client wants a response (e.g within days/months), and (b) the grade of skin-lightening required – light brown, "half cast" white like Dencia of the "Whitenicious" fame. (See the chapter on "Where are the products manufactured /purchased")

Adverse effects of the 'Body works/Exfoliation' Chemicals used

Salicylic Acid is well-documented to have keratolytic action on normal human skin. Because of the possible use of this ingredient as an exfoliating agent, a concern exists that repeated use may effectively increase exposure of the dermis and epidermis to UV radiation. It was concluded that the prudent course of action would be to advise the cosmetics industry that there is a risk of increased UV radiation damage with the use of any exfoliant, including salicylic Acid and the listed salicylates, and that steps need to be taken to formulate cosmetic products with these ingredients as exfoliating agents so as not to increase sun sensitivity, or when increased sun sensitivity would be expected, to include directions for the daily use of sun protection.[6,7,8].

Salicylic acid when absorbed into_the system is nephrotoxic and fetotoxic. Tretinoin are genotoxic¯teratogenic. Salicylic acid when absorbed into the system also causes acute Salicylism. The symptoms and signs of salicylism are nausea and vomiting, occasionally with gastritis. Moderate intoxication is characterized by hyperpnea (deep and rapid breathing), tachycardia, tinnitus, and elevated anion gap metabolic acidosis. Serious intoxication may result in agitation, confusion, coma, seizures, cardiovascular collapse, pulmonary edema, hyperthermia, and death. The prothrombin time is often elevated owing to salicylate-induced hypoprothrombinemia.

Use of penetration enhancers

The human skin barrier is an important part of the skin's intactness and its functionality is a precondition for healthy skin. Ingredients in cosmetic formulations, especially penetration enhancers, can influence this barrier function as they transport active agents into deeper skin layers. Penetration enhancers can increase skin hydration, increase percutaneous absorption of chemicals and amplification of toxic effects[7]. Furthermore, exfoliation in traditional cosmetology is meant to be used for facials alone not total body surface as is used on skin bleachers

Consequences of body works

Unequivocally, all the above factors involved in the "body works" / "Exfoliation" promote percutaneous absorption of the chemicals in skin lightening products for the following reasons:

1. Steaming causes (i) Hydration of the skin which promotes percutaneous absorption of Toxic chemicals.

(ii) Dilatation of all the cutaneous blood vessels
(iii) Extra load on the heart and hyperdynamic heart failure in the vulnerable

2. Exfoliation disrupts the skin's integrity as it removes the protective barrier function of the skin – the horny keratin tissue. Scrubbing a steamed skin may even traumatize the skin and inflict some abrasions for the chemicals to have direct access to the blood stream, and also penetration of infective organisms which may also cause infection of the skin and septicemia (infection of the blood).
3. Expose the client to the adverse effects of the chemicals discussed above and more importantly, the notable active ingredients in bleaching products—mercury, hydroquinone and corticosteroids.
4. Even without the 'body works,' the environmental heat and humidity prevalent in a tropical country like Nigeria, promote percutaneous absorption, a phenomenon enhanced by steaming in body works.
5. Total body surface immersion in the bleaching chemicals implies maximum percutaneous absorption and predisposition to toxic effects of the chemicals.
6. Total body surface, exfoliation leads to loss of iron and protein from the skin scales and may result in chronic iron deficiency anemia and hypoproteinemia.
7. As regards the complications of the methods and ingredients used by the poor and rural dwellers, the additional complications are unimaginable.

References

1. Olumide YM- Personal observation of procedure (Unpublished data)
2. Olumide YM. Akinkugbe AO et at. Complication of chronic Use of Skin Lightening Cosmetics. *International Journal of Dermatology* 2008; 47:344-53.
3. Dr Delle. Interview with Sylvia Arthur for TB WT. Ghana web, General News of Thursday, 7 March 2002 http://www.ghanaweb.com/GhanaHomePage/NewsArchive/artikel.php?ID=22240
4. Lewis Kelly et al, Investigating motivations for women's skin bleaching in Tanzania. *Psychology of Women Quarterly*. 2011; 35 (29): 29-37.
5. Rashida Lawal. Interview with AL Jazeerahttp://www.aljazeera.com/indepth/features/2013/04/201345148459
6. Cosmetics ingredient Review Expert Panel.Safety Assessment of Salicylic Acid, Butyloctyl Salicylate…*Int J Toxicol* 2003; 22 Suppl 3:1-108 http://www.ncbi.nih.gov/pubmed/14617432
7. CMDT current Medical Diagnosis & Treatment. Edited by Lawrence M. Tierney, Jn. Stephen J McPhee, Maxine A Papadakis. 2005 LANGE. McGraw Hill

8. Heinrich K, Heinrich U, Tronnier H. Influence of different cosmetic formulations on the human skin barrier. *Skin Pharmacol Physiol* 2014; 27 (3): 141-7http://www.ncbi.nlm.nih.gov/pubmed/24434680

Duration of use of the skin lightening products

In a study done by Adebajo[1] among traders in Lagos, Nigeria, the duration of use of the skin lightening products is shown in the Table 4:18.

Table 4.18 Duration of use

Duration of use	Female	Male
<6 months	(5.2%)	(9.5%)
6-12 months	(22.9%)	(24.6%)
1-3 years	(39.6%)	(48.8%)
3-5 years	(8.3%)	(8.7%)
>5 years	(24.0%)	(8.3%)

A 35 year old lady who was interviewed by Al Jazeera[2] said she was 12 years old when she started using the skin bleaching product, which meant that she had used it for 23 years. 3% of patients in Ajose's[3] study had used the products for over 10 years and some of them claimed they could not stop the products because each time they wanted to stop the skin complications got worse. Nnoruka's[4] patients had used the products from 3 months to 30years. Some people bleach their skin for special events, e.g the wedding day; others as a lifestyle hence everyday practice. The fact is that once introduced into the practice, skin bleachers have to continue to use the products because the skin repigments when they stop using the products or the skin lesion gets worse (a rebound phenomenon). A woman said she bleached because she wanted to look beautiful when she is laid in-state at her death before burial.[5] This implies that some skin bleachers continue to bleach till death. Hence the duration of bleaching depends on the ***age*** at which the bleacher starts bleaching and when she eventually dies. Therefore, the duration of bleaching is for several decades a lifestyle. Sometimes the bleacher changes to another product when she develops an adverse reaction to a particular product. Rarely they are forced to stop when criticized by relations/friends or deserted by the spouse.[3] It has also been observed that the frequency of the adverse complications of skin bleaching is often related to the duration of use of the products.

References

1. Adebajo BS. An epidemiolocal survey of the use of cosmetic skin lightening cosmetics among traders in Lagos, Nigeria. *West African Journal of Medicine* 2002; 21:51-5.
2. Interview by Aljazeera http://www.aljazeera.com/idepth/features/2013/04/201345148459
3. Ajose Frances OA. Consequences of skin bleaching in Nigerian men and women. *International Journal of Dermatology*. 2005; 44 (suppl.1), 41-3.
4. Nnoruka Edith, Okoye Obiefuna. Topical steroid abuse: Its use as a depigmenting agent. *Journal of the National Medical Association* June 2006; 98 (6): 934-9.
5. Penangnini Toure. Skin bleaching on rise in Africa REUTERS NEWS AGENCY the Toronto star March 10; 1997.

Further notes on the prevalence and demographic characteristics of skin bleachers in Nigeria

Skin bleaching in Nigeria cuts across all demographic characteristics. People from all ethnic groups in Nigeria bleach. All age groups, single / married / widowed, all educational levels—from the analphabetic to university professors, teenage secondary school students, students of tertiary institutions; all professions and occupational groups—including janitors, teachers, police officers, market traders, engineers, lawyers, doctors and nurses, high court judges, politicians and wives of politicians, movie actresses, models, television news casters and presenters, even men and women of God—pastors, Christians, Muslims and traditional religionists, some domestic staff (e.g cooks and stewards) , some 'high profile' street beggars, and those who work in the sex trade. Some men also bleach including some traditional rulers, state governors etc. (See the section on MEN ALSO BLEACH).

The World Health Organization has adjudged Nigeria as the country with the highest number of women who use skin-lightening products in the world! In Nigeria, a growing number of men and women are using skin whitening creams because they believe a fairer complexion will help them succeed in life. According to reports,[1-4] the market for bleaching products to produce a lighter skin color among Nigeria women is booming. But the beauty trend involving harsh chemicals comes with health consequences.

According to a report from World Health Organization (WHO) released in 2012 women in Nigeria topped the list of countries using lightening products with 77 percent of the female population applying them regularly. The Economist reported in September 2012 that in the country's capital of Abuja a store's cosmetics section had two aisles devoted to skin-bleaching products exclusively and that they are expected to be a $10 billion industry worldwide by 2015. It's so popular in Nigeria, the Economist reported, that there's even local lingo for people who only use products on their face, while the rest of their body stays darker. They're called "Fanta face, coca cola legs." Al Jazeera's report stated that the very nature of calling it bleaching has been rebranded as "toning" now as well.

In a recent skin bleaching snap survey conducted by N0I Polls[5] from February 3-5, and published on March 18, 2014 in Abuja, the polling agency said the assessment result confirms the submission of WHO on the endemic nature of skin bleaching among Nigerian women as 83 percent of respondents affirmed the high prevalence of skin bleaching in Nigeria.

Various researchers in Nigeria revealed ***consistently*** high prevalence of skin bleaching practices. Adebajo[6] studied the prevalence among market traders in Lagos metropolis. She gave an overall prevalence rate of 77.3%; 72.4% among women and 27.6% among the men. Ofondu[7] studied the prevalence rate among university students in Enugu. She found an overall prevalence rate of 62.4%; 71.9% among the women and 53.3% among the men. Ajose[8] studied the prevalence rate in a skin clinic at the Lagos State University Teaching Hospital. 92% of the women and 5% of the men claimed to have used the skin bleaching products in the past, but at the time of study 40% of the women and 2% of the men were bleaching the skin. The figures dropped as a result of adverse effects, desertion by spouse, or inability to continue funding the cost of the products. Ofili et al[9] studied the prevalence of skin bleaching among University students in Benin. The overall prevalence rate was 64.9%; 70.7% prevalence among women and 52.2% among men.

In the study of the prevalence of the use of skin lightening agents amongst university of Benin Undergraduates in Benin City[9] Nigeria, it is interesting to note that almost everyone denied **"bleaching"** (95.3%), yet 16.3% agreed that they **"tone".** Only 4.7% correctly said that toning is the same as bleaching. The investigators asked the respondents to **show** the cosmetics being used. There was a great disparity between the presence of bleaching agents in their cosmetics and the denial that they did not bleach (95.3%). This means that if prevalence was collated simply by asking the respondents to answer "yes" or "no", only 4.7% will be bleachers, whereas the actual percentage of **forensically proven** bleachers was 64.9%. Furthermore, if the word "toning" was used, the actual (true) figure of bleachers would be nearer the figure of forensically proven bleachers. The lesson to be learnt from this study is that statistics on prevalence of bleaching should not be collated simply by asking questions which require negative/positive answers. There is need to **sight** the actual cosmetics used by respondents. Further, sighting the cosmetics may not solve all the problem because most of the cosmetics carry no ingredient labeling or are deceptively labeled in content (misbranded).[7] The brand name of the product is no guarantee either because of the rate at which the brand names and packaging are copied by backyard industries. For example, the constituents of "Clear Essence" in the USA may not necessarily be the same as "Clear Essence" in Nigeria.

I believe the above figures may even be an understatement because, from personal experience in the clinic, patients who present with the skin complications of bleaching creams often deny that they are deliberately bleaching due to a guilt complex, because the bleaching habit has been variously denounced, particularly among religious organizations, along immoral connotation. The following scenario is often the pattern in the skin clinic of the Lagos University Teaching Hospital.

Doctor: "Why do you bleach your skin?"

Patient: "I am not bleaching. I use just a normal body cream"

Doctor: "Bring the cream next visit, I just want to see if it is good for you"

At the next visit, on sighting the cream

Doctor: "But see what is clearly written on the cream – "fade cream", "Complexion cream". What else can it mean?"

Patient: "I don't know it bleaches."

Doctor: "Even if you don't know the meaning of "fade" or "complexion" cream, you can see for yourself what it is doing to your skin, that you are getting lighter"

Patient: (now wearing a guilty smile)

"I don't bleach, I just tone";

"I am normally light skin, I just want to be sure I don't get darker in the sun! I am sure the cream I am using is not the cause of my problem, because I have been using it for several years without any adverse effect!"

The denials of bleaching may either be due to ignorance of the functions of the chemicals in the cosmetics or a guilt complex generated by the opprobrium visited on bleachers. The latter is more likely to be the reason. The study by Ofondu[7] revealed that many women particularly those living in the rural areas, were not even aware that the cosmetic body creams they were using contain bleaching agents. The danger from denial of skin lightening products is that many of the symptoms and signs of the complications of skin lightening chemicals are **not** specific to the skin lightening chemicals. The unpleasant sequelae of denial often leads to failure in making prompt diagnosis of the adverse health consequences, and delays in appropriating effective medical interventions and management. For example, I know a chronic skin bleacher suffering from intractable and incapacitating vertigo who has not been helped by the ear specialist nor the neurologist. She found it difficult to believe that the skin bleaching product containing mercury/hydroquinone could be the cause of her vertigo.

Furthermore, there are various levels of skin tones 1-7. Most people do not wish to get to the extreme level 7 as Dencia of Whitenicious fame; they are content to achieve the mid-levels of 3-5 so as not to make it too glaring that they are bleachers. Therefore, a simple questionnaire designed for Yes/No answers in a field survey is likely to give lower figures from the **true** state of affairs. In clinical practice, we do prescribe benzoyl peroxide for acne; and one of the side effects of benzoyl peroxide is mild bleaching of the skin. Some patients who **genuinely** do not want to bleach find the bleaching effect objectionable and they quickly return for a change in prescription once they observe this undesirable side effect of benzoyl peroxide. Doctors in the skin clinic are so familiar with the characteristic features or stigmatas of an artificially bleached or partially bleached skin, at whatever level, hence we know the liars even if they deny the truth. Nigerians and many Africans in Diaspora also bleach. See the chapters on (i) THE CHEMICALS (ii) COMPLICATIONS OF CHRONIC USE OF SKIN LIGHTENING COSMETICS, (iii) UNITED KINGDOM, (iv) USA —Chapters 13,14,15.

References

1. Nigeria's Booming Skin Bleaching Market.*Hope for Nigeria.* Nigeria's No.1 Community Platform. April 6, 2013.http://www.hopefornigeriaonline.com/nigerias-booming-skin-leaching...
2. Nigerians, Top Users of Bleaching Cream‾ WHO-Health. (3) – Nairaland. Thursday, 05 February 2015. http://www.nairaland.com/970754/nigerians-top-users-bleaching-cr..
3. Mohammed Adow. Nigeria's dangerous skin whitening obsession.http://www.aljazeera.com/indepth/features/2013/04/201345148459..
4. Uduma Kalu. Nigerian women lead in skin bleaching WHO. *Vanguard.* June 03, 2013. http://www.vanguardngr.com/2013/06/nigerian-women-lead-in-skin-.
5. NOI Polls. Jide Ojo. Nigeria as the world capital of skin bleaching March 26, 2014 http://www.punchng.com/opinion/nigeria-as-the-world-capita-of-skin.

6. Adebajo SB. An epidemiological survey of the use of cosmetic skin lightening cosmetic among traders in Lagos. *West Afri J Med.* 2002; Jan-March 21(1):51-5
7. Ofondu Eugenia Ogugua. Cosmetic use of bleaching creams in Enugu. *National Postgraduate Medical College of Nigeria Dissertation* 2003.
Study at the Enugu State University of Science and Technology (ESUT) between February and October 2001.
8. Ajose FOA. Consequences of skin bleaching in Nigerian men and women. *International Journal Dermatol.* 2005; 44 (Suppl 1) : 41-3.
9. Ofili AN, Eze EU, Onunu AN. Prevalence of use of skin lightening agents amongst University of Benin undergraduates in Benin City, Nigeria. *Nigeria Medical Practitioner* 2006; 49(1/2):24-7

The motives for skin lightening among women in Nigeria. Why Do Nigerian women bleach their skin?

Several studies have been done to decipher the motives/reasons for skin lightening by women in Africa. Some of the results in tabular forms are listed in Tables 4.19-21.

Table 4.19 Reasons for the use of skin lightening cosmetics[1]

Reasons	Frequency Male	Female
Makes one more attractive	(19.8%)	(34.1%)
A fashionable trend	(17.7%)	(11.9%)
To treat skin blemishes	(34.4%)	(30.2%)
To cleanse/skin tone of the face and body	(22.9%)	(20.2%)
To satisfy the desires of the opposite sex	(5.2%)	(3.6%)

Table 4.20 Reasons for skin bleaching[2]

Reasons for using the product/s	Total	Female	Male
For smoother skin	60 (20.13%)	29	31
For lighter skin	53 (17.78%)	30	23
Fashionable/treat blemishes	27 (9.03%)	16	11
Other reasons	118 (39.60%)	44	74

Table 4.21 Reasons why people bleach by respondents[3]

Reasons why People bleach	Percentage of respondents
To be attractive	77.9

As a result of complex	19.2
Do not know	1.3
Medical reasons	0.8
No response	0.8
Total	**100.0**

The desire to look beautiful and attract the attention of the opposite gender

Light skin tone can be transformed into social capital (social networks), symbolic capital (esteem or status) or even economic capital (high-paying job or promotion). Various motives have been given during interviews for lightening the skin; these are: (1) to look more beautiful and attractive, (2) to improve self esteem, (3) to look younger, (3) to appear important, (4) to belong to a higher social class, (4) to be fashionable, (5) to improve better job opportunity, (6) to increase chances of getting married because men consider light complexioned women more beautiful and (7) due to advertisements that promote white ideal (8) to treat some skin diseases.

Unquestionably, the primary motive why women lighten their skin in Nigeria is to attract the opposite gender. In a recent skin bleaching snap survey conducted by NOI Polls[4] in Nigeria from February 3-5, and published on March 18, 2014 in Abuja, the poll revealed that despite the negative effects of skin bleaching affirmed by 83% percent of respondents; the top reasons why people still engage in the practice of skin bleaching are the need to "look beautiful" (35 percent) and to "look attractive to the opposite sex" (32 percent). Nearly 8 out of 10 Nigerian women bleach their skin and the business is booming. Zainab from Kuddy Cosmetics said: "Lightening creams is the biggest for cosmetics because we could bring in like Jergens or normal body lotions but they always ask. 'Does it lighten?' So if it doesn't they don't want to buy it." Amaka, who has been bleaching her skin for years despite the cost, said she is pleased to be several shades lighter. "Its quite expensive but I just have to do it because I am concerned about my face, because I have spots on my face. I can't go on a natural look,"[5] she said.

Skin-lightening beauty parlors have also sprung up across the city. Dr Felix Ajara of Dr Therapy Beauty and Spa said: "Being Lighter is more attractive. I know a lot of women that come to us, they just want their skin smooth". He said his clients did not feel inferior but "they want to tell people out there that I could look more better. My colour can come out good but generally, every woman believes that when your skin is beautiful people admire you."[5]

Another woman said: "It is clearly a societal issue in Nigeria. If a woman is very rich and dark skinned, whatever she does, she doesn't get noticed, so I feel they just want to get polished so their wealth would show on them. I think it's because a lot of men want fair ladies and the darker ones actually have an inferiority complex."[5]

A 32 yr old lady, said she has been bleaching as a daily routine for the past 15 years. Now several shades lighter she says her new skin makes her feel more beautiful and confident. "Bleaching just makes me feel special, like I'm walking around in a spotlight", she told **Al Jazeera**[6]. "I am not seeking to be totally white. I just want to look beautiful. I cannot stop using the lightening agents" she adds. She believes fair skin could be her ticket to a better life.

Another cosmetic shop owner and "beauty therapist" on a radio talk programme, said most of her clients are in a hurry. "Some of them will come in today and say: "I have a very important party next week and I want to urgently whiten my skin before the day of the party". When the beauty therapist asked the reason for the undue haste in having a light complexion, the client said "because each time I attend parties with my light-complexioned friends, they get noticed **instantly** by the men and get all the attention, which I don't enjoy". The young lady added, "it is not that I believe that those light–complexioned friends of mine are more beautiful, but I want to get married. How do I get a husband if I am not attractive to men simply because of the dark colour of my skin?"

Compared with non-users, people who use skin lightening products are more likely to believe that lighter skin tone has a positive role to play in self-esteem, perception of beauty and youth, find marriage, and employment opportunity compared with non-users. The Nigerian-American rapper Kingsley "Rukus" Okafor[7] says "they bleach possibly to gain "more respect, increased desirability . . . finding a well-to-do husband/sugar daddy is a priority and women are willing to do what they have to fit standards of beauty".

A status symbol and sign of sophistication

Some view the regular simple body creams and toiletries as cheap and not befitting their status. They then patronize the more expensive skin-lightening creams to boost their ego as "modern", "civilized," "sophisticated" and "fashionable".[8] Many of the skin bleachers truly or falsely claim they were normally light-skinned but only use the skin lightening products to "tone" their skin and prevent the skin darkening effect of chronic exposure to sunlight.

Bleaching before important events

Some people bleach their skin before important events. The most notable event for skin bleaching is before the wedding day. Indeed, there is a skin bleaching product called *"before the wedding."* In Nigeria, a well known TV presenter bleached her skin to vampire white when she was to be a member of the team of journalists to interview the then President of Nigeria on National issues. A known male TV presenter bleached his skin just before the last general election in Nigeria because he was the main anchor person for the election discourse and commentaries in one of the popular TV channels in Nigeria. After all the media storm on the election, it has been observed that his skin has gradually changed to ash-brown. Some people bleach their skin before they attend a job interview.

Bleaching for "cleansing"

Some others view the removal of the brown pigment as a form of "cleansing" the skin. I recall several years ago while on vacation in Togo, a young teenage girl who was hawking the products in the market place, confidently walked up to me, offered me her tray of bleaching products and with a commanding voice said "nettoiyer!" which means "clean-up" in French. Some market women in Nigeria actually encourage themselves to "clean up" and ask a woman who has not bleached why she has not "washed" herself. Some of the women actually perceive the cushionoid steroid-induced bloatedness as a sign of affluence and one can hear them encouraging each other in the Yoruba language "maa..wu" which means "swell on"!.

A lady so obsessed with skin lightening would not only bleach herself with the most toxic of agents but persuaded her husband to bleach and also "treated" her baby's skin! Some mixed race people bleach to appear more white and worse still, they only marry people who are the lighter shade of mixed race because "No one wants a dark skinned baby… they aren't cute!" said one of them.

Private parts bleaching

Prostitution is another significant factor which could be responsible for skin bleaching practice. The concept of the body, especially the female body, as a commodity may also be traced to prostitution. In the past, the tendency to bleach was known primarily as the preserve of prostitutes and women who worked in the local sex trade.

Private parts bleaching involves the bleaching of the sexually sensitive parts of the body in order to become lighter. The private parts, which may be involved, include the breasts, penis, the vagina, the buttocks and the thighs. The purpose of private parts bleaching could be for sexual attraction of the opposite gender, which is popular among commercial sex workers. Indeed, in the skin clinic, commercial sex workers constitute a notable group of people who bleach their skin. They brand themselves as "fashion designers" to hide the identity of their sex trade. It has also been observed that some female students in secondary and tertiary institutions sell sex to be able to fund the cost of the skin-bleaching products. Once initiated into the practice of skin bleaching, they have to sustain it so that the skin does not revert back to its original dark color. Moreover, they need the light skin tone to attract clients in the sex trade. This factor was dominant during the rage of HIV/AIDS because many of our HIV/AIDS positive young girls seen in our clinic were bleaching their skin.

Why older married women bleach

A 57-year-old woman, Madam Sibe, as she's fondly called, is known for her heavy make-ups and exotic dresses, but one thing baffles her neighbours and on-lookers ‾ she still bleaches at her age. When asked "What would make an older woman bleach?" She responded thus: *"That which makes a younger lady bleach."* Continuing, she said, *"Anyway, I've to look good and to spice it up, I have to top up my cream."*[9]

There are women in their fifties, sixties and seventies – mothers and grandmothers who still use the skin lightening agents. There are several reasons for this:

(i) Some of them have been bleaching before marriage when their husbands met them. They have to **continue** to bleach so that their husbands, family, friends, and the general public and colleagues at work may never know the secret of their light skin. If they discontinue bleaching, the skin progressively becomes darker. Indeed the secret is usually revealed to the gossiping public when such a person celebrates landmark birthdays and prints a commemorative photo-gallery reflecting what she looked like from childhood, teens etc up to their present age. Then it becomes clear that the dark skinned school girl has metamorphosed into a "half cast" in adulthood!

(ii) Bleached mothers usually encourage their daughters to use the same skin-lightening products with them. It is therefore a common sight to see, on the daughter's wedding day – bride and mother as

hardcore bleachers. So much has been preached to condemn and question the morality of skin bleaching along religious ethical values, that an unbleached daughter serves as a constant reminder and indictment on the moral authority of the mother. Inorder for the mother to rid herself of the burden of a guilty conscience, she ensures that her daughter looks like her, and even deceive her husband and the public that her light skin was genetic. Another reason for encouraging her daughter to bleach is to attract attention from men and enhance her daughter's marriage prospects.
(iii) With the very high prevalence of bleached seductresses on the prowl in work places, churches and recreational clubs, some married women find it **expedient** to bleach and remain "attractive and youthful" to prevent their husbands from being snatched by another woman!

It is not an exageration to say that the **dominant** stories acted out in the Nigerian movies are all about witchcraft and light skined actresses successfully seducing married men and snatching other peoples' husbands. When criticized for always acting out film messages that do not add morally nor spiritually edifying values in the minds of the people, the film producers have always defended themselves by saying the scripts acted out truly reflect the happenings in the society and that they are simply producing what feeds the African market. Regrettably, these acted-out messages are highly suggestive, and a married woman, with no strength of character, would succumb to bleaching her skin to appear attractive enough to prevent losing her husband to a light-complexioned seductress outside her home.

This threat to the stability of homes makes some married women continue to bleach to remain attractive to their husbands. I know of a man whose wife, a Nigerian socialite, is milky white bleached, always dresses in a most outrageously loud manner with blond Caucasian wig, long, voluminous artificial eye lashes accentuating her bulging eyeballs, heavy make-up, jet red lipstick, revealing dresses in shimmering bright colours, bedecked in heavy jewelry, and other accessories. This lady is such a moving bill board that whenever she appears at social events and even in church, everyone turns to look at her in utter amazement that someone's wife and mother could be so distastefully vulgar in taste. A family friend of theirs said when her husband was asked if he could not get his wife to tone down her appearance, her husband's reply was that he was always proud to see his wife the cynosure of all eyes in public! It is truly common place to hear or read about men of base values describing their wives, approvingly, as "yellow and fine"! I dare say, without any equivocation, if the Nigerian men suddenly develop an avertion for bleached skin, the prevalence of skin bleaching in women will crash for good.

Susan Maxwell, a heavily bleached Nigerian Nollywood actress, who makes her own brand of bleaching skin care business has this to say

"Black is beautiful, but I have no qualms with enhancing your complexion. 80% of Nigerian men want their women to be fair. They want a lady that draws attention to them. I've worked with many married women who complain of their men staring at fair women and they say to me, Susan, make me fair, I want to be attractive to my man!" Some women have said their sons want them to visit their schools because they want to show off their fair mother. Clients all over the world have asked for my products. Black is beautiful but there is nothing wrong with enhancing your complexion."[10]

Hence if you want to secure a boyfriend and you don't want the boyfriend snatched from you by other **bleached** girls; if you want to marry and you don't want to lose your husband to **bleached** seductresses always on the prowl, you have to bleach your skin!"

Even the Federal Government of Nigeria consciously or subconsciously, appointed a milky white biracial Nigerian lady to head the agency that promotes **tourism**! This lady, donned in the Nigerian colours of green and white, enjoys high visibility in the print and electronic media. The lady is not to blame in any way as she is simply doing the work for which she was appointed, but a visiting tourist to Nigeria would wonder the paradox of a white-skinned lady representing the identity of Nigeria, a 100% black community! Even Nigerian children of impressionable age may get the wrong signal that they need to be light-skinned for the country to be so proud of them as to appoint them as front-line representatives of Nigeria to tourists! Most hotels and public institutions usually appoint light complexioned ladies as receptionists to man the client / front office desks!

Even young teenage girls bleach to enhance their marriage prospects

A study was conducted to investigate the perception of female secondary school students on skin bleaching practice in Ibadan metropolis.[11] These were young girls between the ages of 11-14yrs (85.3%) and above 14yrs old (14.7%). The 3 top reasons for bleaching are related to finding and securing a marriage relationship. The major findings revealed that young girls engaged in skin bleaching as a method of receiving desired attention and relationship from the opposite sex and attract the desired marriage partners. The findings of the above study among school girls was therefore not surprising in a society where some mothers have indoctrinated their daughters to see marriage as the ultimate goal in life for the girl child!

Skin bleaching as a "Cry for help"!

The phenomenon of bleaching of the skin among women in Nigeria can also be seen as a "cry for help." One of the commonest skin ailment I see in my skin clinic is acne (pimples) – breakouts – in women in their 30s and 40s. Since this is not the age for physiological acne (the teens), I always want to find out the root cause of the breakouts in the women. This could be due to stress, hyperprolactinemia, polycystic ovarian syndrome and even adverse reaction to corticosteroid-based skin lightening products. The sources of stress could be at home or at work. Stressors arise in ones private life and home e.g from pain, sorrow, conflict, marriage problems, family discord, fractured relationships, bereavement, barrenness/childlessness, loneliness, rebellious children on drugs, ill health in the family, sexual abuse etc. Some stressors arise at work e.g. fear of failure, desperation to deliver projects on time and to budget, fatigue, loss of job, blowups of business partnership, business collapse, burden of financial debts, perennial trade disputes, poverty due to national or natural circumstances, robbery and cheating, worry over position or status etc.

A **notable** characteristic of several of these **professionally successful women** in their 30s and 40s with breakouts is that they have **bleached** the skin and whenever I ask searching questions to elucidate any source of stress they invariably **break down in tears** – the reason – they are not married at that age and have experienced some failed relationships. The pressure the society puts on them for being single is immense. Usually they are taunted with such comments by family, friends and foes with such unkind comments as "your biological clock is ticking" – which means you will soon reach menopause. Some mothers harass such unmarried daughters to produce grandchildren for them before they (the mothers) die and even advise an unmarried daughter, who is advancing in age, to seduce a married man so that she can get pregnant for him. Such bleached patients also develop social hypersensitivity as they suspect that they are not accorded the level of respect enjoyed by married women of their age. Even former female friends, when married, try to keep their unmarried friends at arms length so that they do not seduce their husbands. The churches also harass them with incessant, often spurious programmes for "singles" with the objective of match-making and giving them opportunities to meet single men to marry. These bleached unmarried women often confess to me that that they have low self-esteem and are suffering from depression which was serious enough to interfere with their ability to work, sleep, study, eat and enjoy life. Atimes they feel dehumanized and traumatized. **Worse still they are suffering in silence and not getting help for their depression** because of the stigma surrounding mental health or even being seen consulting a mental health professional.[12] Some have confessed to having suicidal ideation. It is noteworthy that some of these women are high profile professional women, yet because they are unmarried, they suffer from feelings of sadness, hopelessness, and nothingness, at times feelings of self-blame that in the past they had shunned possible suitors.

Furthermore, depressed people have negative thoughts and feelings of anger often playing themselves in their minds. They feel restless, irritable and often lash out at the people closest to them. This makes it even more difficult to develop or sustain heterosexual relationships. An irritable unmarried woman is often ridiculed by co-workers and colleagues as an angry woman who is irritable because of the frustration from being single and childless!

Whatever the reason chronic bleachers give for lightening their skin, in Nigeria, the overarching drive is the desire to be noticed and appreciated by men. The reality is that at that stage they have experienced some failed relationships, developed extreme social hypersensitivity, loss of self-esteem, and have become emotionally distraught. The desperation becomes acute once they reach the age of 40 and above as they dread the menopause when they can no longer bear children. They then become seductresses in their bid to get pregnant through a married man and have one or two children of their own.

It is critical to note that most young physicians and dermatologists will not discover this phenomenon of bleaching as a "cry for help" because it is a closely guarded secret in the minds of the victims. They break down in tears and open up to me to tell their whole story because of my age and mother figure. I therefore devote greater attention to counseling them than drug therapy. At the end of the counseling session they feel so relieved that one of them actually said "I came for medications for my facial breakout but you have succeeded in doing something else." The nature of the counseling given to them will be highlighted under the chapter on BIBLICAL PERSPECTIVES ON MARRIAGE; SELF WORTH AND SELF ESTEEM—Chapter 20.

Nigerian women are generally self-assured people. It is not usual to find a woman of great professional/career achievements admitting, even to friends or relations, that she still feels a void in her life because she is not married, until one finds such a woman later in life entering into a polygamous relationship with a man. Indeed a culture is gradually evolving where Nigerian women are secretly having their eggs (seeds from the ovaries) frozen by the gynaecologist for future child bearing, when they painfully find that they are advancing in age and yet no suitor is in sight. Such a woman **suffers emotionally in silence** dreading menopause or the birth of a mongol if she eventually bears a child of her own at a late age.

Nigerian couples have not yet fully embraced the culture of adopting children, although there are homes for motherless babies waiting for couples to come forward and adopt some of the children. The parents of the husband, in a childless marriage, also tend to discourage their son from adopting a child whom they regard as a "bastard"!

Perhaps one of the greatest tragedies to befall a woman in Nigeria is to be childless after even a few years of marriage. If a wife is found not pregnant by the first anniversary of the wedding, the societal pressure starts, particularly from the relations of the husband, and of course from the mother of the bride who is, understandably, concerned about the happiness of her daughter with her husband. If after several years the wife is still unable to conceive, the husband is pressurized to get another women to father his children. In Nigeria, there is a rich repetoir of bleached unmarried women desperate to boast of a relationship with a man of high social standing, and who would readily trap him with a pregnancy (even if he is not the biological father of the baby in her womb!).

Gynaecologists tell us that the rate of infertility among married couples in Nigeria is on the rise and currently is about 40%; and that the cause of infertility among married couples is about 50:50 between husband and wife. Judging by the frequency of prayers for "the fruit of the womb" in our churches in current times, the prevalence of infertility among couples in Nigeria is certainly a cause for concern. Regrettably, the pressure is more on the wife. People hardly apportion any blame on the man nor even suspect that the husband contributes to the childlessness in the husband/wife relationship. Urologists and Gynaecologists admit that the commonest cause of infertility among men is chronic epididymo-orchitis from sexually transmitted infections acquired through having multiple sexual partners. Also the commonest cause of infertility in the woman is chronic pelvic inflammatory disease which may have existed before marriage or which she may have acquired **after** marriage from the promiscuous husband!

There is no doubt that unfaithfulness of a husband weakens the relationship between a husband and his wife. It is worthy of note that in several instances, the "other woman" (mistress) is not hidden from the legal wife of the man. The wish of the mistress is to send the legal wife out of her matrimonial home. Hence if this fails to happen and the legal wife decides to remain in her home inspite of the adulterous life-style of her husband, the other woman may decide to taunt the legal wife by ridiculing her on the phone or even face to face with the comment "you keep the wedding ring while I keep the man"!

Even after the husband has bolted out into a full-blown relationship with another woman or other women, **the only weapon left in the wife's arsenal to retain a semblance of marriage may be a tube/jar of bleaching cream which costs just a few dollars!**

Why the desperation to marry and *remain* married?

To a Nigeria woman, a husband is expected to confer on the wife all forms of capitals—*social* capital (social network), *symbolic* capital (esteem or status) and even *economic* capital (provision of other resources). In the African culture a wealthy high profile husband could be a real vehicle of economic capital to the wife's extended family as he is expected to fund the education of the siblings of his wife, fund and provide shelter for her ageing parents if they are not economically empowered. In the African culture, a husband means much more than a companion— he is a veritable vehicle of socio-economic privileges.

In Nigeria, unfaithfulness in marriage by a woman is rightly called adultery, according to biblical injunction, and a sin that may merit dissolution of the marriage. The Islamic law even prescribes stoning to death. However, where a husband is even a pathological serial adulterer—it is referred to as "having an affair" which is not considered a grave matter but something to be expected and tolerated by his wife. **Hence, the wife is left in the lurch by the society to seriously work at her marriage to salvage it, by doing whatever it takes (like bleaching her skin) to prevent her husband from being completely lost to seductresses.** This desperation to **remain** married has even led women to suffer in silence, endure and remain in the most dehumanizing and abusive relationships with their husbands. Therefore, the skin bleaching phenomenon cannot be dissociated from the issue of women empowerment in Africa.

In some cultures in Nigeria, women have no inheritance rights. Furthermore, it is not uncommon to find a man who has abandoned his wife, after several years of separation, **initiating** divorce proceedings in court (at the instigation of the other woman who now has a stronghold on him as the mother of his only child/children). The court in Nigeria, instead of charging the man for bigamy, gives the man **all** the property acquired in marriage because his wife has produced no child from the relationship! The abandoned wife is therefore condemned to a life of wretchedness, except she is economically empowered. Even when the husband has not instituted any formal divorce proceedings and the legitimate wife decides to tolerate it all and remain with her husband till death, it is a common sight to read full page advertorials in the Newspapers (in form of obituaries) where "the other women", boldly and shamelessly, announces for all to know that she has a child/children for the deceased man. This serves as a forewarning that she and her child/children are geared up towards taking legal actions for their own share in the dead man's property, if perchance he died intestate! If a wife who has **only** female children abandons her marriage, or her husband dies she and her daughters will walk away empty-handed as the husband's relations will cart away all the family property, moreso if her husband has identified his brother/uncle/father as his '*next of kin*' in his official documents. See Appendices 9, 10 and 11 on (i) THE MARRIAGE LAWS IN NIGERIA, (ii) POLYGAMY, (iii) BIGAMY, and the section on THE MARRIAGE PRESSURE—Chapters 5,6.

It is worthy of note that the strange phenomenon of African men having a special affinity for light complexioned women is not peculiar to Africans alone. The same dominant driving force for women bleaching their skin to find marriage exists in several other countries. Therefore, if perchance a divine alchemy is performed in the hearts of African men today to develop an aversion for the bleached skin, the manufacturers of the skin-lightening cosmetics would cease to have a market for their products in Africa except in countries with **institutionalized colorism**.

Conclusion

It is easy to pathologize women for taking "unnecessary risks" with their health, and sometimes, the health of their children, and that they are simply hoodwinked, drowning in their own self hatred or vanity. Poor women, in particular, are castigated as either "brainwashed" or "too illiterate to know better." The fact is that in sub Saharan Africa, marriage prospects carry a host of socioeconomic implications for women and their families, such that what is socially perceived as beauty can produce tangible economic payoffs. No woman wants her marriage ruined by another woman, for whatever reason, let alone for a skin tone which she can also acquire from a tube of cosmetics. If Nigerian men appreciate and admire their dark skinned women as beautiful and attractive for courtship and marriage, if the women are confident and have the strength of character to stand their ground and not let the men nor media to define the parameters/checklist for beauty, if the societal pressure on women to see marriage as the ultimate goal in life is lifted, if all women are economically empowered, if the men are not reduced to bread crumbs at the sight of light skinned seductresses, if a level playing ground is given to all (irrespective of skin tone) in search for jobs, it is my sincere conviction that the menace currently posed by the use of skin lightening cosmetics and toiletries will gradually wear off.

This bleaching syndrome is propelled by several factors: an arresting desire to be appreciated and loved by the opposite gender, a jaundiced feeling of inferiority complex, ignorance/crisis of identity, need for visibility and attention, a desire for beauty as defined by the gatekeepers of beauty in the magazines and adverts that valorize the light-skinned models and celebrities as the ultimate beauty! Hence in the context of the Nigerian culture, three words describe the motives for skin bleaching among women in Nigeria: **'Security', 'self worth'** and **'significance'.** See the chapter on RECOMMENDATIONS PART II—Chapter 20.

Do skin bleachers truly enjoy advantage in Nigeria?

As regards the possibility of gaining job advantage, the most important factor that facilitates securing a job for women in Nigeria is **merit** – that is possessing appropriate relevant qualification and skills. Another factor is when the employing organization has a policy of reserving a certain quota for the female gender. Atimes the issue of "State balancing" or "Federal character" comes into play in securing a job. This is a deliberate institutionalized policy of ensuring even geographic spread of job opportunities. However, when there are many women with merit applying for the same job, and there are limited vacancies, the other factor that may come into play is having influential interventions – what is referred to in local parlance as "long leg" or "man know man". Indeed, except a skin bleacher has outstanding qualifications and merit, she is **not** likely to be taken seriously by serious minded employers, as she would be assumed to be a possible seductress/sex object suitable for jobs like marketing or public relations. Indeed a bleached woman conveys the image of an empty headed person seeking for notice from the opposite gender. No doubt, there are highly intelligent and professionally qualified women who bleach, and who would secure a job because of their brain but not because of their skin tone. Invariably such women are those still in search of a male partner or who do not feel secure at home with their husbands, and such women are often the object of ridicule and gossip in their places of work. However, a bleacher is likely to stand a better chance of being engaged as a receptionist, Front office staff, public relations job or a sales agent—e.g marketing services—securing investors for commercial banks and securing patronage of advertisers for Television houses. In such services women are given ***measurable targets*** which must be delivered within a time frame, and they are blackmailed that they have to do whatever it takes to attain the targets by whatever means—even if they have to sell their bodies—to avoid being sacked from their jobs! I have often seen young girls at the clinic admitting that they resorted to bleaching their skin so as to attract investors for the banks where they work or advertisers to place commercials at the TV houses of their employers. It is poignant to also know that some of these organizations encourage their staff to bleach in order to lure customers; some of them are even given 'bleaching' allowance.

It is pertinent to note that these young girls, blackmailed with often unattainable measurable targets, suffer in silence for fear of being perceived as prostitutes on their jobs. Furthermore, there is an unwritten rule that you need a light skin to be employed in the movie industry and to get casted for high profile roles in Nollywood.[1] (See the chapter on THE CELEBRITY DISCOURSE—Chapter 6)

Is skin bleaching truly linked to "success," "power" and high mobility" in Nigeria? To the **"*impressionable minds*"—**the answer is "Yes". One only needs to look at the prevalent fair skin complexion of highly visible women e.g. TV News anchors and presenters, wives of politicians, politicians e.g female members of the House of Assemble (Senate and House of Representatives), State Commissioners and Federal Ministers, female Company Secretaries, even some nurses and doctors etc. The predominant shade of skin is the *light* skin—mostly acquired through chemical bleaching—and even if the light complexion is marginally natural with some of them, they still find the need to enhance the whiteness or prevent tanning through the use of skin bleaching products. Furthermore, these women belong to the socio-economic class that can afford the expensive high-end skin lightening products and methods, hence they do not show the tell-tale signs of skin bleachers e.g exogenous ochronosis. This class of women constitute veritable bill boards for the skin bleaching culture. The responses of those teenage girls in the study by Durosaro *et al*[11] confirm the impact of this class of women on the minds of young impressionable girls in search of "success" and "power" in Nigeria.

In Nigeria, for the same position, men and women earn the same salary as there is no gender-based differential in salary structure in public institutions. However, when it comes to being noticed by the opposite gender and securing a boyfriend/husband, bleached women stand a better chance of being noticed by men who have a special affinity for light-complexioned women. Hence, in Nigeria skin bleaching does **not** always confer any economic capital. It only confers social capital which may translate into economic capital, among people with like minds. Therefore, whatever perceived job advantage bleachers believe the light skin confers on them is an illusion as the skin tone is only relevant in certain jobs where the skin tone is perceived to be an enhancer (rightly or wrongly) at the job.

It is noteworthy that nobody claimed she bleached to enhance her chances of employability in the job market in **all** the studies in Nigeria, except Nollywood actresses![13]

References

1. Adebayo SB. An epidemiological survey of the use of cosmetic skin lightening cosmetics among traders in Lagos, Nigeria. *West Afri J Med* 2002 Jan – March 21(1): 51-5.

2. Ofondu Eugenia Ogugua. Cosmetic use of bleaching creams in Enugu. *National Postgraduate Medical College of Nigeria Dissertation* 2003.

Study at the Enugu State University of Science and Technology (ESUT) between February and October 2001.

3. Ofili AN, Eze EU and Onunu AN. Prevalence of use of skin lightening agents amongst University of Benin undergraduates in Benin City, Nigeria *Nigerian Medical Practitioner* 2006; 49 (1/2): 24-27.
4. NOI Polls Predominance of Skin Bleaching Linked to Search for Beauty and Attractiveness. Noi-polls.com/root/index.php?pid=182&parented=14&ptid=1
5. Nwangu Liwewe video: eNCA Nigerian tops list for skin-lightening products Tech Report. AFRICA Thursday 29 August 2013 http://www.enca.com/africa-life/nigeria-tops-list-skin-lightening-product
6.Interview by Al Jazeera http://www.aljazeera.com/indepth/features/2013/04/201345148459
7.Kingsley "Rukus" Okafor http://www.xojane.com/issues/nigeria-as-theworld-capital-of-skin
8. Olumide Y.M. Unpublished data
9. Lara Adejoro. What would make an older woman bleach? http://www.dailytimes.com.nig/article/what-would-make-older-wom... Daily Times NG. Article May 10, 2014
10.http://naijahomeandaway.blogspot.com.ng/2015/05/i-bleached-because-80-of-nigerian-men.htm/#.Vfvsk32sxDf.
11.Durosaro AI, Ajiboye SK, Oniye AO. Perception of Skin Bleaching Among Female Secondary School Students in Ibadan Metropolis, Nigeria. *Journal of Education and Practice.* 2012; 3:7):40-46. ISSN 2222-1735 (Paper) ISSN 2222-288X (Online)
12. http://www.youbeauty.com/mind/depression-data-from-cdc-notgetting-help.
13. 5 (five) Reasons Nollywood Celebrities Bleach their Skin/…http:www.nigerianbulletin.com/threads/5-reasons-nollywood-celebr…

======================================

Perspectives about skin bleaching in Nigeria

Women's perception of the benefits and risks of skin lightening

Some studies have been done on the benefits and risks of skin lightening in Nigeria.

Adebajo[1] in a study among traders in Lagos twelve years ago asked how respondents felt about their new look after bleaching.

As regards user satisfaction, 64.1% felt they were more attractive hence, they were more confident about their new look. Only 13.2% claimed they were relieved of their skin blemishes while 9.5% claimed they were better appreciated by their spouses; and 13.2% were indifferent to the outcome of their new look.

In a study among University undergraduates[2], respondent were asked what they knew about the meaning of toning. The result is given on Table 4.22.

Table 4.22 Respondents knowledge about the meaning of toning

Respondents knowledge About toning	Percentage
Less degree of bleaching	53.0
Not the same as bleaching	28.0
No response	14.3
Same as bleaching	4.7
Total	100.0

Ignorance about the adverse effect of skin-bleaching

Ignorance, to some extent, may be responsible. For example, the Cushinoid bloatedness, a complication of long-term use of corticosteroid creams, is being glorified and appreciated as a sign of "affluence" particularly among the market women. They deliberately encourage themselves to intensify the use of the corticosteroids to achieve the desired effect.[3,4] Some people actually regard the brown melanin pigment as "dirt". Some years ago, while visiting a neighboring French-speaking African country, a young girl who was hawking the skin–bleaching cosmetics in the market, walked straight to me offering me a tube of bleaching cream to purchase because I stood out of the crowd with an exceptionally dark skin, and blurted out "nettoiyer" which means "clean up"! This experience made clear the depth of ignorance among **some** of the bleachers, who may continue to see anyone who hasn't bleached as old fashioned for retaining a "dirty" pigment. "Fade Cream" is a popular skin lightening product in Nigeria and its name clearly defines its function to make the tone of the skin paler/lighter by gradually removing the brown /black melanin pigment. Out of ignorance about the meaning of fade, some Nigeria (particularly the Yoruba speaking market women and illiterates) pronounce it as "Fade" (as if it were a French word). Hence, they perceive 'Fade' as a brand name not as a name describing its function of bleaching the skin.[5]

However, the reality is that even when they are aware of the health hazards, the hard core bleachers are not likely to stop. See Table 4.2. Several efforts have been made by various people, journalists in the print and electronic media, and corporate bodies – for example, the Medical Women's Association of Nigeria (MWAN), Nigerian Association of Dermatologists (NAD), the Nigerian Medical students Association, and some religious organizations to educate the public about the inherent dangers of these products. Indeed MWAN has written a small book on the subject,[6] while NAD has always carried the campaign and annual pre-conference awareness rallies with the slogan "I'm proud I'm black" to the grassroots in the market place etc. In Nigeria, respondents in a survey[3] identified some of the negative effects associated with skin bleaching to include "skin cancer" (35%) and "skin damages" (25%).[7] Furthermore, these women interviewed have added that although skin whitening products may have harmful effects, they would still use these products to **look** and **feel** more beautiful.[8] The response from this undergraduate Law student in a University in Lagos sums up the pervasive attitude:

> "With all the warnings from the health sector, people still smoke. The same goes with campaigners against HIV/AIDS. People still engage in promiscuity'. People will still bleach, no matter what. "What I am concerned with is how to maintain my skin tone."![8]

Kpanake[9] in phone interviews with three doctors – a Nigerian practicing in Baltimore, another from Dominican Republic practicing in New York, and a doctor practicing in Pennsylvania and New York, said many Africans know about the medical dangers associated with skin bleaching, but disregarded them because the desire of many Africans to have light skin is just too intense.(See the chapter on UNITED KINGDOM—Chapter 15).

Skin bleaching in Nigeria: perspectives among teenage girls in Nigeria

Durosaro et al[10] investigated the perception of female secondary school students on skin bleaching practice in Ibadan metropolis. The sample comprised six hundred female students across ten secondary schools in Ibadan metropolis. These were young girls between the ages of 11-14yrs (85.3%) and above 14yrs old (14.7%). The instrument employed for the study is titled "Perception of skin Bleaching Questionnaire" (POSBQ), designed by the researchers.

In this study, the rank order (by the mean scores) of responses to items on perception on skin bleaching are as follows:

Table 4.23 Expectations from skin bleaching

Skin bleaching helps to:	
Gain the attention of the male fold	1st
Get desired marriage partners	2nd
Successfully maintain pre-marital relationship	3rd
Get connected with high caliber in the society	4th

Attain high social standard	–	-	-	5th
Become more successful in life	-	–	-	6th
Look fashionable	–	-	-	7th
Express positive self-worth	–	-	-	8th
Compete adequately with males	–	-	-	9th
Gain public support	–	-	-	10th

The data collected were analyzed using percentage, mean and t-test statistical measures. The major findings revealed that young girls engaged in skin bleaching as a method of receiving desired attention and relationship from the opposite sex and attract the desired marriage partners. The study revealed that religions have no significant influence on the perception of the respondents as regards skin bleaching while age has significant influence.

The above major ranking of motives shows that major reasons why people bleach their skin are, to build heterosexual relationships and become public figures. The major findings revealed that young girls engaged in skin bleaching as a method of receiving desired attention and relationship from the opposite sex and attract the desired marriage partners.

What privileges does fair skin afford Nigerian women in particular? It was found that the teenage girls already perceived skin whitening as a route towards achieving a range of social and economic benefits. In addition to enticing men romantically, they believed bleached skin products would enable them to "enter into connection with high calibers, attain high social standard, become more successful in life, look fashionable, express positive self-concept and be able to compete well with their male counterparts. Additionally, marriage prospects carry a host of socioeconomic implications for women and their families, such that beauty can produce tangible economic payoffs. Whether real or imagined, the perceived benefits of fair skin expand far beyond one's appearances. For further detailed discourse on this subject see the chapters on (i) DETERMINANTS FOR SKIN BLEACHING (Chapters 5, 6) and (ii) COLORISM IN SUB-SAHARAN AFRICA: NIGERIA AS A CASE STUDY (Chapter 11).

The authors conclude that counselors should enlighten female students on best practice in body beautification and guide them on life building skills such as assertiveness, decision making and healthy living.

NOI Polls

Against the background, that Nigeria has the highest prevalence of skin lightening practices in the world, NOI Polls conducted its recent poll on skin bleaching to seek the views of Nigerians regarding the predominance, possible reasons and the negative effects of skin bleaching.[10]

NOI polls is the No1 for country-specifics polling services in the West African region, in technical partnership with Gallup (USA) to develop opinion research in Nigeria. NOI Polls, is a platform where the voices of ordinary Nigerian can be collated and used to support decision making across the different facts of the economy.

Respondents to the poll were asked six specific questions
Q1.Do you agree or disagree that light-skinned people are more attractive than dark-skinned people?
Q2.In your opinion, how predominant is skin bleaching in Nigeria?
Q3. Amongst what group of individuals do you think skin bleaching is most predominant?
Q4. Are you aware there are negative effects of skin bleaching?
Q5. In your opinion, what are the negative effects associated with skin bleaching?
Q6.Why do people still engage in skin bleaching despite its negative effect?
The responses were as follows:

Q1. Do you agree or disagree that light-skinned people are more attractive than dark-skinned people?

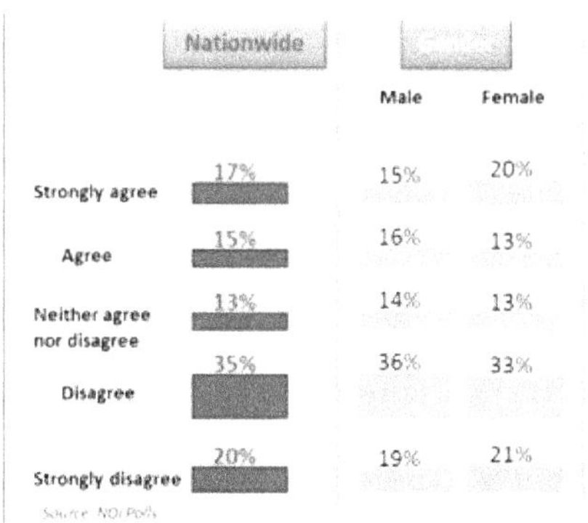

Q2. In your opinion, how predominant is skin bleaching in Nigeria?

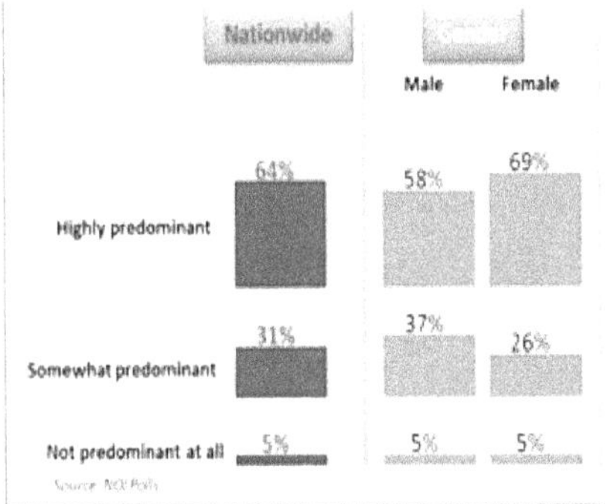

Q3. Amongst what group of individuals do you think skin bleaching is mostly predominant?

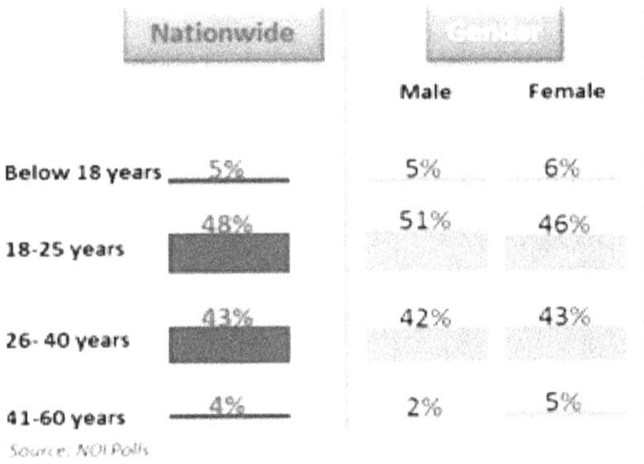

Q4. Are you aware there are negative effects of skin bleaching?

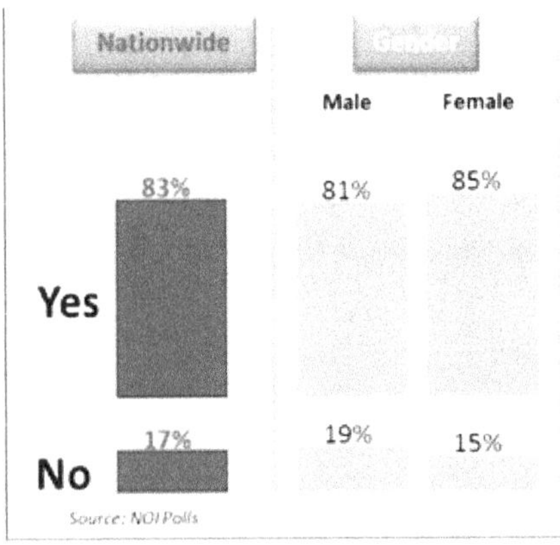

Q5. In your opinion, what are the negative effects associated with skin bleaching?

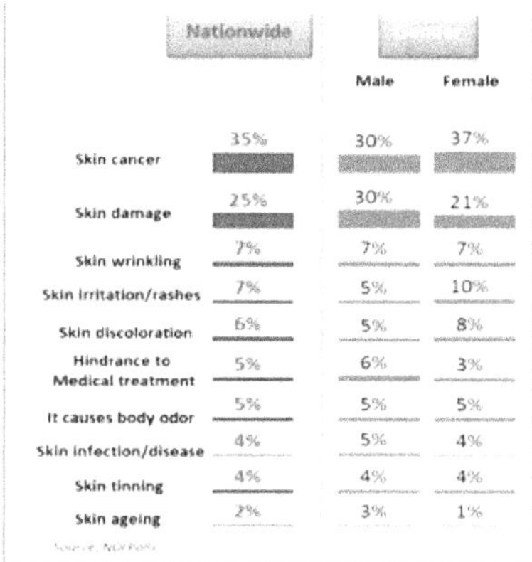

Q6. Why do people still engage in skin bleaching despite its negative effect?

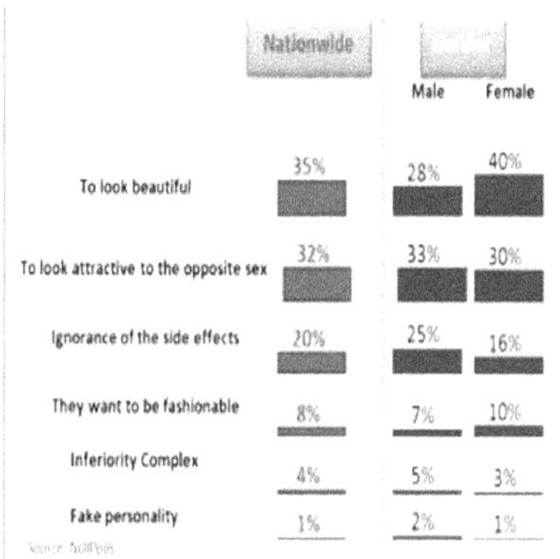

Summary of NOI Polls

Latest snap poll results released by NOI Polls have revealed that **64%** of Nigerians are of the opinion that skin bleaching has become highly predominant in the country, especially amongst Nigerian females **(97%).** This finding supports the claim by the World Health Organization (WHO) that Nigeria has the highest number of women that use skin-lightening products in the world. The poll further revealed that despite the negative effects of skin bleaching affirmed by **83%** of respondents; the top reasons why people still engage in the practice of skin bleaching are the need to "look beautiful" **(35%)** and to "look attractive to the opposite sex" **(32%).** Skin bleaching was also reported as being mostly predominant amongst Nigerians within the age groups of **18–25** years **(48%);** and **26-40** years **(43%).** In addition, respondents identified some of the negative effects associated with skin bleaching to include "skin cancer" **(35%)** and "skin damage" **(25%).** These were the key findings from the *Skin Bleaching Snap Poll* conducted in the week of **February 3rd 2014.**

Recommendations of NOI Polls

Finally, public enlightenment championed by health campaigners may be a key to highlighting the negative effects of skin bleaching and re-orientating the public about contentment with their natural skin colour; particularly amongst youths of between ages 18 – 25 years, campaigns across tertiary institutions may be organized. However, we do understand that for some Nigerians, the perceived benefits of beauty and attraction may outweigh the actual risks of skin bleaching, thus supporting Maslow's hierarchy of needs which highlights that certain attitudes are motivated by the need "to belong", gain self-esteem and confidence in the society.

References

1.Adebajo BS. An epidemiological survey of the use of cosmetic skin lightening among traders in Lagos, Nigeria. *West African Journal of Medicine* 2002; 21:51-5.

2. Ofili AN, Eze EU, Onunu AN. Prevalence of use of skin lightening agents amongs University of Benin Undergraduates in Benin City, Nigeria. *Nigeria Medical Practitioner* 2006; 49 (1/2):24-27.

3. Olumide YM, Akinkugbe AO, Altraide Dan, Mohammed T, Ahamefule N, Ayanlowo S, Onyekonwu C, Essen N. Complications of chronic use of skin lightening cosmetics.
Int J Dermatol 2008:47; 344-353

4. Olumide YM. Editorial: Use of skin lightening creams. Lack of recognition and regulation is having serious medical consequences. *British Medical Journal* (BMJ) 2010; 341:c6102 (published 23 November 2010)

5. Olumide YM. Unpublished data

6. *BLEACHING OF THE SKIN (What everyone should know)* Publisher: *Medical Women's Association of Nigeria* 1988; 37 pages.

7. NOI Polls. Predominance of Skin Bleaching linked to Search for Beauty and Attractiveness http://www.noi-polls.com/root/indexphp?pid=182&parentid=14&ptid=1

8. Tunde Alao. Staff Reporter. Lagosians and the bleaching scourge. *The Guardian.* Thursday, February 6, 2003.

9. The "NCUR 2012 Research Survey". *Kpanake*, and Expert Interviews.
Nina-Belle S. Mbayu. Skin Bleaching in Western and Central Africa: A Critical Analysis Utilizing the Social Learning and Colonial Mentality Theories. Proceedings of The National Conference On Undergraduate Research (NCUR) 2012. Weber State University, Ogden, Utah March 29-31. 2012.

10. Durosaro Al, Ajiboye SK, Oniye AO. Perception of Skin bleaching among female secondary school students in Ibadan metropolis, Nigeria. *Journal of Education and Practice* 2012; 3 (7): 40-6.

"Whitenicious" and responses to the motives for bleaching

A controversial skin lightening product range which was release by a Cameroonian-Nigerian musician sold out within a day of being launched, according to reports. Whitenicious, by Dencia, which is sold online for $150 per 60 ml and is advertised as a Knees and Elbows moisturizing cream and skin lightener, defied heavy criticism to prove a hit in Nigeria. Dencia posted on twitter: "What just happened? Whitenicious just sold out. Wow, restocking and will have more products by January 10th but you can place orders."

But Nigerian blogger, Myne Whitman, said skin bleachers are not just being used by black women who feel inferior because of their dark complexion. Admitting that she has used products similar to Dencia's Whitenicious, she made the point that often women use bleachers to even their skin tone and remove spots. She said: "My face is much darker than my body and back in my late teens, I wanted an even look. My face actually got to the same tone as my quite fair thighs at some point, but I stopped when I realized I was becoming a slave to those creams and had got into a vicious cycle ̄from using them on only my face, I began using them all over as my face got lighter than my body." Whitman claimed she stopped using the products after being enlightened about the possible side-effects of long-term use. But she says she understands why women use skin lighteners, not because they are ashamed of their colour but as a beauty aid.

The following are some of the reactions on twitter to the Nigerian blogger, Myne Whit-man

Xavibee-Lydia De Angel from Kenya Utalii College, Nairobi says:

"Sometimes bleaching is something you are forced to do for example eczema makes the skin look bad and one can't wear sleeveless tops or cleavage bearing clothes I think one can bleach out if its the only thing that can return their confidence"

Ari Tiamiyu says:
"That's so shameful that the melanated peoples of the world most importantly from the birthplace ***of the entire world*** *feel it necessary to keep up with the beauty standards of European and white America."*

Ray Peters, a Top commentator says:
"hahahaha a beauty aid?!
Just another excuse as I see it. When women African women throughout the world wear weaves is that a beauty aid too?!"

"Come on ladies, you are not fooling anyone, clearly you have issues with self and the pressures of how you think you're supposed to look. These creams/lotions clearly damage yourselves in the long run. Self esteem classes are needed, a counteraction is needed for all this madness that is happening to African women worldwide"

Sandra Grant from Hertford, Hertfordshire says:
"The ironic thing about these ladies having such low self esteem is that they feel compelled to lighten their skin. They haven't been observant enough to realise, the lighter your skin, the quicker you appear to age, so in time, they will have more low self esteem hang ups when the wrinkles start to show up (which they would never have had if they kept their beautiful youthful melanin), and believe me they definitely will show up. Only then will they realise just how beautiful and age resistant their skin tone was in the first place, and it may be too late to reverse the damage. But of course I also realise they may be forced to do this because of social pressure, which is why I don't judge them but pity them."

Sandy Lawrence from Syracuse University says:
"scary, scary, scary"

Stephen Thomas from Nottingham, United Kingdom says:
"Shameful"

Paul Pinnock Twyford Church of England High School says:
"Ladies if it's not Johnson & Johnson Baby Lotion you a'salt Mackerel out'a barrel"

Nnedi Uzowihe from Washington, District of Columbia says:
"Does this help prolong aging? I mean what I mean ... Lmfao!!! Interesting!!!

In response to serialized publications on the subject of skin-lightening, by Gbenga Adebambo[2] several responses on perspective were received.

The problem is more than just cosmetic, it is culturally destructive. It encroaches on our culture, values and heritage. We might really have gained independence from the 'whites' but we are really in dire need of mental emancipation and Bob Marley had in a prophetic way delivered this message succinctly long time ago in one of his songs.

Redemption song, "Emancipate yourself from mental slavery, none but ourselves can free our mind. Have no fear for atomic energy, 'Cause none of them can stop the time… Won't you help to sing, these songs of freedom? 'Cause all I ever had, Redemption songs…These songs of freedom."

The Black Pride movement celebrating heritage, personal pride, authenticity and afrocentricism needs to be consciously and actively injected into expressions of pop culture by artists, musicians, film-makers, writers and media practitioners. In the face of acute self-degradation, we must not allow our sense of self to be distorted through a white lens.

"We should stop buying into the myth that a lighter skin means a better life. It is a blatant lie; your mind and not your skin should be the object of enlightenment. It is appalling to see in Nigeria how people are addictively desirous to bleach their skin to look like the white man but will never go any length to upgrade their spoken English! When I see people paying for bleaching creams, I pitiably get angry because they are paying for their ignorance and doomsday. Unfortunately, the elite and respected people in the society who are supposed to speak against this degrading and self-inflictive act are gradually bleaching themselves into oblivions
— Gbenga Adebambo
Editor in Chief, Maximum Impact Magazine
and Columnist YOUTHMAGAZINE, THE GUARDIAN

"I strongly believe in my 'naturality' and appearance. I don't need to impress anyone, because what I see in the mirror is my reflection not anybody else's. My advice is this: be proud of your natural skin colour, be on a good diet and take loads of fruits to retain that awesome colour you have got"
— Oluwatosin. (Student, Dept of Chemistry FUTA, AKURE)

"It is high time we all build and developed ourselves from within…our self-worth."
— Gbemisola. (Educator at Chrisland Schools, Lagos)

"Bleaching is only a form of reflection of lack of confidence. One of many, we need to believe in ourselves and what we are." — Samuel (Edo State)

"Those who bleach must learn to accept their skin colours and be proud of being black. 'BLACK is BEAUTY' is not about the colour but the content the person carries. False appearance or wearing of mask keeps one in perpetual bondage. I sum this up with a stanza from Chara Nyashia Sanjo's poem (Beautiful To Be Black): "It's beautiful to be black, it is the colour of strength and pride. I will say it out loud. I don't have to hide." — J. Oyasotie. (Edo State)

"Wow!... I am imploring Nigerians to desist from this 'heinous' crime against their skin…Be comfortable in your skin." — Adeola (Medicine & Surgery, University of Ibadan).

'Well, from my own point of view, I felt bleaching your body isn't good. So many people bleach their skin colour mostly because their skin is black and they believe having a black skin isn't good. But actually, having a black skin is one of the best gifts you can ever receive from God. Stop paying others to damage your skin! Even, Guinness Africa launched their newest **ad** *with the made of black* tag to celebrate Africa's uniqueness: Black is not a colour. Black is an attitude. It's a mindset, it's a way of life.' #MadeOfblack#. — Olujimi (Lagos State).

"The chemicals present in bleaching creams are very harmful to the body; most of them penetrate into the skin to cause irreversible damage to the skin tissue. This piece is an eye-opener to the real reason behind this self-destructive act." — Oghenekome (Warri, Delta State)

"What a world! I think those indulging in this shameful action need proper orientation because I don't think I need to spend a whole month's salary on cream all in the name of trying to look attractive or beautiful. God bless you sir for raising this crucial topic." — Damilola (Ronk New Age, Ibadan)

"Bleaching creams are not just life-threatening; they can affect the user's offspring whether male or female." — Johnson (Ajah, Lagos).

"It is appalling how brainwashing has turned us to be modern slaves." — Akpobome (Warri, Nigeria)

"But Godliness with contentment is a great gain (1 Timothy 6:6). I assume that anybody that is not content with his or her natural skin colour cannot be contented with anything in life. All that God created are beautiful as I am dark and beautiful."

— Funke (CEO Passion Designers, Ibadan)

"There is need to value our identity in connection with our skin colour. I therefore appeal to every youth out there to embrace their skin colour, their identity and be very proud about it. I am proud to be one of "...the African queens that have vehemently refused to join the mad and demented race of skin bleaching... It begins with you!"
— Ogunmodede (Ogun State).

"This dangerous act of bleaching is tunneling deep down to the psyche of our ladies. We are not good enough, we are not beautiful enough, so we now bleach and wear other women's hair and now we are beautiful. So, so sad! We are telling the Almighty that he was not good enough in his creation of my sisters. We are made in his image and likeness. But we want or desire to be someone else!" As a medical doctor, I must add that the health effects of the chemicals in the cosmetics are very troublesome. Anything you put on your skin goes in through the skin into your

body. Once in, the blood will help it circulate to other organs. Many of the chemicals are toxins and are linked to hormonal problems, abnormal menses, fertility problems, ovarian problems, mood disturbances, bowel problems, fibroids, and cancer, examples are parabens and phthalates. Many of these chemicals are being found in blood, even of new-born babies. How did they get there? The cumulative effect with daily use in small quantities. Let us stop destroying God's Perfection!

— Dr Patrick Ijewere (Internal Medicure

Consultant at Johns Hopkins University and Radio Host of Wellness Half-hour on Inspiration 92.3 fm, Lagos)

References

1. Natricia Duncan. Skin bleachers are often used to remove spots and even skin tone, says user New Nigeria skin lightening range sold out in a day/ *The Voice Online* http://www.voice-online.co.uk/article/new-nigerian-skin-lightening-r... 15/01/2014.

2. Gbenga Adebambo. Stop Bleaching Away Your Destiny. # Say No To Bleaching. I, II, III. *YOUTHMAGAZINE. THE GUARDIAN.* May 7, 14, 21, 2016.

Should skin bleaching cosmetics be available on prescription by doctors?

Case Study

A 35 yr old densely bleached, single lady was seen at the skin clinic in Nov'14. Her primary reason for consultation was that she was having recurrent eruptions of "greenish patches" on her thighs which she believed was "allergic" in nature and she wanted to identify the allergen in her life e.g food, drugs, etc. "The greenish patches" were not present on the day of consultation and I was not aware of any type of allergic reaction that presents as "greenish patches". However she had extensive gaping striae (stretch marks) on the inner surfaces of the upper third of the thighs including the crotch. Indeed it was one of the most severe types of striae I have seen in decades of clinical practice as it was highly inflamed and sore with oozing serum and excruciatingly painful. The patient claimed the lesion was so painful that she found it difficult to walk about when the thighs rubbed against each other. See Figure 4.3 below.

I asked her for the type of cosmetic she was using but she told me not to bother about that as they were **"prescribed by a doctor hence they were medicinal"**. She willingly gave me the name of the doctor, (Dr MC) and described him as a Caucasian, who was the "President of the Association of Laser **s**urgeons in England".

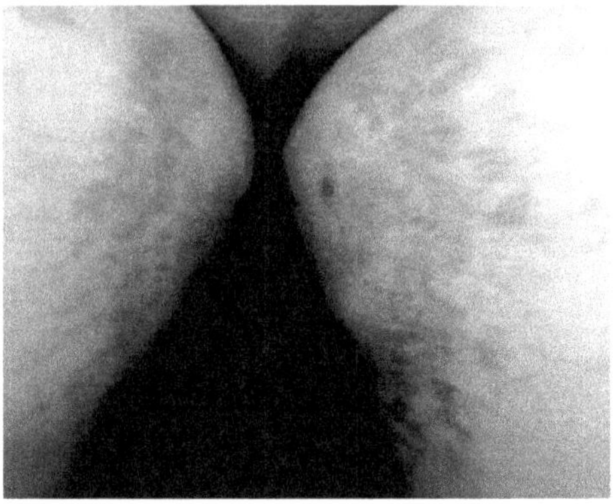

Fig 4:3 Extensive inflamed striae on the inner surfaces of the upper thighs

She also said she had an appointment to return to him sometime in 2015 for Laser surgery to eliminate the extensive striae on her thighs. When asked how she got to know about Dr MC before she traveled out of Nigeria to consult him in London, she said she identified him through internet advert and booked an appointment online to see him. She offered the information that she was suffering from depression for which she was being treated with antidepressants. I asked her to bring all the cosmetic products to me the following day so that I could identify the possible cause of her "allergy". She complied, and I was nonplussed to see the battery of creams—**seven** different products—some of which were "for morning" and some "for night" application according to the doctor's instructions. The list of creams are given below.

i. ZO SKIN HEALTH
by ZEIN OBAGI, MD
ORASER Emulsion
Anti-aging formula

ii. OBAGI
Nu-derm Toner; PM, 2 (restores skin's natural pH)

iii. OBAGI
Nu-derm Blender
Skin Lightening and blending cream
Hydroquinone USP 4%; Rx only

iv. OBAGI
Nu-derm Exfoderm forte; 4
AM Exfoliation enhancer

v. NeoStrata SKIN ACTIVE
Advanced Comprehensive Antiaging
Firming Collagen Booster

vi. NeoStrata TARGETED TREATMENT
Intensive treatment for specific concerns
HQ Skin Lightening Gel

vii. SKINCEUTICALS
Body Tightening Concentrate
Firming and smoothing Cryo-fluid
for gravity-fighting zones

Struck by the recklessness of the prescription, I decided to follow up and gave the name of the doctor to a practicing physician in London to help investigate the credentials of the doctor and if the products were indeed available on prescription in England. The response from the investigator is stated below.

"Dr MC is not on the General Medical Council registered doctor list, neither does 'Association of Laser surgeons of UK' exist! I checked under British Medical Laser Association which is the closest to the Association he represents and he's definitely not on their board of directors nor president. I found of As regards the prescribed cosmetic products, the enquiry was uncovering more and more issues about the treatments.

1. *The Skin ceutical products I couldn't locate at all on the official website on Skinceuticals.co.uk which lists all their products.*
2. *Obagi products also I couldn't locate and that particular product has another very closely linked named product which Obagi has officially dissociated from ... so similar names but not the original Obagi. However I still couldn't locate it online. I asked a pharmacy friend of mine who said there were lots of 'off market' seller underground which means products were outside the control of Medicine and drugs regulator. As I said these are not prescription drugs so outside medical regulation as well. Cosmetic medical treatments are not considered medical treatments*
3. *Cost of erbium laser cosmetic surgery starts from £1500 for a 5cm radius area for treatments and upwards depending on size and what the skin disorder is.*

I hope this is helpful. In fact my discovery suggests this can be an unholy grail with complications....infection, scarring, neuralgia etc for the unweary."

Conclusion from the above findings

It becomes clear that, if this level of quackery can exist at this time in the history of health care services in a nation like the UK, that can boast of having one of the best practices anywhere in the world, it is unimaginable to comprehend what can happen in a country like Nigeria or indeed most African countries where quacks may even outnumber ethical medical practitioners and where any purported prescription can easily be obtained for a fee!

Quackery abounds in medical practice in every country

However, the fact that quacks exist is no justification for not putting in place measures to curb the misuse and abuse of cosmetics. Corticosteroid creams are drugs and they should be made prescription drugs (not over-the-counter) as is the case in developed countries. Hydroquinone and mercury in cosmetics should remain banned. If there are no laws to regulate the availability, then there will be no justification for prosecution. I recall that several years ago in 1991, an importer of some cosmetic products sued the Federal Government department of Customs for confiscating a huge consignment of contraband cosmetics at the point of entry into Nigeria. I was invited by the Dept of Customs to help testify in court. The impounded contraband was sent to a credible independent (not FDA) laboratory for analysis and it was found to contain 4% hydroquinone. The importer lost the case because there was an existing law prohibiting the manufacture and importation of any cosmetic product with hydroquinone. If there had been no law in place, the Federal Dept. of Customs would have lost the case as there would have been no justification for impounding the imported dangerous cosmetics.

Other notable findings on prescription issue and medical practitioners

Should skin bleaching products be made available only when prescribed by medical doctors?

Jarrell Minyard[1] says: A survey carried out by the British Skin Foundation found that 16% of dermatologists believe skin lightening are 'completely unsafe' and 80% feel they are only safe when prescribed by a dermatologist.

"During my research for this paper, I came across countless websites owned and operated by dermatologists and medical doctors who sell skin-bleaching creams as panacea for plethora of skin conditions such as "aging spots", "freckles", "wrinkles", acne and similar skin ailments".[2]

Several dermatologists and non dermatologists in Africa already have their own product lines and are making huge money from skin lightening products.[3]

Dr Melanie Miyanji, a dermatologist in Kenya says she treats dozens of women of all ages who have abused skin lightening creams, and are now suffering the visible consequences. Among the reasons she gave "*some physicians are known to give out concoctions with no known formula of contained ingredients. Strict prescription products are readily given out by pharmacies on demand without prescription and sold in back streets*".[4]
In Nigeria, some doctors hold consultancy services in some cosmetics beauty parlors and spas. They give the skin bleaching injections in these beauty parlors and they run clinics where they dispense concoctions for skin bleaching as this is a money-spinner for them.[5]

References

1. http://ukzambians.co.uk/home/2011/07/07/rampant-abuse-of-skin-lightening-creams-by zambian-women/ July 7, 2011

2. Mire Amina. Skin-Bleaching: Poison, Beauty, Power and the Politics of the Colour Line. *Resources for Feminist Research* 2001; 28[3-4]: 13

3. Josephine Mogiti. SKIN DEEP. Destination Magazine. http://www.eadestination.com/investigative-journalism/467-ski-deep 6/3/2015

4. Josephine Mogiti. SKIN DEEP. Destination Magazine. http://www.eadestination.com/investigative-journalism/467-ski-deep 6/3/2015

5. Melanie de Souza. The concept of skin bleaching in Africa and its devastating health implications. *Clinics in Dermatology*. 2008; 26: 27-9

6. Olumide YM. Unpublished data

Recommendations

The Medical and Dental Council of Nigeria is the body responsible for Regulating doctors and ensuring Good Medical Practice. The Pharmacists Council of Nigeria is an Agency responsible for regulating and controlling the education, training and practice of pharmacy in Nigeria.

The above two agencies should revisit, as a matter of urgency, the respective laws monitoring ethical professional practices, scrutinize the activities of doctors and pharmacists as regards the above unethical practices and mete out appropriate sanctions to erring doctors and pharmacists. Doctors are not trained to compound drugs nor cosmetics and really are not legally covered to prescribe their own concoctions for skin lightening. Pharmacy shops constitute a major outlet for marketing of skin lightening cosmetics. There is need for regular inspection of pharmacy shops to ensure that cosmetics containing contraband ingredients like mercury and hydroquinone are not available for sale in their facilities, nor should they sell corticosteroid products without prescription.

Chapter 5

Skin lightening Culture In Africa
Determinants I

Story highlights I, II, III

Why women in Africa are more susceptible to skin-lightening than men?

The marriage pressure

Dominant signals from highly visible women

The desire to create an identity that is perceived as more socially acceptable

Roots in colonization and slavery; the belief that lighter skin tone is seen as a means of achieving upward social mobility

Effects of agents of socialization such as Eurocentric educational system, media and popular culture—cultural migration

Media images which glorify lighter skin tone and disseminate images of white beauty

The effect of celebrity endorsement

Accessibility, availability, affordability and effectiveness of cheap, lowend skin lightening products

Commodity racism: the law that permits the manufacture of dangerous creams in Western countries for export to Africa

Ineffective and inadequate legislations, regulatory agencies and policies

Ineffective and inappropriate health education on skin bleaching practices

Cultural love for light skin tone

Advances in the technologies of the body, global economics and huge growth in the cosmetic industry

Marketing and selling of white ideals by cosmetic manufacturers

Polyvalent claims. The concept of multi-tasking/multi functional beauty products

Aggressive marketing strategies

Skin bleaching as a sign of non acceptance of one's cultural background

Skin bleaching as a sign of body dysmorphic disorder

Story highlights I

- Light skin tone can be transformed into social capital (social network), symbolic capital (esteem or status) or even economic capital (high-paying job or promotion).

- The cultural ancestry/memes and institutions which though not codified have nonetheless continued to undergird, guide, define and propel otherwise rational people to want to change their physicality by bleaching their skin, in spite of the overwhelming risks to their health.

- Women are judged much more heavily on the basis of appearance. Men are more likely to be considered valuable when they have wealth, education and other forms of human capital, while women are considered valuable when they are physically attractive, even if they lack other capital.

- Skin-lightening is of utmost importance in attracting most men. Women bleach so that they are not trapped in spinsterhood because most African men valorize light complexioned women since they find such women beautiful and sexually attractive. Even while married, women need to continue to bleach their skin to sustain the attention of their husbands so that they are not lost to bleached seductresses always on the prowl.

- Women associate fair skin tone with elegance, beauty and a higher social status.

- The dominant signal from highly visible women (celebrities) is that fair skin is associated with success
- The desire to create an identity that is perceived as more socially acceptable drives the bleaching culture

- Ignorance about the function of the brown melanin pigment promotes skin bleaching; it is perceived as 'dirt' among some people, and some women encourage themselves to "clean up" by bleaching. Also the Cushinoid bloatedness, a complication of long-term use of corticosteroid creams, is being glorified and appreciated as a sign of "affluence" particularly among the market women.

- In some countries parents approve of skin bleaching and actually fund the cost of the products for their teenage daughters. In Sudanese culture, if you want to remain natural and love your skin tone you are seen as a radical woman instead of a woman who is proud of whom she is.

- In some countries women have taken it upon themselves to lighten their skin tone after experiencing the bullying and discrimination of not "fitting in". Women who refuse to bleach often find themselves regarded as second class citizens and are ostracized.

- In South Africa, for instance, skin bleaching is one of the psychological scars of colonialism and apartheid—some of which are self-hatred and low self-esteem. These negative psychosomatic influences often push people to alter their physical appearance to feel better about themselves.

- Agents of socialization such as Eurocentric educational system, media and popular culture have been found to influence people to internalize Eurocentric standards of beauty. The desire to bleach one's skin is similar to the obsession to acquiring Eurocentric beauty ideals such as a thin figure, aquiline nose, long straight hair.

- Media images which glorify lighter skin tone and disseminate images of white beauty drive the skin bleaching culture by portraying "whiteness or lightness" as a symbol of what is attractive, adorable, desirable, pure, loveable and competent. Women with lighter complexions are regularly used to advertise on the electronic and print media a broad spectrum of consumer products. Women have only to watch television commercials, read print and digital advertisements, or drive past huge billboards to internalize the message that light skin is to be desired.

- Easy accessibility, availability, affordability and effectiveness of cheap, lowend skin lightening products drive the skin bleaching culture. Corporations have created product lines in a wide range of price categories, such that whiteness is financially accessible for both rural villagers and white-collar urban professionals.

- With the advent of online marketing, the products can be ordered and delivered, same day, at your door steps just by the click of the mouse!

- The various bans on the skin bleaching culture have been ineffective for the following reasons: a) the bribery culture and corruption in most African countries, b) cross border smuggling, c)thriving Black market for the products, d) bootleg versions abound, e) illegal vendors and desperate marketers, f) easy accessibility, availability and affordability of cheap products, g) the role of Websites—skin lightening products can be purchased through the internet, h) ineffective and outdated regulatory policies, i) failure to enforce the ban, j) lack of political will to enforce the ban, k) the population of skin bleachers has reached a critical mass for the ban to make any meaningful impact as the continued manufacture and sale of the products are demand-driven.

- Advances in the technologies of the body, global economics and huge growth in the cosmetic industry drive the bleaching culture.

- Polyvalent claims. The concept of multi-tasking/multi functional beauty products in a world where every minute is rationalized, a simpler life becomes the Holy Grail. In order to appeal to the powerful discourse of "natural beauty" in many societies, most products claim to *restore* the natural beauty of skin (if it is lost), *reveal* the natural beauty of skin (if it is hidden), or *create* a natural beauty (if the consumer never had it to begin with).

- Skin bleaching can be a sign of non acceptance of one's cultural background due to the belief that the *only* standard of beauty is those defined by European ideals.
-
- Skin bleaching may be simply a personal choice like tattooing or it may be an indication of more pathological problems such as Body Dysmorphic Disorder.

Story highlights II

Ineffective and Inappropriate health education on skin bleaching

- Educational content on adverse health effects is generally sketchy and grossly inadequate.

- The public health discourse has the effect of maintaining silence around the structural benefits of light skin, and pathologizing women for taking "unnecessary risk" with their health, and sometimes, the health of their children.

- Findings in Ghana, Nigeria, and some other African countries, show that even doctors and nurses bleach. Can these people be regarded as ignorant of the health risks of bleaching?

- The very real social and economic disadvantages attached to dark skin around the world feed into a compromised psychological sense of self. Disrupting this psychological damage requires addressing the large system by which dark skin comes to symbolize a lack of life opportunity.

- What privileges does fair skin afford women in particular? Light skin tone can be transformed into social capital (social network), symbolic capital (esteem or status), or even economic capital (high-paying job or promotion). Whether real or imagined, the perceived benefits of fair skin expand far beyond one's appearance.

- Interventions to reduce the burden from skin lightening practices have to be a multi-agency approach, pursued in concert and synergistically. Therefore, each component of the DETERMINANTS has to be studied and analyzed so that the various governments of each country can galvanize all the relevant stakeholders to formulate and articulate the methodology of activities of interventions before any meaning impact can be achieved.

Story highlights III

Commodity Racism

- Toxic skin bleaching creams made in the UK have been found in dozens of countries, including Nigeria, Ghana, Tanzania, Zimbabwe and South Africa.

- The law allows companies in UK to make the products even though they contain substances banned in Britain as long as they are for export.Clearly this type of legislation is race-or ethnicity-based capitalism.
- *"We know it is illegal. We used to sell it to the Middle East and North Africa where it is perfectly legal. We have no control over what happens to it after that.,* said Eric Dupont of General Healthcare UK.

- These creams are easily available over the internet, and as long as the demand is there will be somebody to sell them.

- The skin bleaching market is similar to colonialism in that the promotion of white superiority allows a few powerful and wealthy groups to become increasingly wealthy and powerful at the cost of masses of other people.

- The hypocrisy is stunning: In the U.S., Unilever, the parent company of the brand Dove, sells products to women by promoting "real beauty." But in other parts of the world, Unilever sells the skin lightener Fair & Lovely.

SKIN LIGHTENING CULTURE IN AFRICA: DETERMINATS I

Introduction

Skin bleaching/lightening is a growing trend in Africa and may be defined as the removal of skin melanin to achieve lighter skin tone. It is done through the use of homemade products, cosmetic products and dermatological products. Skin bleaching in Africa goes across age cohorts, gender, marital stratus, social class, race and the rural-urban dichotomy. Skin bleaching is a phenomenon that cuts across **all** socioeconomic strata—from the analphabetic to the most learned professional—academics, legal luminaries, even "men of God", doctors and nurses! Skin bleaching practices in Africa spans class levels, though the use of such products is concentrated in urban areas.

Skin bleaching is fraught with several hazards—physical, emotional, psychological and involves serious economic implications—both in physical cash and in time—man hours devoted to the practice. Several questions have been asked—why do people with dark skin find it compelling to remove the natural dark (melanin) pigment from their skin? What are the driving forces? What are the motives? And what benefits (real or imaginary) are derived from lightening the skin colour?

Several scenarios or thought processes have been posited as to why dark skinned people consciously or subconsciously find it compelling to bleach their skin? Some of these paradigm are the self hate thesis, the colorism perspective, the identity thesis, the complex personhood explanation, the colonized mindset, the post traumatic colonial African syndrome, mental slavery, Stockholm Syndrome and Bleaching Syndrome. These paradigms shall be fully described. Light skin tone can be transformed into social capital (social network), symbolic capital (esteem or status) or even economic capital (high-paying job or promotion). Hence, the issue of **motives** also merits a separate discourse on its own. Therefore see the general section on MOTIVES—Chapter 6 and the discourse under each individual countries. It is noteworthy that some people have **consciously** refused to lighten their skin in spite of societal pressures to comply and bleach their skin. This issue has also been highlighted under the individual country discourse, when identified—for example, religious conviction was a strong deterrent among some communities in Ghana and Rwanda. In Sudan some men divorced their wives for daring to bleach their skin; while in Nigeria some men deserted their wives only after the disfiguring complications of exogenous ochronosis have set in.

The phenomenon of skin bleaching is like a bad dream that one would wish away; but skin bleaching is a reality which appears to have come to stay. However, before any meaningful and efficacious interventions can be proffered and activated, it is critical to clearly define the cultural ancestry/memes and institutions which though not codified have nonetheless continued to undergird, guide, define and propel otherwise rational people to want to change their physicality by bleaching their skin, in spite of the overwhelming risks to their health. The primary objective of this chapter is to elucidate those factors.
Another section has been devoted to the topic PARADIGMS FOR SKIN BLEACHING—Chapter 6. These are thought processes/theses that have been theorized or conceptualized to explain why people of colour have consciously or subconsciously internalized the need to change their physicality by bleaching their skin. That chapter is complementary to the present chapter.

(i) Why women in Africa are more susceptible to skin-lightening than men?

If women in Africa are more susceptible to skin bleaching than men, it is merely because women are judged much more heavily on the basis of appearance. Men are more likely to be considered valuable when they have wealth, education and other forms of human capital, while women are considered valuable when they are physically attractive, even if they lack other capital. Flick through those magazines and you'll find that the women featured are almost always a few shades lighter than the men. Black men don't need to be light-skinned to be worth paying any attention, but black women do.

In one Tanzanian study, women claimed Tanzanian men preferred white, soft-skinned girls. Thus, skin-lightening was of utmost importance in attracting men. And once you've got a guy, you want to hang on to him. Another woman in the study explained that she used skin-lightening products to prevent her husband from being attracted to other girls, while yet another, a 25 year old, reported that she *"started bleaching to be beautiful and to look like Arabians or Europeans and attractive to people, especially men." "We are all competing for mates, and we do whatever we can to give ourselves an advantage over the next person."* Men would probably be content to live in caves if they didn't have to acquire the trappings necessary to compete for the most desirable women, and there would be less incentive for women to lighten their skin if men didn't keep valuing lighter skinned sisters over darker skinned ones. The women in the study also said they lightened their skin to enhance opportunities in life (especially job opportunities), and to reduce the experience of negative stereotypes that are applied to dark skinned people. It puts one in mind of the associations with skin colour drawn out from black American kids by black American filmmaker Kiri Davis when she recreated the 1940's "doll experiment" a few years ago in *A Girl Like Me*.

Another study found that women in Senegal associate fair skin tone with elegance, beauty and a higher social status. And in the Tanzanian study, many participants felt that their lighter skinned peers have higher status, income, education, job opportunities, as well as more friends. These women are not deluded; misguided definitely, but not deluded. They see the evidence around them. It is not surprising then that some "darker skinned people are often envious of those with lighter skin and attempt to achieve the same status by engaging in skin-lightening practices." (See the sections on "MOTIVES FOR SKIN BLEACHING" and "THE MARRIAGE PRESSURE"—Chapter 6).

(ii)The Marriage Pressure

Some women claim they lighten their skin so that (i) they are not trapped in spinsterhood because most African men valorize light complexioned women since they find such women beautiful and sexually attractive. Secondly, even while married, women need to continue to bleach their skin to secure and continue to engage the attention of their husbands so that they are not lost to bleached seductresses always on the prowl. (Read the section on SKIN BLEACHING: A CRY FOR HELP in the chapter on NIGERIA—Chapter 4).

(iii) Dominant signal from highly visible women

Some highly visible women—'celebrities'—such as politicians, e.g female national assembly members, Hon. Ministers and Commissioners, female deputy governors, local government chair persons, wives of State governors and local government chairmen (assorted 'first ladies'), women in the entertainment industry (Nollywood Movie stars and women in the modeling industry), Television presenters and newscasters, Company Executives (CEOs), Company Secretaries or the wives of such people, Client Services/Front Office Desks staff/Receptionists in companies, hotels, hospitals, public institutions etc, some "men and women of God"—female pastors or wives of pastors who mount the pulpits to preach the word of God. Some of these groups of people enjoy high visibility in the print and electronic media.

It may not be an exaggeration to state that the vast majority, about 70 percent of "celebrities" in Nigeria are light skinned. For example, the proceedings of the National Assemble are sometimes covered on TV. Curiously **black skinned** female politicians appear to be in the **minority.** It is pertinent to note that the word **"celebrities"** is often used in Nigeria, not in the sense of a **famous** person as defined in the Oxford Dictionary, as some of these 'celebrities' are really **not** famous, but **notorious,** because of their low morals and ethical standards such as corruption and embezzlement of public funds. Therefore, "celebrities", in this context, simply describes people who enjoy high visibility and publicity by the very nature of their work and/or in the print and electronic media. The undiscerning minds see such people as role models, "achievers", and symbols of "success" and may want to be like them by bleaching their skin. Hence light skin, acquired through bleaching, is gradually metamorphosing into a symbol of success in Nigeria. Hitherto, up till the early 1960s, light skin was associated with the Fulani people of Northern Nigeria, some ethnic groups in South Eastern Nigeria, albinos, and biracial people. **Genetically** light skinned people were not common in other parts of the country, but today in Nigeria, dark skinned women are gradually going into extinction—this observation inspired the title of this book—**THE VANISHING BLACK AFRICAN WOMAN**.

(iv) The desire to create an identity that is perceived as more socially acceptable

African's traditional beauty standard of full bosom, wide hips and dark skin like ebony has metamorphosed into Caucasoid features of light skin, thin figure and aquiline nose. Indeed some time ago in the past, among some African communities, a thin bride was a source of concern to her in-laws as it raised doubts about her reproductive potentials. For example, in some communities in Nigeria, prospective brides are fattened up before marriage and kept indoors to avoid the tanning effect of the sunrays. Hence at the time of marriage they are light skinned voluptuous brides. Further in Nigeria some mothers indoctrinate their daughters to see marriage as the ultimate goal for a woman. Therefore young teenage girls claim they bleach their skin to enhance their chances in the marriage market. (See the section on MOTIVES and PERSPECTIVES in Nigeria—Chapter 4).

In Nigeria, and some African countries the brown melanin pigment is perceived as 'dirt' among some people, and some women encourage themselves to "clean up" by bleaching. Also the Cushinoid bloatedness, a complication of long-term use of corticosteroid creams, is being glorified and appreciated as a sign of "affluence" particularly among the market women. They deliberately encourage themselves to intensify the use of the corticosteroids to achieve the desired voluptuous effect. Ezinne Ukoha says[1]

> "It has never been a secret that Nigerian men prefer their wives, light, bright, and voluptuous. Anytime a man picks his future wife, there is high praise if she happens to be lighter skin than him. I remember attending several weddings as a kid, and hearing the grown-ups relentlessly discuss how gorgeous the bride was with emphasis placed on her light skin. A bride with a darker complexion never gets the same amount of attention."

In Mali, 53% of women in Bamako use bleaching agents. Women who refuse to bleach often find themselves regarded as second class citizens. A woman who did not bleach her skin said she is often not offered a chair at baptisms, and is asked to make herself scarce when group photographs are taken at marriages." (See the section on MALI—Chapter 7).

In the Republic of Benin, 70% of parents approve of skin bleaching and actually fund the cost of the products for their teenage daughters. In Sudanese culture, if you want to remain natural and love your skin you are seen as a radical woman instead of a woman who is proud of whom she is. Even within the same Sudan, some men find skin bleaching a most disgusting practice, some even divorced their wives for daring to bleach the skin, while some secondary schools suspended female students for bleaching their skin. In Zambia, some men severed relationships with their fiancés because they bleached the skin. In Rwanda, some adolescents indicate that they knew about the practice but are restricted by family, religion, and Rwandan culture (See the sections on REPULIC OF BENIN, SUDAN, ZAMBIA and RWANDA—Chapters 7, 8, 10).

In Zambia, some men severed relationships with their fiancés because they bleached the skin. In Rwanda, some adolescents indicate that they knew about the practice but are restricted by family, religion, and Rwandan culture (See the sections on REPULIC OF BENIN, SUDAN, ZAMBIA and RWANDA—Chapters 7, 8 , 10).In Zimbabwe some people have taken it upon themselves to change their looks after experiencing the bullying and discrimination of not "fitting in". Drugs are even advertised to "enhance the hips and the breast" – curvy hips and a rounded bottom. (See the section on ZIMBABWE—Chapter 8).

In a study among women of Bolgatanga municipality of Ghana, 39.2 percent of the women were skin bleachers. Those who did not bleach their skin gave the following reasons for noninvolvement—"fear of critics", "cannot afford the cost," "not interested." The researchers conclude that this could be attributed to the fact that most of them are very religious and perceived the act as a violation to their belief system. (See the chapter on GHANA—Chapter 7).

> Josephine Mogiti[2] says: "The opinions of most Kenyan's on skin lightening is best described as ambivalent. Light skinned or dark skinned, Kenyans dissect every aspect of a woman's beauty routine; if she's in a weave, she is too Westernized; if her hair is kinky or nappy, she is not paying enough attention to her looks. From head to toe, from her make-up to her choice in shoes, the Kenyan women is always under scrutiny for how she balances Kenyan-ness and the Western beauty ideals that are being adopted there. And this is unlikely to change. Skin lightening has been a part of the Kenyan culture since the 60s, and it's most likely here to stay. What we have to decide is whether or not women should have to use chemical treatments." (See the chapter on EAST AFRICA: KENYA—Chapter 9).

References

1. Ezinne Ukoha. This is forty: I bleach my skin. 21 Jan 2014. *https://thsppl.comthis-is-forty-i- bleach-my-skin-52baf1479.*

2. Mojiti Josephine. SKIN DEEP. DM Destination Magazine *http://www.eadestination.com/investigative-journalism/467-skin-deep*

(v) Roots in colonization and slavery; the belief that lighter skin tone is seen as a means of achieving upward social mobility

Europeans, who enslaved and colonized people primarily from Africa and India, exploited the region on the basis of racism. They believed that they were superior to the indigenous people and to people brought to work on plantations. The belief that whites were superior was partially attributed to their skin tone and indoctrinated into the minds of Africans, Asians, and other racial or ethnic groups in the

Caribbeans. The complexion consensus is that lighter skin is superior and often privileges light-skinned individuals with more opportunities for success and prestige. However, this is mediated by factors such as level of education and talent.

In South Africa, for instance, skin bleaching is one of the psychological scars of colonialism and apartheid¯some of which are self-hatred and low self-esteem. These negative psychosomatic influences often push people to alter their physical appearance to feel better about themselves, and one of the most common methods of doing so is by bleaching the skin. South African women are more affected by the stigma left by colonialism and apartheid than men. During colonialism, black women were treated in a most dehumanizing way and were viewed as objects of the colony.[1] They were always slaves or servants to their white counterparts leading them to believe that only white was right. For some of these women, the whiteness of a woman's complexion, the more likely she is to get a well-paying job, promotion, spouse, and/or to receive respect. (See the chapter on SOUTH AFRICA—Chapter 8).

Skin bleaching is also a serious problem in Ghana. Ghana the former British colony of the Gold Coast, was the first black African nation to gain its independence from Colonial rule. Ghana is a country known for its explicit Pan-African history and positive representation of blackness. It is clear that Ghana already has its own built-in challenge to wholesale white supremacy, particularly its racial values. Unlike some other places throughout the African diaspora where racially black populations are often only a subset of the larger population, Ghana boasts a nominally racially homogenous population. However, there is the history of prominent mixed-race families in the eighteenth and nineteenth centuries who were distinguished from the local community through education, dress, cultural practices, class, status, and who articulated a distinctive racial identity based on ancestry and their positions in society. Alongside state sponsored Pan-Africanist cultural events and politics advocating a black racial renaissance, for instance, there is also a predominantly white expatriate community who, because of their attachments to multinational corporations and foreign agencies, occupy elevated position that often tie whiteness to racial privilege.[2,3] (See the chapter on GHANA—Chapter 7).

The truth is that dark-skinned men and women of Africa descent continue to suffer the legacy of White world Supremacy. The desire to bleach one's skin is similar to the obsession to acquiring Eurocentric beauty ideals such as a thin figure, aquiline nose, long straight hair. Congo was a Belgian colony and the Belgians were really colorist and favored the light skinned Congolese with thin noses just like they did in Rwanda. A racist society devalues women of African descent and market women of European descent as beautiful, intelligent and powerful. Male and female skin bleaching is a highly prevalent practice in Congo. (See the section on CONGO—Chapter 10).

References

1. Julien Nahomie. Skin Bleaching in South Africa. A result of Colonialism and Aparthied? DISCOVER: *Georgia State Honors College Undergraduate Research Journal:* 2014; Vol 2, Article 4 *http://scholarworks.gsu.edu/discovery/vol2/iss1/4*
2. Pierre Jemima. 'I Like Your Colour!' Skin bleaching and geographies of race in urban Ghana. *Feminist Review.* 2008; 90:9-29.
3. Pierre Jemima. The predicament of Blackness: Postcolonial Ghana and the Politics of Race and White Women. *Skinner, Elliot. University of Chicago Press Amazon.com.* 2013:110-2.

(vi) Effects of agents of socialization such as Eurocentric educational system, media and popular culture—cultural migration

Western standards of beauty are influencing cultures across the globe and impacting personal, professional, romantic and familial relationships. Processes like skin lightening in India, hair smoothing in Black America, eyelid reconstruction in China, and plastic surgery worldwide continue to rise in popularity for men and women facing discrimination from both within and outside of their own increasingly fluid ethnic groups. Agents of socialization such as Eurocentric educational system, media and popular culture have been found to influence people to the practice of skin bleaching.

Although countries in Africa secured their independence from colonial masters at different times, when it comes to exposure to agents of socialization such as Eurocentric educational system, media and popular culture, the countries in Africa may be regarded as coeval in the skin bleaching practice though the rate of progression of the practice may vary.

In Sudan, war caused displacement that sent waves of people to urban areas where they were introduced to new colours and new standards of beauty that Sudanese had to live up. (See the section on SUDAN). Lewis Kelley *et al* examined the historical and cultural influence of skin bleaching in Tanzania.The authors took an exploratory look at the institutions of slavery, colonization, westernization, and neocolonialism in East Africa and argue that these institutions may have placed Tanzanians in a colour-conscious society. This also may have fueled potent skin-color ideals that have resulted in efforts to assimilate to dominating groups. In their attempt to understand the demography of skin bleachers in Tanzania, Lewis *et al* found several common characteristics among users. Findings suggest users are typically older (20+ years), higher income earners, married, and from the southwest region of Tanzania (a higher income-earning region due to tourism, and with increased access to manufactured mercury skin-bleaching products due to gold and copper-lead mines. Lewis *et al* also found that skin bleachers in Tanzania have higher internalized Eurocentric standards of beauty as well as political affiliations with the Civic United Front party (CUF) – a nationally based liberal political party that is heavily represented by Zanzibaris of mixed ancestry. Lewis *et al* argue that individuals possessing these common characteristics, likely have greater access to resources such as higher quantities of more potent skin-bleaching creams and possess more widespread idealized beliefs that lighter skin is better than darker skin, possibly due to influences of westernization and neocolonialism on subordinate groups. Some others confessed they started bleaching to be beautiful and look like Arabians or Europeans.

Skin lightening in east Africa has more to do with globalization of European ideals than with colonialism. The 60s, as Kenya gained Independence and Pan- Africanism was all the rage, saw the initial surge of East African women using skin lightening products – an era that also saw the rise of television and American media, where the practice of preferential treatment for light-skinned black Americans was well established, and the black stars exported were Chuck Berry, Diana Ross and Jimi Hendrix. But as this idea grew, so did the forces against it, with postcolonial African politicians deeming it racial betrayal. On the insistence of medical professionals, who were also opposed to skin lightening, Tanzania became the first country to ban the practice in 1968, followed by Uganda in 1972. While Kenya never enacted a total ban, it prohibited ads for Ambi soap, one of the most popular products at the time, on the basis that it insinuated that modern, post-colonial Africans were light skinned. However in 2001, Kenya banned a list of products listed in APPENDIX. 12.

However, it wasn't a clear-cut case of racial pride versus globalisation, as the many social revolutions occurring during that time also included feminism. Audrey Wipper, a Canadian sociologist who was living in Kenya in 1972, criticised the range of bans in East Africa, arguing that "prohibition of Western fashions and beauty aids were efforts by postcolonial male politicians to use urban African women as scapegoats for the nation's problems." Skin lightening and, beyond the practice itself, the desire for light skin, had become contentious issues in the country, and women who used the products did so discreetly. (See Chapter 9 on EAST AFRICA: TANZANIA, KENYA).

The issue of cultural migration is not only manifested by skin bleaching but also through the assimilation of other practices permissible by the Western culture. For example, the practice of cohabitation between unmarried men and women, and having children outside wedlock were considered abominations in the African cultures a few decades ago, but today men and women show no inhibitions nor shame as the society has become permissive like the Western countries. Another evidence of cultural migration is the rising rate of divorce among married couples in Africa. For example, in Nigeria in the 1950s and 60s cases of divorce were extremely rare, but today the divorce rate has sky rocketed.[3-6] Unsuccessful marriages have become a norm in the society and courts are thriving on cases of divorce between couples. An investigation by the News agency of Nigeria identified approximately 50 divorce applications filed at two 'customary' courts in the city of Ibadan in western Nigeria, between January 2014 and Dec 2015. 'Customary' courts operate according to traditional tribal practices. Meanwhile, at least five divorces a day are filed at the local civil court. Single parenthood is now very common and male adultery and unemployment are the commonest causes of divorce. Adultery is one of the reasons women claim they want to prevent by bleaching their skin to engage the attention of their husbands. Increasingly, financially comfortable women seem content to have babies fathered by married men as single mothers; while some unmarried men and women simply want to enjoy the companionship by cohabiting "with no strings attached." All the above used to be abominable practices in the past in Africa but are now the norms due to cultural migration.

References

1. Lewis KM, Harris S, Camp C, Kalala W *et al.* The historical and cultural influences of skin bleaching in Tanzania. In: The Melanin Millennium. Skin Colour as 21st Century International Discourse. Publisher Springer Netherlands 2013 pp 19-38.

2. Josephine Mogiti. SKIN DEEP. *Destination Magazine.* '*http://.eadestination.com/investigative-journalism/467-skin-deep6/3/2015*

3. Amazon Kindle. Unemployment blamed for Nigerian divorce rate. *Marilyn Stowe Family Law.* January 4, 2016. *www.stowefamilylaw.co.uk.*
4. Blessing Ukemena, Stanley Uzoaru and Aronke Olayiwola, Usman Ahmed. Adultery: The Reason behind High Divorce Rate. Feb 1, 2014. *http://leadership.ng/news/342464/adultery-the-reason-behind-high-div...*
5. Rita Onauoha. Reasons for high dovorce rate in Nigeria. *NEWSNG Current Nigerian News. http://newsng.com/nigeria-news/2015/03/reasons-for-high-divorce-rate*
6. Nigeria: High Rate of Divorce Catholic Bishop of Lafia. *Daily Independent (Lagos).* 6 February 2015. *http://allafrica.com/stories/20150260895.html*

(vii) Media images which glorify lighter skin tone and disseminate images of white beauty

When interviewed by news outlets, many African women have expressed that media images portraying white women as beautiful greatly influenced their decision to whiten their own skin. Furthermore, these women have added that although skin whitening products may have harmful effects, they would still use these products to look and feel more beautiful.

The mass media, particularly television, contributes to this perception by portraying "whiteness or lightness" as a symbol of what is attractive, adorable, desirable, pure, loveable and competent. Lighter skin tone is thus portrayed as a standard for attractiveness and competence. In Nigeria about two out of every three female newscasters and television presenters are bleached light skinned ladies. Hence television is a veritable medium for promoting skin bleaching.

Women with lighter complexions are more often used to advertise on the electronic and print media. A wide range of products including alcoholic beverages, toiletries and cosmetics (that are not even skin lightening agents), telephone handsets, textile materials, home and office furniture items and doors etc are advertised using light complexioned/bleached women. Massive, well lit bill boards adorn the streets of various cities in Nigeria using light-complexioned women to advertise a broad spectrum of consumer products.

Graham Busfield, a General Practitioner in Reading – England, in a reaction to my Editorial in the British Medical Journal, wrote to me:

"One driver to skin lightening that I believe exists but you did not mention was the technical difficulty of photographing or film dark faces against bright backgrounds. To produce images that portray all subjects equally within the field of view cameras have to adapt and adjust their exposure particularly for very dark or shadowed objects against bright backgrounds. Less technically proficient film makers will therefore select lighter coloured subjects. More proficient film-makers or

those with technically more advanced equipment can overcome such difficulties. Of course most technology has been developed chiefly for the richer, Northern, world. We view so much of our surroundings through a lens that may be this issue should receive more attention because of its public health benefits".

During an interview with me on this subject of skin bleaching, I showed Vladimir Duthiers, a CNN Correspondent, the letter from Graham Busfield. Vladimir debunked the excuse given by Graham for the preference of light complexioned people for adverts. Vladimir said any professional photo-journalist can produce very good and clear images of dark complexioned people and achieve the desired effect on adverts.

The effects of media that promote skin bleaching among women and children have been studied in Ghana and some other African counties.[1] Women see that the ideal skin complexion represented in the media is of fair skin tones. They have only to watch television commercials, read print and digital advertisements, or drive past huge billboards. The media portrays "whiteness or lightness" as a symbol of what is attractive, adorable, desirable, pure, and lovable.

Akua Djannie[2] says:

> "Africans need to redefine what beauty is and not sit passively while fashion houses in Milan and Paris tell us what is beautiful. We can no longer leave the definition of beauty in the hands of international, non-African movie makers, advertising agencies and music video directors. As Africans we have to accept whatever shade of black we are."

The powerful role of the MEDIA in promoting skin bleaching and in defining BEAUTY is so important that a whole section has been devoted to the discourse. (See the discourse on "THE MEDIA AS A MAJOR DRIVING FORCE OF SKIN BLEACHING"—Chapter 6, (ii) "BEAUTY"—Chapter 17).

References

1. Jessica Edmond. PROJECT. Skin Bleaching in Ghana: Media and Cultural Impact. *http:pulitzercent.org/reporting/Africa-ghana-skin-bleaching-women-…*
2. Akua Djannie. Skin Bleaching is a sin against God. *Ghanaian Chronicle/ All Africa Global Media.* September 18, 2007.

(viii) The effect of celebrity endorsement

See the section on CELEBRITY DISCOURSE—Chapter 6

(ix) Accessibility, availability, affordability and effectiveness of cheap, lowend skin lightening products

In the gritty slums of several countries in Africa, skin lightening phenomenon has reached dangerous proportions. Beauty has been democratized and is no longer considered the birth right of only the wealthy or fortunate women. Corporations have created product lines in a wide range of price categories, such that whiteness is financially accessible for both rural villagers and white-collar urban professionals. Poor and working-class women more often use concoctions that are more likely to include mercury and other ingredients that make the products more physically dangerous than high-end products.

Ijeoma who works at God First Cosmetic shop in Lagos, said, "*bleaching creams sell these days and we have varieties almost everyday. I'm not an expert on cream but by the time people come here, especially ladies, to ask for a particular cream or soap often, I know it's to bleach and so, I recommend it for others too who come looking for bleaching cream or soap and they say, it works. Most of these soaps and creams are not costly, anyone can easily buy them.*"

Skin lightening is fueled by the widespread availability of a plethora of cheap, purported skin-whitening products. Many of these are homemade, but others flood in across the borders from various African countries as well as from India and Japan. It doesn't take long to copy a cream from a big cosmetics house that promises to remove dark spots, pigmentation etc, and sell it at five or ten times cheaper for a much poorer market. The problem is that a lot of these creams have been tainted because of chemicals and compounds added in unscrupulously, without a scientific base. While the wealthier segments of African society can afford to buy better quality, properly regulated products, and can avail of dermatological guidance for their proper usage, the lack of education that prevails in many nations on the African continent, couple with the over-arching goal of lightening the skin, results in a gross abuse of cheap creams, and the disastrous consequences of this, is one of the biggest problems Africa as a whole faces today.

Products are also available in a variety of price ranges from a few cents per ounce to over one hundred U.S. dollars per ounce. The prices of the products make them affordable to the poor and the rich. The cost of a tube of bleaching product range from as little as $1US or less to $600US or more. The reality is that the size of every pocket has been catered for. In addition to these more expensive products created by multinational cosmetics companies, many small mom-and-pop vendors offer local products in informal markets throughout the Global South and in smaller markets catering to immigrant communities in the West. These products, often created and sold outside of formal regulatory channels, frequently contain active ingredients illegal in many nations, or legal chemicals in illegal doses[4]. Many skin-whitening products with dangerous chemical ingredients are manufactured in Europe or the United States, sent to Nigeria, and then distributed throughout Africa in both formal and informal markets. The bleaching products often make their way back to Europe and the United States for sale to the African and Asian immigrant communities there.

Skin lightening products are readily available from the roadside vendors, flea markets, supermarkets, drug stores, bodejas etc. Scheduled medicines are sold from unauthorized outlets. With the current technology, the products can be purchased online and delivered same day just by the click of the mouse. Furthermore, there are products suitable for the size of each pocket. There are very cheap products that cost just about a dollar or less manufactured at backyard industry by mixing dangerous chemicals; and there are very expensive high-end products that cost hundreds of dollars often used by the wealthy elite. Roadside vendors sell tubes and plastic bags of powders and ointments from cardboard boxes stacked along sidewalks in market places. Many of the tubes are unlabeled as to their actual ingredients. Some contain toxic chemicals like mercury. Some impoverished people resort to homemade concoctions of dangerous products. Some of these concoctions contain battery acid, potash, tooth paste, pulverized naphthalene (camphor balls) a moth proofing agent, peroxides and chlorates used in hair dyes, detergents, hair relaxers, tooth paste, shampoo, laundry bleach, cement, brake fluid etc. In short anything that has a corrosive effect on the skin. The above are mixed with over-the-counter products that invariably contain mercury and/or hydroquinone at dangerous concentrations.

Over the last few years this 'product pandemic' has led to a flood of cheap and affordable over the counter (OTC) products touted to be the "next best thing" for lightening the skin. The products are available everywhere, from big shops in the elite areas of Victoria Island, Ikoyi and Allen Avenue, to the local markets in the neighbourhoods of Mushin, Oshodi, Agege, Oyingbo, Ajegunle, among others. Street hawkers also peddle them, as well as the various types of medicated soaps and similar items which have come within easy reach of residents in the metropolis. With the advent of online marketing, the products can be ordered and delivered, same day, at your door steps just by the click of the mouse! The impact of online marketing is so serious that it is discussed under a special heading. (See the chapter on EPIDEMIOLOGY: WHERE ARE THE PRODUCTS MANUFACTURED; WHERE CAN THE PRODUCTS BE PURCHASED—Chapter 3).

(ix) Commodity Racism

The law that permits the manufacture of dangerous creams for export

Evelyn Glenn[1] writes about how skin lightening is "interwoven into the world economic system and its transnational circuits of products, capital, culture, and people" and about the "media and message, cultural themes and symbols, used to create the desire for skin lightening products". These products are manufactured in some countries and exported or smuggled into others. The media messages are conceived and created by a few individuals and are projected throughout the world. In fact, distribution of mercury soap has been illegal in the EU since 1989, but it's manufacture has remained legal as long as the product is exported.**Clearly this type of legislation is race-or ethnicity-based capitalism.** If it were merely capitalism, then they would allow the mercury soap to be sold anywhere, including Europe. However, the governments and the manufacturers in those countries know the dangers of mercury and want to protect their own people, but are quite willing to make a profit at the expense of people's health in other nations.

According to Glenn, "the desire for lighter skin and the use of skin bleaches is accelerating in places where modernization and the influence of Western capitalism and culture are most prominent. And so, the new face of imperialism can be seen in magazines, on billboards, and on Movie, TV, and computer screens around the globe. **The skin bleaching market is similar to colonialism in that the promotion of white superiority allows a few powerful and wealthy groups to become increasingly wealthy and powerful at the cost of masses of other people.**

Britni Danielle[2] is a regular contributor to **TakePart,** writes on a variety of subjects for Clutch, Ebony, Jet and others. In an article titled **"Proof We're Not Post-racial: People are Paying $10 Billion a year to be lighter,"** she comments on the Ethical aspect of the continued exploitation of people of color worldwide by the western countries and the need to contextualize colorism within White

supremacy. Yaba Blay, an assistant professor of African Studies at Drexel University submits that "failure to contextualize colorism within White supremacy, leads to pathologizing black women and make it seem like we're silly and we fight."Britni Danielle further writes to explore the unethical aspect of the continued manufacture of skin lightening products for export and the use by people of color.Skin beaching can be a *dangerous undertaking*. Burns, permanent damage, scars, infections, and cancer are just some of the risks of skin lightening. The products often contain dangerous chemicals, which have been banned in several countries. Despite this, American and European skin care companies are set to earn $10 billion by 2015 from sales of the products, according to a recent report by *Global Industry Analysts.*
"Most of the ingredients in the skin-bleaching products are banned in the United States and European countries because they recognize the harm it does to skin," says Blay. "But these products are banned for use, not manufacture. A lot of these products are made in the U.K., Italy, and in European spaces specifically for export, and they dump them in Africa, the Caribbean, and in Latin America."

The hypocrisy is stunning: In the U.S., Unilever, the parent company of the brand Dove, sells products to women by promoting *"real beauty."* But in other parts of the world, Unilever sells the skin lightener fair & Lovely. The Anglo-Dutch consumer goods company unilever sells the world's most popular skin-whitening product, a cream called Fair & Lovely. It is heavily advertised across Africa, Asia and the Middle East and boasts on its website that "250 million consumers across the globe strongly connect with Fair & Lovely as a brand that stands for the belief that "beauty that empowers a woman to change her destiny." Blay writes: White supremacy is insidious, if you don't recognize all of the entry points and all of the ways it remixes itself to attack us, we're always going to be on the receiving end of an attack." That "attack" extends far beyond America. Communities of color around the world struggle with colorism, which manifests itself in caste systems, discrimination, and unequal access to social and economic mobility based on skin color." "This is why you have bleaching in every single community where there are people of color," says Blay.[2]

Antony Barnett and Zoe Smith wrote an article entitled "Toxic creams for sale as thousands seek whiter skin."[3] They describe how young black and Asian women are using illegal and harmful skin bleaching creams in an effort to follow fashion. Antony Barnett and

Zoe Smith report "An Observer investigation has uncovered a booming multi-million-pound market in illegal and highly toxic skin-bleaching creams being sold across Britain to black and Asian men and women. Many are manufactured and sold to Asians, Africans, and the Caribbeans in the UK and exported to Africa."

"The law allows companies here to make the products even though they contain substances banned in Britain as long as they are for export. The products are then smuggled back into the UK. One of the skin-lightening creams containing hydroquinone is named Zarina. It is made by Fairtrade International, based in Barnet, north London. Another, Rico Complexion Cream, is made by General Healthcare based in Hayes, west London. Spokesmen of these firms claim they make their creams for export and that it is not up to them to police the trade. 'We have never sold one tube containing hydroquinone in the UK. We know it is illegal,' said Eric Dupont of General Healthcare. 'We used to sell it to the Middle East and North Africa where it is perfectly legal. We have no control over what happens to it after that.' Pride editor Dixon said: 'How can it be that a British company is allowed to make a product that can seriously damage somebody's health and would be illegal to sell here, but be allowed to export it to developing countries knowing not only that it will be used by people not aware of the dangers, but also that there is a fair chance of it ending up back in Britain?'

Toxic skin bleaching creams made in the UK have been found in dozens of countries, including Nigeria, Ghana, Tanzania, Zimbabwe and South Africa. Dermatologist Sujata Jolly has treated many women whose skin has been damaged from using the banned creams. Although Jolly was instrumental in getting hydroquinone made illegal, she fears that, whatever action is taken by the authorities, it will not shut off the supply. **'These creams are easily available over the internet, and as long as the demand is there there will be somebody to sell them."**[3]

References

1. Glenn EN. Yearning for lightness transnational circuits in the marketing and consumption of skin lighteners. *Gender & Society*. April 2008; 22 (3): 281-302.
2. Blay Yaba. in: Britni Danielle. Proof we're Not Post-Racial: People Are Paying $ 10 Billion a year to Be Lighter. *http://www.takepart.com/article/2015/01/23/beauty-companies-are-making-bank-selling-skin- lighteners-around-globe*
3. Antony Barnett and Zoe Smith. Toxic creams for sale as thousands seek whiter skin *the guardian* UK, Sunday 16 October 2005. http://www.theguardian.com/uk/2005/oct/16/health.healthandwellbeing

(x) Ineffective and Inadequate Legislations, Regulatory Agencies and Policies

Why the various bans have been ineffective

Some of the countries that have banned the products and years of ban are as follows:

Tanzania	—	1968
Uganda	—	1972
South Africa	—	1990
Gambia	—	1995
Nigeria	—	1995
Kenya	—	2001
Ivory Coast	—	2015

Most of the governments of the African countries have legislated against the manufacture, importation and sale of skin lightening products in their countries. However these bans have been completely ineffective as the products are still available in **all** African countries and the use of the products have continued to rise unabated. Some notable reasons for these apparent failures are as follows:

a) The bribery culture and corruption in most African countries.
b) Cross border smuggling
c) Thriving Black market for the products
d) Bootleg versions abound
e) Illegal vendors and desperate marketers
f) Easy accessibility, availability and affordability of cheap products. (already discussed above)
g) The role of Websites. Skin lightening products can be purchased through the internet. (See the chapter on EPIDEMIOLOGY: WHERE CAN THE PRODUCTS BE PURCHASED?—Chapter 3).
h) Ineffective and outdated regulatory policies and failure to enforce the ban. Lack of political will to enforce the ban.
i) Inadequate health education methods and content.
j) The population of skin bleachers has reached a critical mass for the ban to make any meaningful impact.
k) The continued manufacture and sale of the products are demand-driven. The bans can only be effective when the people are able to see the products on the market and refuse to buy them – not because it is illegal or dangerous but because it is bad, and they are satisfied with and proud of

the colour of skin they are **born** with— black or white. There is a voracious demand for the products (See the sections on PREVALENCE for the different countries)

l) The various motives for bleaching and determinants responsible for bleaching (which have been documented), need to be addressed with objective and culturally acceptable interventions.

a). Bribery and corruption examples

- **The Gambia**:

Gambia government enacted the Skin Bleaching Decree in 1995 and extended the ban in 2002. Under the Law people caught bleaching their skins are arrested and fined. Indeed the government went further and instructed security forces and police to arrest and detain anyone found with such products. As repressive as the law appears, however, this control remains extremely difficult ***"with the bribe culture in Gambia".***

Reference

Gambia Extends Ban on Bleaching of skin. BANJUL, Gambia Military authorities in the West African State of Gambia have decreed a total ban on skin bleaching. News.google.com/newspapers?nid=1350&dat…id…

- **Kenya**

Kenya banned skin bleaching products in 2001 *"..the skin lightening products and injections are gaining particular popularity on Nairobi's River Road—a busy market place notorious for its black market commerce and* ***bribed law enforcement."***

"When I first went to River Road and started to talk to people about taking photographs, the sellers harassed me, asking me what I wanted, and even pushed me into a room where they could quiz me about what I was doing. They demanded over $ 500 US to tell their story then kicked me out onto the street with dirty looks when I refused to pay it. Skin bleaching is a sensitive topic in a conservative and religious country like Kenya, and operating unlicensed salons that offer injections is against the law. ***It only survives through institutionalized bribery and if any of the skin bleachers get into trouble, it's likely they'll need to make a hefty payout to avoid jail."***

Rich Kenyan's have been receiving skin whitening injections containing a mixture of mercury containing creams and alpha hydroxy acids, particularly from vendors operating on River Road. Pancholi, a medical practitioner says **"skin bleachers operating on River Road make regular payments to the police, and a crackdown on their businesses is unlikely "It is illegal for a non-medic to inject a client, but bribery allows the trade to continue**." He says.

References

Annabel Fenwick Elliott. 'Kenyan men like women with whiter skin': The rise of wealthy Nairobi women illegally INJECTING themselves with skin-lightening creams.' *Mail Online* 6 June 2014 http://www.dailymail.co.uk/femail/article-2650766/Kenyan...

Celeste Hibberts/Al Jazeera. Kenya's backstreet # bleachedBeauty trade. http://www.aAlJazeera.com/indepth/features/2014/06/Kenya-backstreet-bleachedbeauty-trade-2014623134683 81417.html

- **Nigeria**

Discovery by African Business (AB) investigator, Lucy Hannan (an investigative journalist) reports. "While AB was unable to determine who the actual importers were, the thriving success of the trade at Balogun West was evident. It was also evident that the operation was not on a small scale, ***as new stock constantly arrived in vans carrying "Government Licensed Imports" labels— suggesting that the smuggling and trading involved corruption at a high level."*** Lucy Hannan 1988. (Read the chapter on NIGERIA: HISTORY—Chapter 4). In Nigeria, the Federal Government Department that enacted the law banning skin bleaching and responsible for enforcing the ban currently has members of staff (including some doctors, nurses and pharmacists) who are either heavy skin bleachers themselves or have spouses who are heavy skin bleachers! Can such and Organization be taken seriously? This is clearly an example of loss of credibility.

Reference

Lucy Hannan. Companies still make hazardous cosmetics for Africa Feature: Hazardous Cosmetics. *Africa Business May 1988.*

b) Cross border smuggling

A lot of cross border smuggling is ongoing. For example the East African Custom Management Act of 2006 banned the import of all soaps containing mercury. Products like Mekako soaps are readily available in Uganda having been smuggled in before being re-exported to neighboring Kenya, Tanzania and Rwanda. "They are smuggled in jerricans disguised as water while others come in through ordinary containers but are declared as cosmetics, when (in reality) they are drugs that fall under the NDA mandate," says Gyavira Musoke, Head of Imports Inspection at Uganda's National Bureau of Standards (UNBS). Ready marketers for these highly valued cosmetics suggest that smuggling won't stop any time soon. In Rwanda only administrative measures are taken for contravening the ban—that is, the vendors either receive a warning, the products are confiscated or the business closed. Noone is prosecuted.

Zambia boarders Congo and bleaching is part of the culture in Congo which was a Belgian colony who were really colorist and favoured the light skinned Congolese with thin noses just like they did in Rwanda. Skin bleaching is illegal in Zambia because of how badly it affects skin but there are still loads of Congolese people who smuggle in bleaching creams from Congo.

"In Zimbabwe, medical authorities can ban the sale of these products from registered pharmacies but they cannot completely ban their use as the demand is very high on the black market—managing illegal vendors and sellers is where the major issue is."

In South Africa, Dr Imraan Jhetam, a private dermatologist in Durban says that the rise in international travel has increased smugglers'opportunities to respond to a voracious demand for skin lighteners. Mamy Pony, a marketer of skin-lightening products, gets most of her creams from a shop up the street called Aegis, where a bus driver smuggles them from the Democratic Republic of Congo. But the illegal skin bleaching preparations are smuggled in by road, sea and air from all over the world. (See the chapters on SOUTH AFRICA; and EPIDEMIOLOGY: WHERE CAN THE PRODUCTS BE BOUGHT—Chapters 3, 8).

c) Thriving Black Market

The sale of over-the-counter skin-bleaching creams containing hydroquinone was banned in South Africa in 1992. (See the section on INTERVENTIONS in SOUTH AFRICA—Chapter 8). However the products have continued to circulate on the black market. Recently, spice shops and newly opened India and Pakistani beauty parlous have been doing brisk business with 'fairness' creams. Scheduled drugs are sold at unauthorized sites. (Read the chapter on KENYA: MARKET SURVEY—Chapter 9). In Kenya, Nairobi's River Road is a busy place notorious for its Black market commence. In Nigeria, there is actually nothing called Black market for skin bleaching products as the products are sold in the open "White market" in Pharmacies, Departmental stores, SPAS, marketplace, grocery stores—indeed everywhere and anywhere where there is buying and selling and the products are openly displayed in such shops. (See the chapter on EPIDEMIOLOGY: WHERE CAN THE PRODUCTS BE BOUGHT—Chapter 3). Indeed in every country in Africa where there is skin bleaching the products are available for sale and the users know where to purchase the products.

d) Bootleg versions abound

Writing under the title—The dark side of skin lightening, Niyanta Singh wrote that Durban-dark skinned people wanting skin lightening products are the basis of multibillion-rand industries. Some products claim to be totally natural, while many contain potentially harmful ingredients that could scar and cause permanent damage to the skin. Lester Davids says in South Africa, skin bleaching in fueled by the widespread availability of a plethora of cheap, purported skin-whitening products. Many of these are home made, Davids says; but others flood in across the borders from various African countries as well as from India and Japan. ***"It doesn't take long to copy a cream from a big cosmetic house that promises to remove dark spot, pigmentation etc, and sell it at five or ten times cheaper for a much poorer market.*** The lack of education that prevails in many nations on the skin, results in a gross abuse of cheap creams, and the disastrous consequences of this, is one of the biggest problems Africa as a whole faces today.

In the USA and European Union over the counter sales of products containing hydroquinone are banned. Over-the-counter versions of Fair & White contain 1.9 percent hydroquinone, but bootleg versions are being sold with 4 percent to 5 percent. Mercury is the most harmful culprit found in products like lemon herbal Whiting Cream (misleading!), Lulanjina, Diana and Fasco. There are a host of misbranded and counterfeit skin lightening products on the market that will cause harmful and permanent damage to the skin and internal organs. Hence 'fair and white' cream in the USA does not contain the same chemical in an African country.

References

1. Niyanta Singh. The dark side of skin lightening. Durban-Dark-skinned people want to be lighter. Light-skinned people want to be darker. *http://www.oil.co.za/lifestyle/beauty/the-dark-side-of-skin-ligh...*

2. Pumza Filani. Africa: where black is not really beautiful. *BBC News, Africa Johannesburg*. 1 January 2013. *http://www.bbc.com/news/world-africa-204447983*.

3.Skin bleaching/African Science Heroes. *http://afrischeroes.wordpress.com/tag/skin-bleaching/*

e) Illegal and desperate vendors and aggressive marketing strategies

The sale of over-the-counter skin bleaching creams containing hydroquinone was banned in South Africa in 1992. Yet they are still being sold by street vendors, like at the stall on the corner of President and Diagonal Street in Joburg. Mamy Pony who is one of the many hawkers in the Joburg city centre who sell the bleaching creams and ointments says

"I am surviving because of this thing."

Aniece, a refugee from the Democratic Republic of the Congo, supports several children with the profits she makes from selling skin lighteners.

"You see people here, some of them eat out of the garbage. I don't want to eat out of garbage. I am surviving because of this thing."

For example, in Jamaica, Kayja, (a retailer of the products) analyzed the market and found that bleaching products would prove to be a wise investment as skin bleaching was a popular and fashionable trend. Her motivations are obviously to capitalize on the popularity of the products. She explained that while she may not be in full support of people bleaching their skins, she would keep selling the products as she had bills that needed to be paid. Further, she clarified that she has in the past discouraged people from bleaching, if she noticed that they were overdoing it and causing severe problems to the skin,but soon admitted that she would not be insistent as she needed the business.Some so-called celebrities have their own product lines which they concoct and market under specific brand names, hence they proselytize more people who admire them to engage in skin lightening. (See the section on CELEBRITY DISCOURSE—Chapter 6).

Gift packs at girls & women events

Manufacturers and sales agents of these skin-lightening products have devised clever and surreptitious ways of promoting their products – a deliberate ploy. They give out **free** samples of their products in take-away gift packs or conference bags for participants at women and girls events e.g conferences, society meetings, churches mother's day celebrations, varieties of beauty pageants etc. Undiscerning women and girls are often **initiated** into the regular use of skin lightening products through such methods. They then recommend it to their friends and family members at home and in the villages. Rural village family members readily welcome such products as sharing in the goodies of "civilized" and sophisticated city people.

Text messages into mobile phones

Another method of marketing cosmetic products is by disseminating text messages through mobile telephone handsets. One of them which I received reads thus:

"HAPPY NEW MONTH". We pray it shall be a month of Joy, laughter and an unending celebration (Amen). We appreciate your support all through the year. We urge you to always make . . . . cream your products of choice" Tel: ....

Received 1st Dec '14

I know I have never heard of the specific named product nor used it. However the strategy of praying for the recipient and acknowledging, with thanks, the purported patronage of the products, are sufficient incentives for an undiscerning mind to either try out the product or continue to use it

i) Inadequate health education methods and content

There are some reasons why healh education efforts have been unsuccessful. In the vast majority of cases documented in various countries, the adverse health consequences are not well articulated. They appear as an afterthought, very sketchy, perfunctorily done and not likely to be taken seriously.

In response to the growing numbers of women and men using skin bleaching creams in Africa and throughout the Diaspora, many governments have spoken out through their ministers of health to dissuade people from using the products. Often leading government officials will release a formal statement, hold a press conference, and sometimes launch a nation-wide public health campaign informing people of the dangers of the skin-bleaching products. Because these state-sponsored messages come largely from public health entities within the government or NGOs, their focus tends to be on the physical danger of using such products. The government can ban the sale of skin bleaching products in pharmacies but they cannot completely ban their use as the demand is very high on the black market. Instead of discussing the side effects and dangers—users are ignoring the message and continuing anyway.

For example, the Ghana Health Service asks, why do women bleach? "It is centered on vanity"[1] they argue. The public health discourse has the effect of maintaining silence around the structural benefits of light skin, and pathologizing women for taking "unnecessary risk" with their health, and sometimes, the health of their children. They berate women for taking "unnecessary risks." Although women bear the brunt of the health costs associated with bleaching (though some men bleach too), women have been constructed as villains and at fault for succumbing to vain beliefs about beauty and risking their health to attain these standards.[2] A psychology professor from Uganda, when asked to comment on why people continue to use such dangerous bleaching products, he explained, "Such a person lacks self-esteem, has low self-efficacy and a perception that she or he looks ugly. It is common among women who are not educated" Another psychologist in Uganda says "Do something positive to counter your low self-esteem. Take advantage of the good parts of your body or talents."[2,3] The public health professionals in Jamaica and Uganda employ a discourse common among other government largely by altering individuals' attitudes. They assert that many people have misguided beliefs that light skin is better and higher in status, but this is not actually true in countries where colorism is the norm. The inability of many public health professionals to publicly acknowledge the real benefits of light skin, especially for women, has hampered their effectiveness.

Studies conducted on skin bleaching in two different geographic areas among **University students** in Nigerian revealed prevalence rates of 71.% in women and 53.3% in men; and 70.7% and 52.2% respectively.[4,5] Illiteracy or lack of education is therefore not the dominant factor contributing to skin bleaching. **Findings in Ghana and Nigeria show that even doctors and nurses bleach. Can these people be regarded as ignorant of the health risks of bleaching?** The demographic data of bleachers have shown that the level of education, social class, marital and employment status do not have any relevance to skin lightening practice in Africa. **Furthermore, bleachers hardly claim ignorance about the health risks of bleaching–Notable quotes from Nigerian bleachers are as follows:**

"Bleaching just makes me feel more beautiful and confident; "bleaching just makes me feel special, like I'm walking around in a spotlight "I am not seeking to be totally white. I just want to look beautiful. I cannot stop using the lightening agents" She believes fair skin could be her ticket to a better life.

"I have a very important party next week and I want to urgently whiten my skin before the day of the party because each time I attend partieswith my light-complexioned of friends, they get noticed ***instantly*** *by the men and get all the attention, which I don't enjoy." "It is not that I believe that those light complexioned friends of mine are more beautiful, but I want to get married. How do I get a husband if I am not attracted to men simply because of the dark colour of my skin?"* This shows that this lady does not perceive herself as ugly nor does she suffer from low self esteem **before** she bleached.

A young lady in Ghana whose life ambition is to become an actress in the film industry was told by the director when she presented herself for audition:

"You see that girl over there? The only difference between you and her is that she is fair-skinned. Actually, that's not true. You are a better actress, but we like to work with fair skinned women in our films.

Now, if you can tone your skin, we can consider you for future films."

A law student in a University who bleached said

'With all the warnings from the health sector, people still smoke. The same goes with campaigners against HIV/AIDS, people still engage in promiscuity. People will still bleach, no matter what.

What I am concerned with is how to maintain my skin tone."!

In an article titled "Ahoofe Kasa! Skin Bleaching and the Function of Beauty Among Ghanaian women," Blay describes that in Ghana beauty via light skin gained through skin bleaching allows the bleachers across to social capital, and for many, their new found light skin color becomes a "bartering tool" negotiable for economic capital. "Ahoofe Kasa" is a popular Ghanaian aphorism, which literally means "beauty talks"! It becomes clear that beauty acquired via light skin has a language which, though not vocalized, is nonetheless very powerful as a means of achieving upward social mobility.

Read the section on "**Skin Bleaching: A cry for help** in the chapter on Nigeria—Chapter 4). Read Chapter 6 on **THE MARRIAGE PRESSURE,** and the dehumanizing statements and experiences vocalized by the women in various countries. Read the sections on **Perspectives**, **Determinants** and **Motives** for skin bleaching in Kenya in Chapter 9. Kenya is a country which UNICEF says more than half the population lives on less than US$1 a day, yet women are lining up to pay US$70 per shot of serialized skin lightening injections which can result in HIV, Hepatitis C, Tetanus, Tuberculosis, permanent disfigurement and other very serious complications from mercury, corticosteroids, hydroquinone and other chemicals already highlighted in the chapter on COMPLICATIONS—Chapters 13, 14).

Kpanake,[3] Tunde Alao[7] and also Dorkenoo[8] also found that awareness on the health hazards of bleachers is no deterrent to bleaching.

The Public Health Partnership Forum in Zambia urged the government to ban the sale of skin-bleaching creams. The publicity secretary of the organization said, "skin-bleaching, being a psycho-social and health problem, needs to be addressed with interventions aimed at changing the user's perceptions of themselves and educating people on its consequences.[9] Skin-bleaching is defined as an individual problem that can be solved with education on a new attitude. Sentiments such as this are common throughout the discourse is emblematic of an individualist, attitude oriented perspective on bleaching.

> **Many female bleachers observe the acute correlation between race, skin colour and socioeconomic class and want to improve their opportunities in the local employment and marriage markets, as well as adopt a cosmopolitan, modern identity. It would be both unfair and inaccurate to assume that such women are simply hoodwinked, drowning in their own self-hatred.**
> Margaret Hunter[10]

As a function of living in a color-conscious society where people of darker skin tones are systematically and socially regarded as less desirable, individuals who fall within this group may begin to develop feelings of inferiority and internalize negative beliefs about themselves, come to value lighter skin tones, and reject themselves. The very real social and economic disadvantages attached to dark skin around the world feed into a compromised psychological sense of self. Disrupting this psychological damage requires addressing the large system by which dark skin comes to symbolize a lack of life opportunity. Given that the power attached to white skin globally has deep historical roots and is reiterated by contemporary popular media, this is not an easy paradigm to shift. It would be naive to expect women of color in the developing world to simply embrace their dark skin in the name of self-love and abandon skin-lightening practices.

> **A sustainable solution for countering the fundamental motivation behind skin bleaching requires disrupting the**

> **perceived link between disproportionately high life opportunity and fair skin—Colorism!**

What privileges does fair skin afford women in particular? Light skin tone can be transformed into social capital (social network), symbolic capital (esteem or status), or even economic capital (high-paying job or promotion).[10]

> **In a study of female school students in Ibadan, Nigeria, Durosaro[11] found that the girls perceived skin whitening as a route towards achieving a range of social and economic benefits. In addition to enticing men romantically, they believe bleached skin would enable them to "enter into connection with high calibers, attain high social standard, become more successful in life, look fashionable, express positive self-concept and be able to compete well with their male counterparts. Whether real or imagined, the perceived benefits of fair skin expand far beyond one's appearance.[10,12,13]**

> **Interventions to reduce the burden from skin lightening practices have to be a multi-pronged approach, pursued in concert and synergistically. Therefore, each component of the DETERMINANTS have to be studied and analyzed so that the various governments of each country can galvanize all the relevant stakeholders to formulate and articulate the methodology of activities of interventions before any meaning impact can be achieved.**

> **Bleachers want to be accepted within their circle of society; they want to be attractive to the opposite sex; they want career opportunities. But we are saying there are side effects and risks; we are saying is it worth the risk? We are saying must we adopt Eurocentric standards to achieve the above objectives? Surely there are excellent alternative pathways. These social, cultural, moral, psychological, economic and ethically acceptable pathways are discussed and proposed in the last chapter of this book entitled RECOMMENDATIONS —**Chapters 19, 20**.**

References

1. Delle Edmund. In: Dying to be white by Sylvia Arthur. *http//www.clutchmagonline.com/2008/01/dying-to-be-white.*

2. Gwaravanda, Ephraim Taurai. "Shona Proverbial Implications on Skin Bleaching: Some Philosophical Insights." *The Journal of Pan African Studies*, June; 29(3): 114. *http://www.jpanafrican.com/docs/vol4no4/Shona_Proverbial_Implications_on_Skin_Bleaching.pdfhttp://www.jpanafrican.com/docs/vol4no4/Shona_Proverbial%20I implications_on_Skin_Bleaching.pdf*

3. The "NCUR 2012 Research Survey" *Kpanake*, and Expert Interviews. Nina-Belle S. Mbayu. Skin Bleaching in Western and Central Africa: A Critical Analysis

Utilizing the Social Learning and Colonial Mentality Theories. *Proceedings of The National Conference On Undergraduate Research (NCUR)* 2012. Weber State University, Ogden, Utah March 29-31, 2012.
4. Ofondu EO. Cosmetic use of bleaching cream in Enugu. [*Nigeria FMCP dissertation*] National Postgraduate medical College, Nigeria, Nov 2003.
5. Ofili AN, Eze EU, Onunu AN. Prevalence of use of skin lightening Agents Amongst University of Benin Undergraduates in Benin City, Nigeria. *Nigeria Medical Practitioner.* 2006; 49: 24-7.
6. Olumide YM. Unpublished Data
7. Tunde Alao. Staff Reporter. Lagosians and the bleaching scourge. *The Guardian.* Thursday, February 6, 2003.
8. Tom Dorkenoo. In : Dying to be white by Sylvia Arthur. *http//www.clutchmagonline.com/2008/01/dying-to-be-white.*
9. Enock Kaputula. Ban sale of skin-bleaching cream—PHPF. *Zambia daily Mail.www://lusakatimes.com/2010/03/31/ban-sale-skinbleaching*
10. Hunter Margaret. Personal interview with Imani Franklin. Nov 2012.
11.Durosaro AI, Ajiboye Sk, Oniyo AO. Perception of skin bleaching among female secondary school students in Ibadan metropolis, Nigeria. *Journal of Education and Practice* 2012; 3(7): 40-6.
12. Imani Franklin. Living in a Barbie world. Skin Bleaching and the preference for fair skin in India, Nigeria and Thailand. Senior Honors Thesis Standard University. May 14, 2013.
13. Thomas Lynn. Phone interview with Imani Franklin. March 15, 2013.

xi) Cultural preference for light skin tone

See the chapters on:

(i) SKIN COLOUR PREFERENCE IN SUBSAHARAN AFRICA—Chapter 11.

(ii) NIGERIA: HISTORY OF SKIN BLEACHING —Chapter 4

(iii) COLORISM IN SUB-SAHARAN AFRICA—CASE STUDY NIGERIA—Chapter 11

(iv) COLORISM AND BLEACHING OF THE SKIN IN AFRICA—GENERAL COMMENTS RETRIEVED FROM SOCIAL MEDIA—Chapter 11.

xii) Advances in the technologies of the body, global economics and huge growth in the cosmetic industry

There is no doubt that there has been tremendous improvement in the **visible cosmetic** end result of the art of skin bleaching. At the inception of the bleaching syndrome in Nigeria, bleachers could only lighten the facial skin effectively, while the covered trunk, the arms and legs, the knuckles and the extensor surfaces of the elbows and knees remained dark colored. This glaring disparity in color gave birth to the derisive appellation – "Fanta face and Coca Cola legs." At that time also, the unsightly, waxy, dirty brown pigmentation of exogenous ochronosis (EO) on sun exposed areas and the offensive fish body odour due to the excretion of the chemical trimethylamine in the breath, urine, sweat, saliva, and vaginal secretions in exogenous ochronosis due to hydroquinone in the bleaching creams, were enough deterrents to make some people have a rethink before embarking on skin bleaching. (See the section on HYDROQUINONE AS A BLEACHING AGENT—Chapter 13).

However at the current stage of development in the art and science of skin bleaching, those who can afford it have access to better formulated products with sunscreen which do not cause EO. Furthermore, there are now available injectable forms and tablets of bleaching products which are used systemically and give a uniform, disseminated effect. This systemic bleaching agents and the "body works" in Spas, which have been described, give a rapid and universal body bleaching like the Nigerian-Cameroonian pop singer Dencia, whose cream "Whitenicious" was a sellout hit.[1] Surgical (Laser) depigmenting procedure is also available to give instant result. Laser depigmenting procedure leaves the skin permanently bleached without the need for repeated application of topical products. Although these latter procedures are very expensive, the wealthy women are able to afford them. Hence while the cheap old fashioned art of bleaching gives the face a sallow look like one wearing a mask of dirty clay, the current technology makes the bleachers skin atimes flawless like Caucasian dolls on display!

With increasing purchasing power and disposable income, the rapidly growing middle class in countries such as South Africa, Nigeria, India, and China no longer view the human body as "given," but increasingly see it as changeable. Rapid developments of technologies of the body, global economics and the huge growth in the cosmetic industry, have led more people to view light skin tone and Anglo features as traits that can be purchased for the right price.

It should however be noted that improvement in **cosmetic result** does ***not*** always translate into improved **safety** because the nature and long term safety of the new, often customized bleaching products, are not yet well defined, and the new methods of delivery—injections, tablets and highly chemicalized "body works" would clearly increase toxicity and adverse health effects. Details of this have been discussed under COMPLICATIONS AND ADVERSE EFFECTS—Chapters 13, 14.

Many young women perceive skin bleaching as a modern thing, like Botox, to fashion their body in a unique way. Yet in others, skin bleaching may be simply a personal choice like tattooing or it may be an indication of more pathological problems such as Body Dysmorphic Disorder. (See below).

Reference

Britni Danielle. Nigerian Singer Releases 'Whitenicious' Skin Lightening Cream and its sold out. Jan 20, 2014 http://www.xojane.com/issues/nigerian-singer-releases-whitenicious

xiii) Marketing and Selling of White Ideals by Cosmetic Manufacturers

Hegemonic representations of white skin are thoroughly rooted in multiple social institutions including education, religion, mass media, and popular culture.[1] The rise of skin bleaching around the globe can also be attributed to the constant, current mass-marketing of contemporary images of white beauty. Wealthy nations like the United States, Japan, and many European nations create many of the global images of white (or light) beauty.[2] In turn, these same nations are also home to the cosmetics companies that produce some of the top-selling skin-bleaching creams, including L'Oreal, Unilever, Schiseido, Vaseline, Emami and others.

The production and marketing of skin-lightening products offering the promise of lighter, and whiter skin has become a multi-billion dollar international industry.[3] Skin lightening has been incorporated into transnational flows of capital and culture and is implicated in both the formal global economy and various informal, often underground economies. Multinational corporations have jumped on the bandwagon and are spending large sums of money on research and development of both mass and specialised skin-lightening markets.[4]

The global beauty industry has reinvented itself in recent years in the image of multiculturalism. Many cosmetics companies that once exclusively featured white women have added light skinned women of color to their advertisements as spokespersons for their products. Hunter calls this maneuver the "illusion of inclusion".[5] The Illusion of inclusion is a seductive marketing strategy to draw in women of color who might otherwise feel alienated from products marketed exclusively with images of white beauty. By including a few light-skinned, Anglo-looking women of color,cosmetics distributing companies appear to be inclusive of people of color, without their message that white bodies are beautiful. The inclusion of fair-skinned women of color like Halle Berry of the US (Revlon), Aishwarya Rai of India (L'Oreal), Genevieve Nnaji of Nigeria (Lux soap), or Terry Pheto of South Africa (L'Oreal) is designed to lull women of color consumers into buying these products and believing that their bodies and beauty are being valued.[6]

Ironically as the marketing strategies have added a veneer of inclusion, there has simultaneously been a boom of products offered that all claim to lighten, brighten, or whiten the skin. Skin-lightening products are readily available from major cosmetics companies, from local mom-and-pop stores and widely over the Internet.

As this industry grows and more consumers are affected by its devastating consequences, ethical questions abound. Studies report the dumping of substandard products in the global south by overseas industries. Often these products were not passed for human use in their country of origin.[7] Many of the mercury soaps used by Africans are manufactured in the European Union (EU), where they are allowed to be manufactured as long as the product is exported. EU manufactured soaps are reportedly smuggled back into the EU where they are sold to African and Caribbean immigrant communities.[8] A number of third-world countries are believed to be used as off-shore production and distribution sites for Western-based pharmaceutical companies.[9] The South African, Zimbabwean, Gambian, Kenyan and Nigeria governments have banned the import and sale of mercury and hydroquinone products. However, these bans are often poorly enforced and difficult to control due to the fact that they are smuggled in from other African or European nations.[8] Products remain easily available in African cities where they are sold without medical prescription and control, hence fuelling the extensive and uncontrolled use of skin-lighteners. Counterfeit products and adulterations of branded products are commonly sold in backstreets or are even given out by physicians[5]. Scholars are critical of the Western medical community who have failed to intervene in the production and use of these skin-lightening chemicals and who seem to dismiss their use as an exclusively black problem.[9] In India and Pakistan, Fair and Lovely by Unilever still remain a popular brand despite the company being forced by the Indian government to withdraw television advertisements for the product as far back as 2007.[10]

References

1. Hunter Margaret L. Buying racial capital: Skin- bleaching and cosmetic surgery in a globalized world. *The Journal of Pan African Studies.* 2011; 4(4):
2. Burke T. Lifebuoy Men, Lux Women: Commodification, Consumption,and Cleanliness in Modern Zimbabwe. Durham, NC: Duke University Press. 1996
3. "Pell Research" *(https//www.pellresearch.com/cosmetics-and-Beauty-Products-Manufacturing.htm).* Cosmetic Manufacturing Report
4. http://frontiersnews.com/index.php/news/3636 exclusive-bleaching-...
5. Hunter M. 'If you're light you're alright: Light skin color as social capital for women of color. *Gender & Society.* 2002; 16 (2), 175-93.
6. Osuri G. Ash-coloured whiteness: The transfiguration of Aishwarya Rai. South Asian Popular Culture 2008; 6(2), 109-23. Consultancy Africa Intelligence (Pty) Ltd 2013
7. The colour conumdrum: Understanding skin-lightening in Africa.http://www.consultancyafrica.com/index.php?option=com-content&..
8. Glenn EN Yearning for lightness: Transnational circuits in the marketing and consumption of skin lighteners. *Gender & Society.* 2008; 22(3) : 281-302
9. De Souza MM. The concept of skin bleaching in Africa and its devastating health implications. *Clinics in Dermatology* 2008; 26: 27-9.
10. Mire A. Skin-bleaching: Poison, beauty, power and the politics of the colour line. *Resources for Feminist Research,* 2001; 28 (3).

xiv) Polyvalent claims. The concept of multi-tasking/multi functional beauty products

Examples of multi task

"This all-over body emulsion leaves your skin extra soft, extra smooth and extra beautiful, powerful ingredients like retinol, and emollients help boost skins natural collagen production and protects from moisture loss. The result is fully hydrated skin with improved texture and tone. An antioxidant rich complex with lactic acid softens rough patches. Skin feels perfectly hydrated, exfoliated and nourished".

In a world where every minute is rationalized, a simpler life becomes the Holy Grail. Downsizing the number of products needed to cover skin needs should also translate into a neat cost-benefit that may appeal to most people. Polyvalent cosmetic creams promise the following effects – provide moisturization, plus mattifying anti-ageing, soothing and healing properties, sheer coverage, "even effect" on skin tone as well as SPF protection (SPF¯Sun Protective Factor). Such polyvalence allows consumers to minimize the number of products they use and cut on time spent on their daily beauty routine. While some of the skin lightening products are simply marketed as "fairness cream" or "anti ageing cream", polyvalence may be desirable, they sound a bit commercial and opportunistic. More than ever, formulating has become a science with a hint of magic that, when mastered, creates beauty spells in a cream as the majority are extravagant marketing strategies making false, often unsubstantiated claims.

In order to appeal to the powerful discourse of "natural beauty" in many societies, most products claim to ***restore*** the natural beauty of skin (if it is lost), ***reveal*** the natural beauty of skin (if it is hidden), or ***create*** a natural beauty (if the consumer never had it to begin with). All of these claims are supported with compelling before and after photos and promises backed with the discourse of science in phrases like, "clinically tested" or "scientifically developed". Ads use phrases such as, "reveal your natural beauty" to appeal to consumers' need to ***feel*** like their achieved light skin is theirs by birthright. (See the section on SCIENTIFICATION OF SKIN WHITENING—Chapter 6).

Reference

Diane Bilodeau. How do you spell beauty? *Household Personal care (HPC) H & PC Today articles.* Home >H&PC Today > Vol. 9 (5) September / October 2014 *http://www.teknoscienze.com/Articles/HPC-Today-How-do-you-spe...*

xv) Aggressive Marketing Strategies

Advertisements create a need for skin-lighteners by depicting dark skinned women as unhappy, ignored by men and suffer from low self-esteem. Dark skin is presented as a burden or disease that can be cured with the use of skin-lightening products. Light skin is depicted as a necessity to being youthful, beautiful, modern and affluent[1]Hunniya Waseem[1]. Emergency physician, Public Health Solutions. Pakistan, while responding to Olumide on the editorial on bmj.com,[2] said

"In my country, Pakistan, the media plays a very negative role in promoting such cosmetic agents. Dozens of television adverts run day and night promoting creams and bleaches to make women fairer".

Advertising does not represent reality as it is, but as it should be. For this reason, advertising is a good site to observe dominant physical appearance ideals. Advertisements also depict the connections between complexion ideals, conceptions of gender roles as well as moral and aesthetic standards. In 2003-2004, Baumann[2] undertook a content analysis of 2133 individuals appearing in print advertisements. He found that on average women are portrayed as having fairer complexions than men of the same race. These genderdifferences in complexion highlight attractiveness ideals that are gender specific. Baumann also found that female models with darker complexions are more frequently overtly sexualized than the lighter skinned counterparts. They are also more likely to be depicted in intimate contact with a man. Lighter skinned women however, were statistically more conservatively dressed and were more likely to appear alongside other women. (See the section on THE MEDIA AS A MAJOR DRIVING FORCE OF SKIN BLEACHING—Chapter 6).

References

1. Hunniya Waseem. BMJ/12 February 2011; Vol 34:346.
2. Baumann S. The moral underpinnings of beauty: A meaning-based explanation for light and dark complexions in advertising. *Poetics*, 2008; 36:2-23.

xvi) Skin bleaching as a sign of non acceptance of one's cultural background

Skin bleaching can be a sign of non acceptance of one's cultural background due to the belief that the only standard of beauty is those defined by European ideals. Malcolm X once asked, *"Who taught you to hate yourself? Who taught you to hate the texture of your hair? Who taught you to hate the colour of your skin?"*

We were taught to hate ourselves through centuries of the slave trade (Arab and trans-Atlantic) and the colonial period that followed, and we are still being taught to hate ourselves through a Western consumer culture that is sold through today's global media. Many of those who don't go in for skin-lightening also tacitly accept the idea that lighter is better (particularly if it comes with European, rather than African, features), so we're all part of a system that promotes self-hate. When people defend skin-lightening/bleaching by saying what people do to their skin is their own business, it's usually a sign that they too value lighter skin over dark skin, whatever their own skin tone.

Does self-hatred sound too strong a term? What else is one to conclude when you have someone like South African kwaito star Mshoza proudly stating that she started undergoing skin-lightening and plastic surgery because she was "tired of being ugly"?

This internalized form of racism is an invisible presence in our psyches, and some of us don't even realize it's a factor in how we perceive ourselves and others. Thus, for instance, black guys (not only in Africa) think their attraction to light-skinned girls is just a matter of taste, and some who lighten their skin can't articulate why they do so beyond saying that it's just prettier, as though skin lightening were akin to putting on lipstick. It's a matter of identity, self-worth and self-acceptance that, in some respects, is even existential.

Reference

Siji Jabbar. Who taught you to hate your [dark] skin?" *This is Africa. https:thisisafrica.me/who-taught-you-to-hate-your-dark-skin/*

xvii) Skin bleaching as a sign of Body Dysmorphic Disorder

Skin bleaching may be simply a personal choice like tattooing or it may be an indication of more pathological problems such as Body Dysmorphic Disorder.

Body dysmorphic disorder (BDD) is a psychiatric condition in which a disabling pre occupation with a non-existent or slight defect in appearance is the main symptom. Indeed, no such defect is considered to exist by people other than the individual affected. However, these concerns lead to significant disturbance or impairment of daily functions, which differentiate BDD from simple concerns with appearance. Patients may typically be preoccupied with any part of the body, particularly the skin, hair, and parts of the face, such as the nose. Both the subjective criteria, as reported by the patient, and objective criteria, indicating the presence of a slight or imaginary defect, must be met for a diagnosis of BDD. In addition, patients must be free of any other psychiatric disorders that might cause preoccupation.

References

1.Mackley CL. Body dysmorphic disorder. *Dermatol Surg* 2005; 31: 553-8

2.Phillips KA, Mc Elroy SL, Keck PE, *et al.* Body dysmorphic disorder; 30 cases of imagined ugliness. *Am J Psychiatry* 1993; 150: 302-8

Chapter 6

Skin lightening Culture In Africa
Determinants II

Story highlights I-VI
The various paradigms posited for the phenomenon of skin bleaching
Motives for skin bleaching in Africa
The marriage pressure
Celebrity discourse: The good, the bad and the awkward
The media as a major driving force of skin bleaching
The Scientification of skin Whitening

Story highlights I

In order to understand the social, economic and psychological problems/conditions/complexes — *enemy within* — affecting individuals/families/organizations/communities and nations alike, which make people want to change their skin colour, various paradigms have been proposed.

The various paradigms proposed for skin bleaching are:

i. Colorism perspective
ii. Mis-education theory
iii. The Identity thesis
iv. Self hate thesis
v. Complex personhood explanation
vi. Colonial mentality
vii. The colonized mindset: The enemy within the African communities
viii. Post traumatic colonial African syndrome (PTCAS)
ix. Transgenerational trauma
x. Post traumatic slave syndrome: America's legacy of enduring injury and healing
xi. Mental slavery: the most insidious legacy of slavery
xii. Stockholm Syndrome (survival identification syndrome)
xiii. The Skin bleaching Syndrome

- In Africa the **motives** given for skin bleaching can be grouped under the following headings

Aesthetic and Beauty
Social domination
Attraction and Seduction
Fashion
Strengthening the self
Success
Compliances
Pleasure and Sensuality
Medical reasons

Story highlights II

The Marriage pressure

The single most important "social capital" for skin bleaching in Africa is a husband.

In all the countries studied globally, the most consistent motive for skin bleaching is to secure a husband. However this marriage pressure looms large in Africa for the following reasons

> — a woman's status and worth in the society is often tied to her marital status.
>
> — tremendous pressure is often put on single women by their families, churches and society to secure a husband
>
> —a large percentage of African women are not economically and politically empowered; hence they have to depend on their husbands for means of livelihood.
>
> —polygamy and de-criminalizing the law of bigamy make men see their wives as expendable partners in marriage. The onus is on the woman to do whatever it takes, even if it means altering her skin tone, to remain in her matrimonial home.
>
> —in most African cultures women do not have inheritance rights. Hence, if she chooses to divorce her husband for whatever reason, she is likely to be sent away empty handed.

- Some men in many cultures have a desperate desire that borders on manic obsessions for light skin women either as girlfriends or wives
- Undeniably, the burden to be attracted to the opposite gender, find marriage and remain happily married is a common thread that runs through all cultures
- It has been observed that some African men when interviewed about their preference for light-skinned women tend to deny the truth. Larry Modowo in Kenya calls them 'hypocrites'. However Indian men and men in Hong Kong clearly admit their preference for lighter skinned women.

Notable quotes

"Are Ghanaian men unwilling accomplices in promoting the lighter-is-better stereotype?"

"Many Black women were trapped in spinsterhood because Black men were sexually and romantically attracted to light-skinned women, who they took as marriage partners"

"We need to ask all the men out there why are they more attracted towards white women. This tends to create complexity among the darker skin colored women. We need to first of all change the mindset of men; and do not forget how much we all talk about women emancipation and empowerment; unfortunately it will always be a man's world."

"Lastly, we need to examine our African men's obsession with "white skin" or "light skin" women, and how their attitudes and behaviors toward our dark skin women drive our women to bleach their skin. We need African men to support dark skin women by embracing our blackness."

Story highlights III

Female Celebrity Discourse: The good, the bad and the awkward

• Celebrities, in context of Nigeria culture, are "highly visible people in the media. Media is defined as an umbrella term that encompasses television, movies, newspapers, magazines, music and various other forms of commercialized art including digital media e.g facebook, instagram, twitter etc." The celebrities in Nigeria are movie stars, models, female television presenters and news casters, female politicians and wives of politicians, musicians, winners of beauty pageants, leading women in the corporate world, some female Christian pastors and wives of pastors. Skin bleaching is highly endemic among these groups of people.

• The troubling message that the celebrities transmit is that those with fair skin go further. The entertainment industry disproportionately projects and elevates light-skinned women in magazines, films, music and commercials.

• There is no equivocation on the fact that the current wave of celebrity 'bleached beauties' in Africa has been a major driver of the bleaching culture. The media creates ideals in the form of celebrities and models, for women to admire.

- 5 reasons Nollywood celebrities give for skin bleaching are:
  - To look more beautiful/attractive
  - To increase their professional relevance
  - To attract the right suitors
  - The bandwagon syndrome
  - Looking good in photos

- Celebrity endorsements serve four important purposes: (i) when Celebrities endorse a particular product, the public is more likely to believe in its effectiveness and purchase the product; (ii) when celebrities endorse skin-lightening products they also endorse the act of skin lightening itself, suggesting that their own beauty is attainable and that itself, skin lightening is a mainstream, culturally acceptable act; (iii) celebrity endorsement forms a direct association between whiteness and experiencing success; (iv) the celebrity endorsers have a greater influence in reinforcing hegemonic whiteness due to their popularity.
- Some of the celebrities proselytize others to bleach because they use their celebrity status to start their own line of "skin care business" which **consistently** involves skin bleaching products.

- Undue publicity given to some of these bleached celebrities is doing more harm than good to impressionable youths.

• Dencia the popular Cameroonian singer, is a multitalented hip hop video model and an entrepreneur. Her whitenecious skin lightening products are packaged in small quantities for evening out skin tones and not for total body surface bleaching done by Africans. Those who patronize her products are largely African-Americans and Caucasians. She is engaged in philanthropy as she is building an orphanage in her home country. She believes in **inner** beauty, not just physical appearance. She takes her relationship with God seriously and she gives God the credit for her success in all her endeavors.

• Vera Sidika is a highly controversial Kenyan model who came under severe criticism after claiming that she spent $170,000 on skin lightening in the UK. She has also been criticized for acting in strange ways. She modified her boobs and butt and never ashamed to expose nude photos on social media. She has no **visible** source of income to sustain her extravagant lifestyle. Indeed she has been denounced for being a bad example to young impressionable Kenyans. Yet she is not fazed. Orie Rogo Manduli, a former Miss Kenya and an advocate for women's rights, named Sidika "the most despicable woman we have ever had in this country" and called for a media blackout on Vera's activities to protect young girls from her bad influence and misguided ways."

- **The Icons of black beauty are**
  - (i) Ajuma Nasenyana —a Kenyan model
  - (ii) Alek Wek—a South Sudanese British model
  - (iii) Lupita Nyong'o—Kenyan Hollywood actress and the Academy Award-Oscar-winner and Glamour Woman of the year for 2014.

Note!

Bleachers want to be accepted within their circle of society
Bleachers want to be attractive to the opposite sex
Bleachers want career opportunities
But what we are saying is there are side effects and risks with bleaching
We are saying is it worth the risk?
We are saying must we adopt Eurocentric standards to achieve the above objectives?
We are saying must skin color be the only barometer for defining beauty?
We are saying there are great black female achievers, globally, and in each country in Africa, who have retained their dark skin colour.
We are saying there are well known and many brilliant successful dark-skinned women who were the "it" girls in high school and college. They are ascending the corporate ladder while beating off suitors with a stick. We are acknowledging that dark-skinned beauty is not just possible, but actual reality.

We are saying pain has no colour—the fact is that when you're in pain emotionally about your life, the colour of your skin does matter.

Does dark skin prevent Alek Wek, Lupita Nyong'o, Ajuma Nasenyana from being household names today as Icons of black beauty?

Story highlights IV

The media as a major driving force of skin bleaching

The term "media" is an umbrella term that encompasses television, movies, newspapers, magazines, music, and various other forms of commercialized art including digital media e.g facebook, instagram, twitter, blogs etc.

> The media is a pivotal force through which cultural ideals are spread, articulated and internalized.

People who lighten their skin and those who associate light skin with positive virtues and dark skin with negative ones aren't stupid. They just don't have the psychological resources to withstand the deluge of images they are presented with every day.

White/light beauty is communicated through mass advertising, television shows, film, internet images, billboards, and celebrity culture. Images of white beauty do not simply rely on white women with blonde hair and light eyes to sell products. Images of white beauty sell much more than beauty ideals of fashions for women around the globe. Taken as a whole, images of white beauty sell an entire lifestyle imbued with racial meaning. The lifestyle that is communicated through these adverts sells whiteness, modernity, sophistication, beauty, power and wealth.

The media promotes hegemonic whiteness
The media promotes consumer culture
The media promotes cultural migration
The media fosters commodity racism
The media fosters a feeling of inferiority

Upon completing data collection and analysis, three major themes emerged: (1) advertisements use language to equate whiteness to perfection and beauty, (2) advertisements use celebrity endorsement to form a direct association between hegemonic whiteness and experiencing success, and (3) advertisements suggest darkness is a problem.

Story highlights V

The Scientification of skin Whitening

"The Scientification of Skin Whitening" is a term coined by Amina Mire[1] to describe the interlocking strategies of scientific entrepreneurialism and academic capitalism in cutting-edge innovations in molecular biology, biomedicine, and other life sciences deployed in research and the development of high-end skin whitening and anti-aging cosmeceuticals. Skin lightening has come to be associated with health promotion, self-enhancement and the fight against aging—a "disease".

• **Pathologizing** skin colour and ageing as "disease". The conceptualization of bodily imperfections, such as uneven skin tones, age spots, hyperpigmentation, and photo-aging are produced as signs of pigmentation *pathology*. As a "cure"designed to mitigate the signs of aging, skin whitening practice is often conceptualized as a biomedical strategy to *purify, restore*, and *cleanse* the signs of aging from the skin and faces of women.

• Start-up biotechnology firms in the sciences, Giant transnational cosmetics and pharmaceutical corporations, and public universities have entered into the research and development and mass commercialization of anti-aging and skin whitening products.

• Innovation in high-end skin whitening biotechnology are designed to turn academic-based innovations into lucrative spin-off business ventures.

•*Symbolic* prestige and financial rewards have been paired with the productions of proprietary marketable innovations.

• High-end skin whitening products are often labeled under the new quasi-pharmaceutical category called *cosmeceuticals*–cosmetics that provide **additional** health-related benefits so as to **evade** the rigorous premarket testing **before** they could be **legally** mass-marketed.

• One of the latest development in anti-aging and skin whitening discourses is prescribing a popular self-diagnostic device called SkinChip to women to determine the status of their skin(i.e. pigmentation and hydration levels). Another innovation is the introduction of a novel macro- and micromolecular system to increase the bioavailability of active agents%hence these products are **legally** drugs not cosmetics.

• Use of strategies to ensure a cooperative relationship with consumers:

1. Pathologization of dark skin colour and aging
2. Biomedicalization of women's bodies and skin
3. Innovative advertising strategies

• Consolidation of information on pharmaceuticals, food/nutrition, and cosmetics into **one** easily accessible online source. These corporations continue to make claims about how these cosmetics-foods nourish the body and *cure* signs of aging– e.g. "Dove Beauty Milk Chocolate". As a result, leading corporations in cosmetics, pharmaceuticals, and the food industry are already incorporating untested and unregulated nanotechnologies in their latest *skin-whitening* and anti-aging cosmeceuticals and "edible beauty food" and "cosmetic drinks"

- The powerful economic forces at play in the skin whitening anti-aging industry need to be understood and confronted. The manufacturing, advertising and selling of skin-lighteners has become a major growth market for multinational corporations. These corporations play a leading role in the creation and manipulation of needs and desires often overtly or covertly supporting and funding innovations in high end skin whitening biotechnology designed to turn academic based innovations into lucrative spin-off business ventures.

THE VARIOUS PARADIGMS POSITED FOR THE PHENOMENON OF SKIN BLEACHING

Introduction

Skin bleaching in Africa leads to dermatological, medical and neurological effects. Some dermatological effects are stria atrophicae, ochronosis, and various dyschromias, acne, skin atrophy, defective wound healing and fish odor syndrome. There are also reported systemic complications such as hypertension, diabetes, renal damage, adrenal insufficiency, neuropathies, immune suppression, irritability, insomnia, memory loss, vertigo and psychological and emotional complications arising from criticism and ridicule. A surface reading of these negative health outcomes may lead one to assume that skin bleachers must hate themselves because they use toxic products despite these outcomes and the available medical warnings. However, a deeper reading of the phenomenon suggests that there are powerful cultural triggers and institutions that influence the African skin bleachers to alter their physicality. Understanding the skin bleachers as sophisticated multidimensional individuals provides a means by which to engage them with culturally and psychologically appropriate interventions to address the negative health outcomes.

Various reasons have been theorized for skin bleaching. The phenomenon of skin bleaching is not like having a flue which if you treat the symptoms, the flue will eventually go away if the immune system is acute and alert. Several arguments have been theorized to explain the emergence of the bleaching culture so as to understand the social, economic and psychological problems / conditions / complexes—*enemy within* — affecting individuals / family/organizations/community and nations alike, which make people want to change their skin colour from black/dark to white/light. Any meaningful and sustained intervention can only be realistic if people are *truthful* about the reasons for skin bleaching. The utmost need to shun self deception informed the first article below published in **Cosmic Yoruba** entitled "Why are women playing down skin bleaching?

Why are women playing down skin-bleaching?

The point of this exposition is to illustrate that **Cosmic Yoruba** on July 31, 2014, published an exposition to illustrate that admiration of light-skin does not necessarily lead to skin bleaching. The title of the exposition is **"Why are women playing down skin-bleaching?"** The article is reproduced below.

The Daily Telegraph recently posted an article by a Nigerian lawyer suggesting that skin-bleaching is OK because women do it to be more attractive, and that's their prerogative. It's not the first time someone has defended the practice and missed the point. Sede Alonge's recent Telegraph article on the controversial topic of skin-bleaching was a half and half for me: while I agree with some of the points raised I disagree completely with others, and remain stunned by the essay's lack of insight as to why whitening of the skin remains so hot today. I had similar reactions when I read Bibi Bakare-Yusuf's take on skin bleaching among Nigerian women, in which she asserts that people who bleach their skin do not hate being Black and that blaming women's choice to bleach on "colonial mentality" denies their agency. It seems in an effort to boost and/or assert the confidence of African women in themselves and their beauty regimens, the historical roots of skin-bleaching are being pushed to the side. That such essays – written by brilliant and popular women–are published on websites with large readerships sends a dangerously incomplete message to young African women who bleach or are considering skin-bleaching.

African societies hypocritical stance towards skin bleaching

Firstly we must not deceive ourselves, a huge number of Africans prefer light skin. To confirm this, one only has to look at our music videos and the faces of many of our most popular celebrities. The confusing thing about this preference is that these are usually the same Africans who will turn around and chastise people for skin-bleaching. When a woman looks like she is obviously whitening her skin there will be much ridicule directed towards her, however, if a woman is fair-skinned (regardless of whether she is bleaching or not) she will be praised for her beauty. I have witnessed different reactions towards my complexion because of the ease in which I can bounce from one spectrum of the skin tone scale to the other. I get light enough to be considered "fair" in Nigeria during the winter and then go back to being my regular dark tone in other seasons. When I am lighter I never hear the end of compliments on how beautiful my skin looks, but when I'm darker it's "why are you so *black* now?"

Alonge claims that women bleach because that is what men find attractive, which in my opinion misses the point. The mothers who force their children to bleach their skin are not doing this to make their daughters attractive but because of their deep-seated belief that light-skin is aesthetically better. Some women may be bleaching because their mother is light-skinned and they are not, or because they feel that once they have attained a certain socio-economic class they need to "freshen" up their skin a bit. There are myriad reasons why women bleach today, yet these are all linked to the history of colonialism, trans-Atlantic slavery and the continued dehumanization of the African.

There is no such thing as "get over it" (or as Alonge writes "get beyond that") when an issue has remained topical for centuries and may remain so for centuries to come. One of the biggest delusions we suffer as post-colonial Africans is that we can easily get over the devastation of colonisation. Over 300 years of slavery, subjugation and ruthless oppression can apparently be solved in 50 or so years since we were "freed". Bleaching among African Americans started in the late 19th and early 20th centuries, the practice grew popular in African countries during the colonial era, becoming increasingly popular as a cosmetic choice in the 1950s. Today the spotlight is on Vera Sidiki, bleaching her skin and proclaiming that she is proud of the way she looks. Tomorrow it will be someone else doing the exact same thing, and it will generate the exact same response. Who remembers Mshoza and Dencia? The only way out of this conundrum is if those of us of African descent finally wake up and remove our mental shackles, but it is never that easy.

- **Trans-generational trauma?**

It has been suggested that the descendants of Africans who were forcibly enslaved in the United States still suffer from post-traumatic stress linked to the brutal treatment of their ancestors. Put forth by Dr Joy DeGruy Leary in her book *Post Traumatic Slave Syndrome: America's Legacy of Enduring Injury and Healing*, Post Traumatic Slave Syndrome is described as a condition that came about due to the extreme dehumanization of African slaves, leading to mental scars that are manifested in diverse symptoms which are borne by their descendants and passed on from generation to generation. Although Dr Leary's research is uniquely based on the experience of African Americans, when I first came across her work I wondered what kind of trauma could be borne by colonised people and that are manifested in their descendants. We may not have been there to witness directly how our ancestors were made to believe that everything about themselves including the way they look was inferior, yet we deal with confusion in navigating our identities. Could skin-bleaching be considered a manifestation of a kind of self-destructive impulse, especially due to the side effects of using harmful chemicals on the skin? As mentioned above, colonialism is something that is continually trivialised despite the fact that its effects are still felt today. Here we are discussing something that is directly correlated with colonialism and we are still expected to have gotten beyond that.

Imagine that in the pre-colonial past, there were African people who prized light-skin. Amadioha, the Igbo deity of thunder and lightning, is said to be the patron of light-skinned Igbos, and some scholars have argued that Igbo people admired whiteness before they encountered Europeans. Yet Igbo people do not have a tradition of skin-bleaching, at least not that I know of. Now skin-bleaching actually dates back centuries, some would argue that it is even a tradition. Indeed in diverse Asian cultures where light skin was associated with high class and wealthy living, there are traditions related to skin-lightening. A Korean friend once pointed out to me as we were cooking that using rice water to wash the face will make it brighter. I am not aware of any similar tradition among any African ethnic group. The point of this exposition is to illustrate that admiration of light-skin does not necessary lead to skin-bleaching.

Today apparently 77 per cent of Nigerian women bleach their skin. Can we truly believe that the rate would have been this high without the intervention of something catastrophic? The reality is that women of African descent started religiously attempting to whiten their skin upon contact with and conquest by pale-skinned foreigners. For us, preferring fair/light skin cannot simply be a matter of choice or aesthetics. We inhabit a world where white skin and Western European features have been established as the hallmarks of beauty and status. The justification of colonialism came from Europeans convincing themselves (and eventually others) that they were the height of human civilisation, and Africans the lowest. Women bleaching their skins to boost their image and self-worth clearly points to the fact that they regard their dark skin as lacking in some way, as inferior and less beautiful, which is something the generations preceding them learnt from mental colonisation. In a country like Nigeria, someone like Miss World South Sudan 2013, Modong Manuela Mogga ought to attract a similar level of attention as an equally attractive black woman at the other end of the skin-tone spectrum

If only we could divorce ourselves from that pesky thing called history

Considering this history, one cannot simply equate Black women bleaching their skin to white women going to a tanning salon. The only people who have outrightly said they are tanning to imitate Black people are the young Japanese that are part of B-kei (style) which appropriates African American hip-hop culture. Furthermore, white women started tanning their skins as part of a fashion trend, not because someone had colonised them and taught them to believe that everything about them was inferior. European women have a longer history of bleaching their skin than tanning it, in the past they doused their faces with lead to achieve the porcelain complexion that was considered the sign of a woman's modesty and virtue back in the day. White women did not start tanning because they admired the dark skin of African women, and unfortunately the few times white people do darken themselves in imitation of African skin tone is to ridicule us.

Alonge writes that "physical attraction is instinctive and lighter skinned women are bound to attract more attention from men in a dark-skinned society such as Nigeria – just like darker skinned people do in predominantly white societies." This does not make sense. If physical attraction is instinctive, and going by this logic, shouldn't women who are darker than the norm also attract more attention? In a society filled with people the same shade as Omotola Jalede-Ekeinde for example, someone like Eku Edewor would attract attention…but someone like Modong Manuela Mogga ought to attract a similar level of attention. If physical attraction is instinctive there is no reason for only light-skin to be preferred yet this is not our reality. No one has to say "white is beautiful" because there is no need to spell it out, we are told white is beautiful every time we open magazines, turn on the television or spend time online. That is why there is so much excitement from Black women worldwide when women like Lupita Nyong'o and Ajak Deng grace our screens.

The reason skin lightening is regarded as an outright rejection of Black identity clearly has to do with the history. Why should an African woman feel that lightening her skin will make her prettier or more confident? We need to ask ourselves, why do we bleach? Of course it is the prerogative of any individual to bleach or not to bleach, but we should not ignore the deep-rooted reasons we bleach in the first place. I believe that if you are doing something, you should at least be honest with yourself about the reasons you are doing it. If I decided that the reason I am yet to unlock the highest level of my self-worth is because I am dark-skinned, and then choose to bleach, I would be doing so with full knowledge of the history behind this act. I would do so knowing why people of African descent started bleaching their skin in the first place, and I would at least be truthful with myself in admitting that I cannot associate lighter skin with self-worth and in the same breath argue that I am proud of being Black and African.

With articles like Alonge's popping up every once in a while, one has to wonder, why this need to reduce skin bleaching to a matter of choice? Can we just be honest to ourselves and accept the history of this practice while continuing our "aesthetic" beauty treatments? I believe we can. It is not compulsory to view black as being beautiful, but to ignore the historical reasons behind such a view is erroneous.

Reference

Cosmic Yoruba. Why are women playing down skin-bleaching? July 31, 2014. *http://thisisafrica.me/skin-bleaching-post-traumatic-colonial-syndrome/*

Various paradigms for skin lightening

Skin bleaching is not mono-causal. Identity processes are more complex than rigid binaries and the desire for light skin is not necessarily synonymous with the adoption of white values, nor do they want to become white people. Various paradigms have been posited to explain why people choose to modify their skin colour. Thirteen scenarios ot thought processess have been described viz:

i. Colorism perspective

ii. Mis-education theory
iii. The Identity thesis
iv. Self hate thesis
v. Complex personhood explanation
vi. Colonial mentality
vii. The colonized mindset: The enemy within the African communities
viii. Post traumatic colonial African syndrome (PTCAS)
ix. Transgenerational trauma
x. Post traumatic slave syndrome: America's legacy of enduring injury and healing
xi. Mental slavery: the most insidious legacy of slavery
xii. Stockholm Syndrome (survival identification syndrome)
xiii. The Skin Bleaching Syndrome

i. Self hate thesis

Europeans colonized North America, Latin America, the Caribbean, the Middle East, Africa, and Asia-Pacific region through the use of military force and the subjugation of the local populations. Europeans exploited the resources of their colonies to meet their needs and accelerated this process by importing captive Africans to work on plantations in the Americas. The racist ideology that Europeans were "superior" to the "savage" and "backward" races that they subjugated justified their exploitation as "civilizing missions." The ideology of colorism accorded light skinned people in the colonies societal privileges over dark skinned people. Racism discriminated based on race and colorism discriminated based on complexion, and created a racial-complexion hierarchy with Europeans at the Zenith and non-Whites below. The institutional consensus projected that Europeans had "superior" culture, history, societies, intelligence, education, aesthetic physicality, values, and moral worth over non-Whites. The oppression and exploitation of the non-Whites for centuries socialized these people to hate themselves, which is revealed today in their yearning to be like their White masters[1].

This self hate thesis received empirical "support" from the famous doll study conducted in the United States. Black and White children were asked to select the doll that looks like them. Some 14% of the children in the total sample made anti-black statements. This finding was interpreted to mean that the oppression of racial segregation caused Blacks to hate themselves[2]. Since then there have been numerous "replications" of the doll study in many countries. The self-hate thesis explains skin bleaching within this framework of self-hatred: Blacks embrace the bleaching syndrome because they internalize the negative messages about Blackness, thereby hating them selves, and so desire to be like Whites[3]. However, high self-esteem scores of many people who bleach their skin suggest that the self-hate explanation of their behavior is wrong, and numerous subsequent theories have challenged the self-hate thesis as the reason for skin bleaching.

ii. Colorism perspective

Colorism is a persistent problem for people of color in the USA. Colorism, or skin color stratification, is a process that privileges light-skinned people of color over dark in areas such as income, education, housing, and the marriage market. The **colorism perspective** argues that the privileges given to people with light complexion in society influence other people to bleach their skin. The body The body becomes a site of survival in response to the complexion and racial hierarchies the society impacts people's life chances. Non-Whites experience racism across multiple domains, such as during housing purchases, securing loans and jobs, and in the criminal justice system. The influence of colorism which has its origins in colonialism, can be seen in the reasons given for skin bleaching such as beauty, spousal attraction, social status, and social mobility. Light skinned non-Whites earn higher incomes because it is said that they are more intelligent, beautiful, dependable, hardworking and trustworthy; they also possess greater marriage potential and social mobility compared to dark skinned non-Whites. Therefore, the colorism thesis argues that dark skinned non-Whites lighten their complexion to access some of the societal benefits associated with lighter complexion, rather than because of self-hate[4].

iii. Mis-education theory

The mis-education framework theorizes that non-white people bleach their skin because they have been educated about Europe and mis-educated about their own culture, history and the achievements of their race. Skin bleaching is linked to colonialism through mis-education rather than self-hate. The mis-education about non-Whiteness can be seen in the Whites curriculum that non-Whites are given in societies dominated by Caucasians and in the former European colonies. The mis-education of non-Whites is reinforced by the White-owned media that negatively frame the news about non Whites and the White-controlled churches that disseminate the view that God is White. Mis-education is pervasive because it has a long history, and the views expressed are often now considered normal.

This position then situates yearning for light skin by non-Whites in society as resulting from mis-education[5] rather than self-hate. The African Americans were being culturally indoctrinated, rather than taught, in American schools.

iv. The Identity thesis

The identity thesis argues that people who alter their complexion do so because they define themselves as light skinned people in the society. This identification with, and attachment to, light skinned people in society is not understood as self-hate, because they use light skin values to make sense of themselves and understand the world. These persons also transact or express their identity with people they interact with daily. This identity transaction occurs through the processes of buffering, bonding and bridging. People who tone their skin confidently buffer against critics by humoring them, cursing at them or ignoring them; people who offer compliments for the bleached skin are treated with warmth. Those who alter their complexion bond with the people who compliment them and bridge with strangers by finding common ground. The identity construction and transactions of people who bleach are theorized not as deficits but as psychological strengths[6].

References

1. Fanon F. *Black skin white masks.* 1967; New York: Grove Press.

2. Clark KB & Clark MP. Emotional factors in racial identification and preference in Negro children. *Journal of Negro Education.* 1950; 19, 341-350.

3. Hall RE The color complex: The bleaching syndrome. *Race, Gender & Class.* Journal. 1995; 2(2) 99-110.

4. Hunter ML. The persistent problem of colorism: Skin tone, Status, and inequality., 1, *Sociology Compass* 2007; 1(1):237-254.

5. Woodson CG. *The mis-education of the Negro.* Reprint. Book Tree, 2006.

6. Cross WE Jr. & Strauss L. The everyday functions of African American Identity In J. Swim & C. Stangor (Eds.), Prejudice: The target's perspective. 1998; pp267-279. San Diego: Academic Press.

v. Complex personhood explanation

The Complex personhood explanation posits that non-Whites who bleach their skin are sophisticated, integrated and multidimensional people who display strengths, resilience, weaknesses, confidence, fears and ambiguities as they go about their lives daily. It understands Non-Whites as having the will and desire to forge their own destiny. This will and desire was seen in slave rebellions, the strikes, riots and liberation wars in the European colonies, and the strong motivation of non-Whites to succeed after emancipation and political independence. The oppressed peoples were not understood as this because they constantly resisted their oppression. In the contemporary era, the people who bleach their skin do not see the definition of themselves as fixed; they see themselves as changeable. The people who modify their complexion are understood as strong and sophisticated people who see light skin as a shade of non-Whiteness, and who make strategic and rational decisions to accrue the societal benefits of light skin. Skin lightening is seen by the people who do it as modern expressions of body fashion and style. Persons who bleach live wholesome lives by having intimate-partner relationships, working, engaging in recreation, interacting with friends, raising children attending religious services, and serving their communities.[1]

Christopher Charles[2] argues that self hate is just one of the many reasons for skin bleaching and the majority of the skin bleachers do not hate themselves. He posits that the notion of complex personhood liberates skin from the mono-causal self-hate explanation. Identity processes are more complex than rigid binaries and the desire for light skin is not necessarily synonymous with the adoption of white values.

There are other works that also validate skin bleachers as complex persons. Blay[3] finds that skin bleaching in Ghana can be best understood by unpacking the social history and culture of the country. The motivational loci embedded in the narratives of the study participants revealed that skin bleaching is caused by colorism with its attendant symbols and functions. Skin bleaching is an expression of a cultural memory anchored in colorism and its antecedent colonialism; self-hate was not found to be a factor in Ghana. According to Blay, the source of skin bleaching lies in the cultural memes and institutions which guide the behavior of the skin bleachers. She posits that skin bleachers were trying to gain some social capital from lightening their skin.

Ajose[4] reveals some of the colorized cultural triggers in Nigeria. The reasons articulated by the skin bleachers for their action all point to the motivational loci anchored in colorism where light skin people are valued over those with dark skin in African societies. Skin bleachers report that they bleach their skin because they desire light skin, they want to even out their skin tone; and their male partners on whom they depend economically have a preference for light skin women.

Some skin bleachers reported stopping the practice because of unacceptable side effects, disapproval of family and peers, pregnancy and the financial cost of engaging in the practice. The skin bleachers' ways of speaking reveal that there are perceived social pressures and benefits that guide the behavior of the skin bleachers, which all point to the high social status and rewards of having light skin. Also, the fact that some skin bleachers were able to stop the practice for the varied reasons reported suggests that they did not suffer from the mental pathology because they seemingly have control over the self

In Charles, previous work in Jamaica,[5] the participants in Jamaica said that they bleach their skin to look "cool," become beautiful, and to attract a partner. They also reported that skin bleaching is popular and they like light skin, which is revered a "higher color." These reasons suggest that there are perceived social and physical benefits driven by the high status of light skin over dark skin in the society
Some research participants in Jamaica have low self esteem, a form of self-hate, but the majority does not. It is important to critically review some of the classic self-hate literature which informs the international discourse on skin bleaching. Self-hate is defined as a person's hatred for the self. Low self esteem which is defined as a person's low evaluation of the self is a form of self-hate.[6,7] Psychological scars that result from being members of a minority caste that is separated from the dominant White majority group. Case studies of Negroes reveal the mark of oppression, which is the internalization of caste and its effects.
The mark of oppression or self-hate is the legacy of slavery spurred by discrimination in the post-slavery era.

Negroes internalize an inferiority complex because of the colonial aberrations they experience. Likewise Memmi,[8,9] writing about the colonial relationship, argues that the colonizer manufactures the colonized, thus producing a dominated man. The colonizers circulate the cultural myths of the "inferior", "lazy", "wicked" and "backward" subjects which are internalized by the patriotic colonial subject. Memmi[10] argues that the self hating dominated man lingers as the new citizen in the post-colony which serves the formal colonial powers. There is cultural lethargy and the dominated man has been unable to solve society problems in the post-colony.

Ogbu and Simmons[11] and Ogbu[12,13] argue that there are two kinds of minorities in the contemporary United States: (1) immigrants who are *voluntary* minorities that migrate for better opportunities, and (2) *involuntary* minorities that have been conquered, colonized and enslaved and thus migrated against their will. Discrimination triggers *different* cultural interpretations between the two minority groups which influence their behavior. Voluntary minorities develop a positive dual frame of reference. This frame of reference sees opportunities for socioeconomic advancement because acquiring education leads to success. The comparative base of the voluntary minorities is their home country and they behave in accordance with the positive frame of reference. This positive behavior occurs in contrast to the pathological behavior of involuntary minorities whose negative dual frame of reference, based on their oppressive social conditions, tells them that America is not a land of opportunities where education leads to success. Thus, they engage in self destructive behaviors.

It is the *miseducation* of Blacks which emphasizes European values and achievements and ignores Black history, culture and achievements[14] and the diffusion of colorism globally[15] that links skin bleachers to the colonial past, not self-hate. The self-hate thesis is an inadequate construct to explain the problems of Black communities, including that of skin bleaching. Complex personhood is a useful construct to understand the practice of skin bleaching among Blacks.

Several Black African countries have banned skin bleaching creams and have embarked on public education programs to educate their populations about the negative dermatological, medical and neurological effects of skin bleaching. The banning of the skin bleaching products is a challenge to colorism. It is therefore not true that there is cultural lethargy in post-colonies.

The critique of the self-hate argument in the academic literature does not mean that European colonialism and plantation slavery does not influence Blacks who bleach their skin in Africa and the Diaspora. However, the links between the past and present must be clearly delineated which the self-hate thesis fails to do. *It is the miseducation of Blacks which emphasizes European values and achievements and ignores Blacks history, culture and achievements and the diffusion of colorism globally that links skin bleachers to the colonial past, not self hate.* The self-hate thesis is an inadequate construct to explain the problems of Black communities, including that of skin bleaching. Complex personhood is a useful construct to understand the practice of skin bleaching among Blacks.

Complex personhood argues that identity construction, negotiation, and maintenance are more sophisticated than the Black/White binary. Non-Whites who construct their racial identity by manipulating their skin color know that they cannot become physically white, and that they would not be socially accepted as whites, so these people are not striving to attain biological and social whiteness. These non-whites modify their skin color to make use of the complexion continuum that is salient in their culture. This use of the color continuum reveals lived complexities and intricacies and the analytical redundancy of a strict Black/White binary with which to understand racial identity. Recall that there are also whites who bleach their skin. Non-whites' use of the complexion continuum to create their version of who they want to be does not necessarily mean that these people have internalized white values, accents, dress, taste, or worldview (psychological whiteness). Many non-white who modify their skin color do not display the Eurocentric characteristics of whiteness.[16,17] The counterfactual argument also supports complex personhood because whites who tan their skin and braid their hair do not necessarily desire Blackness. Many minorities who assimilate into white dominated countries have low salience to Blackness rather than negative feeling and/or low evaluation of Blacks and other minorities.[16]

Complex persons do experience vulnerabilities. The deficit captured in the minority of skin bleachers who displayed low self esteem, a form of self-hate, could be due to major life events in the post-slavery environment that are unrelated to slavery. Some of these possibilities are the skin bleachers being unemployed for a very long time, experiencing a bitter divorce, experiencing trauma, experiencing abuse in a difficult relationship, etc. Therefore, a skin bleacher having low self esteem does not mean that this form of self-hate is linked to slavery.[5]

Despite the above appearances of vulnerabilities, contradictions and ambiguities, skin bleachers display inner strength. They defend or buffer the self by ignoring or cursing those who criticize them on the streets for altering their physicality. The power of language (the verbal defense of skin bleaching) and action (the goal-directed behavior) maintains the multidimensional self of the skin bleachers. Skin bleachers also bridge (talk with) and bond (treat like friends) with people who compliment them on the street for altering their physicality. Complex personhood argues that skin bleachers have agency and personal autonomy to alter the self and the psychic strength to defend publicly their choice of a lighter shade against their critics, while embracing warmly persons who support their personal autonomy.

Finally, complex personhood holds that despite the use of colorism to organize a self that varies from the hegemonic cultural expectations, careful scrutiny of the skin bleachers' daily lives reveal that the majority live integrated multidimensional (well-adjusted and fulfilling) lives as functioning members of their society. Skin bleachers by and large behave in relationships, social groups, organizations and cultural institutions in much the same way as do non-bleachers.

Charles concludes that one of the most popular causes posited for skin bleaching is self-hate. The notion of complex personhood seeks to deconstruct the complex lives of skin bleachers and liberate them from mental pathology. Complex personhood suggests a multidimensional integrated life and voice that display contradictions, vulnerabilities, ambiguities, purpose, fear, confidence, weaknesses, resilience and strengths as the person subjectively embraces the totality of his or her psychological deficits. *Complex personhood argues that self-hate is just one of the many reasons for skin bleaching and the majority of the skin bleachers do not hate themselves.*

The bleaching syndrome has not been empirically verified. The concept does not deal with the physical bleaching of the skin and the sophisticated and varied ways of constructing the non-white self. It should be noted that people have agency and many who bleach their skin do not want to become white as the self-hate thesis suggests. The power of colorism cannot be ignored. International cosmetic companies strategically market their products globally via the internet by tapping into colorism. *It is the pervasive nature of colorism and miseducation rather than self-hate that drives skin bleaching globally. In Africa the power of colorism is evident in the popularity of skin bleaching despite the known dermatological, medical and neurological consequences.* Colorism also drives skin bleaching in Jamaica where the self esteem studies refutes the self-hate thesis.

Thus, it is important to note that it is colorism and miseducation which links the skin bleachers to the past and not self-hate.

The notion of complex personhood liberates skin bleachers from the mono-causal self-hate explanation. Identity processes are more complex than rigid binaries and the desire for light skin is not necessarily synonymous with the adoption of white values.

Conclusion

Complex personhood states that skin bleachers have functional and multidimensional goal-directed selves with strengths, weaknesses, ambiguities, contradictions and resilience. This personhood liberates skin bleachers from mental pathology argument by (1) rejecting rigid identity binaries, (2) accepting their vulnerabilities which are separated from the trauma of slavery, (3) highlighting their black identity, (4) revealing their psychic strength and autonomy in their defense of their body modification and (5) articulating their daily optimal psychological functioning.

Complex personhood argues that self-hate is just one of the many reasons for skin bleaching and the majority of the skin bleachers do not hate themselves. It is the pervasive nature of colorism and miseducation rather than self-hate that drives skin bleaching globally. In Africa the power of colorism is evident in the popularity of skin bleaching despite the known dermatological, medical and neurological consequences. The notion of complex personhood liberates skin bleachers from the mono-causal self-hate explanation. Identity processes are more complex than rigid binaries and the desire for light skin is not necessarily synonymous with the adoption of white values."

References:

1. Charles CAD Representations of colorisms in the Jamaican culture and the practice of skin bleaching. Ph.D. Dissertation; Graduate School and University Center of the City University of New York. 2010.

2. Charles CAD. Liberating skin bleachers: from mental pathology to complex personhood. *JENdA: A Journal of Culture and African Women Studies* 2009; 14 : 86-100

3. Blay YA. Yellow fever: skin bleaching and the politics of skin color in Ghana. PhD. Dissertation. Temple University. 2007

4. Ajose FOA. Consequences of skin bleaching in Nigerian men and women. *International Journal of Dermatology* 2005; 44: 41-3.

5. Charles CAD. The Crowning of the Browning: Skin Bleaching and the representation of black identity in the context of dancehall music. *MA Thesis,* Hunter College of the City University of New York. 2006

6. Charles CAD. "Skin Bleaching, Self-hate and Black Identity in Jamaica," *journal of Black Studies,* 2003; 33: 711-28.

7. Rosenberg M "Old Myths Die Hard: The Case of Black Self-Esteem," *Revue internationale de psychologie Social.* 1989; 2: 355-65

8. Memmi A. *The Colonizer and the Colonized.* Boston: Beacon press. 1965

9. Memmi A. *Dominated Man. New York*: Orion Press. 1968.

10. Memmi A. *Decolonization and the decolonized.* Minneapolis: University of Minnesota Press. 2006.
11. Ogbu J & Simons HD. "Voluntary and Involuntary Minorities: A Cultural-ecological Theory of School Performance with Implications for Education," *Anthropology of Education Quarterly.* 1998; 29: 155-188.
12. Ogbu J Differences in Cultural Frame of Reference, *International Journal of Behavioral Development*, 1993; 16: 483-506.
13. Ogbu J. Collective Identity and the Burden of Acting White in Black History, Community and Education. *The Urban Review.* 2004; 28: 13-38.
14. Carter G Woodson (1875-1950) The Mis-education of the Negro. 1st Edition 1933 by Carter G Woodson.
15. Hunter M. The persistent problem of colorism: skin tone, status, and inequality. *Sociology Compass*, 2007; 1: 237-54.
16. Cross W E Jr .*Shades of Black.* Philadelphia: Temple 1991
17. Charles CAD. Skin bleaching, race and political identity in Jamaica. Unpublished Manuscript. 2005.

vi. Colonial mentality

A **colonial mentality**[1] is a conceptual theory around feelings of **inferiority** within some societies post-European **colonialism**, relative to the values of the foreign powers which they became aware of through the contact period of **colonization.** The concept essentially refers to the acceptance, by the colonized, of the culture or doctrines of the colonizer as intrinsically more worthy or superior. The subject matter is quite controversial and debated. Colonial mentality in men can be displayed in how a brown man places higher or lower value on a woman as a partner based on skin color or race. It can also be displayed in the brown person's insecurity about the way that they look as a brown person. Such as being ashamed of skin color, facial features, and if the ethnic group has curly hair, also being insecure about their curly hair. People who suffer from a colonial mentality, often times do not realize that they have one and could become defensive when confronted on it. A colonial mentality usually affects people of color and can also be found amongst biracial people. It's psychological damage as a result of the society they live in. One way for the person who suffers from this mentality, to overcome this mentality, is to realize that they have it, and work towards self love and overcoming their inferiority complex.

Origins

Throughout human history, nations and peoples have continuously colonised and been colonised. It is said that when a foreign **colonial** or **imperial** power is too strong to be effectively resisted, the colonised population often has no other immediate option than to accept the rule of the **foreigners** as an inescapable reality of life. As time progresses, the colonised **indigenous people**—natives would perceive the differences between the foreigners and themselves, between the foreigners' ways and the native ways.

This would then sometimes lead the natives to mimic the foreigners that are in power as they began to associate that power and success with the *foreigners' ways*. This eventually leads to the *foreigners' ways* being regarded as the *better way* and being held in a higher esteem than previous indigenous ways.

In much the same fashion, and with the same reasoning of *better-ness*, the colonised soon equates the foreigners' racial strain itself as being responsible for their *superiority*. The native soon strives to that strain to give their children a *better* standing in life than just their native genes.

United States; Black America

The **race-**conscious society of the United States is often cited as a prime example of colonial mentality. Numerous examples included the "**one drop rule**" and practice of the "**Paper Bag Test**", where **African Americans** were allowed or denied entry in Black-only social institutions (bars, night clubs, cinemas, sororities, fraternities, etc.) based on how light the skin tone was when compared to a brown paper bag. Those African Americans with skin tones the same or lighter than the paper bag were allowed entry. This practice of institutionalized **colorism**, favoring degrees of "whiteness", was exemplified more so by "**The Blue Vein Society**".

Black is Beautiful

In the late 20th century, the "Black is Beautiful" movement attempted to counteract the colonial mentality among African Americans by promoting dark skin and African features as ideals, with varied success.

Physical consequences

One of the more adverse physical consequences in the idealization and acceptance of the racial concepts of colonial mentality can be seen in the high rate of consumer demand for **skin bleaching** products used by some indigenous women, also with a smaller percentage of indigenous men and brown-skinned mestizas and mestizos, in the Philippines.[2,3] Skin-whitening creams have for a long time been popular and widely used in much of the Philippines for the lightening of the skin tones in order to achieve the so-called "**Mestizo** look".

The products are believed to be used primarily by women who have succumbed to the Filipino ideal and colonial doctrine of the idealization of mestizo beauty to the greatest extreme. The consumers of these products, whether conscious or subconsciously, are following the dangerous edict on beauty by continuing to use those products despite the extremely hazardous side effects to their health, including a high risk of various cancers due to many of its active ingredients, including **mercury**, and most important cancer, skin cancer, because of the lack of melanin that is the natural skin protection from the ultraviolet rays.

These skin products' sale and demand in the Philippines and in some other tropical countries continues to be widespread.[4] Another thought to achieve the so-called "Mestizo look", some indigenous Filipino men and women of all classes dye their hair auburn (reddish-brown), **golden brown**, or **blond**, and/or **changing their noses** to **aquiline**, and/or **enlarging their eye shapes**

References

1. Colonial Mentality.
https://en.wikipedia.org/w/index.php?tittle=/Colonial_mentality&oldid=682327962
2. American Chronicle l Brown is Beautiful
http://www.americanchronicle.com/articles/viewArticle.asp?articleID=11261
3. Counter S Allen. Whitening skin can be deadly.
http://www.boston.com/news/globe/health_science/articles/2003/12/16/whitening_skin_can_be_deadly/ Boston Globe. 16 December 2003
4. The Beauty in Me. *http://www3.niu.edu/ptaa/beauty-in-me.htm*

vii. The colonized mindset

The colonised mindset: The enemy within the African communities.[1]

The writer is going to put forward an argument that unless the slave/colonial mindset is recognised as the active enemy, within the African communities world-wide, attempts to understand the social and economic problems will be useless. This mindset has been affecting the individual/family /organisations/community and nations alike. From an early age, adults have been referring to people as having "being colonial or slave minded" in a most benign way. It is as if having this mindset is like having a flue. You treat the symptoms and eventually, it should go away, if the immune system is acute and alert. ***In reality, the colonized mindset is the most virulent***

psychological condition prevalent amongst African communities.[1]

History[1-7]

The disastrous effects of slavery and colonialism on the physical aspect of the Africans in the Americas, the Caribbean and on mainland Africa have been well documented by a host of European and African-American historians including Basil D Davidson, Walter Rodney and Professor Jeffries. Few writers have focused on the debilitating effects of the mindset on the emotions and the psychology as Carter G Woodson(1875-1950)[6] who was probably a pioneer when he addressed this condition in his book - **The Mis-Education of the Negro**. Later, Dr Na'im Akbar painstakingly outlined the psychological effects in his book–**Chains and Images of psychological slavery**.[2]

According to Peter D'errico,[8] The interesting—and complicated—thing about colonialism is that it encompasses not just politics and economics, but consciousness. Critical theorists such as Frantz Fanon and Paulo Freire have pointed this out. Fanon, a black man born in the French colony of Martinique, became a world-renowned psychoanalyst and philosopher, working in Algeria. He wrote, "*For a colonized people the most essential value, because the most concrete, is first and foremost the land: the land which will bring them bread and, above all, dignity*" [The Wretched of the Earth]. Fanon's study of psychology and sociology led him to the further conclusion that colonized people perpetuate their condition by striving to emulate the culture and ideas of their oppressors. He wrote, *"Imperialism leaves behind germs of rot which we must clinically detect and remove from our land but from our minds as well."*

Patrice Lumumba, the first indigenous leader of the Republic of the Congo, called for mental decolonization in his speech to the 1960 Pan-African Congress, saying we have to *"rediscover our most intimate selves and rid ourselves of mental attitudes and complexes and habits that colonization … trapped us in for centuries."* Lumumba thought it possible to work together with the former Belgian oppressors; for their part, they saw him as an enemy and facilitated his assassination.[8]

Examples of the colonized mind[1]

This mindset certainly has a blindfolding effect e.g African girls aspiring to be like their "blonde Barbie dolls". African men dream of marrying "a Barbie doll" type of woman as soon as they arrive in

Europe and or UK/USA/Canada, so as not to have "too black" children. The mindset nutures self-hating, self-destruction and confidence lowering. This is evident in the practice of self-harming through bleaching the skin, straigthening the hair and looking to Europe and European institutions as saviours. It also makes killing each other almost acceptable.

What do we begin to do?[1]

The logical place for decolonisation to begin is in the home, with parents taking the lead. The early years 0-11 is the crucial time to inculcate the Afrocentric values. It means that, we have to be prepared to build our own nurseries and create our own culturally inclusive and sensitive curricula. The parents must be re-educated. It is almost pointless waiting until a child becomes an adult, when he may or may not be exposed to Pan-Africanism. All the research available would agree that, the pre-natal and early years are the most important educating years. Ideally, the decolonisation ideals should be embedded in the early years curricula, The Community leaders and families should make attempts to discuss post trauma syndrome and it's effects openly and proactively put into place some short term and long term remedies.

Comment posted in response to the above article[8]

Interesting article with certain assumptions that, in my opinion, miss the point of "how to be free." The argument that there are only two choices (oppressor/oppressed) is incomplete. "Colonialism" is a fact of life in the world at large, within nations, within communities, within families, within tribes, within corporations, within awareness organization, within universities, within political groups...any human organization. "Colonialism" meaning domination of one over the other. The most critical ingredients of freedom are *truth*, *justice* and *righteousness* (responsibility) otherwise one oppressor is traded for another.

References

1. What is the colonized mindset? The enemy within the African communities. July 23, 2006. http://answers.yahoo.com/question/index;-ylt=AOLEVw7bLg5WTRU

2. Cheryl Sanchez mailto:sanchez-@hotmail.com sendmey-@earthlink.net . July 23, 2006.

3. Akbar Na'im. Chain and Images of psychological slavery- *Winston-Derek, Nashville, TN.* 1992.

4. Blumm W. Rogue State: Chapter 17. *Zed Books London UK.* 2003.

5. Brittain V Death and Dignity: Angola's Civil War. Chapter 2. *Pluto Books. London UK.* 1998.
6. Woodson Carter G. (1875-1956). The Mis-education of the Negro. *Africa World Press NJ USA.* 1937. 1st Edition 1933.
7. Wright BE.The psychopathic racial personality and other essays. *Third World Press Chicago, Ilinois USA.* 1984.
8. Peter D'errico. What is a colonized mind*? Indian Country Today Media Network.com.* Dec 12, 2011. http://indiancountrytodaymedianetwork.com/2011/12/12/what-coloniz..

viii. Post Traumatic Colonial African Syndrome—PTCAS

The Post Traumatic Slave Syndrome (PTSS)[1] is, " a theory that explains the etiology of many of the adaptive survival behaviors in African American communities throughout the United States and the Diaspora. It is a condition that exists as a consequence of multigenerational oppression of Africans and their descendants resulting from centuries of chattel slavery. A form of slavery which was predicated on the belief that African Americans were inherently/genetically inferior to whites. This was then followed by institutionalized racism which continues to perpetuate injury."[1]

Racial Theory[2]

In 1735, Carl von Linneaus (1707-1778) released "Systema Naturae," a book of nomenclature creating biological classifications. In the book, Linneaus also classified various races of people, and at one point argued that Black-Africans were inferior to other races. In 1786, Thomas Jefferson, who studied Linneaus' work, wrote "Notes on the State of Virginia." Having adopted Linneaus' thoughts on the inferiority of Black- and Native-Americans, Jefferson used these ideals to promote the institution of slavery. Jefferson's work used both physiological and anatomical characteristics of Blacks as evidence to support his belief of inferiority. Jefferson further commented on the mental capacity of Blacks, saying:

Comparing them by their faculties of memory, reason, and imagination, it appears to me, that in memory they are equal to whites; in reason much inferior, as I think one could scarcely be found capable of tracing and comprehending the investigations of Euclid; and that in imagination they are dull, tasteless, and anomalous.

Colonialism[3] is the establishment, exploitation, maintenance, acquisition, and expansion of colony in one territory by a political power from another territory. It is a set of unequal relationships between the colonial power and the colony and often between the colonists and the indigenous population.

The *European colonial period* was the era from the 16th century to the mid-20th century when several European powers established colonies in Asia, Africa, and the Americas. At first the countries followed mercantilist policies designed to strengthen the home economy at the expense of rivals, so the colonies were usually allowed to trade only with the mother country. By the mid-19th century, however, the powerful British Empire gave up mercantilism and trade restrictions and introduced the principle of free trade, with few restrictions or tariffs.

As Post Traumatic Slave Syndrome (PTSS) exists, an observer in Bamako propose in Bamako Journey Post that **Post-Traumatic Colonial African Syndrome (PTCAS)**[4] exists as well. As I traveled throughout West Africa, I've noticed a willingness to embrace Westernized concepts while outwardly demonizing traditional African concepts. The very justification for colonialism and slavery are embedded in dehumanizing traditional African culture and concepts.

Colonization and Slavery were the most inhumane, brutal and uncivilized acts in world history and the trauma still exists in many of the descendants of these atrocities.

In my opinion, one extreme form of the Post-Traumatic Colonial African Syndrome would be skin bleaching. Just imagine the internal hate that one possesses to actually risk their health by bleaching their skin.[5]

According to a report published by the World Health Organisation (WHO) in June, 77% of women in Nigeria use skin-lightening products, the world's highest percentage. That compares with 59% in Togo, and 27% in Senegal.

It became an increasingly popular practice among African women in the late 1950s. And it is a lucrative business. The industry is set to be worth $10bn globally by 2015, according to a recent report by Global Industry Analysts. In Nigeria, skin lightening can cost anything from a few dollars for a cream or soap to hundreds of dollars for a treatment in a beauty parlour, and the increasing westernisation of young Nigerian women has bolstered the demand for more expensive products.

But the trend comes with hazardous health consequences. Many products contain mercury and hydroquinone, which can lead to kidney damage, skin rashes, discolouration and scarring. Excessive use may even cause psychological problems, according to the WHO report.

While in Bamako, I saw a lady with dark brown toe and finger knuckles and very bright skin, signs of bleaching. As Fela says, "You dey Bleach o You dey Bleach, Yellow Fever, Stupid Thing, Ugly Thing." It's time for us to wake-up.

References

1. Joy Degruy Leary. Post Traumatic Slave Syndrome: America's Legacy of enduring injury and healing. *Uptone Press* 2005. ISBN 978-0963401120
2. Excerpt from: Linneaus to Lewis: A Brief Examination of Racial Theory (Rachel D. Maree, M.P.H. / 2012 M.D. Candidate, Medical University of South Carolina). *http://jsnma.org/2010/09/from-linneaus-to-lewis-a-brief-examinition-of-racial-theory/*
3. Colonialism. *https://en.m.wikipedia.org/wiki/colonialism.*
4. Post Traumatic Colonial African Syndrome. *Bamako Journey Post # 3 http://www.ibeafrikanoriginal.com/?p=250*
5. Excerpted from The Economist.com *http://www.economist.com/blogs/baobab/2012/09/beauty-nigeria.*

ix. Transgenerational Trauma

Transgenerational trauma[1] is trauma that is transferred from the first generation of trauma survivors to the second and further generations of offspring of the survivors via *complex post-traumatic stress disorder* mechanisms. **Enslavement and slavery, civil and domestic violence, sexual abuse, and extreme poverty are also sources of trauma that can be transferred to subsequent generations**

History

Soon after descriptions of the so-called *concentration camp syndrome* (also known as survivor syndrome) appeared, clinicians observed in 1966 that large numbers of children of Holocaust survivors were seeking treatment in clinics in Canada. The grandchildren of Holocaust survivors were overrepresented by 300% among the referrals to a child psychiatry clinic in comparison with their representation in the general population.[2]

The phenomenon of children of traumatized parents being affected directly or indirectly by their parents' post-traumatic symptoms has been described by some authors as *secondary traumatisation* (in reference to the *second generation*). To include the *third generation*, as well, the term intergenerational transmission of trauma was introduced. Building upon the clinical observations by Selma Fraiberg, child trauma researchers such as Byron Egeland, Inge Bretherton, and Daniel Schechter have empirically identified psychological mechanisms that favor intergenerational transmission, including dissociation in the context of attachment, and "communication" of prior traumatic experience as an effect of parental efforts to maintain self-regulation in the context of post-traumatic stress disorder and related alterations in social cognitive processes.[3,4,5,6,7]

Both survivors and immediate witnesses of traumatic events in family history have traditionally been treated by family therapists. The first-generation experiences of combat veterans, hostages, prisoners of war, and the civil population who was victimized at the hands of war criminals from genocidal organizations such as the German Nazi Party, Italian Fascist party, and similar organizations and their (para-)military arms, have been dealt with within the confines of political arena and international law, however the descendants of both immediate witnesses and victims of genocide, colonial suppression, slavery, political totalitarian control, clerical abuse in religious organizations, and many survivors of terrorism had to deal with the victimization symptoms themselves, without the transfer of original trauma being recognized and help offered.

Trauma transmission

Previous research assumed that the trauma transmission was mainly caused by the parents' child-rearing behavior, however, it may have been also epigenetically transferred.[8]

References

1.Transgenerational trauma—Wikipedia, the free encyclopedia. *https://en.wikipedia.org/wiki/Transgenerational_trauma#Trauma_trans,,.*

2. Fossion P, Rejas M, Servais L, Pelc I, & Hirsch S. "Family approach with grandchildren of Holocaust survivors," *American Journal of Psychotherapy,* 2004; 57(4): 519-527.

3. Fraiberg S, Adelson E, Shapiro V. Ghosts in the nursery. A psychoanalytic approach to the problems of impaired infant-mother relationships. *Journal of the American Academy of Child & Adolescent Psychiatry.* 1975; 14 (3): 387-421.

4. Egelan B, Susman-Stillman A. Dissociation as a mediator of child abuse across generations. *Child Abuse Negl.* 1996; 20 (11):1123-32.

5. Bretherton I. Communication patterns, internal working models, and the intergenerational transmission of attachment relationships. *Infant Mental Health Journal,* 1990; 11(3): 237-251.

6. Schechter DS. Intergenerational communication of maternal violent trauma: Understanding the interplay of reflective functioning and posttraumatic psychopathology. In SW. Coates, JL. Rosenthal and DS. Schechter (eds.) *Trauma and Human Bonds. Hillside, NJ: Analytic Press, Inc.* September 11, 2003; 115-42.

7.Schechter DS, Zygmunt A, Coates SW, Davies M, Trabka KA, McCaw J, Kolodji A, Robinson JL. Caregiver traumatization adversely impacts young children's mental representations of self and others. *Attachment & Human Development,* 2007; 9 (3): 187-205.

8.Kellermann N. Epigenetic Transmission of Holocaust Trauma, *Isr J. Psychiatry*, 2015; 50, (1): 33-9.

Further reading

- Coffey R. Unspeakable truths and happy endings. *Sidran Press.* 1998. ISBN 1-886968-05-5
- Danieli Y. (Ed.). International handbook of multigenerational legacies of trauma. *New York: Plenum.* 1998
- Daud A, Skoglund E. & Rydelius P. Children in families of torture victims: transgenerational transmission of parents' traumatic experiences to their children. *International Journal of Social Welfare.* 2005; 14: 23-32.
- Degruy J. Post Traumatic Slave Syndrome: America's Legacy of Enduring Injury and Healing. *Uptone Press.* 2005. ISBN 978-0963401120
- Fossion P, Rejas M, Servais L, Pelc I. & Hirsch S. Family approach with grandchildren of Holocaust survivors. *American Journal of Psychotherapy.* 2003; 57(4): 519-27.
- Herman JL. Trauma and recovery: The aftermath of violence from domestic abuse to political terror. *New York: Basic Books.* 1997
- Schwab G. Haunting Legacies: Violent Histories and Transgenerational Trauma. *Columbia University Press.* 2010
- van der Kolk BA, Roth S, Pelcovitz D, Sunday S, & Spinazzola J. "Disorders of extreme stress: the empirical foundation of a complex adaptation to trauma". *Journal of Traumatic Stress.* 2005; 18: 389-99.
- Plaskon Kyril D. Silent Heroes of the Cold War. 2015. ISBN 1507884664. https://www.createspace.com/5303636

x. Post Traumatic Slave Syndrome (PTSS): America's Legacy of Enduring Injury and Healing[1]

(PTSS) is a 2005 book by Joy DeGruy (formerly Leary)[2] *PTSS* describes a set of behaviors, beliefs and actions associated with or, related to multi-generational trauma experienced by African Americans that may be inclusive of but not limited to undiagnosed and untreated Post Traumatic Stress Disorder (PTSD) in enslaved Africans.

PTSS is an explanatory theory which posits that centuries of slavery in the United States, followed by systemic and structural racism and oppression, have resulted in multigenerational maladaptive behaviors, which originated as survival strategies. The syndrome continues because children whose parents suffer from PTSS will often be indoctrinated into the same behaviors, long after the behaviors have lost their contextual effectiveness.

The author states that PTSS is not a "disorder" that can simply be treated and remedied clinically but rather must necessarily require a profound social and structural change in Americans and American institutions that continue to promote inequalities and injustice.

Reference

Post Traumatic Slave Syndrome: Retrieved from
https://en.wikipedia.org/w/index.php?title=Post_Traumatic_Slave_Syndrome&oldid=68381603

xi. Mental Slavery: The Most Insidious Legacy of Slavery

"Mental slavery is a state of mind where discerning between liberation and enslavement is twisted. Where one becomes trapped by misinformation about self and the world. So someone can claim to be conscious, they can read all the books, they can recycle the popular rhetoric but still be unable to balance real-world priorities and self-interest"

- *"Mental Slavery is far more sinister than physical slavery because the chains are invisible and are transmitted across generations."*

If African slavery was only physical, African people would have within one generation been able to skip the plethora of socio-economic issues which plague African people globally the second the chains came off.

Slavery, and other institutionalized forms of targeted race-based oppression has caused certain symptoms of dysfunction in the African community, which has been reinforced in each generation. The legacy of slavery has promoted and nursed the direct association between being African and being inferior, being African and being unequal, incapable and less worthy. It also promotes ways of thinking which continue to impede growth and development. Such as cultivating dependence and reactive behaviors. More content to be at best an observer complaining about the world, as opposed to being a change agent in the world Content to be histories permanent victim. Every possible solution is dismissed with yet another trite excuse.

- *"Emancipate yourselves from mental slavery. None but ourselves can free our minds"* **Bob Marley**

Mental slavery affects how people see their own reality. This manipulation has always been through mainstream media, religion, and education. So the opinions about reality are sourced—without any suspicion—from the very same people that said Africa was bursting with primitive cannibal savages; a place of no history, a place of no humanity—the dark and savage continent. And via these mass indoctrination devices the very same imperialistic colonial powers are still (without change in strategy) stating that; without Western "help" you have no hope, our ways are the best ways, our goods are the best goods, and our 'human rights' (aka quest for more oil) is good for you, you are better off with us, than with your own people. People remain gullible to the "gospel" of their former enslavers—despite all the sordid history in evidence. So the root of mental slavery is ignorance resulting in a poor grasp of information about self and the world, to function to one's full human potential.

When someone is mentally enslaved they do not understand the guys dressed in fire protection gear, with fire hose, breaking down their door to rescue them from the fire and saving them. That is why mental slavery is worse than physical slavery. Because, at least during Physical slavery, if you got on board the slave ship and start breaking the chains and taking people back to Africa they would all thank you and call you a liberator. Today, trying to free people mentally enslaved you get called names while they run away from you deeper into oppression.

It is critical that we understand the slave mind: not the slave mouth. You can train someone to say anything; they can say "I am 100% for transforming African people" but deep inside the mind is that little slave who only wants "a more comfortable cage". So when African agency and African economics hit reality they freeze up and go into slave attack mode to preserve the cage environment.

During slavery the scraps and leftovers of food and apparel went to the enslaved Africans. Today the crumbs, the fat from the used bones of Western propaganda still are staples of the diet of the subaltern. Blind allegiance to a system which has no recourse to any sort of higher human values. Copied aped, celebrated and applied by free men and women under 'independent' flags and anthems all over the world; almost oblivious to their re-applying the machinery of oppression.

- *"Mental slavery blocks the connection between us and liberation"*

So what being oppressed means in the broadest and most salient terms is the occupation of ethics, logic, and culture, thought process, long term thinking, critical thinking, and paradigms by those of the oppressor's. So the beauty standard which is applicable to the European aesthetic is transferred, without modification, regardless of the incongruous state of beauty that is to the oppressed. These models of beauty are desperately adopted—at all cost. Mental slavery created an inability to make reference to self, so that in both the contemporary and historical context identities, even those under the banner of "liberation," are corrupted and sit upon the very platform of their oppressors paradigms, for the benefit of that oppression. Liberation within the structures that created the African "Other" is therefore relative—not absolute. The discourse on post-traumatic slavery syndrome, popularized by Joy Leary, is part of the study of mental slavery. While that study looks for biological connectivity to the genetic ancestors of African people, this study reports on the patterns in human behavior, which includes economics, socialization, formal and informal relationships, ideology, work ethos, and all other related areas of people activity.

- *"When you show a mental slave freedom they are more likely to turn and attack you for disturbing their paradise: Liberation is their chains, and liberators their enemies"* **Alik Shahada**

More than the film Roots, of lives on a plantation exposed to inhumanities, the most violent product of chattel slavery is mental slavery. It expresses itself by creating, among other things, dependency and an inferiority-complex. It infects every concept from notions of beauty, values, and even the preference of "renting" over the prospect of "buying." Many Africans globally, especially in areas heavily influenced by European domination, continue to wear their wealth on the outside (shoes, clothing, cars), while other groups wear their money on the inside (educational development) first. Mental slavery, also impacts African discernment. Because failure to know oneself also means failure to identify self-interest; it is often in this confused state the offense of oppression cannot be located in the minds of the mental slaves. It is no wonder they are given to attack the seat of their own liberation for minutia issues.

- *"What I hate is ignorance, smallness of imagination, the eye that sees no farther than its own lashes. All things are possible …Who you are is limited only by who you think you are"* **Book of Coming Forth by Day**
- *"No longer was reference made to African culture,it became barbarism. Africa was the 'dark continent'. Religious practices and customs were referred to as superstition. The history of African society was reduced to tribal battles and internecine wars."*

Steve Biko

- *"The essential problem that Kwame Nkrumah faced was how to transform a neo-colonial outpost of Western imperialism, into a real country and a modern one also. Initially once African countries gained political independence they looked up and discovered that they did not have economic independence, they did not have psychological independence. Ghana got a flag and an anthem in 1957 it didn't get real independence. [Nkrumah] realized that he needed economic independence and when he moved for economic independence to re-organize the country he realized that he couldn't move in the direction of economic independence with the old colonial state apparatus. And even though you may succeed in transforming the state apparatus to something which is more forward-looking, you also had to tackle the minds of the people, certainly the so-called educated people."*

Kimani Nehusi

W. E. B. Du Bois, the great Pan ***Africans*** intellectual worker, activist and academic, said that the problem of the last century would have been the problem of the colour line. The greatest battle of the new century, and indeed of the entire new millennium, is the battle for the African mind.

In chattel slavery Africans could not own anything; you could not have long term investment plans in your family (they could be sold away at any moment). Myopic thinking is a vestige of slavery, as no enslaved African had the luxury for over 300 years of thinking beyond the moment. So today a flashy car (instant gratification) takes the place of any long-term wealth (like owning a house). The need to sate the superficial is not exclusively created by mental enslavement but is heavily augmented by it.

Investment in education was futile in slavery and still this legacy continues. Mental slavery also impacts most of all value of self, value in seeing African stories. How else can we explains why the Jewish story in film and print is everywhere in the world despite Jews only being a World population less than the city of Lagos. And why is it the story of Africa (more than 1 billion people) is rarely told, and when it is told it is at the hands of European agents. Some Africans are so mentally confused that they are active agents of whitewashing and escaping from slavery, they will state "I am sick of hearing about slavery the past is the past." The African voice, the African woman and man, the African relationships and African films and media have no value in the minds of those who have no value of self. And this pervasive legacy washes not only this contemporary African generation, but future generations waiting to be born.

Mental slavery is a medical disorder

The Diagnostic and Statistical Manual of Mental Disorders (DSM) is the American Psychiatric Association's standard reference for psychiatry includes over 400 different definitions of mental disorders. They define a mental disorder as a psychological pattern or anomaly, potentially reflected in behavior, which is not considered part of normal development in a person's culture. Mental disorders are generally defined by a combination of how a person *feels*, *acts*, *thinks* or *perceives*. The first thing an afflicted person says? I do not have a problem. Despite all the empty alcohol bottles and the empty credit card balance—they are not sick. Denial. Redirection, are all medical signs of a mental disease.

If someone was beautiful and started to tear their beauty apart they would be diagnosed as having a mental condition. Agoraphobia, Bipolar, Anorexia, Dyspareunia, Bulema, and. If someone destroys their beauty to achieve something which is not naturally beautiful is it not possible that person is suffering from a mental disease—like skin bleaching and extreme chemical treatment of hair. If a mother rejects a child, is that not listed under a mental condition? If someone acts outside of their own self-interest but in the self-interest of another person, clearly that is a brain misfiring. And that is exactly how mental slavery should be treated. Like Stockholm syndrome and all other mental diseases. **Diagnosing the condition**

"He lacks the power of organization, and is conspicuously deficient in the management and control alike of men or business. He loves the display of power, but fails to realize its responsibility... He has the courage of the fighting animal, an instinct rather than a moral virtue... In brief, the virtues and defects of this race-type are those of attractive children, whose confidence when it is won is given ungrudgingly as to an older and wiser superior and without envy...perhaps the two traits which have impressed me as those most characteristic of the African native are his lack of apprehension and his lack of ability to visualize the future" **Lord Frederick John Lugard**

Like all mental defects or diseases, mental slavery is very hard to define. Bipolar disorder, despite all the medical technology, eludes detection by any know medical test. Likewise there are no instruments that can calculate the percentage of mental enslavement a person is suffering from. A person might be affected in one area, but not in another. It might subside for a while and later reoccur under certain stresses—like when a marriage breaks down, or when financial circumstances change.

Part of the criteria of diagnosis has to take into account patterns in group behavior—the group being African people. On an individual level you will find Europeans suffering for low self-value, they may have poor image of self, but this is very different because while on an individual level they have an inferiority complex due to inadequacies of their local self, they have zero racial inferiorities as a collective. They do not look at their racial station in the world and wonder, like Africans do, what have my people contributed to modernity. They are in the extreme opposite set-up by every single thing—not dealing with if it is true or false—reaffirms their "superiority" station among the races of human kind.

In some cases, like the capitalist greed running rife in South Africa, is a problem born of two mothers; the legacy of low self-worth created during apartheid, and the naturally occurring bling bling culture of a people who were isolated from consciousness. Apartheid, in this case, modulated a pre-existing condition. An entire dynamic range of discussion now emerges. What is what and what belongs where? When is it mental slavery and when is it plain old garden variety human stupidity?

Many use the term mental slavery as a political device for labelling all behaviors which are outside of their political "solutions." So it has become a catch all box for a wide range of behaviors some of which are totally unrelated to mental enslavement. Not every bad habit seen in African communities is the legacy of mental enslavement. Not every instances of crime in Detroit by an African American male is due to mental slavery, not every negative urban culture is due to mental enslavement. And it is critical to distinguish where possible between these things. There are behaviors which arise, independent of slavery, from poverty. While in the case of many African people, poverty may have its roots in slavery, that slavery factor might be replaced by just the poverty factor. And one way to test it is to look at other situations where groups or communities have not endured slavery but display identical behaviors in similar circumstances. So poverty and poverty alone may be the consequences of obesity in America. Hence European-Americans, who have never experienced slavery—but experience poverty display identical habits. In this case we cannot list obesity in unprivileged communities as a direct legacy of slavery in America. We must accept a multi-rooted possible in all of our analysis without resting all the symptoms on one agent. So our treatment of the subject will attempt to tie the contemporary behavior to a behavior directly related to something passed on through the generations, up from slavery.

Mental States (Theory)

To assist in a better understanding of mental slavery, we will posit 4 mental theoretical states.

- **NIGGERS:** The Nigger, or Nigga as they preferred to be called, is the end product of White supremacy infected with the full strain of **Willy Lynch** syndrome to the point where they will burn their own body for food. Feed off their communities. Represent the most immoral pits of human existence. They are a liability to humanity period. And some mutated forms of the Nigger mind speak hot rhetoric and appear to be revolutionary as a cover for insecurities. They are antisocial walking bigots, who use words like "black supremacy" as a ruse to be thugs, ignorant and irresponsible.
- **NEGROES:** The Negro is more productive in assisting the White supremacy system and well behaved and contained, he is the perfect companion if ever a white person needed a trusting friend. Even a rebellious Negro services slavery, for their rebellion is always first and foremost profitable to the system of oppression.
- **BLACKS:** The Black recognizes the problems with the aforementioned groups and is striving to be more, they are *still* doing this within the framework of the slave world and with the tools of their enslavement. The African connection is generally nascent and skin deep. Confidence and knowledge of self are the barriers to the state of being African.
- **AFRICANS:** The African is a fully liberated being with identity, culture and purpose, with paradigms of his or her own agency. The African is a continuous journey which builds on the past to construct a new future of possibilities. And while the Black mind-set is still searching, the African is at his or her intended ideological destination and busy with the business of growing.

Reference
'Alik Shahadah. MENTAL SLAVERY. The Most Insidious Legacy of slavery. MENTAL SLAVERY/Legacy of African Holocaust. http://www.africanholocaust.net/html_ah/mentalentslavement.html

vii. Stockholm syndrome: The Negro Madness Disease.

Most blacks involved in exclusively white relationship are suffering from Stockholm Syndrome. Stockholm syndrome is also known as *Survival identification syndrome.*

Stockholm syndrome refers to a group of psychological symptoms that occurs in some persons in a captive or hostage situation. It has received considerable media publicity in recent years because it has been used to explain the behavior of such well-known kidnapping victims as Patty Hearst (1974) and Elizabeth Smart (2002).

The term takes its name from a bank robbery in Stockholm, Sweden, in August 1973. The robber took four employees of the bank (three women and one man) into the vault with him and kept them hostage for 131 hours. After the employees were finally released, they appeared to have formed a paradoxical emotional bond with their captor, they told reporters that they saw the police as their enemy rather than the bank robber, and that they had *positive feelings toward the criminal.*

In order to survive in this oppressive and maddening white-dominated society where you are constantly being told you are: worthless, ugly, lazy, no-good, disease-ridden, and a scourge to all society, it is imperative to dissociate one's mind from the constant abuse and develop "***coping mechanism.***"

The **"survival identification syndrome"** leads to skin lightening which is regarded as one of the manifestations of "negro madness disease."

Like most illnesses—"negro madness"— the first step is admitting that you have a problem. Then second step is admitting what the problem is: "**White supremacy**."

All blacks in the system are **reacting** to their environment. That's the key word: ***react*****.** **Whites *act*; Blacks *react.***

In conclusion, skin lightening is an **adverse** response to White supremacy

Reference

Observations of an Invisible Woman. *Stockholm syndrome: The Negro Madness Disease.* Diaryofanegress. 15 Nov 2012 (87 comments.) *http://diaryofanegress.com/2012/11/15/stockholm-syndrome-the-negro...*

xiii. Bleaching Syndrome

Ronald Hall suggests that 'the bleaching syndrome' the internalization of a white aesthetic ideal, is the result of the historic legacy of slavery and colonialism around the globe. He argues that many African Americans, Latinos, and Asian Americans have internalized the colonial and slavery value systems and learned to valorize light skin tones and Anglo facial features. He understands this deeply rooted culture values as a cause of psychological distress and socioeconomic stratification

References:

1. Hall Ronald E. The Bleaching Syndrome Among People of color. Implication of skin color for human behavior in the social environment. *Journal of Human Behavior in the social Environment.* 2006; 13: 19-31.

2. Hall Ronald E. The Bleaching Syndrome. African American's Response to cultural domination Vis-à-vis skin color. *Journal of Black Studies.* 1995; 26:172-84

MOTIVES FOR SKIN BLEACHING IN AFRICA

Preamble

The worldwide use of skin-lightening products is driven by an indelible belief that the lighter gradation of skin tone results in more prestige and opportunities. So much so that this belief has led to the growing epidemic of the consumption of skin-lightening products, both within and between racial/ethnic groups. Not only is a lighter skin complexion seen as a form of symbolic capital, it has also been implicated as a sign of attractiveness and desirability, particularly among females. Far from being an out-moded practice or legacy of past colonialism, the use of skin lighteners is growing fastest among young, urban, educated women in the global South[1] (p181). This is not unexpected, because for hundreds of years there has been an embedded proclamation for white supremacy, which sees white skin as the essential skin and black skin as not only inferior but less important in defining humanity. (See chapter 2). Such views have been expressed by Western philosophers such as Kant and Hegel[2] (198).

The strong influence of the need for a lighter skin tone is shared globally in both Western and non Western societies with the view that practice of skin bleaching has more to do with the modern outlook as opposed to black inferiority[2]. International cosmetic companies have capitalized on this market using different marketing strategies, including the use of the internet by capturing racial and colorized norms and values and the class and gender differences within the White and non-White market[3] (p200).

References

1.Glenn EN. Yearning for lightness: transnational ciruits in the marketing and consumption of skin lighteners. *Gend Soc* 2008; 22:281-302.

2.Gwaravanda TE. Shona proverbial implications on skin bleaching: some philosophical insights. *J Pan Afr Stud* 2011; 4:197-218.

3.Charles CAD. The derogatory representations of the skin bleaching products sold in Harlem. *J Pan Afr Stud* 2011; 4:117-41

While there are many works on the dangers and popularity of skin bleaching, few offer plausible solutions to help decrease the spread of the practice. The objective of this chapter on **motives** and analysis of the motives is to elucidate the **true** reasons for bleaching from analysis of existing studies on motives in Africa. Further details are discussed under the chapter on individual countries. Possible interventions shall be proffered in subsequent chapters to help make this dangerous practice obsolete. Further, there is hope that the analysis of motives will help inspire other researchers to find possible solutions in order to makeskin bleaching unattractive.

Bleaching for beauty

What makes it worth the risk?

"I bleach my skin for "beauty" and for making my skin "smooth." For women to look beautiful, they need to have smooth light skins" (Sibamba, Zambia) (See chapter 8 on ZAMBIA)

Winnie, a Kenyan, is adamant that being light skinned has its perks, especially when it comes to beauty. *"How long did it take the modeling industry to accept dark skinned models like Alex Wek and Ajuma on their runways*? She asks. *"Most people will not want to admit it, but light skin is more appealing, it's a sign of purity."* While many will cite standing out or preferential treatment as an easier time finding employment, Winnie is honest about the fact that she was motivated by appearance. *"The recognition is a plus, but I used to think that I would be prettier if I was lighter. That is why I decided to lighten my skin. "When you… walk into the modeling agencies, the girls there who get picked up for jobs are usually fair-skinned".*

In Kenya, the lighter "brown" girls are usually considered to be more beautiful than "black" girls–and the more successful prostitutes are invariably "brown."[1]

Kenyan socialite, Vera Sidika says she's already seen an increase in demand for her services after bleaching her skin. (See the chapter on CELEBRITY DISCOURSE— Chapter 6).

Sylvia Arthur,[2] in her brief story titled "Dying to be white" wonders why Ghanaian women desperately continue to use most dangerous chemicals to bleach their skin in spite of persistent warnings by dermatologists that other adverse effects from skin-bleaching methods and technology are deadly/life threatening. Why would one risk dying to acquire "beauty"?

In an article titled "*Ahoofe Kasa*!": Skin Bleaching and the Function of Beauty Among Ghanaian Women," Blay describes the "*function*" of beauty in Ghana[3]. In the article, Blay explores the politics of beauty among women in Ghana, particularly those who currently use or at one time have used skin lightening agents. The study relies primarily upon qualitative data to investigate the relationship between gender, skin bleaching, light skin, and beauty. Although the participants interviewed indeed express that their use of skin lightening agents is fueled by their desire to be perceived as more noticeably beautiful, critical analysis of the data reveals that what they are seeking is not an arbitrary beauty or "abstract beauty", but one that is **functional** and **materializes** via light skin. In this way, beauty via light skin gained through skin bleaching allows participants across to social capital, and for many, their new found light skin color becomes a "bartering tool" negotiable for economic capital. "Ahoofe kasa" is a popular Ghanaian aphorism, which literally means "beauty talks"! This means that skin bleachers have a "hidden agenda." It becomes clear that beauty has a language–a language which though not vocalized is nonetheless very powerful.

Both journalistic and scientific literature have repeatedly documented the existence, in various cultures, of social hierarchies where skin tone is an important factor. For example in the United States, Brazil, Mexico, and in West Africa, lighter-skinned individuals are more likely to be employed in occupations with higher status and they are more prone to upward social mobility compared to darker-toned counterpart.[4] (See the sections on COLORISM—Chapters 11, 12, 17)

A former beauty queen in Ghana[5] bleached her skin. When critized about her action she replied thus: "In life we are all entitled to what we want to do…I choose to tone my skin and I don't think it's a problem because if it were a problem to me, I won't do it. When asked if she was aware of the adverse health effects she said "In life, every thing comes with the bad aspect of it… when you are doing something, sometimes you don't really need to think about the bad part of it. I am just doing it because I am comfortable with it and I don't even think about the negative part of it."

A recent report in the Washington Post on the emerging phenomenon of skin-bleaching among mainly poor black women in Kingston, Jamaica, backs up this point. When the reporter asked a 17-year-old young black woman why she was willing to take serious health risks to make herself appear lighter, she answered, "When I walk on the streets you can hear people say, 'Hey, check out the brownin.' It makes you more important." In the same report, a 22-year-old black woman responded: "I want people to think I am more than a ghetto girl…. I want to walk into dance halls and feel like a movie star, a white one". It is clear that from the perspectives of these women, who stand to risk their health and cause themselves unspeakable pain, gaining a few shades of whiteness is worth all the pain and suffering they go through in the process. (See Chapter 15 on JAMAICA).

Malangu Ntambwe and team from the National School of Public Health at Madunsa has shown "that the quest for fairness" in skin colour through the use of skin lighteners is based on many 'unfair' problems and in the long term has very unfair and unhealthy results. He argues that the practice of skin lightening is a public health issue with social, psychological, socioeconomic and environmental determinants. The root cause being a response to a deep-seated need for individual to cope with the suffering they perceive or experience resulting from social norms. In this sense, skin lightening could be regarded as a disease in the broader definition of health which is defined as a "state of mental and social well-being".[6]

The general pervasive belief is that people of colour lighten their skin in order to fit within the larger society's definition of beauty. It is also believed that skin bleaching symbolizes more complex psychological issues such as self perception and self-esteem that have plagued people of color since the advent of international slavery especially in the Americas. For instance, African-Americans are often coerced through the mass media to believe that lightening one's skin through bleaching products brings greater acceptance into the larger North American society.

There are many reasons why black, dark-skinned people resort to skin lightening and these reasons may be grouped in two kinds–The first are personal reasons–beauty and its pursuit are universal. The face is viewed as the mirror of the soul, therefore a person's self-esteem, self-hate, self-image is a determinant factor in the quest for beauty. The second factor is social norms and environmental, that is, socioeconomic and environmental determinants. For example Blay finds that skin bleaching in Ghana can be best understood by unpacking the social history and culture of the country. The motivational loci embedded in the narratives of the study participants revealed that skin bleaching is caused by colorism with its attendant symbols and functions. Skin bleaching is an expression of a cultural memory anchored in colorism and its antecedent colonialism. According to Blay, the source of skin bleaching lies in the cultural memes and institutions which guide the behavior of the skin bleachers.[7]

Interviews conducted on skin bleachers in sub-Saharan African countries highlight many factors driving this practice. A desire to lighten skin colour is cited as a **primary** motivating factor for skin bleaching.[8] This is because in some countries, white skin is still perceived to be associated with social privileges, including better job and marital prospects. However, some skin bleachers may not desire white skin, but instead desire radiant skin.[8] Up until recent years there was limited choice with regard to the types of cosmetic products available in Africa and Europe especially for individual with Fitzpatric skin phototype VI.[9] In the absence of such products, bleaching the skin may be perceived as an alternative method of enhancing one's beauty, especially prior to important social events.[10] Other reasons cited by individuals partaking in skin bleaching include imitation of others and dependency on the products[10,11] —the rebound phenomenon when the user attempts to discontinue use of the product. Furthermore, the higher prevalence of dyschromias in people with skin phototypes IV to VI may be another factor that initiates, promotes, and/or excuses the practice of skin lightening.[12,13] The lack of understanding about the appropriate use of depigmenting agents, coupled with negative cultural perceptions about dark skin, may lead to cutaneous depigmenting agents being subsequently intentionally or inadvertently misused.

Some examples of studies done

Nina–Bella S. Mbayu[14] of Howard University Washington, uses the social learning theory to examine the reasons why skin bleaching is still rampant in West and Central Africa, despite all scientific research showing it is very harmful to one's health. The aim of the study is to see what can be done to reverse the increasing popularity of this trend.

The Social Learning Theory states that people engage in specific behaviors because of (1) what they witness in their environment (2) the ability to reproduce the behavior, and (3) a higher probability for a positive outcome. Therefore, it is hypothesized that an increasing number of Africans continue to engaged in skin bleaching because (1) it is what they see their peers practice (2) the products are readily available and (3) the possibility of becoming more attractive and powerful is highly favorable and luring. The Colonial Mentality Theory suggests that peoples of nations which were formerly colonized still feel inferior to the peoples of the nation(s) that colonized them and still strive to be accepted by these former foreign powers.

The majority of answers by respondents revolve around the concept of increased beauty: that is, skin bleaching is practiced because people believe it will make them more beautiful. "Western perceptions of beauty" and the presence of "a negative stigma that comes with being African/dark skinned" were two of the answers given that support the Colonial Mentality Theory having a part in the popularity of skin bleaching. One respondent answered that in her country (Cameroon), men are more attracted to women with lighter skin, thereby fueling its popularity among Cameroonian women. Another respondent believed that skin bleaching is done because lighter skin has the effect of "opening doors to a higher status" in Central Africa.

After thorough research of qualitative and quantitative data, both hypotheses have been supported by this study. That is, the popularity of skin bleaching within nations of Africa is ever-increasing due to its accessibility and desirable outcomes (including increased beauty, salary, and social status). Mbayu finally submits that Black Africans continue to lighten their skin with the hope of obtaining a fairer, more "metisse" (mixed) appearance, because in these regions, a lighter skin tone is tied to

1. a higher level of beauty
2. increased chances of obtaining work and
3. overall power, and higher status.

Other studies indicate that a desire to lighten the complexion is the main reason why people use these products. Women in ***Senegal*** associate fair skin tone with elegance, beauty and a higher social status.[15] The expected result of "xessal" in Senegal is to clear the skin to obtain the so-called "taint Clair," which is supposed to "improve appearance" and is considered by women as "a standard of elegance, beauty, and higher social level." A study conducted in ***Tanzania***[16] found that many Tanzanians have embraced Eurocentric beauty ideals and feel pressured to look white. In this study, a 25 years old lady reported that she "started bleaching to be beautiful and to look like Arabians or Europeans and attractive to people, especially men" Other reasons for using skin-lightening products include a desire to even out skin tone/improve the texture of the skin, treatment of skin blemishes, to remove the adverse effects of extended skin bleaching, to satisfy one's partner or attract male companions, to satisfy or impress peers, to enhance opportunities in life (especially job opportunities), to reduce the experience of negative stereotypes that are applied to dark people, for the enjoyment of light-coloured skin, fashion and dependency–undesirable worsening of the skin rash (rebound phenomenon whenever one attempts to stop usage of the skin lightening agent. Lewis *et al* identify six key motivations behind why Tanzanians bleach their skin (1) to remove pimples, rashes, and skin diseases, (2) to have a soft skin (3) to be white, "beautiful", and look more European: (4) to remove the adverse effects of extended skin bleaching use on the body, (5) to satisfy one's partner or attract male mates, and (6) to satisfy oneself.

Lonzozou Kpanake *et al*[17] studied the motives for skin bleaching among women in **Togo**. Four motives appeared as clearly dominant. Participants practiced skin bleaching on a regular basis mainly (a) to appear important, (b) to look attractive, (c) because they enjoyed their lighter-colored skin, and (d) because skin bleaching was fashionable. They did not practice skin bleaching as a demonstration of opposition to African culture or to their relatives or as a demonstration of compliance with others' wishes. They also sometimes practiced skin bleaching as a means of securing a job.

In **Mali**, Joan Baxter, in an article titled "The heavy cost of light skin" describes how women who refuse to bleach are discriminated against and ostracized in Mali. Women who refuse to bleach often find themselves regarded as second class citizens. A woman who did not bleach her skin said she is often not offered a chair at baptisms, and is asked to make herself scarce when group photographs are taken at marriages[18]

In **Rwanda,** a survey in Kigali market shows that 35% of the study population were skin bleachers but only 27% claim they use the products purely to lighten the skin colour; and some adolescents indicate that they know about the practice but are restricted by family, religion, and Rwandese culture.[19]

In **Uganda**, consumers of bleaching cosmetics claim they want to enhance their beauty. One woman who declined to be named, explains, "One has to look good, by having fair, lighter skin." Unfortunately, her skin is now multi-colored from bleaching. For this woman, the condition of her skin has only brought her shame; she now tries to cover most parts of her body in an attempt to conceal the damage done by the products she thought would enhance her beauty.[20]

A study was conducted in **Nigeria**[21] to investigate the perception and motives of female secondary school students on skin bleaching practice in Ibadan metropolis. These were young girls between the ages of 11-14yrs (85.3%) and above 14yrs old (14.7%).

In this study, the rank order (by the mean scores) of responses to items on perception on skin bleaching are as follows:

The above major ranking of motives shows that the major reasons why these young girls bleach their skin are, (1) aesthetics (2) find and sustain marriage (3) upward mobility. (4) heterosexual relationships and become public figures.

Another study was done among Nollywood celebrities in Nigeria to identify the motives for skin bleaching. The reasons given are as follows:[22]

1. To look beautiful and attractive
2. To increase their professional relevance
3. To attract the right suitors
4. The bandwagon syndrome
5. To look good in photo

In a study in **Jordan,**[23] there was no difference in the prevalence usage among women from the lowest and the highest economic status. On the influence of lighter skin tone on women's perception of self-esteem and age, 60% of the skin bleachers associate lighter skin tone with self esteem and youth. 55% of bleachers believe that lighter skin tone contributes to a better employment opportunity. This points out that job opportunities/employment is a significant factor promoting skin bleaching. 71% of bleachers believe that a lighter skin tone is more attractive to men and increases a woman's chances of getting married. 77% of respondents believe that TV advertisements contribute to the practice of using skin-lightening products by presenting models with light skin tone as being more attractive and more likely to achieve success in their life (i.e employment opportunity and mate selection).

In **Saudi Arabia**, the prevalence of women bleachers in a study was 38.9%. Only 26.7% of the bleachers used bleaching agents for medical purposes to treat localized abnormal skin hyperpigmentation. 56.8% of the skin bleachers believed that lighter skin colour made them more beautiful, whereas only 15.9% believed that lighter skin colour made them more self-confident.[24]

References

1. Mc Vicar KG. *Twilight of an East African Slum.* Ann Arbor, University Microfilms (UCLA Dissertation 1968). 1969.

2.Sylvia Arthur. Dying to be white *http://www.clutchmagonline.com/2008/01/dying-to-be-white.*

3. Blay YA Ahoofe kasa!: Skin bleaching and the function of beauty among Ghanaian women *JENda: A Journal of Culture and African Women Studies* 2009b: 14: 1-10

4. Fokuo J. Konadu. The Lighter Side of Marriage: skin bleaching in post-colonial Ghana. *African and Asian Studies.* 2009; 8: 125-46

5.Ghana News–'I am confortable bleaching my skin–*Ghana-Most Beautiful's Nasara.* Source, *Ghana/myjoyonline.com/Ernesty Dela Aglan http://myjoyonline.com/entertainment/2013/December-17th/i-am.comfo...*

6. Ntambwe M. 'Mirror mirror on the wall, who is the FAIREST of them all?' *Science in Africa.* March 2004. *http://www.scienceinafrica.co.za/2004/march/skinlightening.htm*

7. Blay YA. "Yellow fever: Skin Bleaching and the Politics of Skin Color in Ghana". PhD. Dissertation. Temple University

8. Charles CAD. Liberating skin bleachers: From mental Pathology to complex personhood. *Jenda: A Journal of Culture and African Women Studies.* 2009b; 14:86-100

9. Findlay GH. Ochronosis following skin bleaching with hydroquinone. *J Am Acad Dermatol.* 1982; 6:1092-3.

10. de Souza MM. The concept of skin bleaching in Africa and its devastating health implications. *Clin Dermatol.* 2008; 26:27-9.

11. Traore A, Kadeba J-C, Niamba P, Barro F, Quedraogo L. Use of cutaneous depigmenting products by women in two towns in Burkina Faso: epidemiologic data, motivations, products and side effects. *Int J Dermatol* 2005; 44: 30-2.
12. Keane FM, Munn SE, Taylor NF, du Vivier AW. Unregulated use of clobetasol propionate. *Br J Dermatol.* 2001; 144:1095-6.
13. Taylor S. Skin of color: biology, structure, function, and implications for dermatologic disease. *J Am Acad Dermatol.* 2002; 46: S41-S62.
14. Mbayu Nina-Belle S. skin Bleaching in Western and Central Africa: A Critical Analysis Utilizing the Social learning and Colonial Mentality Theories. *Proceedings of the National Conference On Undergraduate Research* (NCUR) 2012. Weber State University, ogden, Utah. March 29-31, 2012.
15. Pascal del Guidice and pirier Yves. The widespread use of skin lightening creams in Senegal: a persistent public health problem in West Africa. *Int J Dermatol.* 2002; 41: 69-72.
16. Lewis KM, Harris S, Camp C, KAlala W et al, the historical and cultural influences of skin bleaching in Tanzania. In. The melanin Millennium: Skin color as 21st Century International Discourse. Publisher Springer Netherlands. 2013 pp 19-38
17. Kpanake Lonzozou. Skin bleaching amongst Togolese: A Preliminary Inventory of Motives. *Journal of Black Psychology*. 2010; 38: 350-68.
18. Joan Baxter. The heavy cost of light skin. BBc News. 18 April, 2000. *http://news.bbc.co.uk/2/hi/africa/718359.stm*
19. Léocadie kamagaju, Renato Morandini, Françoise Gahongayire et al. Survey on skin-lightening practices and cosmetics in Kigali, Rwanda. *International Journal of dermatology 2015*; 1-7 doi:1111/ijd.12833.
20. Skin bleaching/African Science Heroes *Http://afrisciheroes.wordpress.com/tag/skin-bleaching/fantaface,cocacolabody:* why do black people bleach their skin? Jan 16, 2012.
21. Durosaro AT, Ajiboye SK, Oniye AO. Perception of skin bleaching among female secondary school students in Ibadan metropolis, Nigeria. Journal of education and practice. 2012; 3(7): 40-6.
22. 5 (five) Reasons Nollywood Celebrities Bleach their Skin… *http:www.nigerianbulletin.com/threads/5-reasons-nollywood-celebr…*
23. Hammed SH, tayyem R, Nimer N, and Alkhatib HS. Skin-lightening practice among women living in Jordan: prevalence, determinants, and user's awareness. International Journal of dermatology. 2010; 49:414-20.
24. Al Ghamdi KM. The use of topical bleaching agents among women: a cross-sectional study of knowledge, attitude and practices *European Academy of Dermatology and Venereology*. 2010; JEADY DOI:10.1111/j1468-3083.2010.03629.x

THE MARRIAGE PRESSURE

Husband: The single most important "Social Capital" in Africa to skin bleachers

After The Temptation and The Fall of Man, one of the consequences pronounced by God on Eve was:

"Your desire shall be for your husband,
And he shall rule over you." (Gen 3:16).

Globally, even across other cultures this, *innate* desire by a woman for mate exists but it does not loom as large as it is in Africa, because other cultures accommodate the single lifestyle, does not put undue pressure on women to marry, and because the women are majorly educated and economically empowered, they are not desperate for a "bread winner"—the husband.

Various motives have been given during interviews for lightening the skin; these are: (1) to look more beautiful and attractive, (2) to improve self esteem, (3) to look younger, (3) to appear important, (4) to belong to a higher social class, (4) to be fashionable, (5) to improve better job opportunity, (6) to increase chances of getting married because men consider light complexioned women more beautiful and (7) due to advertisements that promote white ideal.

Unquestionably, right across the continent of Africa (except perhaps South Africa, Sudan and Liberia where there is institutional colorism), the **primary** motive why women lighten their skin is to attract the opposite gender. Right from early teen-age school years, some mothers indoctrinate the girl child that the ultimate goal for a woman in life is to get married and bear children. For unexplainable reason, most African men have a special affinity for light complexioned women as girlfriends, concubines or wives. Culturally, in Africa, the social status of a woman of marriageable age is defined by her marital status and reproductive capability i.e to bring forth children. Irrespective of a woman's educational, professional or career achievements, failure to marry and bear children, leaves her with a feeling of nothingness. Therefore, most women are willing to change their skin tone to attract a suitor and, preferably, a high profile husband. Furthermore, even after the woman has succeeded in finding marriage, she still has to **work at it to secure** the husband so that she does not lose him to light complexioned seductresses always on the prowl!

The age worn paradigms for skin lightening such as self hate thesis, colorism perspective, mis-education theory, the identity thesis, and complex personhood explanation— of course do exist in some cases, but do not loom large in cases of ***black Africans living in Africa***. The vast majority of Skin bleachers do **not** wish to be Caucasians nor do they want to marry Caucasians, but deep down in their hearts, there is a yearning for, a vacuum which an unmarried woman believes can only be filled by a husband. Therefore, if there is any deliverable 'social capital' for skin lightening in Africa, it is a **husband**!

Women bleach their skin to *find* a husband and *secure* the husband
Quotations from women in several countries and responses from other women and men.

- Gambia — West Africa
- Ghana — West Africa
- Mali — West Africa
- Nigeria — West Africa
- Senegal — West Africa
- Sierra Leone — West Africa
- Kenya — East Africa
- Rwanda — East Africa
- Tanzania — East Africa
- Zimbabwe — East Africa
- Sudan — Central Africa
- South Africa — Southern Africa
- Zambia — Southern Africa
- UK (Africans in diaspora)
- Jamaica
- India

1. Gambia

"We need to examine our African men's obsession with "white skin" or "light skin" women, and how their attitudes and behaviors toward our dark skin women drive our women to bleach their skin. We need African men to support dark skin women by embracing our blackness". Anonymous–Gambi

Reference

Anonymous. (A concerned Gambian). President Jammeh's ban on skin bleaching. *Freedom Newspaper online.* *http://www.freedomnewspaper.com/Homepage/tabid/36/newsid/367/9...* concerned Gambian.

2. Ghana

"Men are accomplices in the bleaching culture".

According to one African specialist, men encourage women to bleach by considering light-skinned women to be more attractive, intelligent, moral desirable and chaste. In contrast, dark-skinned women are said to look mean, evil, stupid and untrustworthy. This opinion is consistent with the results of a survey among Ghanaian women. Most of the respondents thought that men prefer light skin in a women. *"Sometimes if you really want to marry a particular man, you have to bleach".*

Fokuo recognizes that skin color plays a significant role in the lives of Ghanaian women. Many Ghanaian women's feelings about beauty, attractiveness and the marriage market are associated with skin complexion. Using sixty Ghanaian students and thirty market trading women, Fokuo investigates skin colour (i.e its lightness-darkness) as a function of social capital in the marriage market. A skin Color Assessment Procedure was administered to all participants. The study showed:

> "lighter skin has also been found to be a valued quality in the contemporary Ghanaian marriage market and the popularity of skin bleaching… this study showed that although participants were satisfied with their skin color, they believed that Ghanaian men found lighter-skinned women more attractive."

> "When we were growing up most men of our time preferred fair-coloured women to those who were black. Even just listen to some of the songs our musicians compose; they are always glorifying fair ladies so I decided to change my colour."

References

1. Ntambwe M. Mirrow mirror on the wall, who is the FAIREST of them all? Science in Africa 2004 March. *http://www.scienceinafrica.co.za/2004march/skinlightening.htm*

2. Fokuo J Konadu. The lighter side of marriage: Skin bleaching in post-colonial Ghana. *Research Review NS* 2009; 25(1): 47-66

3. Mali

> "Many of the women who use these products say they do so because Malian men prefer women with bleached skin". But male musician Al Hassan Soumali disagrees. "I don't think Malian men like bleached women" he says. "It's better for Malian women to change their minds".Dr Gindo

Reference

Joan Baxter. The heavy cost of light skin. *BBC News.* 18 April, 2000. *http://news.bbc.co.uk/2/hi/africa/718359.stm*

4. Nigeria

"80% of Nigerian men want their women to be fair. They want a lady that draws attention to them. I've worked with many married women who complain of their men staring at fair women and they say to me, "Susan make me fair, I want to be attractive to my man!" Susan Maxwell– a bleached actress.

They thought they were more attractive, yes. But in a way you can't blame them. It's the society. They've got men and women praising light skin as the ultimate ideal/sign of beauty. The girls want to look beautiful. But more importantly, with so many being fairly uneducated & poverty stricken. THEY NEED A MAN to survive. Marriage= shelter, food etc. So they do their best to fit the ideal."

> "It has never been a secret that Nigerian men prefer their wives, light, bright, and voluptuous. Anytime a man picks his future wife, there is high praise if she happens to be lighter skin than him. I remember attending several weddings as a kid, and hearing the grown-ups relentlessly discuss how gorgeous the bride was with emphasis placed on her light skin. A bride with a darker complexion never gets the same amount of attention.[1]

Ajose, while revealing some of the cultural triggers of skin bleaching in Nigeria writes

> "Some bleachers reports that they bleach their skin because they desire light skin, they want to even out their skin tone; and their male partner on whom they depend economically have a preference for light skin women"[2]

References

1. Ezinne Ukoha. This is forty: I bleach my skin. 21 Jan 2014. *https://thsppl.com/this-is-forty-i-bleach-my-skin-52baf1479*
2. Ajose FOA. "consequences of skin bleaching in Nigerian Men and women. *International Journal of Dermatology*. 2005; 44:41-43.

5. Senegal

Women in Senegal say "they lighten their skin for the same reasons women the world over say they tweeze, squeeze or alter their bodies– in sometimes dangerous ways–to achieve a certain standard of beauty–*to catch a husband*, to stand out in the crowd, to smooth-out imperfections, to get ready for a special event"

Reference

Anne Look. In Senegal, Skin-Lightening Remains popular despite health risk. *http://www.voanes.com/content/in_senegal_skin_lightening_remain...*

6. Sierra Leone

It is a sad state of affairs when skin tone becomes the defining feature of one's position in life. Speaking to an unmarried, female cousin in Sierra Leone who uses skin-lightening products, she told me that

> "being overweight and very dark skinned is a double curse for her. How will she ever find a husband? It's much better to be the fat light-skinned girl than the fat black one. At least men will say I'm fat but my skin is pretty and yellow."

Reference

Kay Montano. The fairest of them all: Dija Ayodele on the culture of skin-bleaching.
THANDIEKAY 31 July 2014. http://thandiekay.com/2014/07/31/the-fairest-of-them-all-dija-ayodele

7. Kenya

After a TV interview with Vera Sidika, and several men criticized her for bleaching her skin– TV host Larry Madodo describes the reactions on social media;[1]

> "Fascinating", "astounding" "hypocritical" "Many men in Kenya do indeed prefer light-skinned women", "referring to them affectionately as "yellow, yellow". Dark-skinned women are sometimes derogatively called "tinted".

Mercy in Kenya says her dream is to be as white as a European and she will try anything to achieve her objective.[2]

> "My husband prefers half-caste women to darker girls, and he is proud to be mine when we go to the club,"

> "I get far more male attention now I am lighter."

Mercy cries out when the needle pricks her skin but after the injection she seems pleased that she went through with it. Grinning she gives a shrug and says,

> "Nairobi is very competitive and Kenyan men like women with whiter skin."

Rita in Kenya says

> "It was peer pressure, especially the expectations of the opposite sex, that persuaded me that light skin was better. You would really like this boy but he would go for the lighter girl". Boys would say to her. "Okey, you look good but I think you would look better if you were light."[2]

References

1. BBC trending: Is Kenya's Vera Sidika a # BleachedBeauty? www.bbc.com/news/blogs-trending-27768032

2. Annabel Fenwick Elliott. "Kenyan men like women with whiter skin": The rise of wealthy Nairobi women illegally INJECTING themselves with skin-lightening creams. Published: 6 June 2014 | Updated: 7 June 2014. http://www.dailymail.co.uk/femail/article-2650766/Kenyan-men-like-women-whiter-skin-The-rise-wealthy-Nairobi-women-illegally-INJECTING-skin-lightening-creams.html#ixzz3mXa3Twk4

8. Rwanda

> "The use of bleaching creams became common because women with darker skins were shunned by men, while those with lighter skins were always favoured; hence the rise in the use of bleaching creams."

Reference

Koyitenkore Kayitesi. In: women resort to cheap 'mixures' as skinlighteners. *The East African. http://www.theeastaafrican.co.ke/Rwanda/Lifestyle/Women-resort-to...*

9. Tanzania

In various **Tanzanian** studies women claimed Tanzanian men preferred white, soft-skinned girls. Thus,

"skin-lightening is of utmost importance in attracting men.
And once you've got a guy, you want to hang on to him".
Another women in the study explained that she used skin-lightening products

> "to prevent her husband from being attracted to other girls",

While yet another, a 25 year old, reported that she

> "started bleaching to be beautiful and to look like Arabians or Europeans and attractive to people, especially men." "We are all competing for mates, and we do whatever we can to give ourselves an advantage over the next person". Men would probably be content to live in caves if they didn't have to acquire the trappings necessary to compete for the most desirable women, and there would be less incentive for women to lighten their skin if men didn't keep valuing lighter skinned women over darker skinned ones.

Reference

Lewis KM, Robin N, Gaska K, Njoku L. Investigating motivations for women's skin bleaching in Tanzania. *Psychology of Women Quarterly* 2011; 35(1): 22-37.

10. Zimbabwe

Farai, a 35 years old Harare man, thinks that women who use the creams are delusional to think that all men find light-skinned women attractive; while Cliff a 32 year old, also from Harare, thinks that "**women who do not get adequate attention from men"** are the ones resorting to these "**desperate**" measures. Cliff believes women need more self-confidence, and users of these products are **"short-term investors trying to swindle men".** Another older women who spoke to this publication on condition of anonymity, concurred with Cliff, saying enhancements were for women who saw themselves as "**mere sex objects"**. She also thinks men who bleach their skin are most likely sexual deviants. A social media survey by Robin revealed that people who seek to modify themselves in one way or another have insecurity issues, low self-esteem or identity crises".

Reference

Robin Chaibva. Beauty is in the eye of the skin bleacher. *The Sunday Mail.* June 28, 2015. *http://www.sundaymail.co.zw/?p=37974*

11. Zambia

> "It appears beauty is all about being light skinned. It is not unusual to see many light-skinned women on the streets these days". "If Kitwe could be used as a yardstick for all the other towns in Zambia, one can safely predict that being dark skinned and natural is almost heading for "extinction"

Helen Sibamba, a single mother of twins who has bleached her skin says:

> "dark-skinned women nowadays are left with no choice but to use some skin-lightening lotions. This is necessary to deter men, in particular husbands, from leaving their dark-skinned women or wives in search of light-skinned partners or wives." In her view, "light-skinned women are more desirable by men!"

Lizzy Chansa, a trader at Chisokone market and a mother of six says:

> "Men are to blame for the increase in the number of women who are using lightening lotions because we fear that if we don't lighten our skins, our husbands will go after those who are light skinned. You will find that men leave their dark-skinned spouse in their homes and go after the light-skinned ones, so what are women expected to do?"

A number of men spoken to disagree with the views that they indirectly encourage skin bleaching by going after light-skinned women. According to Farley Musonda, a businessman of Kitwe, most men hate skin bleaching. "There was one time my wife used a lotion that started to lighten up her skin. I ordered her to stop using the lotion because I just like her being natural...I wonder what kind of husband would encourage his wife to bleach." Musonda says it was nonsense for women to believe that men could leave their wives if they were not bleaching. And Peter Chibomba of Kitwe discloses that he quit a four-year relationship with his fiancé after she came back from University of Zambia with a lightened skin. "She went to the University of Zambia as a natural beauty but I was surprised that when she came back, she was looking like a Cape-Coloured, so I told her that 'it's either you quit this bleaching or there will be no marriage' and that was it," he said.

Responses to the question by Mwila Chansa @gmail.com in Zambia

"Should beauty or Love really be a justification for women to bleach"

- *Never in my life will I bleach my skin, I would rather not get married if one of the conditions is to bleach for a man to marry me. Black is beautiful; that's what I call myself.* (Mofya Chisenga Mukunta 9/9/2010).
- *Black is beautiful* (Terry Oreilly 9/9/201).
- *I prefer unbleached woman. Bleaching women are inferior and usually not confident.* (Michael Chipande 9/92010).
- *I think each person has the rights on her body, because some men appreciate women with bleached skin and some don't!. It's just like smoking. Some*

appreciate husbands like that and other don't! that's my point of view anyway. I haven't bleached my skin and I,m proud of myself!! (Haulie Temb 9/9/2010).

- *The Malakoz are dark. Natural women are the best, whether dark or light.* (Obinna Chuma Onukogu 9/9/2010).
- *I can say, BEAUTY is what we all possess; confidence is all it takes to bring it (beauty) out. I,ve seen girls who still lack confidence even after having bleached their skin. I guess it is because they feel strange in some sort of a borrowed skin. Be proud of your natural beauty girls!!* (Mwich grace Kangwa).
- *It really amazes me why women want to destroy their faces with these harsh creams. The government has also not done their part in ensuring that this skin bleaching is stopped.* (Ella Mwinji Zkonde Zulu 10/9/2010).

References

1. Brighton Sinkola. Should women bleach their skin? *http://www.facebook.com/peralink.php?story-fbib=138030709574...*
2. Mwila, chansa@gmail.com
The Post Newspaper Zambia

12. UK (Africans in diaspora)

Skin bleachers defend the manufacture and sale of skin lightening products

In July 2015, High street health store Holland & Barrett came under fire for selling a legal skin-whitening product called **Dr Organic Royal Jelly Skin Body Whitening Cream**, which retails £9.99. The sale of the product provoked outrage, with some accusing the chain of encouraging racist ideals. Yet Irene, who's 34 and lives with her husband and four children in a kent mansion, claims that

"in some communities the pressure on women
to use such products is overwhelming".

Former model Irene Major is a wealthy women who knows all about looking after her skin. The wife of a Canadian oil tycoon Sam Malin, has tried everything from super-expensive **Crème de la mer** moisturizers to the services of the most exclusive Harley street dermatologists. But Irene, who is originally from Cameroon, West Africa, has a shocking admission; she also regularly uses skin-lightening creams to alter the color of her complexion. "*when my skin is lighter, I just feel prettier*"; she admits with startling candour. '*It's a taboo subject, and people get judgmental about it, but that's how I feel.*'She says

> "*A skin-lightening regime has been part of my life practically since birth." 'There are many different types of African skin–from dark*

> *charcoal to a lighter version–and you grow up knowing that the lighter ladies are the prettier ones. It's just a fact."*

Her younger sister, Elsa, 27, agrees, explaining how disturbing hierarchies of skin colour are still influencing African girls.

> *"Being lighter shows you belong to a different place on the social ladder.* ***All the rich, successful black African men marry either a white or a very light-skinned girl because they too grew up thinking that the lighter is the most pretty. It doesn't matter how dark a man is, of course–the pressure is all on women."***

Reference

Rebecca Ley. As Holland and Barrett come under fire for selling a controversial skin lightening cream…The women who'll do anything to have whiter skin. *Mail Online* 27 November 2014. *http://www.dailymail.co.uk/femail/article-2850927/As-Holland-Barret...*

13. Jamaica

Henriques[1] and Ellis[2] found that many upper class men sought fair-skinned wives because of the socioeconomic advantages of marrying women with this complexion. Many women were trapped in spinsterhood because Black men were sexually and romantically attracted to light-skinned women, who they took as marriage partners. The educated Black women refused to marry lower class, uneducated Black Men. The foregoing was a part of the cultural context within which, in the last decade before Jamaica received independence from Britain, the *Gleaner* Newspaper carried numerous skin bleaching advertisements. The labels on the products suggest that light skin is sexy and attractive, so Black women who bleach their skin will be flocked by men who find them beautiful and sexually attractive. The advertised bleaching creams gave the Black women the opportunity to escape spinsterhood and enter romantic relationships with men who want light skin partners through the alteration of their black skin.

> "People [women] do it purposely for husbands. They want to get married: they want to get attractive to men".[3]

References

1. Henriques F. Color values in Jamaican society. *British Journal of Sociology*. 1951; 2:115-21

2. Ellis RA. Color and class in a Jamaican market town. Sociology & Social Research 1957; 41:354-60.
3. Robinson Petra Alaine. Skin bleaching in Jamaica: A colonial legacy. *PhD Dissertation* May 2011.

- **India**
  All the men out there why are they more attractied towards white women? This tends to create complexity among the darker skin coloured women. We need to first of all change the mindset of men and do not forget how much we all talk about women emancipation and empowerment. Unfortunately it will always be a man's world".

Madhumati Napal. (See chapter 16 on INDIA).

Reference

Dan Morrison. Has India Skin-Lightening Obsession Reached the Final frontier?-… *http://voices.nationalgeographic.com/2012/04/12/has-indias-skin-lig...*

The burden to find marriage

Men valorize light skin tone

A lot of men have a desperate desire that borders on manic obsessions for beautiful fair skin. Studies show that men from all races prefer fairer skinned females. Fair skin is subconsciously linked to "innocence, purity, modesty, virginity, vulnerability and goodness". The preference for light skinned women has remained prevalent over time in all cultures: Asians, Europeans, Africans, Caribbeans and Americans. However, there are exceptions like the Maasai in Kenya who associate light complexions with being cursed or witchcraft.[1]

In Europe, during the industrial revolution, light skin was associated with high social status as those with tanned skin were the poorer classes who worked outdoors. Colonization and racism, perpetrated the idea that light skin slaves were more beautiful, smarter and cooperative and they often got jobs working in the house "house Negros" while their darker relatives slaved in the fields "fields Negros". Lighter skin amongst blacks still retains its elevated status to the point that studies have associated blackness with low self esteem.

Undeniably, the burden to be attracted to the opposite gender, find marriage and remain in marriage is a common thread that runs through all cultures. See sections on MOTIVES in country specific chapters.

If women in Africa are more susceptible to bleaching the skin than men, it is merely because women are judged much more heavily on the basis of appearance. Men are more likely to be considered valuable when they have wealth, education and other forms of human capital, while women are considered valuable when they are physically attractive, even if they lack other capital. Flick through those magazines and you'll find that the women featured are almost always a few shades lighter than the men. Black men don't need to be light-skinned to be worth paying any attention, but black women do.

In **Sudan**[5,6], a woman is a "girl" until she is married and marriage has become so incumbent on looks. Women carry a heavy burden.[5] The sad thing in the culture is that when you want to remain natural and love your skin you are seen as a radical women instead of a woman who is proud of whom she is. To be happy with whom God made you is to be seen so odd in this generation. To be proud of yourself is a rare thing yet a very rebellious thing in a society where people behave like sheep waiting on their shepherd to tell them what to do"[6]

Skin color plays a significant role in the lives of **Ghanaian** women.[7] Many Ghanaian women's feelings about beauty, attractiveness and the marriage market are associated with skin complexion. Using sixty Ghanaian students and thirty market trading women, a study investigated skin color (i.e. its lightness-darkness) as a function of social capital in the marriage market. A Skin Color Assessment Procedure was administered to all participants. The study showed that although participants were satisfied with their skin color, they believed that Ghanaian men found lighter-skinned women more attractive. This project expands existing scientific and scholarly literature concerning skin bleaching by presenting the implications of skin bleaching from a psychological perspective.

As regards **Senegal**, Dr Pierre-Andre Aka from Ivory Coast says that the predominantly Muslim Senegal, where polygamy is prevalent, rival wives lighten their skin to compete for their husbands favor.[8]

In **Kenya**, wealthy Kenyan women are injecting themselves with dangerous chemicals to lighten their skin because Kenyan men like light complexioned women. This dangerous practice costs $70 US dollars per shot. This is a very lucrative black market practice in Kenya. Wealthy Indian and Somalian women also engage in this practice[9,10,11].

As regards **Jordan**,[12] The role of lighter skin tone in mate selection and the potential perception by men that a lighter skin tone is more attractive are two important reinforcing factors for the use of skin-lightening products. The majority of respondents believe that lighter skin tone is perceived by men as being more attractive and increases a woman's chances of getting married (62.6%). This belief is as expected, more common among skin-lightening products users (71.5%)

In **South Africa**,[13,14] Indian women bleach their skin to enhance their chances of finding marriage. A distinct example revealed itself through marriage advertisements. Indian newspapers, the ethnic weeklies in the US, and South African marriage websites all contained adverts seeking light-skinned partners. Five advertisements on one South Africa website have skin-colour designations ranging from "wheatish" to "very fair".

India's Matrimonial advertisements

Skin color preference in matrimonial matters is something certainly not unique to India; however the way it gets expressed is most certainly distinctive from that in any other society. Whether it is sticking to the tradition of 'arranged marriages' but evolving from the use of matrimonial columns in newspapers to websites like shaadi.com, bharatmatrimony.com or evolving to the system of 'love marriages'; *people still prefer their partners to be light.*

Example: "I am a TV journalist and working in no.1 news channel of India. I want to be the most dynamic and popular news anchor of India. I want to earn a lot of money in my life through my occupation. *My wife 'must be very fair' and beautiful, who can understand and respect my feelings".*[15]

See chapter 8 on SOUTH AFRICA: Motives. Nomazulu says; "*Our men find lighter women very attractive.*" She says skin lightening creams are popular among her friends as they want to brighten their skin. Her husband and other people even compliment her on her complexion now and again."

References

1. Skin bleaching/Africa Science Heroes
http://afrisciheroes.wordpress.com/tag/skin-bleaching

2. Lewis KM, Robin N, Gaska K, Njoku L. Investigating motivations for women's skin bleaching in Tanzania. *Psychology of Women Quarterly* 2011; 35(1): 22-37.
3. Lewis KM, The need for interventions to prevent skin bleaching. A Look at Tanzania. http://jbs.sagepub.com/content/43/7/786.abstract.
4. Lewis KM, Younge S, Njoku LC, Andrews E and Young L. The case of skin bleaching in Tanzania: Who does it? *International Journal of Africana Studies* 2010; 15(2):1-18.
5. Nyabuoy Gatbel. Skin bleaching and the South Sudanese Community. http://www.nyabuoygatbeldeng.com/blog/skin-bleaching-and-the-south-sudanese-community. 10/2/2014
6. Women in Sudan: What the 'ugly' debate tells us about Society. http://www.theguardian.com/world/2014/dec/10/-sp-sudan-ugly-wo..
7. Fokuo JK. Marriage: Skin Bleaching in Post-Colonial Ghana. http://www.ajol.info/index.php/rrias/article/view/44933
8. Penangnini Toure. Skin bleaching on rise in Africa REUTERS NEWS AGENCY. The Toronto Star March 10, 1997. http://www.biyokulule.com/viewcontent.php?articleid=5534
9. Siji Jabbar. Who taught you to hate your [dark] skin? This is Africa. http://thisisafrica.me/who-taught-you-to-hate-your-dark-skin/
10. Celeste Hibbert / Al Jazeera. Kenya's back street #Bleached Beauty trade. http://www.aljazeera.com/indepth/features/2014/06/Kenya-backstreet-bleachedbeauty-trade-201462313468381417.html
11. Celeste Hibbert and Wil Crisp. Rick Kenyans are injecting themselves with Black Market creams to become white. May 29, 2014http://www.vice.com/read/rich-kenyans-bleach-their-skin-white
12. Hamed SH, Tayyem Reema, Nimer N. and Alkhatib HS. *International Journal of Dermatology* 2010;49:414-20.
13. Niyanta Singh. The dark side of skin lightening. http://www.iol.co.za/lifestyle/style/beauty/the-dark-side-of-skin-ligh...
14. Pumza Fihlani Africa: Where black is not really beautiful. BBC News, Johannesburg 1 January 2013http://www.bbc.com/news/world-africa 20444798.
15. Discrimination based on skin color. http://en.wikipedia.org/wiki/Discrimination_based_on_skin_color#cite_note-22

FEMALE CELEBRITY DISCOURSE

The good, the bad and the awkward

Definition

Celebrities, in context of Nigeria culture, are "highly visible people in the media. Media is defined as an umbrella term that encompasses television, movies, newspapers, magazines, music and various other forms of commercialized art including digital media e.g facebook, instagram, twitter etc." The celebrities in Nigeria are movie stars, models, female television presenters and news casters, female politicians and wives of politicians, musicians, winners of beauty pageants, leading women in the corporate world, some female

Christian pastors and wives of pastors. Skin bleaching is highly endemic among these groups of people.

To what extent is the entertainment industry to blame for the fact that so many young women choose to bleach?

It is hard for average people to resist changing their skin tone when they see celebrities looking lighter. Former Major League Baseball player Sammy Sosa's complexion has undergone a drastic change since he retired, but he claims he did not bleach his once-dark skin. When asked what happened, a representative of Sosa said he'd had "skin rejuvenation" and was "surprised he came out looking so white." Pop stars Beyoncé and Rihanna have both been accused of altering their complexion in an attempt to appear whiter. Neither woman has admitted to changing her skin tone.

The troubling message that the entertainment industry transmits is that those with fair skin go further. The entertainment industry disproportionately projects and elevates light-skinned women in magazines, films, music and commercials. If there's a fair girl in it then it's most likely she'll be the lead—affluent, attractive, desired, rich and successful. One is not against light-skinned ladies being centre-stage or in the spotlight. The recommendation is that lead roles should not be because of the shade of their skin, but because they have the right talent for the project. In an ideal world, opportunity should always come down to how good you are at what you do, not how light your skin is. This 'fair girls go far' belief is so deeply engrained in Africa's entertainment industries that a generation of impressionable young people are being driven to seek brighter future by lightening their skin.

A huge bone of contention in west Africa's entertainment hubs—Ghana, Nigeria—is that it is much harder for dark-skinned girls to get decent on-screen roles.[1,2] This was confirmed by Akua Djannie, a Ghanaian writer,[3] who says:

"Not too long ago, a young lady whom I shall call Yaa, came to me with what was for her a very serious dilemma. You see, Yaa's one true desire is to act. In films. O yes, those that know her say from the day she was born, that has been Yaa's only destiny. Anyway, recently she went to audition for a new Ghanaian film and left the place so distraught. The reason? Maybe if I put it in the words of the director, it would be easier to explain. "You see that girl over there? The only difference between you and her is that she is fair-Skinned. Actually, that's not true. You are a better actress, but we like to work with fair skinned women in our films. Now, if you can tone your skin, we can consider you for future films." And there, dear reader was the reason for Yaa's dilemma. Here she was, a very dark skinned woman. Following her heart's desire, yet, it looked like for as long as she maintained her natural God given colour, she would not be able to pursue her dreams. So this young lady came to me for advice. What should she do? Should she tone a little?

Jane 'Efya' Awindor,[4] a practitioner in the entertainment industry writes:
"I have never had to directly deal with this bias so far—not to my face at least (although who knows whether I have missed out on other opportunities due to discussion held behind closed doors where my skin tone was a factor in someone else's discussion-making process). But if someone were ever to suggest to me that I could, say. Conquer the US and win a Grammy if I were to just lighten my skin a little, I would stand my ground and shut them down. Period. I am fine as I am and, more to the point, I have total faith in my talent. I would rather reach my career goals through working hard, working smart, and developing my gifts."

In the Nigerian film industry, a study was done to identify the reasons for the high prevalence for bleaching among the actresses.[5] It is notable that one of the top 5 reasons they gave was "To increase their professional relevance." Not many actresses who bleach their skin would openly agree with this but the truth is that the bold minority have argued in the past that being light skinned has helped them secure more jobs especially in the Nigerian movie industry adding that a broad section of Nollywood producers and film makers have expressed their preference at getting more professionally involved with actresses who are light skinned in comparison with their dark-skinned counterparts.

References

1. Jessica Edmund. Skin bleaching in Ghana: The next generation? Pulitzer center. http://pulitzercenter.org/reporting/africa-ghana-feature-youth-skin-bleac...
2. Siji Jabbar. "Who taught you to hate your [dark] skin? This is Africa http://thisisafrica.me/who-taught-you-to-hate-your-dark-skin/
3. Akua Djannie. Skin Bleaching is a Sin Against God. September 18, 2007 *Guadian.co.uk*. http://www.biyokulule.com/view_content.php?articleid=5534
4. Jane 'Efya' Awindor. Skin lightening strikes at the heart of young women. *Onliris* Sunday, 30 November 2014. http://www.onliris.com/blog/item/27-skin-lightening-strikes-at-the-he..

5. 5 (five) Reasons Nollywood Celebrities Bleach their Skin/…http:www.nigerianbulletin.com/threads/5-reasons-nollywood-celebr…

There is no equivocation on the fact that the current wave of celebrity 'bleached beauties' in Africa has been a major driver of the bleaching culture. The media creates ideals in the form of celebrities and models, for women to admire, Most of them are movie actresses who also feature in the modeling industry. In Nigeria, another group of notorious skin bleachers are some television (TV) news casters and presenters. Because news reading is an everyday, indeed every 30 minutes affair (at the top and bottom of the hour), the people are continuously bombarded with disgustingly yellowish looking faces of bleached news presenters. Curiously, the TV news casters have an unexplainable "halo effect" around them, as they are hardly the subject of overt criticism as their counterparts in the movie and modeling industry. Some of the male news-casters also bleach—it is just that the men are not bold enough to go the whole spectrum like the women. Worse still, some of these celebrity bleachers are **covertly** proselytizing impressionable women—both young and old—by developing and marketing their own range of "skin care" products which are veritable skin lightening products branded, "skin **restoration**" products!

At the other end of the spectrum are **true** celebrities who have **resolutely** decided **not** to bleach their skin and are veritable role models worthy of being celebrated in the ***true*** sense of a celebrity.

It is very useful to examine the lives and life-styles of these two groups (skin bleachers and non bleachers) of celebrities along the following discourse.

1. Who are the notable female celebrities in Africa?
2. Why do they bleach their skin?
3. What methods do they use to lighten their skin?
4. What lessons can we learn from the interviews granted by some of them?
5. No doubt among the skin bleachers Bioncé and Vera Sidika stand out of the crowd as the most vilified. What lessons can we learn from reading details of their life styles and the interviews they have granted?
6. As regards the non-bleaching celebrities—Alex Wek, Lupita Nyongo's and Ajuma Nasenyana stand out. What do we know about them?

The effects of celebrity endorsement

The most lucrative skin-lightening products are increasingly likely to have celebrity ndorsements serve four important purposes: (1) when Celebrities endorse a particular product, the public is more likely to believe in its effectiveness and purchase the product; (2) when celebrities endorse skin-lightening products they also endorse the act of skin lightening itself, suggesting that their own beauty is attainable and that itself, skin lightening is a mainstream, culturally acceptable act; (3) celebrity endorsement forms a direct association between whiteness and experiencing success; (4) the celebrity endorsers have a greater influence in reinforcing hegemonic whiteness due to their popularity. The latter point is particularly important because skin-lightening is still shameful in some cultures either because one should "naturally" have light skin, not chemically derived light skin, or because some believe that lightening the skin implies a shame of one's race or ethnic identity, and that bleaching women are trying to get something that is not naturally theirs. Overcoming these powerful narratives of "natural beauty" and "racial pride" are crucial for the success of cosmetics companies.

A classical example of celebrity endorsement is Whitenicious by Beyonce, the Nigerian-Cameroonian pop musician. Whitenicius promises to help users rid themselves of pesky dark spots by gradually lightening the hyper-pigmented areas of their skin. However, from the looks of Beyonce own skin, she's been using it (or something more powerful to transform her complexion from deep mahogany to vampire white. According to its website, Whitenicious (priced between $50-$150 US), was instantly sold out! For her efforts Beyonce has been inundated with criticism (and praise) about her skin-toning line via Twitter, but she isn't fazed. Along with re-tweeting links to mentions her product, she's been taking on critics who deride her for promoting and capitalizing on self-hate.

One of the most controversial celebrity endorsements came in 2007 when mega-successful Bollywood actor, Shah Rukh Khan endorsed the skin-lightening product, "Fair and Handsome." Created by the British company, Unilever, and marketed as the masculine companion product to best-selling Fair and Lovely, Fair and Handsome became the first major skin-lightening product mass-marketed exclusively to men. Khan's endorsement was read by the Indian public as an endorsement of skin-bleaching itself and as an endorsement of a strongly colorbased system of privilege in India. Similarly, U.S. baseball star Sammy Sosa, originally of the Dominican Republic, recently attracted international media attention when he appeared at the Latin Grammy Awards with notably lighter skin than he had during his career in Major League Baseball. Sosa has suggested that he is negotiating an endorsement deal with the cosmetic company that manufactured his skinlightening cream (which he has refused to name in public). His de facto celebrity endorsement of skin-bleaching elicited significant feedback including a televised ridiculing from former NBA basketball star, Charles Barkley. Despite the media furor, Sosa's actions reinforce the idea that skinbleaching is a mainstream route to building racial capital.

Meanwhile, Jamaican celebrities continue to line up to endorse these products. In 2013, the music of black origin (MOBO)-nominated artist of the year Vybz Kartel launched his own range of men's cosmetics including a variety of "skin-brightening" items.

References

1. Charles CAD. Skin bleaching, self-hate, and Black identity in Jamaica. *Journal of Black Studies*, 2003; 33 (6): 711-18

2. Britni Danielle. . Nigerian Singer Releases 'Whitenicious' Skin Lightening Cream and its sold out. Jan 20, 2014 http://www.xojane.com/issues/nigerian-singer-releases-whitenicious

3. Parameswaran R & Cardoza K. Melanin on the margins: Advertising and the cultural politics of Fair/light/white beauty in India. *Journalism & Communication Monographs*. 2009; 11 (3), 213-74

4. Mitchell F. Sosa says he's preparing to endorse skin product. *Huffington Post*. Retrieved from http://www.chicagobreakingssports.com/2009/11/sosa-says-hes-preparing-toendorse-skin-product.html.

Five Reasons Nollywood Celebrities Bleach their Skin

Below are 5 reasons most light skinned celebrities in Nollywood bleach:

To look more beautiful/attractive

This is perhaps one of the biggest reasons women who allegedly bleach their skin fall into the trap of losing their darker skin tone as they have mentally come to believe that a lighter skin tone automatically translates into a more beautiful and far more attractive outlook. Not that they do not consider themselves beautiful but they consider a lighter complexion a tad more beautiful and of course a bigger element of attraction to the opposite sex.

To increase their professional relevance

Not many actresses who bleach their skin would openly agree with this but the truth is that the bold minority have argued in the past that being light skinned has helped them secure more jobs especially in the Nigerian movie industry adding that a broad section of Nollywood producers and film makers have expressed their preference at getting more professionally involved with actresses who are light skinned in comparison with their dark-skinned counterparts.

To attract the right suitors

Cut out the minority population of Nollywood actresses who have established a notorious reputation as feminists especially those who have resolved never to get married and what we have left are those who look forward to that moment in their lives when they have a family they can happily call their own. Apparently, the first hurdle to cross is that of getting the attention of handsome, confident, wealthy and powerful men who will woo them and besiege them with romantic offerings that offer a promise of exotic locations, comfort and a secure matrimonial future. It is no longer news that some Nollywood practitioners hold a warped belief that being light skinned automatically delivers them into the minds and thoughts of men who have everything it takes to make a woman financially, mentally and emotionally happy for the rest of her life.

The bandwagon syndrome

The fear of being left behind by peers or missing out of what is hypothetically believed to work has just enough mental drive to make a Nollywood actress move from being dark skinned in July 2014 to becoming light skinned in February 2015 and we have had several cases of this in Nollywood's history. First, one person does it, the second person does it, then a third, a fourth, fifth, sixth and then we lose track of the numbers.

Looking good in photos

Take a look at these two facts - First, as at December 2013, over 31 million images tagged #selfies (predominantly by ladies) had been posted on the popular photo-based social media website, Instagram. Secondly, some studies have shown that an amazing population of women are obsessed with their own beauty to the point of always capturing images of themselves no matter how many they already have - When we add these two permutations, the result we have on our hands cannot be far off from the motive behind most Nollywood celebrities who opt to become much lighter than they already are.

Images of these glaring transformations are not farfetched with certain names resonating across the walls of our memories.

Reference

5 (five) Reasons Nollywood Celebrities Bleach their Skin/…http:www.nigerianbulletin.com/threads/5-reasons-nollywood-celebr…

How celebrities lighten their skin tone

Several black celebrities have been accused of bleaching[1]. Notable among them are Diana Ross, Halle Berry, Iman, Lark Voorhies, Latoya Jackson, Lil Kim, Michael Jackson, Nomasonto Mshoza' Mnisi, Rapper Trina, Sammy Sosa, Tamar Braxton, Tempestt bledsoe, Trina McGee, Vybz Kartel, Yvonne Nelson and Beyonce.

Celebrities lighten their skin tone through intensive skin regimens involving a host of different procedures performed by dermatologists and aestheticians. These methods are not permanent and need to be kept up to maintain benefit.[2]

It is possible to lighten one's skin shade by one or two tones. The first level involves minimizing something known as delayed pigmentary tanning for patients with darker skin types. This is done through a combination of the following methods: Skin lightening surgery or skin bleaching plastic surgery, Microdermabrasion, chemical pills, Mesotherapy, LED light devices, Fraxel laser treatment. In addition to all of the above, skin care regimens containing hydroquinone, retinoic acid, arbutin and kojic acid are used at night and protective serums (e.g vitamin C serums) + rigorous sunscreen use in the day time.

Lastly a lot of editing is done to pictures published in magazines which makes the skin of celebrities look super smooth, flawless in many cases. However this is not what their skins would look like without make up and photoshop.

References

1.http://www.docshop.com/education/dermatology/facial/mocrodermabrasion

2. Atlanta Blackstar. 15 Black Celebs Caught Whitening their skin *http://www.atlantablackstar.com/2013/08/19/15-black-celebs-caught-white…*

3. Dr Nair. How do celebrities lighten their skin tone? *http://www.justanswer.com/dermatology/77tvh-celebrities-lighten-skin..*

Dencia—Interview

Dencia Wants to Set the Record Straight on Whitenicious

Reprudencia Sonkey, better known as Dencia, is a Cameroonian artist and business woman. She is a pop singer, hiphop video model and entrepreneur. She is currently based in Los Angles, California. She makes $20 million per year from whitenicious.

The pop stars says her product is not a skin bleach—and that African Americans are the ones rushing to buy it

In early January, 2014, Cameroonian pop singer, Dencia, launched a new skin care line, Whitenicious. Within 24 hours, it sold out—and "before" and "after" pictures of the entrepreneur set the internet ablaze. Three weeks later, sales approach 20,000 units and show no signs of slowing down. Although the product promotes itself as a "7 day fast acting dark spot remover," many have criticized Dencia for not only promoting skin lightening, but self-hatred among women of color and more specifically, African women. Despite the backlash, Dencia stands behind Whitenicious and believes that she is in fact helping women overcome an obstacle. Here, Dencia tells her side of the story.

Ebony: So you know there's been a lot of buzz about you on the internet here lately. Everybody's talking about your new skin care line, Whitenicious. Tell me how you came up with it.

Dencia: And I'm happy that they're talking because my sales are skyrocketing. Anyway. A few months ago, I was coming back from Switzerland. I sat by this chemist. He's from Switzerland. We started talking about all these things and he was like "You have really nice skin." He asked me if I was Puerto Rican by the way. I was like "No, I'm African." We started talking about skin care and stuff and then I told him how I've been doing all these things, going to dermatologists for the problems. Every woman does that. Like when you have a little spot on your face. I know I do. I'll be running from dermatologist to dermatologist trying to find something to get rid of the dark spots. Unfortunately, all dermatologists will give you hydroquinone 4%. It don't matter if you're as dark as Alek Wek or you're as White as a blonde girl from Malibu. They'll give you the same thing. So he was telling me that he makes some products and that he has a line. He asked me if want to be the face of it. And I was like you know what? We'll talk about it. I had come up with this mixture of things that I've been using, not for my skin but for my face for like when I had dark spots or when I hyperpigmented anywhere on my body. And so I sat down with him, we tested it, we looked at it, we added stuff and then we came up with the product. I tested it on me and on my sisters. I have a sister that has suffered with acne for a long time and she had dark spots. So she used it and it worked really good. And I went on Facebook and I asked my Facebook friends if they wanted to try it. They tried it, and it worked really well. And mind you, this product doesn't have hydroquinone, it doesn't have steroids, and it doesn't have mercury.

So, when the time came to pick out the name for the product, I was talking to my best friend and she was telling me, if you're picking out a name you have to look at something that is attractive. When you see Whitenicious, you see the container, you see the product, obviously you're thinking this is gonna work, right? That's what you're thinking. We came up with different names. You know, I was coming up with all these glamorous things and my best friend was like "Nah, 'Whitenicious' is good." And when she gave me the name, I was looking up definitions of white. Ok let me define how I see white. (reads) "The color white affects the mind and the body by aiding in mental clarity, promoting feelings of fresh beginnings and renewal assisting in cleansing, clearing obstacles and clutter and encouraging purification." And guess what? Dark spots is obstacles. Hyperpigmenation is obstacles.

Ebony: Is dark skin an obstacle?

Dencia: No. Dark skin is beautiful. Actually, I will send you pictures of when I was 16. I'm not that lighter from when I was younger, I'm not. The picture they're passing around where I'm wearing the animal print underwear, that picture was three years ago and that was a tan. If anybody looks at that picture and you look at the oil on my skin, you would know it's a tan. And it's funny because one of my friends who was at the photo shoot with me that actually oiled me up with the tan sent me a message yesterday. She was like "Why are people going crazy about this picture when you were tanned on this picture?" I was never that dark in real life and I can send EBONY pictures of me when I was like 15, 16. And guess what? I don't even care because they're bringing me business. Because when you take that picture and you put a picture of Dencia darker, this is what you're telling people – the product really works. And guess what? People really want to buy it. It's what it is. I don't really care.

Ebony: So…you haven't bleached your skin, is what you're saying? You were tan in the before pictures?

Dencia: Have I…Has my skin lightened from when…like from the past five years? Yes it has. It has. Has it drastically lightened? No it hasn't. Is it what people are saying? No it's not.

Ebony: Okay. But do you understand people's response to the pictures? Because many people have become aware that skin bleaching is a big phenomenon around the world, particularly in West Africa where you're from. And so then we see one picture of you or a few pictures of you where you look browner and then we see this new picture of you, and not just that it's a picture of you per se, but an advertisement for a product called Whitenicious. And then it says "Say goodbye to pigmentation and spots forever."

Dencia: First of all when I did the photoshoot…let me tell you something, I did the Whitenicious photo shoot on the 13th of December, 2013. I just came back from Paris. I was in Europe for a month and I was indoors. I don't go outside a lot generally. If you're light skinned and you stay indoors a lot it's gonna give you that pale look. And then I had just been going back and forth to the hospital because I was not feeling too good. My health is not very stable and it's not because of anything with this, it's something that I've had since I was a little girl. I was dehydrated and they gave me the drips to hydrate me. And when you come out with all those things, it makes you fresh and it gives you that pale look because you've not been out in the sun. That is why those pictures look like that. And everybody, even my sister said "Are you okay?" because they knew I was not feeling good. So it's not about being pale because I'm bleaching my skin. It's just because I stay indoors a lot and I take a lot of vitamins. Lots. And all those things have effects on your skin. And in the past I've probably taken medications that… you know there's a lot of medications that have side effects of lightening your skin too.

And anyway, the picture clearly says "Say goodbye to dark spots and hyperpigmentation." I'm not saying "say goodbye to your Black skin and try to be like Dencia." That's not what I'm saying. I'm saying "say goodbye to dark spots and hyperpigmentation." Now did I choose to do beginning pictures for a reason? Yes, I did. I did that because sexy sells. Period. I have men, White men, Black men, buying Whitenicous. Guess what is attracting them? Those pictures. And guess what they're using it for? Dark spots. Not to bleach their entire skin. I don't think a White man is trying to bleach his skin.

Trust me, I've been running this business for the past three weeks and I've read all these emails from girls telling me about how they have this hyperpigmentation, how they have these dark spots. I have seen so many pictures. These girls are not trying to bleach their skin. They're just trying to get rid of these little things that is making them feel uncomfortable, you know?

Ebony: I hear you, I do. And you're right, many women of African descent, many women of color, we do suffer from hyperpigmentation. So there are lots of products on the market that work to fade out those spots, if you will. But there are also products… and you know this, especially in West Africa. We see the billboards, we see them in the markets, we see the women with all of the damage on their skin – there are products out there that are used to bleach the skin. Your product is called Whitenicious, of course people will buy it because they want to bleach. Ok. Will Whitenicious bleach your skin if you use it on all your skin?

Dencia: Yes, it will. Are we selling Whitenicous for that purpose? No, we're not. Whitenicous comes in 30 ml and 60ml. You cannot use the 60 ml to bleach your whole skin. It's impossible. And that costs about $150 each. 60 ml can't even go on your whole feet. I don't see anybody spending all that money to bleach their entire skin. I don't see that happening. Now, do I have customers who come and buy stuff for over $2000? Yes, I do. Do I ask them what they want to do with it? No, I don't. Do I know what they want to do with it? No, I don't care because it's their money, it's how they want to spend it."

Ebony: Is the success of the line because people want to bleach?

Dencia: "No, that's not how I see it. This is how I see it. Everybody that has something negative to say, (1) doesn't need it and (2) don't have the money to buy it. First of all, let me clear this up. As of now 80% of people that buy my products are African Americans. It's not Africans. People are saying that it's Africans because they think I live in Africa. I go back and forth but I live here. I can send you the stats – it is African Americans. I have to be honest with you – I have TV personalities buying Whitenicious for over $1000. People who work for TV stations like Fox.

I have celebrities buying Whitenicous and all of these people are African Americans, they are not Africans. My African market is just 10% because guess what? They don't have credit cards to buy the products and I'm only taking credit cards or PayPal. And they don't have that access, do you get what I'm saying?

Now, my other 10% is White people – I have White people from Europe, America, and everywhere buying Whitenicious. Now, I'm thinking to myself, what do they want to do with it? Of course they're not trying to bleach their skin. Are Black people trying to get White to be accepted in society? No, I don't think so. Now I can't speak for everybody but first of all, White people love the darker skinned

Africans. They like the African that is **Alek Wek**. There's no in between for them. It's extreme. You're either at A or you're at Z.

Now, do you think Africans are lightening to appeal to the White man? No, they're not because the White man doesn't even like the light Africans. They like the Black Africans. Look at all the Africans that are successful in the world. They are as Black as Alek Wek. And if I was as Black as Alek Wek, I would never ever use anything on my skin. Trust me I wouldn't."

Ebony: I hear Whitenicious could cause cancer?

Dencia: "But guess what? The air you breathe outside causes you cancer. Everything in the world causes cancer."

Ebony: What about those before and after photos?

Dencia: "I've always been a beautiful girl. It didn't matter if I was Black, White, yellow, blue, green. I have always been a very beautiful girl. It didn't matter. Do I look more beautiful than I was before? Did I look more beautiful before than I am now? No. My beauty is who I am inside and out. It's what is in my heart, it's what I do for people, [and] it's what I read in the Bible that makes me a better person. Do you get what I'm saying? I read the Bible a lot and I don't see any place in the Bible that says that "If you bleach yourself, if you change your skin color, it's a sin." I have never seen that so please, if you've seen it let me know so I can go read that part of the Bible."

Ebony: Why did you lighten your skin?

Dencia: "Why did I get a couple of shades lighter than I was? That's a personal choice. That is what I wanted to be. And honestly, I just wanted to. I'm very daring. I like trying things. I'm not doing it because I wanna have boyfriends. And I'm not doing it because I want anybody to accept me. It's because I just wanted to do it."

Ebony: Is the skincare line making you rich?

Dencia: Is Whitenicious making me rich? Whitenicious is putting money in my pocket but it's not as much as the money that I have spent being a celebrity. It hasn't gotten to that point. Trust me I've made a lot of money off Whitenicous in 3 weeks. A lot of money. A lot of money that I didn't even expect. And I'm using it to build an orphanage in Cameroon. I've always wanted to build an orphanage but the only way that I could really realize this project was by starting a business. And then Whitenicious fortunately happened."

Ebony: Do you care about the backlash?

Dencia: "No. No, I do not. I have more important things going on in my life. I have my health, I have my career, I have so many things. I have an orphanage I'm trying to build. Where do I have time to sit and think of these people? I don't. Because I don't really feel bad about everything you guys are saying, I don't. Because "she, me, her I don't care" in my Tamar voice.

Ebony: What is responsible for Whitenicious' success?

Dencia: You know what? It's God. Honestly, I don't know. Like I can't even explain. I think its God. Everything I touch turns into gold. And it's not just today. I have run businesses before. My first I was like 15. I had a hair salon and a clothing store. And it was really successful. I just think some people are born to be what they are. It was really successful. And if you believe in yourself and you believe in something and you pray to God to make it successful it's gonna happen.

It's no way it won't happen. I have other things I could do. I have other things I am doing. Like everything you see me wearing, I make them. I have made stuff for a lot of celebrities in America. I have made stuff for Nicki Minaj, I have made stuff for Christina Milian, I have made stuff for Lil' Mama, I've made stuff for Rihanna. I've made stuff for many celebrities. I do design well. I do hair very well. You see all the hair I have on? The wigs or whatever? I make those wigs. I sew, I make shoes, I do all those things. Now, why didn't I get in with these things to the market? Because it's saturated. Everybody and their mama and their grandmama and grand uncles have clothing lines. Everybody is selling hair. Everybody is doing these things. I don't follow the pack, I lead the pack.

But my clothing line is still gonna come out, my shoe line is still gonna come out. I just do it exclusively for celebrities. I have a really big project I'm working on in America. When that project comes out, I'm gonna be able to market the other things that I have but for right now Whitenicious is a better market. Whitenicious markets itself. I don't need to do nothing."

- **Responses and public reactions to Dencia interview**

(1) *"Having read the comments of Dencia on this thread, there are definitely no prizes for guessing right that most of us Naija people are hardcore fanatical haters. There are over 10 different (billion dollar/Trillion Naira) industries that cause cancer that we don't hear any rumbling about from you. I would have listed them but I will instead spare you the details since you guys are Laboratory Scientists that know too well what causes cancer and doesn't. If you can't be happy for the girl publicly, please do your bashing indoors!! Like she said, instead of wasting your time trying to bring her and her products down, you can either send your NDLEA to seize her cancer inducing CONTAINER when it docks at your port or you guys can do something more positive and create cancer free BLACNICIOUS and go out there and win more ARMY for the Black race! If that makes you feel better."*

(2) *"To the keyboard warriors, try and have a heart and support your people. Her market is predominantly not for Africans as she claims, so just help soften your hate. At least they have competent doctors hospitals to look after themselves even if the cancer comes through from her cream unlike our sorry country."*

(3) **Big sigh* "That's off my chest now!! Thanks be to God!! I was boiling earlier."*

"This is BS. She's talking out of her neck." Miss Sisie

"I don't see the issue. Aren't we for personal freedom? After all, it's your skin. You have the right to apply what to and what not to on your body. There are more important problems in the world, and people are concerned with the cosmetic choices of others."

"It is more than a cosmetic ch oice issue…it is an issue of self-hatred…that affects all of us."

"Do you wear makeup? do you use extension? do you use anything for your blemishes? if you answer yes to any of the questions then you know what you are !!!"

"Lip stick, eyeliner and blush are NOT equivalent to SKIN BLEACHING!!!" Tiara Mari

"Make up does not harm your skin. Bleaching damages your skin forever. You are susceptible to skin cancer which is ugly and expensive to treat. Just like smoking and drug taking, we need to discuss and discourage the young generation from indulging in harmful substances. We should care as a society and that's what we are doing." Vundukai

"She's not the first to sell bleaching cream. Btw I think she sells dark spots remover, not total body bleaching cream. JUST SAYING IN CASE WE MISSED IT. I went to her website and she doesn't sell body lotions. Haven't been on her website until today." www.whitenicious.com

Reference

Yaba Blay Dencia Wants to Set the Record Straight on Whitenicious [Interview] *EBONY* February 2014 http://www.ebony.com/entertainment-culture/dencia-wants-to-set-the-r...

Vera Sidika

Kenyan Socialite, Vera Sidika criticized for spending $170,000 on skin lightening treatment

Popular Kenyan socialite, Vera Sidika is under attack for revealing on TV during an interview, Friday, June 6 that she has spent £100,000 (15 million Kenyan shillings) for skin lightening treatment done in the UK. Vera who is popularly called Kenya's 'Kim Kardashian' because of her **massive behind and curves** is obviously not bothered with what critics think said: *"Looking good is my business, my body is my business, nobody else's but mine"*. Vera who says she's already seen an increase in demand for her services is no doubt gaining popularity for her skin lightening as she made it to BBC Trending News on the morning of 10 June 2014. Meanwhile a hashtag #Bleachedbeauty was created for people to share their opinions on the issue of skin lightening and over 4,000 people have commented. According to some tweets: "#BleachedBeauty is fake. Only those with low self-esteem would do that," one tweeted. Another tweet says: "#Bleachedbeauty Ladies will soon begin bleaching their brains so they come up with bright ideas". While some have criticized, others, however praised her "openness and honesty" in speaking about the issue.

One of who is, TV host Larry Madowo who descried the reaction on social media as "Fascinating", "astounding" and "hypocritical" while saying many men in Kenya do indeed prefer light-skinned women, referring to them affectionately as "yellow, yellow". Dark-skinned women are sometimes derogatively called "tinted". Although skin lightening in Kenya is still confidential unlike India where it is common, experts, however says its on the increase and warned of the dangers of unregulated black market treatments.

➢ **Introducing the new Vera Sidika!...Socialite Extraordinaire!**

A few months ago, socialite Vera Sidika shocked Kenyans and the world at large when she confidently bleached and came out defending herself. She made headlines even on CNN and BBC with headlines such as "Bleached Beauty" trending World Wide because of our very own Vera!

We were among the first few people who came out strongly against her bleaching and the kind of morals she is portraying and showing our young girls. So, to those who don't know how Vera bleached, this is how she did it:

Vera Sidika, being broke and living the **"Fake it till you make it… and make sure you are not caught faking it before you make it"** life went for **cheap** Plastic Surgery from a Certain Dr. Abdullahi Aden, a doctor at Karen Hospital, who also did her Breast implants after the surgery. Vera did not have enough cash to do proper plastic surgery (The Lil Kim, MJ type) so she got cheap "River Road" injections from Dr. Aden.

From a very close Doctor friend of mine, I learnt that the injections are normally taken in a span of 8 to 15 months for you to get the desired looks with minimal or no effects at all. Vera wanting it all PAP!...She took a year's worth of injection in just one week…Yes! One week, which made her transform from "Omo" to "Persil" in just "One Wash".

But as we predicated, the type of bleaching she did would definitely have side effects. What the injections do is that they kill your skin pigment (Melanin) making your dark skin turn white since there is no more melanin to give your skin its color.

A little over two months now since Vera **over** Bleached, the effects have started being felt. Vera has since been in hiding because of shame as she now looks **ugly** and close to an Albino. She has stopped posted update pictures of herself on Instagram, Facebook and Twitter but we were able (as usual) to get exclusive pictures of how Vera now looks.

- **10 Things You Didn't know about Vera**[2]

Vera Sidika is a controversial Kenyan model. She has always been criticized in social media for acting in strange ways. For instance, she was criticized and ridiculed for saying that she never wears underpants.

Nobody knows where she gets her money from. Vera is unemployed. She alleges that most of her money comes from her business in Nigeria. Her critics have been fast to outshine her Nigerian deals by explaining that she only goes to Nigeria to extract money from oil tycoons.

The profile of Vera Sidika is published under "10 things you didn't know about Vera Sidika." Notable among the '10 things' are

- She bleached her body
- She enlarged her boobs
- She contested for the Big Brother Africa event

Vera has always strived to participate in the big Brother Africa event but she has not been successful. In one occasion during the selection process, she is reported to have removed her underpants in the presence of the judges in order to convince them. When asked why she removed her underpants, she mentioned that the house was hot. Despite her action she was never taken.

- She claims to have the biggest butt
- She is never ashamed

The controversial things that we hear about Vera have not made her feel ashamed. She has always been eager to give reasons and explain why she does what she does. However, she always maintains silence when asked to explain the nude photos of her that are everywhere in the internet.

➢ **"Letter to all my Haters," By Vera Sidika[3]**

This is what the b()()tilicious Vera Sidika had to say to all her Haters.

Message to the haters;
Here's the thing, this is my page & I post whatever da hell I want.

My body-(let me use an easier term for it to flow) If I wanna bleach my skin, brain, intestines, implants, ovaries that's my problem and not yours!

As long as you are not financing it neither do I have debt with any of y'all. Stop complaining! Fake skin, fake boobs oh hell yeah I own it! I'm real about being fake. But one thing for sure, my ass ain't fake. Don't compare pics of my modelling days when I was starving myself to get jobs with the current situation when I'm content with my life. The day I decide to go for surgery for my ass y'all will know it's fake cz I'll get a super round, huge, perfectly smooth no mistake Brazilian butt!!! & will definitely Inform you. My ass is too small to be claiming it's fake & if I gotta pay for surgery has be HUGE N PERFECT."

References

1. BBC Trending #BBCtrending: Is Kenya's Vera Sidika a #BleachedBeauty? 10 June 2014. http://www.bbc.com/news/blogs-trending-27768032

2. 10 Things you didn't know about Vera Sidika. http://buzzkenya.com/vera-sidika
3. Vera Sidika "Letter to all my Haters" GOSSIP NEWS AFRICA: KENYA. http://africagossipnews.com/

GHANA

- **Yvonne Nelson**

Yvonne Nelson, one of the Ghanaian celebrities, is an enterprising and hard working lady. She has her own line of human hair, her boutique and she is currently working on her third movie. However, people have accused her of undergoing a complete 360 degree change, physically. First people were shocked by her drastic weight loss, then people started to talk about her alleged bleaching. When she heard the talks about the bleaching stuff, she decided to release a statement, setting the records straight that she has never bleached and will never bleach her skin!

Yvonne Nelson Addresses Bleaching Rumours......Releases Press Statement

My attention has been drawn to recent media reports that I am bleaching my skin and the continuous nature of this wicked, unfounded and absolutely unnecessary misinformation have compelled me to once again respond. These stories are absolutely not true and do not in any way put food on anybody's table, does not add value to any body's life and can only be described as mischief.

I fully understand the dangers of skin bleaching and would not engage in any such venture. I am a lady and I appreciate my God-given looks. I do not need to change my skin colour for any reason. Truth is that even if I was bleaching, I do not owe anyone any explanation, but I am not bleaching, I have not bleached and I won't bleach. I love my skin just the way it is and I do my best to keep it healthy and nice. If God has remained good to me and continues to make my skin nicer, I do not see how it should be a problem to someone.

In a society that largely frowns on skin bleaching, it would be unfair and very unkind to falsely accuse me of bleaching when I am absolutely innocent of that charge. As an actress I take different pictures under different shades of light and with different shades of makeup depending on what the picture would be used for. It is therefore not strange to find different pictures of me looking different. It does not mean I am bleaching and one does not need to be an industry player to know this. Even in movies, depending on who the director is, there are different lighting angles and brightness levels that can be used to make a character look different and this is no secret. Even a change of weather can have an effect on one's skin.

I want to use this platform to assure all persons who have expressed worry about these reports that there is no cause for alarm because I am not bleaching, have not bleached and would not bleach. There are more prudent and beneficial things to focus on and these frequent distractions are of no use. I should have spent this time focusing on my new movies or memorizing my next script and not responding to false gossips.
Thank you.
Sincerely yours
Yvonne Nelson

- **Miriam Abdul Rauf**

Former Ghana's Most Beautiful winner, Miriam Abdul Rauf, popularly known as Nasara, was dark skinned when she participated in and was crowned Ghana's Most Beautiful, a TV 3 reality show in 2009. Lately she has become fairer sparking speculations that she is bleaching. The mother of twins confirms she is bleaching, speaking an interview with Doloris Frimpong Manson on the Delay. She explains that, "in life we are all entitled to what we want to do… I choose to tone my skin and I don't think it's a problem because if it were a problem to me, I won't do it." She added "I do not regret it. In fact I love it. Unlike those days when the creams were so harsh and cheap now there are better creams that will just tone your body…. And will just befit you." Reacting to assertions that prolonged bleaching could cause skin cancers, Nasara said "In life, everything comes with the bad aspects of it... when you are doing something, sometimes you don't really need to think about the bad part of it. I am just doing it because I am comfortable with it and I don't even think about the negative part of it." Nasara made the headlines in 2012 when she was accused of stealing a mobile phone and make up kit of Miss England during a beauty pageant outside the country ‰an allegation she denied. She was consequently stripped of her Ghana Most Beautiful title.

SOUTH AFRICA

Former kwaito star **Mshoza**, real name Nomasonto Mnisi; **Sorisha Naidoo**, former *Scandal!* Actress who came out with a whitening skin range of her own. Naidoo's ***Pure Perfect*** apparently fixes "colour problems and even out skin tone." Her complexion has become considerably lighter over the years. Singer **Kelly Khumalo** is said to have used a cream called Carolight to become a few shades lighter. Drum magazine reported that Khumalo and her sister, **Zandi**, were allegedly buying the lightening lotion from street vendors. Pop star **Nicki Minaj** has fueled rumours over the years that she had her skin lightened. The rapper's complexion has changed since she first became popular in the entertainment industry.

NIGERIA

The Nigeria-Cameroonian singer, **Dencia**, released a dark spot remover which she titled ***Whitenicious***. The range was released at the beginning of the year and is available online. According to Dencia, 80% of her customers are African Americans, 10% are Africans and 10% Europeans. Some other Nigerian bleachers are **Tonto Dikeh**—the eccentric, brash, actress and singer. She has been accused of a lot of things and bleaching is one of them. Some others are **Thelma O'khaz**, **Pela Tonye** and **Susan Maxwell**.

References

1. Bernice Maune. Gallery: Skin lightening celebrities. 10 September, 2014. http://www.timeslive.co.za/lifestyle/2014/09/10/gallery-skin-lightening-celebrities
2. Nigerian celebrities who have been accused of bleaching their skin… Before and after Pics (Pt1). Yeoal's Blogzine™/Nigerian Urban, Gossip and Entertainment Site.." Ni… Wednesday, 13 February 2013. http://www.yeoal.com/2013/02/nigerian-celebrities-who-have-been_13...
3. Top 5 Ghanaian celebrities accused of bleaching their skin. *Nollywood HardTalk*. 5 May 2012. http://www.modernghana.com/movie/18675/3/top-5-ghanaian-celebrities...
4. Yvonne Nelson Addresses Bleaching Rumous… Releases Press Statement. Friday, 26 October 2012. http://www.yeoal.com/2012/10/yvonne-nelson-addresses-bleaching.html

Susan Maxwell's Interview (naijahomeandaway)

"I bleached because 80% of Nigeria men prefer fair women"-Actress Susan Maxwell

Susan Maxwell is one of Nollywood stars that are ready to take the acting profession to the next level, and she has got a figure that can assist her do just that. The Abia State-born actress has carved a niche for herself in Nollywood, even without learning the ropes from her late uncle, Ashley Nwosu. Today, she is reaping the fruits of her hard labour. Susan, made her foray into acting with Isawuru. Since then, she has acted and produced several other movies. Although acting is her first love, the cankerworm of piracy which has burned many actors forced her to face her other passion, skin care. In this interview, Maxwell tells all about piracy, why Nigerian men prefer light-skinned women and why acting is her passion, but skin care is her life.

Describe your journey into the movie industry.
Movie making has been a part of me since childhood. I started from my church drama group. When I felt it was time to bring out what I had to people who know more than I do in the field, I joined a group in my area at Ipaja. A year later, I shot my first movie, *Isawuru,* in 2007, directed by Murphy Afolabi, and that was the movie that brought me to the limelight. The marketer approached me to do another movie and the same year we shot another movie called *Nkan to ba gba*, directed by Odunlade Adekola. Later on, I got another vision for my skin care business which I started officially in 2010, but started in my house in 2009, and that pulled me out of the industry. Now this business pays me more than acting.

How has piracy affected your career?
Piracy is not encouraging talents. I did a movie recently and after pumping in a lot of money I did not get returns on my investment. Outside money, acting is something I truly enjoy, but piracy is not letting me practice what I enjoy. I shot *Faramade* with one million, one hundred and fifty thousand naira (N1,150,000) and made only seven hundred thousand naira (N700,000). Most people ask us if we are crazy. Why do we pump money into something that doesn't yield returns? Even if it's not giving you any profit, it should give you the capital back, but when you're doing something you have passion for, it looks crazy to people, and yes I'm crazy about what I do.

What solution would you proffer to this problem?
I don't have much of a choice; as they say, 'If you can't beat them, join them'. There is nothing one can do about Alaba pirates for now. The solution is to produce what the marketers can sell at a reasonable price before the pirates produce theirs. I will still press further and hope that the new government will intervene. I also hope God helps us all. Many in the industry have tried their best to beat piracy to no avail. They have tried everything, from rallies, to visiting Alaba market etc, all to no avail. No one knows who the pirates are. My conclusion is that when something is beyond human power, we have no choice but to call on God.

How did you start your skin care business?
When I started my skin care business, I thought it was for people who needed to brighten their skin. With time, I got clients with serious

medical problems. In some cases, I've had to protect myself because of the severity. Some clients came to me after visiting several hospitals. I was their last resort and by God's grace they used my products and the story changed for better. This has spurred me on. I started with a short formal training, and with personal research and talent; I have only had positive results.

Many people are of the opinion that light-skinned ladies are more attractive, and everything they wear shows off better and that is why I am here to help people enhance their complexion. I used to be very dark; I never thought I could become as fair as I am. I did it because I want to practice what I preach. I want them to see me and be blown away, especially those who knew me when I was dark. Because what I'm giving people isn't something that would damage their skin but repair their skin, I use it on myself as well. If I wasn't in this line of business, I probably wouldn't have toned my skin at all. I don't call it bleaching. I call it skin restoration.

They say "Black is beautiful" is that statement overrated?
In Nigeria, people believe our weather doesn't encourage them to maintain their dark complexions, often getting uneven skin tones because of the harsh rays of the sun. Most people believe when they are fair, rain or shine, they have something constant to maintain. Most of my clients are above 18, and if they want to be white, I give them what they want. ***Black is beautiful, but I have no qualms with enhancing your complexion. 80% of Nigerian men want their women to be fair. They want a lady that draws attention to them. I've worked with many married women who complain of their men staring at fair women and they say to me, "Susan, make me fair, I want to be attractive to my man!" Some women have said their sons want them to visit their schools because they want to show off their fair mother.*** Clients all over the world have asked for my products. Black is beautiful but there is nothing wrong with enhancing your complexion.

Acting is my passion, skin care is my life. Acting has helped my business because people recognize me and are relaxed around me because they know I wouldn't want to tarnish my image.

What are the challenges you face?

So far, I haven't had many. I just have those I call stubborn clients who expect my products to act like magic. I tell them, anything that turns you white overnight can damage your skin overnight but many of them are impatient.

Does this line of business bring you fulfilment?
I have tried many businesses. Clothing, hair, makeup etc but skin treatment has brought me a lot of respect.

Are you married?
I am not married. I have a wonderful daughter who is my life and my world, and I would like to have more kids. I am currently engaged to my baby's father, Tokunbo Awoga, a producer/director, although we do not live together. He directed Faramade and we will be working on another movie soon. I named my movie Faramade after my daughter.

Where do you see yourself in five years?
I would like to see my products retailed in different stores.

Reference

1. http://naijahomeandaway.blogspot.com.ng/2015/05/i-bleached-because-80-of-nigerian-men.html#.VfvSk32SXDf

ICON OF BLACK BEAUTY

(1) Ajuma Nasenyana

Kenyan model Ajuma Nasenyana fights skin lightening and European standards of beauty

From **Clutch Magazine** – Like many other parts of the world, Africa is no stranger to European standards of beauty. The practice of skin lightening is becoming rampant in many African countries as some folks go to drastic lengths to shed their dark complexions for lighter, "more acceptable" ones. And from advertising and magazines, to TV and film, the black aesthetics are being pushed out, while European standards of beauty — blonde hair, blue eyes — are becoming more mainstream.

"It seems that the world is conspiring in preaching that there is something wrong with Kenyan ladies' kinky hair and dark skin," Kenyan model Ajuma Nasenyana told *the Daily Nation*. Nasenyana wonders why European skincare companies that push lightening creams are entering Kenya marketing the European standard of beauty.

"Their leaflets are all about skin lightening, and they seem to be doing good business in Kenya. It just shocks me. It's not OK for a Caucasian to tell us to lighten our skin," she said.

Despite her beauty and that of women like her, Nasenyana is dismayed that while she is heralded abroad for her dark skin, at home she is seen as less than ideal.

"I have never attempted to change my skin. I am natural. People in Europe and America love my dark skin. But here in Kenya, in my home country, some consider it not attractive," she lamented.

Instead of simply being disgusted with the growing contempt some have for their own skin, Nasenyana takes every opportunity she has to speak out against skin lightening and discrimination in the modeling world. She is also very critical of the Western media's influence over Kenyans and concedes they are constantly being bombarded by magazines and advertisements that praise lighter skin.

"When you flip through fashion magazines like Vogue and only see white models, then you get the feeling on what is happening to black models. It is not fair," she explained.

But Nasenyana, who has modeled for everyone from Victoria Secret to Carlos Mienes, isn't just speaking out. The reining South African Fashion Week Model of the Year is also thinking of launching a line of cosmetics and natural skincare products for black women. Her hopes? That her products can inspire her peers to love their skin instead of bleach it.

Let's hope it works.

Reference

Britni Danielle Kenyan model Ajuma Nasenyana fights skin lightening and European standards of beauty. *Clutch Magazine.* June 27, 2012. http://thegrio.com/2012/06/27/kenyan-model-ajuma-nasenyana-fights-skin-lightening-and-european-standards-of-beauty/

(ii) Alek Wek[1,2]

In 2007, Alek Wek released an autobiography, entitled *Alek: From Sudanese refuge to International Supermodel*, documenting her journey from a childhood of poverty in Sudan to the catwalks of Europe.[1] It is relevant to study both the early life and career of this great Icon of beauty – to fully appreciate "The larger Story" when anyone ***truly*** believes that beauty and success have no colour!

Alek Wek is a South Sudanese British model and designer who began her fashion career at the age of 18 in 1995. As the first black model whose looks did not conform to Caucasian aesthetics, she has been hailed for her influence on the perception of beauty in the fashion industry. Wek has modeled, either on runways or in print advertisements.

Before Wek came on board, Dark-skinned models were rare, if not unheard of, in the high fashion industry. Wek was "the first black model who didn't conform to a Caucasian aesthetics, the first with an uncompromising sub-Saharan beauty… her industry saw her as new and exotic – a savage beauty. As a result, Wek's mainstream success was celebrated by black women all over the world. Oprah Winfrey commented that "if Wek had been the cover of a magazine when I was growing up, I would have had a different concept of who I was."

While giving a speech on beauty and self-perception, Kenyan actress Lupita Nyong'o mentioned Wek, stating that she had been a self-conscious, insecure teenager before seeing Wek in the spotlight: "When I saw Alek I inadvertently saw a reflection of myself that I could not deny", she added. "Now, I had a spring in my step because I felt more seen, more appreciated by the far-away gatekeepers of beauty."

Notable quotes from Alek Wek on the concept of beauty

- *"I have no problem with whatever the next big look is. Just don't try and tell me that only one look is beautiful"*

These are appropriate words from the striking Sudanese model whose exotic appearance has taken her to the very peak of her profession and challenged the traditional definition of a catwalk model.

- *"When I was growing up, my mother taught me and my sisters to celebrate each other – there was no room in our household for negativity. She taught us to embrace each other and this was empowering for us. She also taught us the value of celebrating our differences."*

Media images need to stress the diversity of **types** of beauty and desirability so that lightness/whiteness as the dominant standard may be challenged.

- **What Lupita Nyong'o Oscar Win Means to me**

"When I first started modeling I realized I was very different from the platform I have in fashion, to champion the ideals of what is beautiful. For me it always goes back to what my mother taught me and my sisters. That all women are beautiful and we should embrace each other. True beauty is born through our actions and

aspirations and in the kindness we offer to others. Beauty should not be culturally relevant, it should be universal."

(iii) Lupita Nyong'o [3,4,5]

Lupita Nyong'o was born in Mexico, to Kenyan parents. She was raised in Kenya and educated in the USA. She is Hollywood actress and the Academy Award for Best supporting Role. She is a Glamour Woman of the year for 2014.

The gracious and talented Nyong'o has created waves everywhere all over the world. She is inspiring African women to stop bleaching. "Who hasn't admired the actress's gorgeous dark skin (which looks amazing against every color in the rainbow) and radiant smile?" says Savita Iyer."(5) Oscar-winner Lupita Nyong'o heartfelt speech on beauty, delivered at the seventh annual Black Women in Hollywood luncheon hosted by Essence magazine in February 2014, moved many to tears. The full speech is reproduced below.

Oscar-winner Lupita Nyong'o's heartfelt speech on beauty, delivered at the seventh annual Black Women in Hollywood luncheon hosted by Essence magazine in February 2014, moved many to tears.

"I wrote down this speech that I had no time to practice so this will be the practicing session. Thank you Alfre, for such an amazing, amazing introduction and celebration of my work. And thank you very much for inviting me to be a part of such an extraordinary community. I am surrounded by people who have inspired me, women in particular whose presence on screen made me feel a little more seen and heard and understood. That it is ESSENCE that holds this event celebrating our professional gains of the year is significant, a beauty magazine that recognizes the beauty that we not just possess but also produce.

I want to take this opportunity to talk about beauty. Black beauty. Dark beauty. I received a letter from a girl and I'd like to share just a small part of it with you: "Dear Lupita," it reads, "I think you're really lucky to be this Black but yet this successful in Hollywood overnight. I was just about to buy Dencia's Whitenicious cream to lighten my skin when you appeared on the world map and saved me."

My heart bled a little when I read those words. I could never have guessed that my first job out of school would be so powerful in and of itself and that it would propel me to be such an image of hope in the same way that the women of *The Color Purple* were to me.

I remember a time when I too felt unbeautiful. I put on the TV and only saw pale skin. I got teased and taunted about my night-shaded skin. And my one prayer to God, the miracle worker, was that I would wake up lighter-skinned. The morning would come and I would be so excited about seeing my new skin that I would refuse to look down at myself until I was in front of a mirror because I wanted to see my fair face first. And every day I experienced the same disappointment of being just as dark as I had been the day before. I tried to negotiate with God: I told him I would stop stealing sugar cubes at night if he gave me what I wanted; I would listen to my mother's every word and never lose my school sweater again if he just made me a little lighter. But I guess God was unimpressed with my bargaining chips because He never listened.

And when I was a teenager my self-hate grew worse, as you can imagine happens with adolescence. My mother reminded me often that she thought that I was beautiful but that was no consolation: She's my mother, of course she's supposed to think I am beautiful. And then AlekWek came on the international scene. A celebrated model, she was dark as night, she was on all of the runways and in every magazine and everyone was talking about how beautiful she was. Even Oprah called her beautiful and that made it a fact. I couldn't believe that people were embracing a woman who looked so much like me as beautiful. My complexion had always been an obstacle to overcome and all of a sudden, Oprah was telling me it wasn't. It was perplexing and I wanted to reject it because I had begun to enjoy the seduction of inadequacy. But a flower couldn't help but bloom inside of me. When I saw Alek I inadvertently saw a reflection of myself that I could not deny. Now, I had a spring in my step because I felt more seen, more appreciated by the far away gatekeepers of beauty, but around me the preference for light skin prevailed. To the beholders that I thought mattered, I was still unbeautiful. And my mother again would say to me, "You can't eat beauty. It doesn't feed you." And these words plagued and bothered me; I didn't really understand them until finally I realized that beauty was not a thing that I could acquire or consume, it was something that I just had to be.

And what my mother meant when she said you can't eat beauty was that you can't rely on how you look to sustain you. What does sustain us... what is fundamentally beautiful is compassion for yourself and for those around you. That kind of beauty enflames the heart and enchants the soul. It is what got Patsey in so much trouble with her master, but it is also what has kept her story alive to this day. We remember the beauty of her spirit even after the beauty of her body has faded away.

And so I hope that my presence on your screens and in the magazines may lead you, young girl, on a similar journey. That you will feel the validation of your external beauty but also get to the deeper business of being beautiful inside. There is no shade in that beauty."

References

1. Alek: From Sudanese Refugee to International Supermodel. (http://www.theglobe and mail.com/life/article 788203. ece)
2. Alek Wek. *http://en.wikipedia.org/wiki/Alek_Wek*
3. Savita Iyer (2014) Lupita Nyong'o Is Inspiring African Women to stop bleaching their skin. www.savitaiyer.net
4. Oscar Winner Lupita Nyong'o's Speech On Beauty that left...*www.upworthy.com/oscar-winner-lupita-nyongos-speech-on-beauty-that...* Lupita Nyong'o deserves all the awards in the universe for this speech
5. .http://www.youbeauty.com/skin/lupita-nyongo-african-skin-bleaching

THE MEDIA AS A MAJOR DRIVING FORCE OF SKIN BLEACHING

Definition

The term "media" is an umbrella term that encompasses television, movies, newspapers, magazines, music, and various other forms of commercialized art including digital media e.g facebook, instagram, twitter, blogs etc.

The monumental contributory role of the media in promoting skin lightening practices globally cannot be overestimated. Therefore, the subject is being featured as a topic on its own. Although the pernicious influence of advertisements has been recognized globally, a few case studies would be highlighted to help in taking appropriate steps to reduce the burden created by the culture of skin lightening.

The media is a pivotal force through which cultural ideals are spread, articulated and internalized. Advertising, in particular has been a strong influence on the production of knowledge, not just in reflecting ideologies, but also in constructing them. Fundamentally, advertising permeates every aspect of life—in the home, on televisions and radios, on the street, and products advertise themselves.

(1) Effect of Consumer culture and the global mass media

Reinforcing the message a thousand times a day

The most powerful way this message is reinforced today, is through consumer culture and global mass media. The mass media form for us our image of the world. The images they choose to present and how these images are presented subliminally and yet profoundly affect the way we interpret what we **see** or **hear.** Even our image of ourselves is greatly influenced by what media **shows** us about our own group. People who lighten their skin and those who associate light skin with positive virtues and dark skin with negative ones aren't stupid. They just don't have the psychological resources to withstand the deluge of images they are presented with every day. Thousands of images from magazines, TV, film, ads, and the news, all equating light skin with beauty, affluence, happiness and success, and portraying dark-skinned black people as aggressive, unintelligent, criminals, crude, lazy, etc.

Even black-owned media do this. There was a brief period during the Black Power Movement of the 1960s and its accompanying Black is Beautiful campaign when dark-skinned women graced the pages of the popular and influential magazine *Ebony*, but by the eighties it had gone back to featuring predominantly light-skinned black stars, and this was particularly so for the women it featured. This practice is common across all media, so dark-skinned women are hugely underrepresented on the catwalk, in the fashion press, in cinema and on TV.

There is no conspiracy that says this is how we want to represent the world, but there is an unconscious mindset of racial superiority that determines what gets promoted as beautiful and desirable, and in that mindset there is no room for the idea of dark-skinned beauty, or hardly any room. Alek Wek (South Sudan/UK),

Ajuma Nasenyana (Kenya), Naomi Campbell (UK) and Eunice Olumide (Nigeria) are among the tiny handful of high-profile dark-skinned models on the international stage, but as Eunice says, "*... it is still rare to see a very dark-skinned model on the cover of a magazine. I'd love that to change.*"

Most of the foreign media and movies consumed in sub-Saharan Africa are from America and Europe, so we take in these images and mimic the practice of colourism in our own ads and magazines. We see which black women are considered beautiful by the mass media, we see that the black models and singers who are making it are mostly lighter-skinned – Rihanna, Beyoncé, etc. We see which actresses get to play love-interest roles and which ones get relegated to bit parts, and we see which ones make it onto those Top 100 lists. We echo the message we receive and perpetuate the system that excludes dark skin from the spectrum of beauty. We see pictures of Obama and we don't just see a black man, but a bi-racial, light-skinned black man. Some argue that the beauty ideal is shifting from white to a more cafe-au-lait-complexion, and that this is demonstrated by the fact that women like Beyoncé, Halle Berry and Jennifer Lopez now routinely top some of these "most beautiful" lists. But what seems to have happened there is that the previous practice of promoting only white women as beautiful was simply not sustainable when a significant proportion of the American population was clearly non-white, so the parameters were widened to include a handful of non-white women who are not too many skin tones away from being white. Now black people everywhere can feel they're included in the international beauty spectrumwithout really being included. When you look at the Nigerian film industry (the largest of its kind in Africa), you find that its lead characters tend to be light-skinned. Fela's condemnation of the practice in *Yellow Fever* (1976) doesn't seem to have done much good. Check the Ghanaian film industry and you'll find the same.

(2) The media as an agent of Socialization.

Furthermore, agents of socialization such as Eurocentric educational system, media and popular culture have been found to influence people to the practice of skin bleaching. African natives have access to cable television and social media and as such are exposed to Eurocentric programming where western culture is glorified. Even local television stations, for example, in Africa, broadcast a lot of western programming. When exposed to European culture from a young age, the idea that one is better off being white may be perpetuated. For example "roast breadful mentality"[2] is a term used to refer to persons who are supposedly black on the outside but white on the inside! This exposure may enable African people to become more familiar and knowledgeable about western culture and such this can result in the idealization of Eurocentric standards of beauty and fashion.

(3) The role of websites

There are websites where whole forums are dedicated to skin bleaching. People search and compare the best creams, lotions and gels, get 'Do it yourself' (DIY) tips on mixing their own lightening agents and exchange results. Some people actively state that they would like to go two or three shades lighter, so they can look good for a wedding or get better jobs. These websites and forums like these are pits of pressure and insecurity sucking away at the diverse beauty of women.

A cursory search on any Internet search engine reveals hundreds of skin lightening websites that provide information for would-be consumers about the "best" skin-lightening products and strategies. Lighterskin.org, whiterskin.com, skinwhitening.org, skin-whitening-products.com, and skinwhitening-experts.com all purport to share with readers the newest information on, and reviews of, skin lightening products.

With the rise of the internet, the world players in the skin bleaching market have become even more connected. Companies have new inroads for marketing and distribution, and consumers have greater access to information and products.

(4) The media promotes hegemonic whiteness

Hegemonic whiteness could be defined as the domination and assumed superiority based on the whiteness of one's skin.[3,4]

Through television commercials, print and digital advertisements, magazines, film, billboards, and the internet, the ideal skin complexion represented in African media is fair-skin tones. This idea that fair skin is better is common among other cultures in the world both in developed and developing nations worldwide. Media representation that equate light skin with beauty results in African women using skin-lightening products. See chapter 17 on BEAUTY.

Using light-complexioned women to advertise both skin-lightening products, assorted cosmetics, and skincare products and other consumer products, make women more aware of the culturally determined advantages of being light-skinned which would include: increased pay in the workforce, marriage, and social acceptance. As a result, they make efforts to look fair.

Before the term 'globalisation' was popularized in social sciences cultural critics and academics were perfectly happy to talk of imperialism as the equivalent process. It is increasingly palpable that a globalised concept of beauty is emerging as dominant and this is defined by hegemonic 'Caucasianisation'/internationalization of beauty concepts. Ideals of skin colour and societal perceptions of beauty are bound up in hegemonic processes of neo-imperialism and globalisation—ideas and ideals spreading from the 'core' (America and Europe) to the 'periphery' (former colonized countries). The neo-imperial war is fought on three fronts: cultural, economic (driven by neo-liberal globalization) and political (persuasive, coercive and aggressive).

The global capitalist system, entwined in cultural imperialism and cultural colonisation, forces those in the 'periphery' to accept western standards of beauty, high consumption and lifestyle. Sklair[3] considers this to be the intentional propagation of western culture via the media and advertising to help sustain economic domination and profits. This is epitomised by European and American beauty product multinationals (such as Clinique) in producing and aggressively promoting fairness products for Asian, African and South American markets. Western economic domination is (in many cases) accompanied by western cultural domination. While this can be examined as an unfortunate byproduct of global inequality that results from symbolic and economic factors, **cultural imperialism exists despite syncretism** and creolisation.

The spread of the ideology that fair skin is better can be attributed in part to new media vehicles such as Facebook, Myspace, Twitter etc. These are social media representation which women see and interact with every day. Charles[5] asserts, "Identity by nature is dual because it is elaborated internally, having been constructed externally. People internalize identity construction, which manifests itself in the appearance of social actions."

Mosocvici[6] states, "Representations are the shared images of the object in the minds of people that arise from social thought, which guides people's behavior." Mosocvici also states, "Hegemonic representation is a widely and deeply held representation by a highly structured community or group, and this representation is coercive and uniform."

White/light beauty is communicated through mass advertising, television shows, film, internet images, billboards, and celebrity culture. Images of white beauty do not simply rely on white women with blonde hair and light eyes to sell products. Images of white beauty sell much more than beauty ideals of fashions for women around the globe. Taken as a whole, images of white beauty sell an entire lifestyle imbued with racial meaning. The lifestyle that is communicated through these adverts sells whiteness, modernity, sophistication, beauty, power and wealth. The mass-marketing of these images of white beauty and a " white lifestyle" build on the long standing European colonial ideologies that valorize white beauty, European culture, and white aesthetics.

Furthermore, the new mass media and communication technologies combine with the old ideologies to compound the message that "white is right".[7] For example, the largest social networking application, Facebook, launched a new "app" sponsored by cosmetics giant, Vaseline, that allows users to lighten their skin tone in their profile pictures. By dragging a vertical bar across their pictures they can create instant before-and- after images devised to sell more of Vaseline's best-selling product, "Healthy White: Skin Lightening Lotion"[6]

Case study 1

Fairness advertisement in India

Kaitlin Sylvia conducted a study titled, "Hegemonic Whiteness: A Qualitative Study of Fairness Advertisements in India."[4] Hegemonic whiteness is defined as the domination and assumed superiority based upon the whiteness of one's skin. The market for fairness products generates over 6.75 billion rupees (USD $ 150 million) each year, and is growing at a rate of 25% per year.

Kaitlin Sylvia, introducing her study writes: "I passed several beauty advertisements selling fairness products during my morning five-kilometer walk from my apartment to the campus of Christ University. The advertisements were displayed in store windows, pasted on building sides, and billboards were posted throughout the city. While I waited to watch my first Bollywood film, commercials for fairness products bombarded the audience before the movie began. The vast amount of advertisements was initially overwhelming, and without a doubt succeeded in grabbing my attention. Studying and travelling for four months through India inspired me to conduct further research on how advertisements for Indian fairness products embody hegemonic whiteness. Working as a participant and an observer in the field, gave me several perspectives on how hegemonic whiteness is conveyed through these advertisements."

Upon completing data collection and analysis, three major themes emerged: (1) advertisements use language to equate whiteness to perfection and beauty, (2) advertisements use celebrity endorsement to form a direct association between hegemonic whiteness and experiencing success, and (3) advertisements suggest darkness is a problem.

The Power of Persuasion: Using Words as Weapons

Theme 1: Advertisements use language to equate whiteness to perfection and beauty. Based on the content analyzed, the product names reflect this theme such as: Pond's White Beauty Face Wash, Loreal's White Perfect Day Cream, and Fair & Lovely. These products advertise the parallels between whiteness and ideal beauty within the product name. In an advertisement for LUX White Glow, the headline states, "Beauty is one attitude women should have every day", beauty is not only a physical appearance, but an attitude of confidence associated with hegemonic whiteness portrayed in advertisements. This type of language appeals to consumer's emotions and demands their attention. These advertisements encourage a person to buy the product and reinforce the relationship between whiteness and perfection.

Success and beauty is achieved if you use fairness Products

Theme 2: The second finding of this study is advertisements use of celebrity endorsement to form a direct association between whiteness and experiencing success. Indian celebrities featured in these advertisements display uncommon phenotypes within the greater Indian population. In addition to celebrities having white skin, they are thin, with stylized hairstyles, bright sparkling eyes, and so on. The celebrity endorsers have a greater influence in reinforcing hegemonic whiteness due to their popularity. Loreal's White Perfect advertisement features Bollywood actress Sonam Kapoor. Underneath her photo there is a quote stating, "On and off screen, my skin looks perfect." Loreal's product is an example of brands creating an association between the success of a celebrity and their fairness. The product sends a message to consumers that they can also have success and beauty if they use fairness products.

Darkness is a problem and fairness products are the Solution

Theme 3: The third finding of Kaitlin's study discovers how advertisements suggest darkness is a problem. Advertisements portray women with dark skin as insecure and unconfident due to their skin tone. The dark skin women have sad facial expressions, their eyes do not look directly at the camera, and their body posture is poor. Women using the fairness product are portrayed as confident and transformed, because of their whiteness. For example, in an advertisement for Fem Herbal Bleach the title of the advertisement says, "Wear a new face." Next to the text, there is a picture of a smiling woman who was transformed by using "the three steps to fairness." According to the advertisements, women should feel ashamed of their darkness and view their skin as an issue, which needs resolution. Fairness products promise whiteness as the solution to the problem of darkness. The examples shown in the advertisements are overdramatized, showing drastic lightening of skin tone in just one or a few uses. The misconstrued images attract women who want to avoid the negative attention of their dark skin. An advertisement presented color watches ranging from white to dark brown, implying whiteness is the goal and darkness is the problem women want to escape. The models place color watches next to their face to prove their transformation from darkness to lightness, and ugliness to beauty. Advertisements associate negativity with darkness making the skin as a problem with negative consequences if they do not seek a solution.

Conclusion from case study[1]

Equating whiteness to beauty and perfection results in the degradation of darkness. The advertisements use of celebrity endorsement to form a direct association between whiteness and success is problematic, because the message conveys that success is achievable through whiteness. The idea of hegemonic whiteness imposes a form of social stratification on Indian women and society based on whiteness. Companies have profited from the fairness product industry by making women feel inadequate about their darkness. They create a message to consumers of hegemonic whiteness by insinuating women are not beautiful, successful, or desirable without achieving hegemonic whiteness through their products.

Case study 2

Unilever Citra Pearly White body lotion

The Thai subsidiary of Anglo-Dutch company, **Unilever**, was recently forced to apologize over a university competition which suggested that scholarships would be offered to lighter skinned entrants.[7] The competition wanted students to send in pictures of themselves alongside *Citra Pearly White UV body lotion*. The advert broadcast on TV showed a dark female student alongside a lighter-skinned fellow student. The former seemed unable to answer the presenter's questions whereas the latter sailed through and described as beautiful—another subtle hint that the darker the skin tone, the less intelligent the bearer.

Case study 3
Photoshop
Millions of image in the media have our perception of attainable physical standards greatly skewed. The supernatural power know as **Photoshop** is a wrinkle-smoothing, cellulite-eliminating, waist-slimming source of insecurity and self-doubt. Unrealistic perceptions of beauty is caused by overuse of Photoshopped and filtered celebrity images which are damaging to women's self esteem.

The Dove 'Evolution' video[10] shows the process a model goes through before and during a photo-shoot and then how the pictures are edited afterwards. The video starts off with a women sitting down while several different people such as make-up artists and hairdressers transform her appearance. After the photographs are taken, editing software is used to change the size of her lips, increase the length of her neck, intensify her eyes and makes her look thinner. Once the picture looks perfect, it is then put on a billboard for advertisement[7]

The model's picture had been modified so much that the end result did not even look like her anymore. Despite this, women will notice these adverts and then want to aspire to look the same by buying the product advertised. The amount of make-up women in today's society hide behind has a very negative impact on both men and women. It is clear that applying many different types of beauty products allows women to become more like the ideals in the media. However, it can create an unnatural look as well as completely altering their own appearance in the process because in reality, even the ideals do not always look like their pictures. Once more and more women define this as beauty, conformity increases and normalization occurs. Furthermore, men will believe that this is the way women look and therefore have increased expectations of beauty, thus changing the norms of society.

Case study 4
Vaginal bleaching products
Dan Morrison of National Geographic Voices asked[11] **"Has Indian's Skin-Lightening Obsession Reached Final Frontier?** Introducing the subject he says cynically, it is not enough for Indian boys and girls

to fear that they won't get a playmate or a spouse or a job because of their "unsightly" skin-tone. It's not enough that ads should tell women they need their underarm deodorant to include skin-lightening cream if they want to go sleeveless. Now comes **Clean and Dry "intimate wash," which promises women "protection, fairness and freshness" below the waistline**. A new ad for the ph-balanced cleanser features an attractive young bride who lacks confidence around her husband, presumably because her vagina is too dark. After one splash of Clean and Dry, however, love blooms anew. The media's reception has been harsh. "This is a wonder product," Manjula Narayan writes in Indian's Sunday Guardian, "It's an itch Guard that promises to bleach my oyster." Writing in the **Wall Street Journal,** Rupa Subramanya points out that intimate skin-lightening got its start in the West.

(5) The media fosters a feeling of insecurity

Blood[12] argues that the cause of body dissatisfaction is located in the minds of women. However, society can influence a women's body image through media representations. The oppressive westernized ideal makes women with darker complexions feel insecure and alienated so as a result, they feel the need to conform to the society standards of beauty in order to feel beautiful and accepted. In the last decade, the development of technology has significantly increased. Smartphones, Tablets and other portable devices enhance the media as they enable constant mass communication amongst members of society. Women can read fashion magazines and tabloid newspapers on the go and these almost always contain images and articles that influence the way women perceive beauty. Additionally, Instagram and Tumblr are two other types of social media that are widely used today and both are concerned with posting pictures.

The media creates ideals, in the form of celebrities and models, for women to admire.[13] These ideals are in front covers of magazines and advertisements. However, the creation of ideals can have a negative impact on women as their perception of beauty is altered to complement the media. "The mass media has been influential and pervasive mirrors for societal standards". This can result in women feeling insecure about their own appearance and then conforming to the media's perception of beauty by buying beauty products such as creams and other products to lighten the skin. Despite this endeavour for social change, women are still continuing to the unattainable high beauty standards set by the media and will even risk their health (e. g the serious adverse effects of bleaching products).

(6) The media fosters commodity racism

The adverts also serve as media for commodity racism.[14] Another manner in which the European/White nationalist legacy continues to impact African realities is in transmission of commodity racism. Although the colonial regime may have physically left African soil, their legacy of colonial hegemonic ideologies remained. Through commodity racism, Europeans continued to assert the power "inherent" to whiteness. First attempting to instill within the psyche of its colonized subjects notions about their inherent inferiority as evidenced by their blackness (read: dirtiness), the colonial order then attempted to exploit the very psyche it created, as well as the markets it sought to dominate, by importing and further promoting commodities (soap, laundry detergent, powder, cosmetics and skin bleaching agents) that promised miraculous transformation—from dirty to clean, from dark to light. Commodities "were by their very nature about the transformation of the 'traditional' African self into something the advertisers argued would be more commensurate with 'modern' society" Blay used examples of advertisements featured in *The Sunday Mirror*, Ghana's most popular women's weekly, to illustrate the continuation of commodity racism.

Case Study

A 1930 French ad for Dirtoff showed a dark African man washing his hands, with the soap washing away his blackness.[14] Such ads were common in the late 19th and early 20th centuries. Blackness had become a pathological condition — there was something fundamentally wrong with you if you were black—while whiteness became the paradigm, the standard, the ideal, and who doesn't want to be ideal?

Advertisement for *Pear's Soap*, 1899[15,16]

The advert caption reads:

The first step towards lightening The White Man's Burden is through teaching the virtues of cleanliness. Pear's Soap is a potent factor in brightening the dark corners of the earth as civilization advances, while amongst the culture of all nations it holds the highest place—it is the ideal toilet soap.

Through its imagery, wording, and connection to Kipling's poem, the advertisement implies that not only does using Pear's Soap purify and protect the White man's body whilst in contact with the Black (read: dirty) natives, but as he shares the soap with the natives, it further "lightens" his burden and thus helps him to "[brighten] the dark corners of the earth" and advance civilization.

In an 1875 advert for Pear's soap, the juxtaposition of "light" (civilized) and "dark" ("uncivilized") is more blatant, making the presumed "magical powers" of soap more readily comprehensible. Amidst the wording of an endorsement "I have found PEAR'S SOAP matchless for the Hands and Complexion," the viewer is again given access into the private, Victorian bathroom. In the left frame (which represents the "before"), a little Black boy sits in the bath, gazing at the water with a look of shear amazement on his face, which suggests that bathing is a new experience for him. A little White boy, wearing a white apron, which suggests that he was preparing to engage in "dirty work," extends his magic tool - a bar of Pear's soap. The manner in which the White boy shows the soap to the Black boy again suggests that this is the Black child's introduction to bathing. In the right frame (which represents the "after"), as the Black boy stands up, the White boy shows him his "new" image in the mirror, which, by the smile and look on his face, is very much pleasing to the Black child. Magically, the Black boy's body has become white, but his face remains black. The message? As the part of the body that more often than not carries the immutable signs of phenotypical/racial categorization, one's face (read: race) cannot be changed, not even with the magic of Pear's soap. All in all still, the viewer realizes that it is through the White boy, a smaller and younger version of the White man, that the Black boy becomes "domesticated," thus reinforcing Whites' position as active agents towards civilization while Blacks remain passive recipients of their "kindness" and "goodwill."

Drawing on the racist iconography of the soap advertising campaign in which the soap washed away the stigma of racial and class degeneration, today's skin whitening cream advertisements can be said to represent **commodity racism**. By removing from the skin the stigma of dark skin, whitening creams correlate light skin with beauty and socioeconomic progress. The discourse of such contemporary advertising incorporates both racism and colorism. The term colorism conceptualized as a privileging of the lighter skinned over the darker-skinned within a community of color is said to happen over time when the predominantly colored communities internalize white superiority, to create socioeconomic hierarchies. While today the soap advertisements cannot be shown, because of their blatant attempt to naturalize the ideology of white superiority, advertisers now employ semiotic manipulations to convey similar messages.

References

1. Jabbar Siji. Who taught you to hate your [dark] skin? This is Africa. *http://thisisafrica.me/who-taught-you-to-hate-your-dark-skin/*
2. Sutherland ME. Towand a Caribbean Psychology: An African Centered Approach. *Journal of Black Studies.* 2011; 42(8): 1175-94.
3. Sklair L. Sociology of the Global System. London: Prentic Hall / Harvester Wheatsheaf. 1995.
4. Kaitlin Sylvia. Hagemonic Whiteness: A Qualitative Study of Fairness Advertisements in India. *Texas State Undergraduate Research Journal.* 2014; 2 (1): 1-5.
5. Charles CAD. Skin bleachers' representation of skin color in Jamaica. *Journal of Black Studies*; 40(2): 153-70
6. Moscovici Serge. Notes towards a description of social Representations. *European Journal of Social Psychology.* 1988; 18(3): 211-50
7. Hunter Margaret. "If you're Light, you're Alright." Light skin color as social capital for women of color. *Gender & Society* 2002; 16: 175-93.
8. Lana Schupback. Vaseline promotes skin lightening through Facebook app. 14 July 2010. *http://thegrio.com/2010/07/14/vaseline-promotes-skin-lightening-throu...*
9. Ayodele Dija. The fairest of them all: Dija Ayodele on the culture of skin-bleaching *THANDIEKAY.* Thursday, 31 July 2014. *http://thandiekay.com/2014/07/31/the-fairest-of-them-all-dija-ayodel…*
10. Piper T. *Dove Evolution.* [video online].2006. Available at: *http://www.youtube.com/watch?v=iYhCn0jf46u* Accessed: 14 March 2013
11. Dan Morrison. Has India's skin-lightening obsession reached the final frontier? http://voices.nationa/geographic.com/2012/04/12/has-indias-skin-lig...
12. Blood S. Body Work: The social construction of women's body image. East Sussex: Routledge. 2005.
13. Nicole James. Society's influence on the perception of Beauty. *http://docslide.us/documents/societys-influence-on-the-perception-of-beauty-nicole-james.html.*
14. Blay Yaba A. Skin Bleaching and Global white supremacy: By Way of Introduction. *The Journal of Pan African Studies.* 2011; 4(4): 4-46.
15.The Advertising Archives. *http://www.advertisingarchives.co.uk*
16. Glenn EN. Yearning for lightness: Transnational circuits in the marketing and consumption of skin lighteners. *Gender & Society* 2008; 22(3): 281-302

THE SCIENTIFICATION OF SKIN WHITENING

"The Scientification of Skin Whitening" is a term coined by Amina Mire[1] to describe the interlocking strategies of scientific entrepreneurialism and academic capitalism in cutting-edge innovations in molecular biology, biomedicine, and other life sciences deployed in research and the development of high-end skin whitening and anti-aging cosmeceuticals. Skin lightening has come to be associated with health promotion, self-enhancement and the fight against aging—a "disease".

Skin whitening products and anti-aging cosmeceuticals are growing, lucrative markets whose globals reaches are greatly facilitated by new scientific innovations and aggressive internet and print media advertism. Skin whitening products are marketed differently depending on the target demography. Thus in 2009, the high-end skin whitening market share for Pacific Asia was estimated to be worth US$18 billions.[2, 3] However, because of the marketing of skin whitening products as anti-aging remedies to white middle-class women in Europe and North America, it is difficult to obtain accurate data on market shares in the West for skin whitening products promoted under the banner of anti-aging products. Nevertheless, in 2010, the worldwide anti-aging product market was expected to reach US $ 115.8 billion[4]. Wellness economics and rhetoric of health promotion are central to the promotion of skin whitening and anti-aging biotechnologies. The conceptualization of bodily imperfections, such as uneven skin tones, age spots, hyperpigmentation, and photo-aging are produced as signs of pigmentation **pathologies**. As a "cure" designed to mitigate the signs of aging, skin whitening practice is often conceptualized as a biomedical strategy to **purify, restore**, and cleanse the signs of aging from the skin and faces of women. However, such biomedicalization discourses depend on the belief in the message that aging in women is a **disease** and that it is women's own moral responsibility to purchase these products to fight the visible signs of aging.

Amina Mire conducted a study to critically explore the social, health, political, economic, pedagogical, legal, and ethical implications of skin whitening and anti-aging as contemporary globalized marketing of biotechnology products that promise youthful and smooth skin to affluent middle-aged white women and brighter skin tones to women of color. Research, development and mass marketing of skin whitening biotechnology require that consumers purchase the health promotion of scientific consumerism and the discursive production of the aging process as a legitimate female pathology. Start-up biotechnology firms in the sciences, Giant transnational cosmetics and pharmaceutical corporations, and public universities have entered into the research and development and mass commercialization of anti-aging and skin whitening products.

The research, development and globalization of skin whitening and anti-aging cosmeceuticals is facilitated by scientific innovations in molecular biology and genomics. Innovations in high-end skin whitening biotechnology are designed to turn academic-based innovations into lucrative spin-off business ventures. In doing so, the institutional structures and traditional goals of higher education have been reconstituted so that increasingly *symbolic* prestige and financial rewards have been paired with the productions of proprietary marketable innovations.

The scientification of skin whitening and anti-aging market

Skin whitening products can be botanical products, biotechnological actives, or chemical agents applied on the human skin to achieve a lighter skin tone. High-end skin whitening products are often labeled under the new quasi-pharmaceutical category called **cosmeceuticals**—a hybrid entity with pharmaceutical and cosmetic properties. Cosmeceuticals are topical cosmetics-pharmaceutical hybrids that enhance the beauty through constituents that provide ***additional*** health-related benefit. This labeling strategy allows promoters of high-end skin whitening and anti-aging products to make both pharmaceutical and cosmetic claims. From a **regulatory** standpoint, this polyvalent labeling as a third separate category that is neither a cosmetic nor a drug blurs the line between cosmetic and pharmaceutical claims, thereby making it easier to overcome regulatory restraints that regulate the boundary separating drug from cosmetics.

If skin whitening and anti-aging cosmeceuticals were to be marketed as drugs (presumably to cure the signs of aging), they would be required to meet rigorous premarket testing targets to verify and ascertain their efficacy and assess their risks to consumers *before* they could be legally mass-marketed. However, products marketed simply as cosmetics do not require the premarket testing. The other notable advantage from the classification as cosmeceutical is that it confers on skin whitening and anti-aging biotechnologies the allure of biomedical potency and therapeutic efficacy which inevitably links these products to cutting-edge scientific innovations and wellness promotion.

Some examples of scientification

The sientification of skin whitening agents can be categorized broadly into two levels

(1) Innovations of powerful biotechnologies that promise to enhance the health and vitality of users as well as reduce the "disease" of aging and thereby increase the longevity of users.

(2) Socio-scientific, political, ethical, and pedagogical implications associated with how skin whitening knowledge is produced and used.

One of the latest developments in anti-aging and skin whitening discourses is the proliferation of expert advice given to women on how to look after their own health and appearance. Another way in which this is accomplished is via the increasing availability of portable self-diagnostic tools. One such popular self-diagnostic device is a silicon-based semiconductor sensory device called SkinChip which women are encouraged to use to determine the status of their skin (i.e. pigmentation and hydration levels)[5].

A novel macro- and micromolecular delivery systems, first developed for the delivery of pharmaceutic agents, are being redeployed in the manufacturing of new powerful anti-aging and skin whitening cosmetics with the capacity to penetrate deep into the skin and transform the appearance and physiology of the skin.[6, 7, 8] Yet these products continue to be promoted and openly marketed as cosmetics in spite of the fact that the use of pharmaceutical drug delivery systems to overcome the natural defense system of the skin to prevent foreign agents from entering the body, supports the idea that these products fit the **legal** definition of pharmaceuticals.

Drug delivery systems increase the bioavailability of active agents. It is in this context that the transfer of pharmaceutical knowledge to the mass production of cosmeceuticals, such as skin whitening products, has also been used increasingly in the production of anti-aging cosmetics. The desire to suppress or eliminate the body's capacity to produce skin pigment, melanin, age spots, and other signs of ageing, makes nanotechnology an ideal candidate for the production of new skin whitening regimens.

Strategies to ensure a cooperative relationship with consumers.

(1) *Pathologization of dark skin colour and aging*

Dark skin and ageing are presented as a burden or disease that can be cured with the use of "scientifically" formulated skin-lightening products. Lights skin is depicted as idealized complexion ideals marker of feminine real beauty and symbol of attractiveness and a necessity to being youthful, beautiful, modern and affluent. These health claims, despite being unverified, facilitate the systematic integration of skin whitening and anti-aging biotechnology to both over-the-counter consumer goods and pharmaceutical products and to skin care biomedicine

(2) *Biomedicalization of women's bodies and skin*
Economic interest ensures that skin–whitening operates within the purview of science—medicine—biomedicalization of women's bodies and skin. By using the language, technologies, and techniques of science-medicine, including medical delivery systems, the skin whitening industry becomes integrated into legitimate scientific research

(3) *Innovative advertising strategies*
Marketing skin whitening and anti-aging products as legitimate interventions to cure and mitigate visible signs of aging requires both institutional and self-biomedicalization and the pathologization of the aging processes. Though men are increasingly enticed to consume these products, the primary target is women. Visual promotions for skin whitening and anti-aging products use discourse to reconstruct visible aging signs as pigmentation pathologies in need of biomedical intervention. These advertising strategies draw on stereotypical representations of women whose bodies and skin are uniquely vulnerable to premature aging. The advertisements claim that prolonged sun exposure, pollution, bad diet, and genetic predisposition facilitate premature aging in women.[9] Online promotions for high-end skin whitening commodities promulgate the superiority of the science-based commodity of whiteness. The Internet appears to be the main medium to disseminate the wellness discourse of skin whitening and anti-aging skin care.[10] Promotional ads for skin whitening often position the ideal consumers of these products as those sufficiently literate in basic sciences who possess computer skills and have access to the Internet. This is because the Internet is fast, relatively cheap, and capable of facilitating the accelerated globalization of skin whitening. Thus, the globalization of skin whitening requires not only industrial research and marketing strategies but also consumers' acceptance of the values and messages promulgated in advertisements for skin whitening.

The term 'scientification' is used as an analytic device to capture contradictory marketing imperatives that entice consumers with the promise of scientific potency and the promotion of health through the use of skin whitening products though the products are not subject to restrictive drug regulatory constraints. As a marketing strategy, scientification appeals to consumers as being rational, well-informed, self-governing agents capable of reading these complex messages and reaching their own decisions as to whether or not to participate in the consumption of skin whitening biotechnology. In addition, scientification marketing invests heavily in the production of visually pleasing promotional literature for skin whitening and anti-aging biotechnologies, both online and in print. Many advertisements for these products use extensive scientific metaphors, visually dazzling images, and verbal rhetoric that seeks to link the research and development of skin whitening biotechnology to the promotion of good health and the prevention of diseases by halting or reversing the natural aging processes in women. Colourful promotional graphics and images of *seemingly* scientific research, e.g of researchers working in the high-tech laboratory, presumably seek to visually assert the "truth" of the "healing" power of skin whitening biotechnology.

By and large the primary target of these skin whitening products is women (women of color in Africa. Pacific Asia and White women in North America and Europe), but the cosmetics industry is increasingly targeting men (especially Asian men). Recently, there was a media outcry[11] after the firm Unilever, the maker of a new Vaseline skin whitening brand for men, posted an advertisement for this brand on the Facebook social networking site. The ad sought to promote skin whitening to dark-skinned Indian men by promising them a few shades of lighter skin tone with the use of the skin whitening creams. The media focused on Unilever's marketing of skin lightening to Indian men as a blatant double standard in the face of the company's well-known Dove advertisement, which preaches the message of self-respect and self-esteem to women in North America and Europe. Critics have also noted that Unilever promotes whiteness and cosmetic fairness as virtues to Asian women in brands such as Fair and Lovely. However, almost all of the Western-based cosmetic firms have been promoting whiteness modernity to Asian men and women in the last 10 to 20 years. Market shares in skin whitening for men in Asia have been rising steadily, particularly in Japan and China, in the last 5–10 years and are expected to rapidly increase.[12, 13, 14]

Major publishing houses are also getting into online marketing of skin whitening and anti-aging products. In June 2009 it was reported that

CosmeticsDesign.com[15]—the biggest online clearing house for cosmetics and a Website that publishes updated information on all things cosmetic—had been acquired by the giant publishing house *William Reed Business Media.*[16] This is significant because *William Reed Business* Media is a leader in publishing information trends in the food, drink, and pharmaceutical industries. The consolidation of information on pharmaceuticals, food/nutrition, and cosmetics into one easily accessible online source points to further consolidation and merging of these industries. Increasingly, similar market trends are taking shape that are designed to blur the lines between cosmetics and food categories and food and pharmaceutical categories. Terms such as beauty food—that is, food that will not only nourish the body but also can make a user's skin glow with health and vitality as visible signs of aging disappear—have been used, and the related products are gaining a sizable share of the cosmetic-food market[17]. It is pertinent to note the extent to which these new ambiguous products have also tried to evade regulatory constraints, and therefore their claims cannot be independently verified, nor can potential risks to consumers be assessed. Yet corporations continue to make claims about how these cosmetic-foods nourish the body and cure signs of aging. The following quote shows the economic imperatives of this kind of globalized rhetoric:

Datamonitor names Masterfoods as one of the leading companies to have recently enterd the beauty from within market. Its Dove Beauty Milk Chocolate is packed with ingredients that are purported to nourish the skin including vitamins C and E along with biotin, zinc and cocoa flavanols.... Nestle also hit the headlines this year with the high-profile launch of the beauty juice Glowelle[18,19]

As a result, leading corporations in cosmetics, pharmaceuticals, and the food industry are already incorporating untested and unregulated nanotechnologies in their latest skin whitening and anti-aging cosmeceuticals and edible beauty foods and cosmetic drinks.[18, 19, 20]

Implications for science education and knowledge production

The research, development and globalization of skin whitening and anti-aging cosmeceuticals is facilitated by scientific innovations in molecular biology and genomics. In this age of the deregulation of public universities and an uncertain economic climate, the interlocking discourses of academic, scientific entrepreneurship and cutting-edge scientific discoveries in molecular biology and the life sciences, see anti-aging and skin whitening as lucrative spin-off sites to commercialize these innovations with the less regulated domain of cosmetic industry. As a result, skin whitening and anti-aging represent new proprietary sites of capital accumulation and sources of knowledge production and knowledge use.

The research and development and globalization of skin whitening and anti-aging cosmeceuticals is facilitated by scientific innovations in molecular biology and genomics. Innovations in skin whitening biotechnology and related anti-aging skin care cosmeceuticals work within the purview of knowledge production both in the name of the public good and in the name of generating marketable knowledge. Innovations in high-end skin whitening biotechnology are designed to turn academic-based innovations into lucrative spin-off business ventures[2]. In doing so, the institutional structures and traditional goals of higher education have been reconstituted so that increasingly symbolic prestige and financial rewards have been paired with the production of proprietary marketable innovations.

This change, in turn, requires closer cooperation between universities and the private sector. Governments, funding agents, university administrators, corporate leaders, and other stakeholders are encouraged to promote the economic imperatives of innovation and entrepreneurship as central features of research programs and funding policies. Through these public/private partnerships, funding, priorities for academic research and knowledge production are closely linked to economic potentials and market opportunities. Mechanisms such as favorable regulatory regimes, proprietary protection laws, and the formation of small high-tech firms *inside* publicly funded universities are some of the strategies used to turn academic knowledge into marketable innovations and ultimately into mass-produced commodities.

One of the outcomes of the restructuring of publicly funded universities into sites engaged in producing commodifiable knowledge is the rise of a new class of academic researchers: ambitious scientific entrepreneurs and leaders of the new knowledge-based industry known as scientific officers, who maintain their academic roles as researchers and knowledge producers in the name of the public good. The figure of someone who is simultaneously a scientific entrepreneur or a scientific officer of industry and an academic researcher for the public good reinforces the neoliberal restructuring of publicly funded research universities as *entrepreneurial* universities. Thus, by engaging in proprietary innovations financed with public money, an academic researcher can become the corporate chief scientific officer without giving up his or her academic position. The additional role of scientific entrepreneur or corporate scientific officer may increase the symbolic power and economic clout of this class of scientific researcher by possibly, among other things, facilitating his or her capacity to procure more external grants for research projects and funds for business ventures. In their dual roles as scientific officers of privately owned start-up spin-off biotechnology firms and as public intellectuals, such academic entrepreneurs have the potential to increase the transformation of publicly funded knowledge into private wealth, benefiting corporations, individuals, and institutions. Though universities encourage their scientists and researchers to become entrepreneurial and discover commercializable proprietary knowledge, they have the greatest stake in fostering university, industry, and government collaborations and an entrepreneurial academic environment. As a result, not only the researchers and scientists themselves but universities strive to discover and patent proprietary knowledge.

This can have *serious implications* for the production of scientific knowledge in publicly funded universities and colleges. For example, by using their increased symbolic capital and economic clout, scientific entrepreneurs may have a greater chance of publishing their findings in academic journals, possibly helping to fast-track their tenure and other promotions. In addition, these scientific officers may have a greater capacity to procure external grants for their research programs and possibly have a greater chance of incorporating *slanted* views into the education curricula taught to students, thereby normalizing the kind of scientific innovations previously discussed as part and parcel of received knowledge in molecular biology or other life sciences. This could lead to the use of their graduate students and contract researchers to do the bulk of the research while retaining unfair economic and symbolic benefits and claiming exclusive proprietary rights over discoveries with economic potential.

As a result, the rise of the figure of privileged academic entrepreneur/scientific corporate officer has *the capacity to weaken the idea of academic excellence in teaching, research, and knowledge production in the name of the public* good.[21] This is not to deny the essential link between scientific innovations and economic developments as a key to social and economic well-being and national security or that funding commercially oriented knowledge with public money is a bad thing per se. However, when public money is used to fund projects with very little proven social benefit and much potential to harm and these projects are conducted by academic researchers working inside publicly funded universities, the neoliberal push for closer partnership between such universities and the private sector can be problematic. As a rule, excellence in teaching, the capacity to procure external grants, and publishing in prestigious academic journals often determine career success in academia. However, the rise of scientific entrepreneurs and the concomitant lucrative academic capitalism and production of knowledge used for poorly regulated commodities such as skin whitening and anti-aging biotechnologies have the capacity to facilitate a climate under which a selective group of scientific researchers gain the necessary economic clout and symbolic scientific capital to determine not only the direction of future scientific research but also what counts as worthy knowledge.

One implication of the rise of scientific officers and spin-off biotechnologies in academic research in skin whitening and similar biotechnologies is the potential to introduce systemic inequity to what can be construed as excellence in academic research. An obvious dimension of inequity is that these academic entrepreneurs could use their increased available capital to purchase cutting-edge research equipment and procure external grants to further their research projects. This would increase their ability to present their findings in national and international conferences, gain greater opportunities for networking and collaborating with other researchers, gain wider readership of their published work, and gain greater peer recognition. *These scientific officers could possibly facilitate the securing of favorable legal frameworks and state support for the promotion of unregulated biotechnologies such as skin whitening.* For example, the following quote is taken from a life sciences news bulletin posted at the federal government's Industry Canada website:

Fytokem Products Inc. (Saskatoon), a leading producer of Functional-Certified TM plant-based ingredients, today announced that the United States Patent and Trademark Office (USPTO) has issued a patent on the use of its Tyrostat TM line of products for the inhibition of the tyrosinase enzyme. This enzyme is a key enzyme involved in the control of the pigmentation of skin. A product able to inhibit production of the tyrosinase enzyme will provide skin whitening ability

Industry Canada's support for the mass marketing of a product that intervenes and suppresses the natural biosynthesis and function of melanin, a protein vital to the skin's ability to protect the body against sun induced photodamage, must be read against the backdrop of skin whitening as a globalizing lucrative emerging market. The following quote demonstrates the way in which economic imperatives play a critical role in the collaboration between industry and government for the commercialization of skin whitening biotechnology.

> The skin whitening market worldwide is a multibillion dollar venture with the greatest potential in Asia. This regional market continues to be anchored by Japan with the fast emerging China market growing at an unprecedented rate. The market in Japan was estimated to be $ 5.6 Billion U.S. dollars in 2001 where over 25% of all personal care products contain skin whitening actives. The greatest growth potential lies in China where the market is estimated at over $ 1.3 Billion. The market in North America is focused on the lightening of age and liver spots.[22]

The above quote demonstrates that economic imperatives play a central role in state support of the academic innovations of skin whitening taking place in Canadian universities. In the academic-based research and development of skin whitening biotechnology, new policies are enacted to justify allocation of precious cash, human skills, scientific capital, and physical infrastructure (such as scientific laboratories) to house these research projects in their earlier phases. New regulatory frameworks, favorable to the smooth integration of these new technologies into existing technologies, are also enacted. Academic-based scientific entrepreneurs work closely with public policy-makers and corporate leaders in the process of drafting and normalizing proprietary laws in order to protect patentable knowledge designed to benefit corporations, universities, and scientific researchers while defending the funding of these research projects in the name of the public good. *It is through this process that neoliberal economic imperatives shape priorities in the expenditure of public money given for the research and development of market-oriented innovations to advance the competitive edge of multinational corporations.*

The powerful economic forces at play in the skin whitening anti-aging industry need to be understood and confronted. The manufacturing, advertising and selling of skin-lighteners has become a major growth market for multinational corporations. These corporations play a leading role in the creation and manipulation of needs and desires often overtly or covertly supporting and funding innovations in high end skin whitening biotechnology designed to turn academic based innovations into lucrative spin-off business ventures.

References

1. Amina Mire. The scientification of Skin Whitening and the Entrepreuneurial University%Linked Corporate Scientific Officer. *Canadian Journal of Science, Mathematics and Technology Education*. 2012; 12(3): 272-91.

2. Montague-Jones G. Datamonitor features beauty foods in top ten trend list for 2009. *http://www.cosmeticsdesign-europe.com/Products-Markets/Datamonitor-features-beauty-foods-in-top-ten-trend-list-for-2009.*

3. Pitman S. In-Cosmetics Asia focuses on skin lightening trend. 2009. *http://www.cosmeticsdesign-europe.com/Product-Categories/Skin-Care/In-Cosmetics-Asia-focuses-on-skin-lightening-trend*

4. *Global Industry Analysts, Inc.* Anti-aging products: A global strategic business report (Report Code MCP-11-7). 2009. *http://www.strategyr.com/AntiAgingProductsMarketReport.asp*

5. Lévêque J L & Querleux B. SkinChip, a new tool for investigating the skin surface in vivo. *Skin Research Technology*. 2003; 9(4): 343-7. *http://www.ncbi.nlm.nih.gov/pubmed/14641885*

6. Gupta K. Topical delivery systems for antiaging and skin whitening agents. 2010. *http://ip.com/patent/US7777073*

7. Nichol K. Aquea Scientific moves ahead with delivery systems technology. *http://www.cosmeticsdesign.com/Formulation-Science/Aquea-Scientific-moves-ahead-with-delivery. system-technology 2010.*

8. *Pharmagel International Inc.* Pharmaceutical grade anti-aging skin care: Nature's prescription for radiant skin...At any age. 2011; 1-10. *http://www.pharmagel.net/pdf/prod_brochure.pdf*.

9. Henning M. In J. Arthurs & J. Grimshaw (Eds.), Don't touch me (I'm electric): On gender and sensation in modernity. In J. Arthurs & J. Grimshaw (Eds), Women bodies: Discipline and transgression. *London, England: Cassell Press*. 1999: pp. 17–47.

10. Newswire PR. Altruis e-business launched with multiple healthcare Websites and 1000 Internet domain names. 2010. *http://www.prnewswire.com/news-releases/altruis-e-business-launched-with-multiple-healthcare-websites-and-1000-internet-domain-names-73186607.html*

11. Sayeed L. Stand up to Uniliver's hypocrisy over skin-lightening. *The Guardian, 1–2.* 2010. *http://www.guardian.co.uk/commentisfree/2010/jul/16/unilever-hypocritical-promoting-skin-lightening*

12. Prance L. Beiersdorf targets Indian males with skin whitening trends. 2007. *http://www.cosmetics design.com/Products-Markets/Beiersdorf-targets-Indian-males-with-skin-whitening-trend*

13. Prance L. Nutricosmetics targets skin-whitening market. 2006. *http://www.cosmeticsdesign-europe.com/Products-Markets/Nutricosmetics-targets-skin-whitening-market*

14. Technology Catalysts International. Cosmeceutical trends & technologies (3rd ed.). Church Falls, April.2002. *http://www.technology-catalysts.com/reports services/cosmeceutical.asp*

15. William Reed Business Medi. CosmeticsDesign.com. June 1 2009. *http://www.cosmeticsdesign.com/Financial/CosmeticsDesign.com-acquired-by-William-Reed-Business-Media*

16. William Reed Business Media SAS. CosmeticsDesign-Europe.com. 2009 *http://www.cosmeticsdesign europe.com/Business-Financial/CosmeticsDesign-Europe.com-acquired-by-William-Reed-Business-Media*

17. Montague-Jones G. Cosmetics industry hides nanotechnology from consumers, 2008a *http://www.cosmeticsdesign.com/Formulation-Science/Cosmetics-industry-hides-nanotechnology-from-consumers-according-to-report*

18. Montague-Jones G. Datamonitor features beauty foods in top ten trend list for 2009. 2008b. *http://www.cosmeticsdesign-europe.com/Products-Markets/Datamonitor-features-beauty-foods-in-top-ten-trend-list-for-2009*

19. Montague-Jones G. National stem cell exploits anti-aging qualities of stem cells. 2008c *http://www.cosmeticsdesign.com/Formulation-Science/National-Stem-Cell-exploits-anti-aging-qualities-of-stem-cells.*

20. Pendrous R. Food industry "too secretive: About research into nanotechnology. 2010 *http://www.foodproductiondaily.com/Quality-Safety/Food-industry-too-secretive-about-research-into-nanotechnology.*

21. Prance L. Nutricosmetics targets skin-whitening market. 2006. *http://www.cosmeticsdesign-europe.com/Products-Markets/Nutricosmetics-targets-skin-whitening-market.*

22. Magnusson J. Universities, corporations, and biotechnologies: New colonialism of the 21stcentury. *International Journal of Applied Semiotics,* 2005; 4(2): 35–47.

23. Industry Canada. Diagnosis and therapeutics update: Skin whitening patent is issued toFytokem. Life Science News Brief, March 5 2003; 3(3): 2. *http://strategis.ic.gc.ca/SSG/ph01564e.htm*

Chapter 7

West Africa

Story highlight I - VII
Ghana
Gambia
Ivory Coast
Mali
Senegal
Togo
Republic of Benin

Story highlights I

Ghana

- The burnt disfigured face from the complications of skin bleaching products is called "na nso eben" in Akan — a rebuke, emphasizing "it serves you right."
- The prevalence of skin bleaching in Ghana has been variously estimated as 30% and 50-60%; but a study conducted in a municipality in Ghana found a prevalence rate of 39.2%.
- Skin bleaching in Ghana cuts across all sociodemographic characteristics.
- Several empirical research have been done in Ghana on the subject which gave credible insight into historical precedents and contemporary practices on skin bleaching in Ghana.
- Generally, lighter skin tone is valorized in Ghana. Colorism is highly favored in the media and film industry.
- The main motives for bleaching is to acquire beauty via light skin through which they gain social and economic capital. Light skin is very powerful as a seductive tool. Many Ghanaian women's feeling about beauty, attractiveness and the marriage market are associated with the complexion. Lighter skin has been found to be a valued quality in the contemporary Ghanaian marriage market and people bleach purposely for husbands.

- Those who did not bleach gave the following reasons "fear of critics," "cannot afford the cost," "not interested," for religious reasons—"bleaching is a violation of their belief system"
- Ghanaian women use all the spectrum of skin bleaching products—creams, soaps, serums, pills, injectables and skin bleaching surgical procedures. Those who cannot afford the products fabricate their own home made products with caustic harsh chemicals.
- A broad spectrum of complications including skin cancers, and disfiguring exogenous ochronosis has been reported in Ghana.
- A group of scientists have analyzed the content of some skin lightening creams in Ghana but have, regrettably, released very dangerous conclusions from their findings.
- As regards credible interventions, some individuals, organizations and the Press have initiated robust intervention strategies. However, the government appears to be rather slow and non-committal on the matter

Story highlights II

Gambia

- Gambia government enacted the Skin Bleaching Decree in 1995, and the law was extended in 2002. Under the Law people caught bleaching their skins are fined. Indeed the government went further and instructed security forces and police to arrest and detain anyone found with such products. As repressive as the law appears, however, this control remains extremely difficult with the bribe culture in Gambia
- The most troubling factors that should be of concern to all of us are the medical/health problems associated with skin bleaching. In its totality, skin bleaching contributes greatly to the decline of women's health in Africa.
- The health issue involved in skin bleaching is that many skin bleaching products cause great harm to customers due to high levels of mercury.
- Some women are also addicted to it so much so that when they are out of pocket to buy the chemicals at the market, they go in for local chemicals at home level that are cheap but dangerous.
- Skin bleaching also symbolizes more complex psychological issues such as self-perception and self-esteem that have plagued people of colour.

- When interviewed by news outlets, many African women have expressed that media images portraying white women as beautiful greatly influenced their decision to whiten their own skin. Furthermore, these women have added that although skin whitening products may have harmful effects, they would still use these products to look and feel more beautiful.
- Every woman's dream is to have a good skin tone that will be the centre of attraction for that 'Lucky Man'. Every woman wants to have good looking skin that is smooth, spot-free and flawless but does this mean that to get such a skin one needs to bleach by using chemicals?
- "Let me reaffirm and validate that African women are absolutely beautiful in all our hues and we must do all we can to uphold, celebrate and cherish our gorgeous God given blackness and be proud of it."
- Women should not forget that there is nothing more beautiful than having and nurturing the Black skin that God has given them. Black is beautiful and it costs you nothing but skin bleaching costs you more than you can afford in a lifetime because the more you use it, the more addicted you are to it and the poorer you become. Stop bleaching today, save money and guard your skin jealously against cancer.
- "Lastly, we need to examine our African men's obsession with "white skin" or "light skin" women, and how their attitudes and behaviors toward our dark skin women drive our women to bleach their skin. We need African men to support dark skin women by embracing our blackness."

Story highlights III

Ivory Coast

- Ivory coast banned skin-whitening creams in 2015 because of the health concerns. The health ministry says "cosmetic lightening and hygiene creams that depigment the skin are now forbidden. The ban affects whitening creams and lotions containing mercury and its derivatives, cortisone, vitamin A and more than two percent hydroquinone.
- "The number of people with side effects caused by these chemicals is really high," Christian Doudouko, a member of Ivory Coast's pharmaceutical authority, told BBC News.

- "In our culture, some people think women with light skin are the most beautiful. This beauty standard push many girls to de-pigment their skin,"
- Ekra, a dermatologist at the Treichville university hospital in Abidjan, says, "What we see in the media is, the lighter ones skin is, the better one's life" referring to advertisements that fill the streets of Abidjan, Ivory Coast's biggest city, showing models with lighter than average skin. "While the craze is most widespread among women, some men use the cream too," Ekra added.
- The major concern was over unregulated products, which may contain ingredients such as mercury or excessive amount of steroids.
- The creams can cause a variety of health issues, such as "acne, thinning of the skin, glaucoma or cataracts if applied near the eyes, or if applied liberally to the whole body, they can cause high blood pressure, diabetes, osteoporosis, weight gain, mood disturbances due to absorption of large amount of steroids" she said.
- In fact, organizers in Ivory Cost have gone so far as to create a new and controversial beauty pageant called, "Miss Authentica. The important criterion for participation in this pageant is natural, non-bleached skin. Although this pageant has taken a creative approach to revaluing African aesthetics, it has not eliminated the premise that women should be valued for their bodies and their physical beauty.
- White beauty is a discourse of white supremacy and patriarchy. So, while efforts like "Miss Authentica" are an important critique of racial beauty regimes, their reliance on the beauty discourse limits their ability for social transformation.

Story highlights IV

Mali

- In Mali, the term **"tcha-tcho"**is used to describe the practice of skin bleaching
- The prevalence of skin bleaching in Mali is 53%
- The use of bleaching creams to lighten complexions seems to have reached epidemic proportions in Mali, despite widespread education campaigns.
- Women who refuse to bleach are discriminated against and ostracized in Mali. Women who refuse to bleach often find themselves regarded as second class citizens. A woman who did

not bleach her skin said she is often not offered a chair at baptisms, and is asked to make herself scarce when group photographs are taken at marriages.

- Dermatologists estimate that more than half the women in Mali are now using these creams to lighten their skin.
- The poorest people are the most at risk, because the cheaper the product, the more dangerous it is.
- But it is not just the poor women who are bleaching their skin. "We have also people who are well educated like lawyers, writers, professors, or people on the TV who bleach their skin—and this is a real problem because if people who are leaders of opinion bleach themselves, you can imagine how deep the problem is."
- Many of the women who use these products say they do so because Malian men prefer women with bleached skin. But male musician Al Hassan Soumali disagrees. "I don't think Malian men like bleached women," he says. "It's better for Malian women to change their minds.

Story highlights V

Senegal

- The first report from West Africa about skin bleaching was by Marchand *et al*, in 1975, in a study in Senegal; other reports soon followed.
- "Xessal is the term used by the Senegalese population to define the various techniques and preparations used to bleach the skin.
- The prevalence of skin bleaching in Dakar, Senegal, in one study was 36%; another study in Dakar, Senegal gave a prevalence of 67.2%; yet another study among pregnant women shows that 68.7% of pregnant women either initiated or intensified bleaching during pregnancy.
- Interestingly, some of the women reported starting or increasing the use of skin lighteners because of the pregnancy.
- Among the female adult population, the use of "xessal" was higher among married women and in those with higher cultural level, possibly due to economic reasons. It is also believed that in predominantly Muslim Senegal, where polygamy is prevalent, rival wives lighten their skin to compete for their husbands favour.
- The most common products used are hydroquinone and very potent corticosteroids e.g clobetasol. Other products contained mercurials but 25% of women used assorted concoctions

containing e,g detergents, hypochloride of sodium, and creams of unknown composition.

- A soap seller mixes together skin-lightening soaps that come from Ivory Coast, Mali and Ghana. She says "this one is called 'three days before the wedding; It is too strong to use alone. You have to mix it with other products. Women complain that products like this can sting their eyes or burn their skin. The harsh chemicals can weaken the tissue, leading to stretch marks and infections, but still they don't stop."
- "Even when they discover the side-effects and want to stop using the creams, they find they cannot stop. It's only when you stop that the skin changes and begins to become completely burned."
- A broad spectrum of cutaneous adverse effects are reported.
- Some women in the capital city Dakar say the risks are simply the price of beauty.
- Interventions
  - "I'm black and proud" movement "Nuul Kuuk" is growing day by day
  - Models who bleach their skin are banned from participating from modeling at Dakar fashion Week
  - Award winning film documentary campaign against bleaching
  - Successful campaign to bring down offensive advert "Khess Petch"
  - Women with damaged skin campaign against skin bleaching

Story highlights VI

Togo

- The prevalence of skin bleaching in Togo is 60%.
- Motives for skin bleaching are grouped into seven main reasons: social domination, attraction and seduction, fashion, strengthening the self, success, compliance, pleasure and sensuality.
- Mercury derivatives are most commonly used. Other products contain hydroquinone, corticosteroids and products of unknown composition.
- Various adverse effects on the skin are reported which depend on length of use, frequency and the simultaneous use of different classes of chemicals.

Story highlights VII

Republic of Benin

- 36.6% of secondary school teenage students practiced skin bleaching.
- The ratio of F:M bleachers was 2:1.
- Motivation for skin bleaching was largely for aesthetic reasons.
- 70% of parents approved of skin bleaching and funded the cost of the products.
- The researchers concluded that skin lightening is a real public health problem in the Republic of Benin. It also poses a problem of loss of core values in favour of artificial values. It is urgent that a true youth outreach program be set up to fight against the scourge, which could contribute to poor academic performance

GHANA

Prevalence of Skin Bleaching in Ghana

According to the 2005 Ghana Health Service report, approximately 30% of Ghanaian women and 5% of Ghanaian men were actively bleaching. This statistics has shot-up, and currently 50-60% of adult Ghanaian women are currently or have at one time or the other actively used bleaching agents.[1] In Ghana, the prevalence of skin lightening practices vary between different cities or rural areas. In James Town a coastal town, bleaching of the skin is very popular among the Gas, because their fishing activities impact negatively on their skin. Due to the high concentration of salt in the sea, their skin often gets discoloured, hence they bleach to keep a brighter skin tone. The truth is that skin bleaching is not only rampant in the Ga communities of Ghana, nor is it limited to people along the coast.[2] In the Ashanti region in the South of Ghana, which recorded the highest number of bleachers, 462 out of 500 people between the ages of 8 and 76 admitted to bleaching and 102 of them were men.

According to Sylvia Arthur[3]— "A quick walk around Makola market in Accra and the Central Market in Kumasi reveals that, at least, eighty percent of women who trade there bleach." The symptom which most betrays an indulgence in bleaching is that while some women are fair-skinned on their faces, their legs and the rest of their body is black, what's known as "Fanta Faces, Cocoa Cola Bodies" because of their kaleidoscopic colour. Some also have rough black and blue patches scaring their faces while most reek of a nauseating smell. A listen-in to the conversations of women around town reveals just how deep-rooted the colour-complex is. Young women speak with envy of other women being "good-looking" because of their fair colour while a new mother tells a friend that she thanks God that she's given birth to a light-skinned child. Mothers have even started to bleach young children. The signs of the practice are painfully visible."

Delle, a dermatologist in Ghana believes that about 30 percent of women in Ghana bleach their skin.[4] Kuffour et al conducted a study on the use of bleaching products at the Bolgatanga municipality of Ghana and found a prevalence rate of 39.2 percent.[5]

References

1. Abdul-Karim Mohammed A. Skin Bleaching: The Silent Killer. *http://www.modernghana.com/news/488197/1/skin-bleachin-the-silent...*
2. Dorcas Efe Mensah. Ghana: Skin Bleaching. *http://infoboxdaily.com/your-world/ghana/item/1723-ghana-skin-bleaching...*
3. Sylvia Arthur for TBWT. The New Skin Bleaching Phenomenon. Ghana Web. General News of Thursday, 7 March 2002. *http://www.ghanaweb.com/GhanaHomePage/NewsArchive/artikel.php?ID=22240*
4. Delle Edmund. In Dying to be white by Sylvia Arthur. *http://www.clutchmagonline.com/2008/01/dying-to-be-white*
5.Kuffour Richard A, Dartey Emmanuel, Owusu Wellington and Dabouh Philip M. Level of awareness of effects of the use of cosmetic bleaching products among women: a case study of Bolgatanga municipality of Ghana. *Research on Humanities and Social Science.* 2014; 4 (11): 57-62.

Demographic characteristics of skin bleachers in Ghana

In the past the tendency to bleach was known mainly to be a routine of prostitutes and women who worked in the sex industry in Ghana.[1,2] It is believed that the current practice originated in the 1960's when a number of skin bleaching products first became widely available. However, nowadays, all kinds of people, including men and children, are engaging in the activity which can prove both time consuming and costly.

Interestingly, having this mentality has nothing to do with one's level of education because people of all social strata bleach—from the high school girl to the market woman, the fisherman to professionals like doctors, nurses, teachers, police officers business people, celebrities, politicians, queen mothers, chiefs and even pastors. In Ghana's Ashanti region, for example, women who want to be queenmothers are pressured into lightening their skin tone just to increase their chance of getting enstooled.[3]

Delle[4] recalls, "I went to an African country and the Head of state bleaches from head to toe and the wife does the same thing. So when I was going to give a lecture on bleaching, I was told that l had to change the topic. What is more disturbing is the fact that people living in rural communities struggling to exist below the poverty line are also bleaching in earnest and are innovating new and dangerous ways to take part in the trend.

Kuffour Richard[5] et al studied the dermographic characteristics of skin bleachers in the Bolgatanga municipality of Ghana. A total of one hundred and twenty women were randomly selected from different houses in ten selected communities of the municipality. The ages of the women range between 15-40. 22.5% are analphabetic, 45% of them have only basic education, 30% have secondary education and 8.3% have tertiary education. 52.5% of them were married. 39.2% used cosmetic skin bleaching products.

References

1. Sylvia Arthur.The New Skin Bleaching Phenomenon. *http://www.ghanaweb.com/GhanaHomePage/NewsArchive/artikel.php?ID=22240*
2. Pierre Jemima. 'I Like Your Colour!' skin bleaching and geographies of race in urban Ghana. *Feminist Review*. 2008; 90:9-29
3. Dorcas Efe Mensah. Ghana: Skin Bleaching *http://infoboxdaily.com/your-world/ghana/item/1723-ghana-skin-bleaching*
4. Delle Edmund. In Dying to be white by Sylvia Arthur. *http://www.clutchmagonline.com/2008/01/dying-to-be-white*
5. Kuffour Richard A, Dartey Emmanuel, Owusu Wellington and Dabouh Philip M. Level of awareness of effects of the use of cosmetic bleaching products among women: a case study of Bolgatanga municipality of Ghana. *Research on Humanities and Social Science*. 2014; 4 (11): 57-62.

Background to skin bleaching in Ghana

On March 6, 1957, former British colony of the Gold Coast, the first black African nation to gain its **independence** from Colonial rule—named their country the state of **Ghana,** after the medieval West African empire.

Jemima Pierre and Yaba Blay have extensively dissected the aetiopathogenesis of skin bleaching in Ghana, a West African country. Jemima Pierre[1,2] ilt-in challenge to wholesale white supremacy, particularly its racial values. Unlike other places throughout the

African diaspora where racially black populations are often only a subset of the larger population, Ghana boasts a nominally racially homogeneous population. Furthermore, independent Ghana, at least, has never had official discourses and practices denigrating blackness and elevating lighter skin colour. At the same time, however, accumulated historical precedents and contemporary practices do reveal the significance of both intra- and inter-racial skin colour differenciation in the struggle over identity and meaning. For example, the racial politics of the British colonial project in West Africa, and the Gold Coast in particular, necessitated the establishment of forms of racial apartheid, even as foreign rule depended on the aid of local actors. Linked to this is the history of prominent mixed-race families in the eighteenth and nineteenth centuries who were distinguished from the local community through education, dress, cultural practices, class status, and who articulated a distinctive racial identity based on ancestry and their positions in society. The identification was always subject to contestation, negotiation, and transformation, especially within local identification around ethnicity, culture and religion. Nevertheless, the cultural and political presence of such communities reveal a unique history of the formation of racial consciousness in Ghana, particularly through the interplay of notion of race, colour, class and aesthetics. In the modern times, there are a number of ways that skin colour differentiation continues to occur with Ghanaian racial formation. Alongside state-sponsored Pan-Africanist cultural events and politics advocating a black racial renaissance, for instance, there is also a predominantly white expatriate community who, because of their attachments to multinational corporations and foreign agencies, occupy elevated positions that often tie whiteness to racial privilege.

Blay, a world renowned Professor, Scholar and Producer, in her dissertation titled *"Yellow Fever: Skin Bleaching and the politics of Skin Color in Ghana"* gave an insight into the rationales and motivations for skin bleaching from the perspectives of Ghanaians who bleach and also from the perspectives of non skin-bleachers.

Blay noted that in Ghana, skin bleaching has reached proportions with upwards of 30% of the population engaging in the practice. She regretted that in spite of the current global popularity and venomous ramifications, skin bleaching is seldom the focus of academic research. Although the medical community and popular press have achieved some level of success in alerting the public to the incidence of skin bleaching, the publications are hardly instructive as to why individuals ritualistically rely upon skin bleaching in spite of the severe health implications.

Utilizing the qualitative methodological design of African-centered/African feminist phenomenological ethnography, she conducted a study to uncover the rationales and motivations for skin bleaching from the perspectives of Ghanaians who engage in the skin bleaching culture, with the purpose of elucidating the meaning they attach to the practice. Additional insight into the phenomenon is gained from the perspectives of members of various facets of Ghanaian society , including individuals who have resisted the practice and government representatives. Thematic analysis of participants' testimonies reveals that the symbolism and consequent functionality of light skin underlies the various motivations to lighten the skin. She investigates the sociocultural/sociopolitical symbolism of whiteness in Ghana during pre-colonial (traditional), colonial, and neocolonial ("modern") period by contextualizing participants' testimonies within a broader historico-cultural framework. Her findings suggest that the symbolisms and functions currently assigned to light skin find their place within Ghanaian culture and social history. Blay therefore argued that skin bleaching manifests contemporaneously not as a result of either tradition or colonialism/ neocolonialism but rather as a consequence of *both* tradition and colonialism/neocolonialism. As such, the dissertation positions the current experience of skin bleaching as the embodiment of cultural memory. In painting this holistic cultural portrait, Blay provides an analysis of how skin bleaching functions not only in the lives of the individuals who practice it, but in the context of the culture and history of Ghanaian society.

Blay[4] says "Skin bleaching has become a lucrative business in Ghana. Advertising of bleaching products is extensive. The propaganda campaign to encourage women to part with their hard earned cash is waged effectively through the print media. There are approximately 27 billboards dotted around Accra alone promoting products like "Faire & White" with by-lines boasting. "For the colour you've always wanted." Blay[5,6] found that women in Ghana who used bleaching products were trying to attain beauty vis a vis light skin. She argues that light skin and beauty were the vehicles through which women attempted to gain "**social** capital". The concept of "racial capital" is distinct from racial identity. Racial capital is more closely related to phenotype and how others perceive an individual, rather than how that individual defines him or herself. Racial capital only makes sence in a racist society where light skin and Anglo bodies are valued over dark skin and African or India/indigenous bodies. The concept of racial capital is connected to the larger systems of racism and colorism—none of which is applicable to Ghana.

Kwame Osei[7] believes that the reason why some Ghanaian women bleach themselves is as a direct result of European enslavement and cultural imperialism. Kwame Osei in his article "Ghanaian women and skin bleaching–did God make a mistake? says that skin bleaching is the result of "brainwashing that the early missionaries inculcated into the minds of African/Ghanaian people when the Europeans changed the image of God/Jesus from black African to white European. When the Europeans came to Africa with their white version of God/Jesus, they literally created a false impression that everything godly was white. The angels were white, the virgin Mary was white; white being associated with purity and so forth." This then meant that beauty was associated with being white and African/Ghanaians who are 100% diametrically opposed to White/Europeans, began to question their God-given black skin. This hatred/questioning was further compounded by the cultural bombardment of beauty as determined by the Europeans. The Europeans through films, TV, fashion magazines, videos, modeling etc were able to promote whiteness as the standard of beauty. As a result of this constant bombardment, Ghanaians/African women have been conditioned into thinking that white/pale is beautiful. This has created a situation now where many Ghanaian/African women have become dissatisfied with their Black/African skin–whether on a conscious or a sub-conscious level. This dissatisfaction has created a multibillion dollar industry in skin bleaching/whitening creams that have exploded on the market due to the Ghanaian woman's insecurity about her African complexion. Kwame Osei says: "These skin bleaching/whitening products have in the past been imported into Ghana by Nigerians and now more recently by Indians, Europeans and Chinese companies. There are an array of bleaching creams on the Ghanaian market, such as "skin white," "skin light," and "carrot light" with slogans like "Ma wo honam enkasa," that are enticing naïve and gullible Ghanaian women to bleach their God given black skin."

Abdul-Karim[8] attributes the skin bleaching phenomenon to **racism**. The Europeans penetration into the land of Africa did not only see the acculturation and proselytizing of Christianity and democracy, but also saw the wanton looting of the rich mineral resources of Africa, slave trade, break down of African values, and even the portrayal of black skin as inferior. Many Africans have, for time immemorial, suffered the constant abuse of being referred to as 'Monkeys'. The worst culprits of such abuse are our sportsmen and women who ply their trade in Europe and other parts of the world. Many African players have in the past been reduced to tears by slurs from on-field opponents and spectators. Players like Mario Balotelli, Kelvin Prince Boateng, Samuel Eto, Julio Ceser, Sule Muntari and many others have had their fair share of the racist taunts. Owing to the constant racial discrimination which many Africans are often subjected to, there has been a mad-rush by many Africans to look just like the whites. Many Africans therefore apply toxic creams that bleach their skins. The craze for a lighter skin is dangerously recording an alarming proportion of which African women are the worst culprits.

Abdul Karim further explores the reasons why people bleach their skins. She claims this may be informed by several factors. Cultural influence precipitated by colonial mentality of beauty as determined by Europeans is a major factor. The Europeans through their incessant racial abuse has informed many African people that black skin is inferior. The Europeans through beauty pageants, fashion, modeling, TV, Magazines etc were able to promote whiteness as the benchmark of beauty, something many Africans are blindly copying today. Abdul Karim says many other African women bleach their skin because of marriage marketability. Many African men are turned on by fair women and therefore many women would prefer to bleach their skin to entice men. The Akan expression, "If a fair skinned lady lies on bed and there are light-outs, the room brightens" has erroneously gotten into the heads of many African women.

Fokuo[9] also corroborates this valorization of women with fair skin by men and that fair skin facilitates the finding of marriage in Ghana. Some men encourage skin bleaching by considering light-skinned women to be more attractive, intelligent, moral, desirable, and chaste. In contrast, dark-skinned women are said to look mean, evil, stupid, and untrustworthy. This opinion is consistent with the results of a survey by Fokuo among Ghanaian women. Most of the respondents thought that men prefer light skin in a woman: "Sometimes if you really want to marry a particular man, you have to bleach."

Dr Delle,[10] a dermatologist in Ghana, says "The reason for this potentially life-endangering practice is purely vanity. Women who bleach do so because they believe that men prefer their lighter-skinned counterparts. Also, in some African societies light-skinned people are perceived to be more intelligent than those with darker hue."

Jemima Pierre[1] in her article "I Like Your Colour!" Skin bleaching and geographies of race in urban Ghana", reports how Yvonne, a second generation Guyanese immigrant from Brooklyn, who has light brown skin complexion, received a great deal of attention from men and women in Ghana because of her colour. She would often complain of being overwhelmed by the constant refrain of "I like your colour". At the same time, coming from Afro-Caribbean families, both Ynonne and Jemima recognized that light skin valorization was not unique to Ghana. Jemima Pierre also demonstrated that one can also find the real cultural value and material benefits attached to lighter skin in urban Ghana. For example it is hardly disputed throughout Ghana, that former president Jerry Rawling's popularity—mostly with women—was based in part on his perceived attractiveness (which in turn was perceptibly linked to his biracial heritage).

Hadiza Nuhhu-Billa Quansah[11] says Ghanaian women have ignorantly copied a lot of things from the western culture and unfortunately skin bleaching is one of such. While some women do it to attract their male suitors; others bleach as a result of low self-esteem or the desire to be accepted within a particular class. Madam Afia Kanadu Bimpong, a trader at Makola in Ghana, who has exogenous ochronosis, told *The Mirror* she had been bleaching for the past 37 years. She says: "When we were growing up most men of our time preferred fair-coloured women to those who are black. Even just listen to some of the songs our musicians compose; they are always glorifying fair ladies so I decided to change my colour", she narrated. It is alleged that casting for Ghana Films requires that one is light-skin complexioned.[12] In Ghana, directors in the film industry discriminate against dark-complexioned girls. Hence if you want to augment your chances of being recruited into the film industry as an actress, you have to bleach your skin.

Jessica Edmund has researched extensively on the impact of the media on the skin lightening culture in Ghana.[13-15] She found that the ideal skin complexion represented in the media in Ghana, whether through television commercials, billboards, print or digital advertisements, is of fair skin tones and this is impacting adversely on women and children. Her project film titled, "Skin Bleaching in Ghana: Media and Cultural Impact", shows that in Ghana, women see that the ideal skin complexion represented in the media is of fair skin tones. In her film, young and old express various views on beauty, fair skin, and the use of skin bleaching creams. They have only to watch television commercials, read print and digital advertisements, or drive past huge billboards. The media portrays "whiteness or lightness" as a symbol of what is attractive, adorable, desirable, pure, and loveable.

As regards media impact on the skin lightening culture, Jessica Edmond's findings were corroborated by Siji Jabbar[16] who writes: "**Skin lightening ad, Kumasi, Ghana.** Most of the foreign media and movies consumed in sub-Saharan Africa are from America and Europe, so we take in these images and mimic the practice of colourism in our own ads and magazines. We see which black women are considered beautiful by the mass media, we see that the black models and singers who are making it are mostly lighter-skinned—Rihanna, Beyoncé, etc. We see which actresses get to play love-interest roles and which ones get relegated to bit parts, and we see which ones make it on to those Top 100 lists. We echo the message we receive and perpetuate the system that excludes dark skin from the spectrum of beauty. We see pictures of Obama and don't just see a black man, **but a bi-racial, light-skinned black man.** Some argue that the beauty ideal is shifting from white to a more café-au-lait-complexion, and that this is demonstrated by the fact that women like Beyoncé, Halle Berry and Jennifer Lopez now routinely top some of those "most beautiful" lists. But what seems to have happened there is that the previous practice of promoting only white women as beautiful was simply not sustainable when a significant proportion of the American population was clearly non-white, so the parameters were widened to include a handful of non-white women who are not too many skin tones away from being white. Now black people everywhere can feel they're included in the international beauty spectrum without really being included. When you look at the Nigerian film industry (the largest of its kind in Africa), you find that its lead characters tend to be light-skinned. Fela's condemnation of the practice in **Yellow Fever** (1976) doesn't seem to have done much good. Check the Ghanaian film industry and you'll find the same."

References

1. Pierre Jemima. 'I Like Your Colour!' skin bleaching and geographies of race in urban Ghana. *Feminist Review*. 2008; 90:9-29

2. Pierre Jemima. The predicament of Blackness: Postcolonial Ghana and the Politics of Race and White women. *Skinner, Elliot.* University of Chicago Press Amazon, com 2013:110-2

3. Blay YA. Skin Bleaching and Global White Supremacy, By Way of Introduction. *The Journal of Pan African Studies.* June 2011; 4(4):4-46.

4. Blay YA. Yellow Fever: Skin bleaching and the politics of skin color in Ghana. http://yabablay.com/yellow-fever/ Publisher: Temple University. 2007

5. Blay YA. Ahoofe Kasa!: skin bleaching and the function of beauty among Ghanaian women. *JENda: A Journal of Culture and African Women Studies.* 2009b; 1 4:1- 10.

6. Blay YA. Editorial: Struck by Lightening: The Transdiaporan Phenomenon of skin bleaching. *Jenda: A Journal of Culture and African Women Studies*, 2009a; 14:1-10

7. Osei Kwame. Ghanaian women and skin bleaching— did God make a mistake? *Women's health special features: Ghanaian women and skin bleaching…* 14 July 2010 http://www.modernghana.com/news/284437/womens-health-specia...

8. Abdul-Karim Mohammed A. Skin Bleaching: The Silent Killer. http://www.modernghana.com/news/488197/1/skin-bleachin-the-silent...

9. Fokuo JK. The lighter side of marriage: Skin-bleaching in post-colonial Ghana. *African and Asian Studies.* 2009; 8 (1-2):125-46.

10. Delle Edmund. In Dying to be white by Sylvia Arthur. http://www.clutchmagonline.com/2008/01/dying-to-be-white

11. Hadiza Nuhhu-Billa Quansah. Black to white to black: Tales of "na nso eben." Ghana News (/index.php/articles-and-opinions-section/item/2282-black-to-white-to-black-tales-of-na-nso-eben) myghanalinks-Displaying items by tag: skin lightening. http://ww.myghanalinks.com/index.php/articles-and-opinion-sectio...

12. Akua Djannie. Skin Bleaching is a sin against God. *Ghanaian Chronicle/ All Africa Global Media.* September 81, 2007.

13. Jessica Edmond. PROJECT. Skin Bleaching in Ghana: Media and Cultural impact. http:pulitzercenter.org/reporting/africa-ghana-skin-bleaching-women-…Launched September 2, 2014.

14. Jessica Edmond. Skin bleaching in Ghana: The cost of beauty. Pulitzer Center http://pulitzercenter.org/reporting/africa-ghana-skin-bleaching-women-... September 8, 2014.

15. Jessica Edmond. Skin bleaching in Ghana: The next generation? Pulitzer centerhttp://pulitzercenter.org/reporting/africa-ghana-feature-youth-skin-bleac... September 2, 2014.

16. Siji Jabbar. "Who taught you to hate your [dark] skin?" *This is Africa http://thisisafrica.me/who-taught-you-to-hate-your-dark-skin/* February 27, 2014.

Motives for skin bleaching in Ghana

Ghanaian women have ignorantly copied a lot of things from the western culture and unfortunately skin bleaching is one of such. While some do it to attract their male suitors, others bleach as a result of low self-esteem or the desire to be accepted within a particular class.[1]

In Ghana, peoples' reasons for whitening their skin are varied. It has to do with the skewed mentality that black skin colour is not attractive. It is believed that people with lighter skin tone are just prettier and have higher chances of winning desirable partners and even other opportunities which may not be readily available to dark-skinned people.[2]

Kuffour *et al*[3] in a study on bleaching practices among women of Bolgatanga municipality of Ghana in 2014, found that 39.2 percent of the women were skin bleachers. Those who did not bleach their skin gave the following reasons for noninvolvement–"fear of critics" (25%), "cannot afford the cost" (19.17%), "not interested" (16.67%). The researchers conclude that this could be attributed to the fact that most of them are very religious and perceived the act as a violation to their belief system. The 39.2% that were involved in skin bleaching gave the following motives%"to attract men" (12.5%), "enhancement of beauty" (15%), "please their men" (9.17%), and "to change skin color" (2.5%).

In an article titled "Ahoofe Kasa! Skin Bleaching and the Function of Beauty Among Ghanaian women," **Blay describes that in Ghana beauty via light skin gained through skin bleaching allows the bleachers across to social capital, and for many, their new found light skin color becomes a "bartering tool" negotiable for economic capital.**[4] "Ahoofe Kasa" is a popular Ghanaian aphorism, which literally means "beauty talks"! This implies that skin bleachers have a hidden agenda. It becomes clear that beauty via light skin has a language which, though not vocalized, is nonetheless very powerful as a seductive tool.

Fokou[5] in a study found that skin color plays a significant role in the lives of Ghanaian women. Many Ghanaian women's feeling about beauty, attractiveness and the marriage market are associated with the complexion. Lighter skin has also been found to be a valued quality in the contemporary Ghanaian marriage market and people bleach purposely for husbands. They want to get married; they want to get attractive to men. Madam Afia Konade Bimpong, a trader at Makola in Accra, who has facial disfigurement from exogenous ochronosis, told *The Mirrow* she had been bleaching for the past 37 years. "When we were growing up most men of our time preferred fair-colored women to those who are black. **Even just listen to some of the**

songs our musicians compose; they are always glorifying fair ladies so I decided to change my colour she narrated.[6]

References

1. Lastest craze—bleaching injections and pills. Citifmonline. *http://citifmonline.com/2014/11/07/latest-craze-bleaching-injections-pills/*
2. Sylvia Arthur. The New Skin Bleaching Phenomenon. *http://www.ghanaweb.com. GhanaHomepage?NewsArthive/artikel.php?ID=22240*
3. Kuffour Richard A, Dartey Emmanuel, Owusu Wellington and Dabouh Philip M. Level of awareness of effects of the use of cosmetic bleaching products among women: a case study of Bolgatanga municipality of Ghana. *Research on Humanities and Social Science.* 2014; 4(11): 57-62.
4. Blay YA. Ahoofe Kasa!: Skin bleaching and the function of beauty among Ghanaian women. *JENda: A Journal of Culture and African Women Studies.* 2009b; 14: 1-10.
5. Fokuo J Konadu. The lighter side of marriage: Skin bleaching in post-colonial Ghana. *Research Review NS* 2009; 25(1): 47-66.
6. Hadiza Nuhhu-Billa Quansah. Black to white to black; Tables of "na nso eben" (/index.php/articles-and-opinions-section/item/2282-black-to-white-to-black-tales-of-na-nso-eben) *http://www.myghanalinks.com/index.php/articles-and-opinions-sectio..*

Perspectives on skin bleaching in Ghana

Generally, lighter skin tone is now valorized in Ghana as people with a lighter skin tone are considered prettier. For example, Dorcas Efe Mensah[3] says "Let a white man land in any Ghanaian community and everybody will stop whatever they are doing to direct an endless, charmed gaze at them; not to mention the giggles from children who will follow them on the streets, shouting "obroni, obroni" (meaning: 'white man', 'whiteman')".

Jessica Edmond, Pulitzer Center student fellow from Southern Illinois University Carbondale, examines the effects of media that promote skin bleaching among women and children in Ghana[2,3,4] In Ghana, women see that the ideal skin complexion represented in the media is of fair skin tones. They have only to watch television commercials, read print and digital advertisements, or drive past huge billboards. The media portrays "whiteness or lightness" as a symbol of what is attractive, adorable, desirable, pure, and lovable. In this film, young and old express various views on beauty, fair skin, and the use of skin bleaching creams.

In the documentary film by Jessica Edmund, young and old express various views on beauty, fair skin, and the use of skin bleaching creams. Among the people interviewed, Dr Otabel, a practicing dermatologist at Ankaful Leprosorium Hospital, said that the practice of skin bleaching in Ghana was not new. "Women have always concocted ways in which to protect their skin from the brutal equatorial sun [with head wraps, dresses, and materials draped across the body]. Otabel says that skin bleaching is not socially considered an acceptable beauty regimen for women in Ghana and that it would be difficult to find women who would truly admit to skin bleaching." Jessica Edmond corroborated this culture of denial by skin bleachers but state that the practice of "skin bleaching is becoming more popular."

While researching "Skin Bleaching in Ghana: Media and Cultural Impact". Edmond found a diversity of views related to physical beauty and skin tone. Darker-skinned women and children tended to have greater complexion dissatisfaction. Edmond asked why, "How much of this is a direct result of viewing media that promotes skin bleaching products?

In her research titled "Skin Bleaching in Ghana: The Next Generation,"[4] Jessica Edmond tries to explore how children perceive their skin. A six-year old girl looks up to her older sisters and says she feels good about her skin. "My sisters are beautiful and everybody says we all look alike, so I think I am beautiful too". Developing a positive self-image starts at home and can have positive effects on young girls. The girls were asked, "Do you think you are beautiful?" A few were confident, and several seemed confused or unsure. Their responses show a range of opinions on the subject of skin bleaching, a practice that has been passed down by older generations. It is embraced by some, rejected by others.

Sylvia Arthur says[5,6] "The skin bleaching industry is big money. Companies manufacturing the bleaching soaps, creams and lotions export hundreds of tonnes of the suspect goods to Africa and make thousands of dollars a year despite the fact that both Nigeria and Tanzania have long since banned their importation, Uganda and Kenya are soon to follow and Britain and France prohibited the export of bleaching products to Africa. However, local government agencies in Ghana whose job it is to regulate the influx of such substances, Customs, The Standards Board and The Food and Drugs Board, are grossly lacking".

Addo[7] recalls a more unusual case. "A woman in her 50s said she wanted to look pretty on the day of her death when she would be lying on public view." Addo says huge profits are made from the products as some users "would rather buy cosmetics than buy food. Some users concoct their own products by mixing illegally obtained chemicals."

Dr Nancy Adams,[8] a Ghanaian skin specialist based in Canada, told *The Mirror* that it is believed that light and pale-skinned people portray beauty, richness and success. "In some parts, dark-complexioned people are considered inferior and so people opt for skin-whitening or bleaching creams, pills and other products" she pointed out.

Former Ghana's Most Beautiful winner Miriam Abdul Rauf, popularly known as Nasara,[9] was dark skinned when she participated in and was crowned Ghana's Most Beautiful, a TV 3 reality show in 2009. Lately she has become fairer sparking speculations that she is bleaching. The mother of twins confirms she is bleaching, speaking an interview with Doloris Frimpong Manson on *the Delay*. She explains that, "in life we are all entitled to what we want to do… I choose to tone my skin and I don't think it's a problem because if it were a problem to me, I won't do it." She added "I do not regret it. In fact I love it. Unlike those days when the creams were so harsh and cheap now there are better creams that will just tone your body…. And will just befit you." Reacting to assertions that prolonged bleaching could cause skin cancers, Nasara said "In life, everything comes with the bad aspects of it... when you are doing something, sometimes you don't really need to think about the bad part of it. I am just doing it because I am comfortable with it and I don't even think about the negative part of it." Nasara made the headlines in 2012 when she was accused of stealing a mobile phone and make up kit of Miss England during a beauty pageant outside the country %an allegation she denied. She was consequently stripped of her Ghana Most Beautiful title.

Akua Djannie[10] gives an insight into the outrage generated by the culture of skin bleaching in Ghana it is reproduced below unedited:

"Not too long ago, a young lady whom I shall call Yaa, came to me with what was for her a very serious dilemma. You see, Yaa`s one true desire is to act in films. O yes, those that know her say from the day she was born, that has been Yaa`s only destiny. Anyway, recently she went to audition for a new Ghanaian film and left the place so distraught. The reason? Maybe if I put it in the words of the director, it would be easier to explain. **"You see that girl over there? The only difference between you and her is that she is fair-skinned. Actually, that`s not true. You are a better actress, but we like to**

work with fair skinned women in our films. Now, if you can tone your skin, we can consider you for future films." And there, dear reader was the reason for Yaa`s dilemma.

Here she was, a very dark skinned woman. Following her heart's desire. Yet, it looked like for as long as she maintained her natural God given colour, she would not be able to pursue her dreams. So this young lady came to me for advice. What should she do? Should she tone a little?

I was aghast. How could she even consider bleaching her beautiful black skin? How? Call it toning, skin cleansing, skin clearing, give it whatever fancy name you want, it is skin bleaching. It is disgusting. It is an insult to all Afrikans worldwide (by Afrikans I'm referring to every black person who accepts their Afrikan heritage). It is a health hazard. But above all, it is a huge insult to our Maker. O yes, a huge insult. Because how can we turn around and tell God we know better the colour we want to be? My goodness, when are Afrikans going to get over this skin colour thing? Look, as Afrikans God created us in a myriad of colours. We come in shades from caramel brown to dark chocolate. We are beautiful in our various shades.

No matter what, I will never advocate skin bleaching. I think it is a weak character that gives in to the social pressure of looking "light". I just don`t get it. I mean, have you ever seen a bleached person? They look like a human tye and dye, a human batik. They look ugly and smell really awful. O yea, it`s true.

No people, we have to change this. We have to redefine what beauty is and not sit passively while fashion houses in Milan and Paris tell us what is beautiful. We can no longer leave the definition of beauty in the hands of international, non-Afrikan movie makers, advertising agencies and music video directors. As Africans we have to accept whatever shade of black we are. But above all, we need to start looking for the beauty in individuals and not in the colour of their skin. It's all nonsense to say just because someone is not as light as another, they are not as worthwhile. It's utter and complete nonsense.

For Africans living outside the continent of Africa, I guess the pressure to look like Beyonce or Tyra is more persistent than those of us here. Right? Wrong. **Because these days in Ghana, we too are being slowly bombarded with images of what is considered beautiful.** I know young girls who want to look like the characters they watch in these B rate Mexican soaps the TV networks insist on pushing down our throats. Admittedly, apart from the stories I've heard about casting for Ghana Films. Skin bleaching is a disease. A mental disease that aims to destroy the black race. O yes, I'm very serious. I mean, how can people hate themselves so much they would want to burn their flesh? The pathetic thing is, no matter how much flesh burning they do, they will never be beautiful. Just look at Michael Jackson. Now tell me truthfully you believe he looks better now than in the "Off The Wall" days yep, you get my point I think? I have yet to see anybody who looks better after bleaching. And no matter what you do, your genes will always remain African. You can burn your flesh as you like, the minute you have a child, believe me, it will be its natural unbleached self. That reminds me of a family I saw recently. There was an African woman, with a white man and a couple of mixed raced children. O my people come see my Afrikan sister. In an attempt to look like her husband and children, this woman had bleached and burned her flesh to such an extent that I couldn't help it. I followed her to the toilet and asked her what bleaching cream she used.

To manufacturers, I know you are making tons of money, but please, stop producing these poisons, especially if you too are African. To young ladies like Yaa , don't even think about it. Skin bleaching is no guarantee you will be considered the most beautiful. And to all the sisters keeping it real .Ayeekoo.

Before I leave, let me remind you, our Creator believes all shades of our black skins are beautiful.

But hey, these are just the reflections of an ordinary Ghanaian woman".

Azera writes[11] —"Our society must admit that skin lightening is a mental and social disease. Whether it is dishwashing liquid, cement water, or window cleaners; a majority of African women are putting themselves through dangerous chemical mixtures all in the hope of getting "lighter" and becoming beautiful. Whatever the reason might be for doing this, it is important to remember that **True beauty comes from within, and that people can radiate the way it should.** Using skin bleach is very DANGEROUS and causes irreversible COMPLICATIONS, so please be sure to pass the message to anyone you know that might be doing this, so that the demands for these products will eventually decrease. As the Dove commercial says, **we must learn to LOVE the SKIN we're IN."**

References

1. Dorcas Efe Mensah. Ghana: Skin Bleaching *http://infoboxdaily.com/your-world/Ghana/item/1723-ghana-skin-bleaching*
2. Jessica Edmond. PROJECT. Skin Bleaching in Ghana: Media and Cultural impact. *http:pulitzercenter.org/reporting/Africa-ghana-skin-bleaching-women-..* Launched September 2, 2014
3. Jessical Edmond. Skin Bleaching in Ghana: The Cost of Beauty. Pulizer Center. *http://pulizercenter.org/reporting/africa-ghana-skin-bleaching-women-...*
4. Jessica Edmond. Skin Bleaching in Ghana: The Next Generation? Pulitzer center. *http://pulitzercenter.org/reporting/africa-ghana-future-youth-skin-bleaching...*
5. Sylvia Arthur. Dying to be White. *http://www.clutchmagonline.com/2008/01/dying-to-be-white/*
6. Sylvia Arthur for TBWT. Ghana Web. General News of Thursday, 7 March 2002. *http://www.ghanaweb.com/ghanaHomePage/news Archive/artikel.php?ID=22240.*
7.Penangnini Toure. REUTERS NEWS AGENCY Skin bleaching on rise in Africa. *The Toronto Satr.* March 10, 1997.
8. Nancy Adams. In Hadiza Nuhhu-Billa Quansah. Black to white to black: Tales of "na nso eben." Ghana News (/index.php/articles-and-opinions-section/item/2282-black-to-white-to-black-tales-of-na-nso-eben) myghanalinks-Displaying items by tag: skin lightening. *http://www.myghanalinks.com/index.php/articles-and-opinion-sectio...*
9.Ghana news-I am comfortable 'bleaching' my skin-ghana-Most Bautiful's Nasara. Source; Ghana/Myjoyonline.com/Ernest Dela Anglanu. *http://myjoyonline.com/entertainment/2013/December-17th/i-am.comfo...*
10. Akua Djannie. Skin Bleaching is a sin against God. *Ghanaian Chronicle/ All Africa Global Media.* September 18, 2007.
11. Azara. Dying to be Light? *http://www.bellanaija.com/2009/03/24/dying-to-be-light/*

Spectrum of skin bleaching products used in Ghana

There is a wide of bleaching products or creams on the Ghanaian market bearing names such as skin toners, carrot light, anti-ageing, lightening bath gels and other steroid soaps. Markets of such products use enticing adverts featuring light skinned women, mostly celebrities, with the aim of attracting buyers. However, the latest and "result oriental" forms of bleaching agents are pills and injections which are taken and injected on the user to lighten the skin and give it a more "radiant look.[1,2]

To achieve a lighter complexion, many Ghanaian women use several homemade as well as over the counter skin bleaching products.[1] Grace Okofu, a 38 year old in Ghana admits that she "occasionally" uses Pure Skin, a skin bleaching product that she explains "makes my skin tingle then burn almost immediately." Grace says that women have learned to mix the products with shea plant butter and aloe vera plant gel to decrease the amounts of irritation to the skin."[3]

Dr Delle,[4,5] a dermatologist in Ghana, says: "What's more disturbing is the fact that people living in rural communities, struggling to exist below the poverty line, are also bleaching in earnest and are initiating dangerous techniques to participate in the trend. Unable to afford sophisticated creams and soaps, they create their own home-made preparations, mixing everything from toothpaste, shampoo and milk to household bleach, cement and brake fluid, anything that has a corrosive effect on the skin. Some women have even developed a new procedure involving the smearing of hair relaxer all over the body.and wearing up to three layers of clothing including socks, gloves, long sleeved tops and wide brimmed hats to protect themselves from the sun's penetrating rays." "Someone wanting to buy an ordinary body cream or lotion would be hard pressed to find one that doesn't contain a bleaching agent among the hundreds that do. And those believed to be non-bleaching are not always so. Dr Delle's research shows that of the 66 beauty products he's analysed, only 11 have adequate labeling specifying that they contain 2% hydroquinone. The remaining, 4 of which are soaps, have no labeling or content specification at all. However, some local individuals have begun manufacturing their own brand of skin creams for the home market, creating a new "backyard industry."

Some of the products identified by Jemima Pierre[6] through advertisement are *Sonet: Popular Facial Cream*, which had a 'before' and 'after' picture of an East Asian woman, where the woman had considerably lighter/whiter complexion in the 'after' representation. Then there was *Skin Light*, which had a description in French as 'La Crème Eclairissante Traitante' (the 'Clearing Treatment Cream'). In a green and yellow tube and packaged like prescription medicine was the *Lemonvate Cream*. Ema's (a lady who bleaches) collection also had the *Maxi Light* cream, as well as a large lotion bottle with a faded top label reading *Body Clear*, with 'skin whitening lotion' written underneath. Jemima was particularly struck by how ironically straightforward the names of these products were in their marketing of cosmetic and, indeed corrective, whiteness. Jessica Edmond[3] featured a wide range of bleaching products in her project on skin bleaching in Ghana.

In Ghana, though mercury has been banned in cosmetics, Ghanaian women can still acquire them. They continue to be imported, often from China and India and are sold illegally in the market or on the street. There is a wide range of bleaching products or creams on the

Ghanaian market bearing names such as skin toners, carrot light, anti-ageing, lightening bath gels and other steroid soaps. Marketers of such products use enticing adverts featuring light skinned women, bleaching agents are pills and injections which are taken and injected on the user to lighten the skin and give it a more "radiant" look.[1]

Ghanaians use the whole spectrum of bleaching agents—creams, gels, lotions, soaps, pills, injectables and surgical methods.[1] An agent on the Spintex Road who spoke on condition of anonymity said pills and injectables, though popular in western cultures, are imported into Ghana on the demand of the customer because of the cost and the different needs, saying one could pay as much as GH¢ 3,000 for the pills and injections. She said though they are not advertised or promoted in the mass media, women, especially the young, contact her for different pills, injections, as well as soaps and creams.

A sample of the injection which she showed the reporter had the inscription: "best whitening, anti-ageing injection, no more dark spots, pimples, uneven tones, blemishes and stretch marks"— with a before and after look photos showing the effect that could be achieved after using the product. The pills had inscriptions which seek to direct the customer to its usage "take two capsules daily with water 10-15 minutes before meal (one in the morning and one at night)." It added "see results within a week and for an effective whitening, use continuously for three months. Not recommended during pregnancy or breast feeding, do not take caffeine whiles taking pills."

In an interview with Mrs Emma Yankey,[1] a cosmetologist at 2nd Image Hair and Beauty Clinic, she said these products though not indicated on them, had a high amount of hydroquinone, lead and mercury chloride or ammoniated mercury. She said the quality of these ingredients determined the time and effect a user could get. Mrs Yankey explained that some women were moving from creams and soaps to injections and pills as these easily diffused into the blood and gave a faster reaction as compared to the creams and soaps. "Once the product is into the body, it enters the bloods steam then the blood circulates it all over the system. Most of the creams and soaps take many weeks or months to achieve results but the injections and pills act faster. So you can inject today and in less than a week, you would start seeing some changes on your skin." she explained.

In Ghana, the words "toning" or "bleaching" are used interchangeably. Mrs Yankey says a lot of women under the cover of "toning" their skin use different bleaching agents. However, she says toning and bleaching are two different beauty processes. Toning is not lightening the skin; it simply means firming your muscles through some form of exercises which is completely different from bleaching. Skin toning has nothing to do with the color of the skin."

References

1. Efia Akese craze—bleaching injections and pills- citifmonline. *http//citifmonline.com/2014/11/07/latest-crze-bleaching-injections-pills/*
http://wwwmyghanalinks.com/index.php/ghana-news/itemlist/tag/skin...
2. Dorcas Efe Mensah. Ghana: Skin Bleaching *http://infoboxdaily.com/your-world/ghana/item/1723-ghana-skin-bleaching*
3. Jessica Edmund. Skin bleaching in Ghana: The cost of beauty. Pulitzer Center. *http://pulitzercenter.org/reporting/africa-ghana-skin-bleaching-women-...*
September 8, 2014.
4. Delle Edmund. In Dying to be white by Sylvia Arthur.
http://www.clutchmagonline.com/2008/01/dying-to-be-white
5. Sylvia Arthur for TBWT. The New Skin Bleaching Phenomenon General News 2002-03-07 *http://www.ghanaweb.com/GhanaHomePage/NewsArchive/The-New...*
6. Pierre Jemima. 'I Like Your Colour!' skin bleaching and geographies of race in urban Ghana. *Feminist Review*. 2008; 90:9-29

Some observed complications of the skin bleaching practice in Ghana

Perhaps no scholar has conducted so much research on skin bleaching in Ghana as Dr Yaba Blay—a Professor/Scholar/Producer. A most recent post "Get Light or Die Trying" is a brief but captivating introduction to the global phenomenon:[1]

"In November 1997, a 58-year old retired female clerical worker presented to the Dermatology Outpatient Clinic of Korle Bu Teaching Hospital in Accra, Ghana "with complaints of dark patches on light-exposed areas of the face, arms, neck, hands, legs and feet of about 10 years duration" as well as a large fungating ulcer on the right side of her neck. Despite a continuous regime of treatment spanning the course of 14 months, her condition failed to improve. In February 1999, the patient died. The cause of death — sun-related squamous cell carcinoma with pulmonary metastasis precipitated by the habitual application of hydroquinone and later steroid-containing creams. Translated – this Ghanaian woman's death was caused by a type of skin cancer, which later spread to her lungs, and was attributed to her ritual practice of skin bleaching for more than 20 years of her adult life".

Doe *et al*[2] studied the pattern of skin diseases at the dermatology clinic of Komfo Anokye Teaching Hospital (KATH), Kumasi, Ghana, and compared the results with the new patients seen at the dermatologic clinic of The William Harvey Hospital (WHH), Ashford, Kent, UK. Doe *et al* concluded that complications from cosmetic skin lightening creams were a frequent problem among women in Ghana.

Sylvia Arthur writes:[3] "Bleaching in some parts of Africa is nothing less than a way of life. Women are known to have strict regimes where they take anything up to half an hour in the morning and evening smearing themselves with powerful soaps and creams in an effort to effect their ideal of black beauty."

A myriad of skin bleaching products are available on the market. Most of them contain active ingredients like mercury, a toxic agent with the potential of causing serious psychiatric, neurological and kidney problems.

The actual process of chemically bleaching one's skin is expensive, labour intensive, often impractical, and medically dangerous.[4] The products that saturate Ghana's market are known to be barely affordable, especially for the poor and working class who often resort to cheaper products in the informal market or household products such as (laundry) bleach, certain shampoos, and even ground bits of glass. Middle and upper classes buy the imported and expensive bleaching products such as *Vantex Skin Bleaching Crème* from African American company Fashion Fair Cosmetics. Next to the expense is the actual intensive process of bleaching. A bleacher's daily ritual, with baths with bleaching soaps followed by the application of a number of creams multiple times throughout the day, demonstrates this. Also, to be effective, skin bleaching products have to be used consistently, and over long periods of time. This affects both cost and increased medical risk. Once a person begins bleaching extensively, she or he has to work diligently to maintain the process. Yet, when used in heavy concentrations the products can cause extreme skin irritation and sometimes the development of 'ochronosis', a disgusting blue-black discoloration of the skin.

Risks abound in whitening one's skin in a tropical country like Ghana. Ghana is geographically positioned very near the equator.[5] Being located along the meeting point of the Greenwich Meridian and the Equator, Ghanaians generously receive sunshine as early as 6am and shines throughout a 12-hour-day till it sets around the same time in the evening. Ghanaians are naturally endowed with very dark skin with the protective melanin pigment to protect against the harmful ultraviolet rays.

Manufacturers of products containing hydroquinone and mercury often warn that consumers stay out of the sun since the exposure will not only make the chemical less effective, but it can also cause the adverse reaction of 'hyperpigmentation' and calloused skin. Because of this key requirement to bleaching chemically, Ghana's hot climate makes it extremely easy to detect a 'bleacher', particularly those who are poor or outdoor working class. For example, in **Makola**, the central, large outdoor market in Accra,[5,6] those who bleach are easily recognizable by their wide brimmed hats, long skirts or pants, with leggings of thick, often woollen socks, and long sleeve shirts underneath their dresses. All this is done to either cover up the damage done to the skin by bleaching, or to protect the skin from the hot sun once one has begun bleaching. As impractical as this may seem, it appears to be common practice among a segment of the bleaching population in Ghana.

The devastating effects of skin bleaching leaves much to be desired and should be abhorred rather than encouraged in the Ghanaian society. Besides the fact that bleaching is on endorsement of self-hatred and mental slavery, most bleaching products and creams on the Ghanaian market contain toxic chemicals like mercury, hydroquinone and corticosteroids. It is not uncommon to see many Ghanaian women and men who have lost their natural skin colour and have exposed their bodies to deformities such as burnt skin, wrinkles, skin blemishes, damaged skin, red spots recalcitrant acne, and striae on the skin — a syndrome normally referred to in Ghanaian local parlance as 'Na nso eben'.[5] In Ghana where many people have disfigured faces due to excessive bleaching, the condition is known as "na nso eben" in Akan; a rebuke, emphasizing "It serves you right." People with this condition are those who use various crude methods of bleaching. For example, they would have spent hours rubbing their skin with harsh chemicals such as hair relaxers, milk mixed with alcohol, sea sand and shells mixed with about 10 different grated medicated soaps. It is very common to see people with such faces at the various market centres and some public offices.

This condition is not only a woman's affair as there are some men who also engage in skin bleaching. The burns are not just limited to their faces; they are found on other parts of their bodies. Some have their necks and shoulder area burnt, to the extent that they always have to wear clothes to cover those parts or their whole body, no matter the weather condition. Nii Amugi, a driver who has also bleached his face and has a disfigured face, said he now feels ashamed when passengers steal glances at him.[5] Ghanaian boxer Percy Oblitei Commey also suffered the same consequences when he lost his national super-feather weight belt to his challenger Smith Odoon in 2001. International report indicated the boxer suffered several punches on his face, opening deep cut on his right cheek, and his nostril bleeding with blood because his skin was too fragile due to excessive bleaching.

Mrs Emma Yankey,[7] a Cosmetologist at 2nd Image Hair and Beauty Clinic said skin bleaching, whether by pills or creams, have several short and long-term effects. She said the chemicals in the bleaching agents weakened the sebum (a natural skin protection and lubricant in the body) resulting in dehydration of the skin, wrinkles, fine lines and breaks the body's ability to heal quickly. She said some people experienced severe headache and eye problems without knowing the cause, adding that excessive use of these products could result in cancer and loss of hair. She advised that anyone who had problems with the skin could see a dermatologist for proper medication.

Tom Dorkenoo,[8] editor of **The Ghanaian Times** newspaper said he began his campaigning journalism against skin bleaching practice when a friend of his, who had been bleaching, died from this very condition. "The shock made me follow up this thing. And I keep on doing it. Every year I write about three editorials on skin bleaching. Dorkenoo stated that the health implications are numerous. Kidney disorders, potential miscarriages and increased susceptibility to common skin diseases and allergies are among the many consequences. Tough, rough, scarred skin; the most serious side-effect, makes it difficult for operations to be performed should surgery be required, since the skin is too thin and too damaged to be stitched up once cut. According to Dr Adams, a Ghanaian skin specialist based in Canada,[5] skin bleaching agents contain certain harsh chemicals that may burn the skin and cause irritation so it is always best to be treated by professionals. She explained that naturally bleaching ingredients like turmeric, yogurt and lemon are mild and better for the face than applying hair relaxers and other harsh chemicals.

There are 'social' hazards as well[9] Obvious 'bleachers' are often openly ridiculed. For example Eazzy was accused and ridiculed after hosting the suffered the same attacks, and she blamed her skin change on use of 'cocoa butter.' Eazzy has to use social media to vehemently deny the bleaching charges but her denial is unlikely to settle the matter since she appears lighter in recent pictures. Poor women, in particular, are castigated as either 'brainwashed' or too illiterate to know better.

Skin bleaching in Ghana is also traditionally attributed to prostitutes who have been known to admit to bleaching for the purpose of attracting more clients.[6] However, it is also an open secret that many of the upper and middle classes—particularly professional women—bleach, a fact that allows for private ridicule and consternation. A most disturbing social hazard is the popular claim that the bleached skin often emits a rancid, rotten odor over time— the fish odor syndrome. (See the section on **Exogenous Ochronosis**)

References

1. Blay Yaba. Get Light or Die Trying. *http://yabablay.com/category/blog/skin-bleaching-why-i-do-the-work-i-do/*

2. Doe PT, Asiedu A, Acheampong JW, Rowland Payne CM. Skin diseases in Ghana and the UK. *Int J Dermatol.* May 2001; 40 (5): 323-6.

3. Pierre Jemima. 'I Like Your Colour!' skin bleaching and geographies of race in urban Ghana. *Feminist Review.* 2008; 90:9-29

4. Dorcas Efe Mensah. Ghana: Skin Bleaching *http://infoboxdaily.com/your-world/ghana/item/1723-ghana-skin-bleaching*

5. Hadiza Nuhhu-Billa Quansah. Black to white to black: Tales of "na nso eben." Ghana News *http://www.myghanalinks.com/index.php/ghana-news/itemlist/tag/skin...articles-and- opinion-sectio...*

6. Sylvia Arthur. Dying to be white. *http://www.clutchmagonline.com/2008/01/dying-to-be-white.*

7. Efia Akese. Latest craze–bleaching injections and pills. Citifmonline. http://citifmonline.com/2014/11/07/latest-craze-bleaching-injections-pills/ http://www.myghanalinks.com/index.php/ghana-news/itemlist/tag/skin...

8.Tom Dorkenoo. In: "Dying to be White" by Sylvia Arthur. *http://www.clutchmagonline.com/2008/01/dying-to-be-white*

9. Gogo Gordon. Tinny, Kan-I against skin bleaching. *News Ghana http://www.newsghana.com.gh/tinnykan-skin-bleaching/*

Responses and interventions to skin bleaching in Ghana

(1) Social Activism through skincare—Grace Amey - Obeng Obeng.[1,2]

An anti-skin-lightening activist in Ghana is successfully reaching rural villages with her message that dark skin is beautiful. Grace Amey-

Obeng was never one to desire the "Cocoa-Cola Body and Fanta Face," referring to African women who use bleaching creams on their faces, leaving their bodies dark with their natural color. Grace's Amey-Obeng for over 30 years has been using social activism through skin care as an intervention tool to stem the tide of skin bleaching in her country. Ghana's Grace Amey-Obeng, is one of West Africa's most successful businesswomen. She made her fortune promoting products which emphasized the beauty of the black skin, at a time when many of her competitors were selling dangerous skin-bleaching formulas. From her earliest days, Amey-Obeng, founder and CEO of the FC Group of companies (makers of beauty products) and the Grace Amey-Obeng Foundation in Accra, Ghana, has been a crusader against the dangers—physical as well as psychological and social—of skin whitening. Today, her efforts are paying off, both in Ghana as well as elsewhere in Africa, and her **Forever Clair** line of cosmetics and skincare products, designed to combat the menace of skin lightening and emphasize instead holistic skin health and well-being, are a huge hit across the continent.

VGMA's. Not too long ago, actress Yvon Nelson Grace Amey-Obeng says:

"The message we want to convey is that we need to preserve our natural skin." "We are also educating people to understand that if you continue to use the wrong products, if you don't protect your skin, this can lead to a vicious cycle, a continual cycle of destruction. What we need more than anything is education and creating awareness." Although there are educational efforts happening across Africa, most of these are centered in urban areas. The bigger problems with respect to skin whitening are in the rural areas, Amey-Obeng says; which is why she organizes groups to make yearly trips to villages to educate people there on the harmful effects of skin bleaching. "I have been doing this for the past 30 years or so, and yes, I can say that in my country, bleaching has gone down tremendously," she says. "People are finding a more refined way of looking after their skin—they understand that 'I need to be black and beautiful' and enhance their natural color, but also they want to make it look youthful and look radiant. That has helped a lot and a lot more people are getting educated and that has changed."

Across Africa today, there's a move toward making skincare products using natural ingredients, in the hope that these will eventually replace more dangerous chemicals. "The Forever Clair line incorporates vitamin C, shea butter, cocoa oil and licorice, among others", says

Amey-Obeng, whose clout has given her a voice at her country's legislative level to ban the use of hydroquinone, corticosteroids and mercury in cosmetics in Ghana.

"Our focus is that whatever you put on your skin should be edible," she says.

Today, Ghana is at the forefront of a movement to change mindsets and practices in Africa, and Ghanians are thrilled by the success that Lupita Nyong'o has achieved internationally.

"Lupita resonates well with what they are hearing locally and trying to achieve and people are citing Lupita as an example not to bleach," Amey-Obeng says.

(2) Intervention by Ghana's Minister of Women and Children's Affairs (MOWAC)

Ghanaians cautioned about skin bleaching

Mrs Juliana Azumah-Mensah, Minister of Women and Children's Affairs (MOWAC), has condemned parents who bleach the skins of their children. She said the act was illegal and amounted to abuse of the human rights of such children, since it exposed their fragile skins to multiple infections and skin disorders. Mrs Azumah-Mensah expressed the worry in a speech read for her by Mrs Evelyn Agyimfra, Director of Administration (MOWAC), at the re-launch of Ghana Society of Dermatology (GSD), in Accra.[3] Mrs Azumah-Mensah said reports reaching the Ministry indicated an increase in reported cases of skin diseases and disorders at the various Out-Patient Departments of health facilities across the country. She said it is shameful that some women would go to every length irrespective of the consequences to enhance the colour of their skins in order to be seen as beautiful. She cautioned that apart from the physical effect of bleaching, some skin bleaching products could be absorbed into the body and result in ailments such as hypertension, osteoporosis, which is the softening of the bones and therefore easily breakable, cancers, liver and kidney disorders. Mrs Azumah-Mensah said since children had very low immune systems and their skins were softer, applying such harsh chemicals on their skins could amount to committing suicide or killing them slowly. She said some Ghanaians continued to bleach their skins with impunity, despite the numerous warnings and education by the Food and Drugs Board (FDB) and other advocates on the use of cosmetics containing harmful chemicals such as hydroquinone. Mrs Azumah-Mensah explained that the persistent use of creams with hydroquinone results in the lightening of the skin, as it removed the outer and protective covering of the skin, and with time leaving such bleached skins with scars and much darker than they were before.

She called on stakeholders including the media to intensify advocacy on the strict enforcement on the ban of cosmetics containing hydroquinone and other harmful chemicals. Mrs Azumah-Mensah said MOWAC would work in collaboration with the FDB to ensure that such products which found their way into the Ghanaian markets were regularly seized and destroyed and vendors punished. Mrs Magaret Lartey, President of GSD, however, said the seizure of such creams, though could minimise the problem was not a panacea to changing the mind set of people, who had become so addictive to the practice. She said such chemicals would always find their way into the country as a result of the free trade system between neighbouring countries. Mrs Lartey said the Society intended to ensure healthy skin for Ghanaians through advocacy, education and training as well as ensure quality treatment of all skin disorders. Mrs Lartey called for the support and involvement of stakeholders including the media to educate and inform the public on the need to maintain healthy skin and support the fight against skin bleaching in Ghana.

(3) Intervention by the Ghana Government

As regards the Ghana's government response to the legality or illegality of the manufacture importation and sale of skin bleaching products in Ghana, the Ghana government appears to be non-committal on the matter as reflected in the excerpts below:

Daniel Pryce says:[4]

"Sadly, the authorities in Ghana have not done enough to curb the importation of these dangerous products into the country. With the vast array of regulatory agencies in the country, particularly the Ghana Standards Board, skin-bleaching products should have been banned in the country by now, as was done in Kenya in 2001 and in several other African nations."

The seeming non-committal stance by the Ghana Government informed the recommendation by kuffour *et al*[5] that:

"The Government should come out with clear policies to regulate the importation and sale of all cosmetic bleaching products in the country. The Government should ban all cosmetic products that contain harmful chemicals such as hydroquinone, corticosteroids, etc."

FDA to ban skin bleaching products in 2016[6]

The Food and Drugs Authority (FDA) says it will ban cosmetic products containing skin bleaching ingredient, hydroquinone. According to the FDA, the ban will take effect from August 2016 in accordance with a directive from the Ghana Standards Authority (GSA). Head of Communication at the FDA, James Lartey, disclosed this at a public forum in the Volta Regional capital, Ho.

"Currently the FDA allows two percent of hydroquinone in skin bleaching products but from 2016, all skin lightening products are supposed to be hydroquinone-free – that means zero percent – and this is going to be enforced".

Some Ghanaians who spoke to *Joy News* were excited about the new directive. They said the directive was long overdue because skin bleaching products are harmful.

"It has taken too long for them to do this but those who are bleaching will have issues with it. Bleaching is not good", one lady told Beatrice Adu.

Another said, "it is good they are banning it, I think black is beautiful and you should be proud of who you are".

(4) Responses and Interventions by others

Kwame Osei[7] describes the women who bleach as "gullible." He says many Ghanaian women who bleach their skin using those toxic creams are not aware of some of the deadly side effects of using them. Kwame Osei, in his special Feature Article titled "Ghanaian women and skin bleaching—did God make a mistake?" writes:

"Apart from the pathetic and erroneous practice of skin bleaching, what Ghanaian/African women are saying on a subliminal level is that God the Almighty made a bad mistake giving them Black skin and that they are bleaching their skin to get rid of what God gave them for a more lighter/fairer complexion —this is grossly insulting to God and an offence to the Almighty of the highest order and is an affront to our ancestors who were proud of their Black complexion. The sad thing about Ghanaian/African women bleaching is that they can never become white. It is about high time that Ghanaian/African women in general recognize the spiritual and historical importance of being African/Black. Black is beautiful and Ghanaian/African women must not allow the European bombardment of beauty to create an inferiority complex in them to believe that being African/Black is ugly. Ghanaian/African women should also remember that it is inner beauty that is much more important than physical beauty."

Alarming as it is, there is hope. A group of celebrities from Ghana have put together a campaign to fight the canker. Actress Ama K Abebrese,[9] along with her industry colleagues Nana Ama McBraown, Paulina Oduro and model Hamamat Montia, is spearheading a crusade dubbed 'Say No To Skin Bleaching and Toning." Through this, they hope to sensitize Ghanaians against the widespread but false belief that lighter skin is superior and more beautiful than dark skin. They also hope to , at least, save those who are willing to receive help. They believe that all skin tones are beautiful and want everyone to love and accept themselves no matter the shade of their skin colour.

Hiplife veteran, Nii Addo Quaynor, popularly known as Tinny, has teamed up with the latest afro pop sensation, Kan-I, to launch a campaign against skin bleaching/toning among black women.[10] The campaign, known as "Bringback our BLACK girls", co-opts the slogan for campaign for the safe return of the kidnapped Nigerian school girls. Both of them are hopping that with this effort, they can create widespread public awareness about the dangers of skin bleaching. He says skin bleaching is a major practice in many African countries and millions of young, impressionable girls have fallen victim to the allure of this sad practice. Kan-I says "Most of us have aunties or mothers or know other women who bleached and they are now having serious regrets because it has affected their skin and their general health. They are spending lots of money trying to reverse the damage done but unfortunately it is too late for them. Tinny and Kan-I are trying to create awareness and warn the young ones about the dangers of skin bleaching/toning, because most of them are clueless about what they are getting themselves into. They see some celebrities on social media flaunting and glorifying their skin tone and they copy them blindly. Tinny and Kan-I just want to help young people realize that "black is beautiful and they don't have to bleach their skin to feel beautiful." They added word of caution thus "Bleaching is bad and once it destroys your skin, there's nothing you can do about it so if you are already practicing it, stop it now. Be proud of who you are and where you are from."

Abdul –Karim[11] also concludes that "Beauty is not defined by only outer looks but the entirety of one's personality and therefore light skin cannot set the benchmark for beauty. Black is beautiful and until we begin to reason like Africans and take pride in ourselves, we would continue to remain mentally imprisoned by this imperialist tactics".

On Monday 2nd September, 2013, TV3 discussed extensively the dangerous effects of skin bleaching in their maiden edition of the rebranded morning show 'Newday'. Government must intensify efforts to educate the public on the dangerous effects of skin bleaching and also pass a bill that would ban hydroquinone-based products that are dumped into the Ghanaian market.

Jessica Edmund[12] says in more advanced jurisdictions, the use of these harmful chemical agents in manufacturing these skin lightening products are banned or strictly controlled, often only available as medical prescriptions. Unfortunately the same cannot be said of Ghana. She noted that the market in Ghana is littered with products containing these ingredients and they are easily available to anyone who wants to bleach. She claims that these lapses in regulatory policies are responsible for the high prevalence of as much 60% of the Ghanaian population who have bleached at some point in their life.

Sena Quashie,[13] responding to the recent ban on skin products in Ivory Coast, released an opinion poll to Ghanaian to vote 'Yes' or 'No' to the question "should bleaching products be banned in Ghana too? She introduced the subject with the question. 'Considering that Ivory Coast, where most of the bleaching products that plaque the Ghanaian market, are being produced has banned bleaching, should Ghana follow suite? The result of the poll is still being awaited.

(5) Ghana Skin Foundation

A non-profit organization, the *Ghana Skin Foundation*,[14] has also started an education campaign.

The Ama K. Abebrese Foundation partners Ghana Girl Guides Association (GGGA) to fight skin bleaching. The Ghana Skin Foundation has as its Motto–"*I Love My Natural Skin Tone*"–a campaign spearheaded by Ama, is against skin bleaching. The Ghana Girl Guides Association has as its Motto "*Free Being Me*". Mrs Alberta Mensah of the Girl Guides Association said:

"We are happy with this partnership and will put in all the efforts we can to project the message of not toning or bleaching their skin". "And since it conforms with our own program '*free Being Me*' we will use her and her ambassadors as mentors to create awareness." "We will have a big walk, a talk and we are still planning more activities that will factor in this message of the girls being themselves in pursuing their goals without toning or bleaching."

Officials of the institution (GGGA) say they agreed to be part of the campaign because they saw in it, a useful social cause that must be supported. They also added that it largely blended in well with their "Free Being Me" campaign.

Ama K said several promotional efforts aimed at whipping up excitement and support for the campaign will go live in December 2014. "It's a self-love campaign and not a judgmental one to point fingers," she says. "The aim is to inform as many girls as possible to partnering with GGGA which is already a big institution, and will give the campaign more ambassadors apart from the celebs we have now. The joint venture will give the foundation a bigger voice and reach across the country." Ama adds: "The rule to avoiding skin bleaching or toning is simple, when in doubt about the content of the cream, use natural shea butter or other products you are certain will not bleach your skin." One thing many of the girls believe is that, when they are two or three shades lighter, they will be beautiful or look better in front of a camera but that is not true."

"The celebs ambassadors of the 'I Love My Natural Skin Tone' campaign will be supporting these girls from time to time whenever the need arises at their events to give it the prominence it deserves." A successful campaign thus far, the ***I love My Natural Skin Tone*** campaign has received great support nationwide. In a sound and silent war against bleaching, it continues to push for women to embrace their natural skin tones.

(6) Recommendations by Kuffour *et al*[5]

As regards the association between level of education and knowledge of the bleaching effects, it is clear that there is a correlation. All (100%) of the analphabetic women claimed they knew nothing about the adverse effects of bleaching products. As regards those with basic education, secondary education and tertiary education, the percentages of those who were ignorant of the adverse health effects were 90.91, 83.33 and 20% respectively. The researchers observed that most of the women in the Bolgatanga Municipality (84.2%) are not aware of the harmful effects of cosmetic bleaching products on their skin and body. The researchers concluded that although 60.8% do not bleach their skin, it is very important that they get much information concerning their health so as to prevent any involvement in the near future–**primary prevention**. The researchers also noted that lack of formal education is a major contributory factor in engaging in skin lightening practices in Ghana. There is need to intervene and create awareness among all the skin bleachers so that they can make informed decision on the matter that would help them discontinue the dangerous habit.

Based on the outcome of the study, the following recommendations were made by Kuffour *et al*:

First of all, the Government should come out with clear policies to regulate the importation and sale of all cosmetic bleaching products in the country. The Government should ban all cosmetic products that contain harmful chemicals such as hydroquinone, corticosteroids, etc.

—Non-governmental organizations and the multi-media organizations via seminars and symposia can help educate the general public about the dangers of skin bleaching.

—Religious organizations should educate their members during meetings on the need to maintain their God-given natural skin colour.

—The authorities of educational institutions, especially High Schools should allocate some amount of time to enlighten the young girls about the adverse effects of skin bleaching.

(7) Some interventions by journalists and others outside Ghana

Tom Dorkenoo,[8] Editor of *The Ghanaian Times*, said he did a study in 1995 with a pharmacologist at the University of Ghana Medical School, and he saw that these creams were destroying the internal organs of women and children. He said in one year alone there were about 140 women who died because they went for surgical operations and they could not be sewn up because the elasticity of the skin had been destroyed by the bleaching products.

Dorkenoo began his campaigning journalism when a friend of his who had been bleaching died from the complications. He said it was a shock to him and made him follow up by writing, at least, three editorial comments on skin bleaching every year. Dorkenoo says he has received little thanks especially from those who are guilty of engaging in the practice, and that he has suffered both physical and verbal abuse as a result of his work, He added "It's not a very comfortable thing because when you write these articles some of the ladies when they see you, they abuse you. A woman spat on me because she bleached and I told people about this. So its not easy because a lot of people in the society are bleaching" Dorkenoo blames Ghana's older generation for being negative role models for the country's youth. "If a child of 11yrs goes to the hospital and sees a nurse sitting before a doctor with bleached skin, that tells the child that it's healthy to do it. If that child leaves the hospital and goes to the classroom and sees the teacher with bleached skin, that too tells the child that it's healthy to do it." Dorkenoo says "the consensus is that the only way to counter the disturbing trend is to wage a multiagency campaign warning people of the dangers of bleaching. But as long as images of Western beauty continue to flood Africa markets and berate the natural black aesthetic, the problem will persist and claim even more lives than ever before."

Daniel K Pryce,[4] who holds a Master's degree in public administration from George Mason University USA, and a member of the national honor society for public affairs and administration in the USA, is a freelance journalist. In his feature article on skin bleaching among Ghanaians: "Exposing the dangers", he regretted that the authorities in Ghana have not done enough to curb the importation of the dangerous products into the country. He believes that with the vast array of regulatory agencies in the country, particularly the Ghana Standards Board, skin bleaching products should have been banned in the country by now, as was done in Kenya in 2001 and in several other African nations. Pryce noted that the unregulated manufacture and distribution of these dangerous chemicals have been on the rise, becoming a very lucrative market for crooks willing to pray on the superficial, unenlightened and naive.

Pryce believes that educating his fellow Ghanaians about the dangers of skin-bleaching might be the way forward in both persuading those currently engaged in the practice to give it up and dissuading those who are contemplating engaging in the practice. Pryce went further to document briefly the history of the use of hydroquinone as a cosmetic skin bleaching agent and lists some of the dangerous health hazards of the use of mercury and hydroquinone. He noted that Mire[16] warns that 2% hydroquinone, the standard "permissible" limit of the chemical in skin-lightening creams and lotions, has not been proven safe in any laboratory so far. Pryce wondered why people engage in the unhealthy practice of bleaching.

De Souza[17] explains that, while the "quest for beauty" is the ultimate goal of most people, skin color seems to play just as important a role in determining what people consider to be the standard of beauty. To this effect, not even a "beautiful, even-toned, blemish-free skin" is enough for some dark-skinned people: these people want to be "white" to be seen as pretty! Ironically, in interviewing a few white people for this article, they told her categorically that they wished they had brown skin, and wondered why people with dark skin would ever want to change their appearance! Yes, race plays an important role in how society "values" a person, especially for those living in white-majority lands, but to think that there is something inherently wrong with our dark skin is nothing short of a disgraceful and bizarrely 'successful' campaign by some non-Blacks to downplay the beauty of the black skin! Roles on television also deceive unenlightened black r children to reject these images, the stronger will be their self-confidence as they grow up!

De Souza believes that the importation of these chemicals must be banned by African leaders because these products are so substandard and toxic, they would never be allowed on store shelves in the originating countries. The twin dangers of flooding African markets with counterfeits and the "adulteration of branded products" should also provide enough reasons to outlaw these commodities altogether. Additionally, passing stricter laws against the sale and distribution of these harmful chemicals may deter would-be distributors.

Pryce then went further to highlight some lessons to be learnt from responses from around the world.

Some lessons from around the world[4]

Australia's Sunday Telegraph: In his February 24, 2008, piece for this August newspaper, Miawling Lam warns Australians about two popular but dangerous skin color-lightening products on the market: *John Plunkett's Superfade Original* and *Thorburn's Whitening Cream*. These products have been known, Lam alleges, to cause "leukemia, liver damage, thyroid disorders and decreases in the formation of melanin."

USA Today: In a January 2006 piece, Sheryl McCarthy, a freelance journalist, decries the worsening of the "black is beautiful" mantra, one which basically states that "African features [are] also attractive." In a society where even black role models and icons, such as Beyonce Knowles and Halle Berry, have many "white" features, it becomes increasingly difficult to convince the full-blooded black girl that she is just as beautiful. McCarthy insists that even some white and Asian girls feel inadequate when comparing themselves with those "Barbie" blondes with long hair, so black mothers are not alone in their quest to convince their daughters that they are just as attractive as other girls out there. As Ghanaians, we need to cultivate a sense of worth in our kids, teaching them that their intellectual capacities essentially dwarf any superficial features they may or may not possess.

London's Daily Mail: Paul Bracchi, writing in the January 13, 2007, edition of the aforesaid newspaper, warns colored people in Harlesden, North-West London, about the introduction to market of a very harmful skin-lightener called, *Maxi White*. Bracchi narrates one person's horror story: "It worked quite well to start with, but as I carried on using it, my skin became thin and dehydrated. My forehead looked like a crinkled up piece of paper it was so cracked. Then, ugly blotches which developed into boils and ulcers started appearing on my face. I was a complete mess." These were the customer's own words! Bracchi concludes: "If hydroquinone which is used in certain industrial processes enters the bloodstream, it can cause fatal liver and kidney damage." So, my fellow Ghanaians, we have been warned.

Pryce concludes thus:
Arguably, many Ghanaian women (and occasionally men) bleach their skins, in order to appear more "attractive" to the opposite sex. Are Ghanaian men unwilling accomplices in promoting the lighter-is-better stereotype? Do Ghanaian women and, occasionally, their male counterparts feel inferior to Asians, Latinos and whites because of these other groups' paler skins? It is saddening to observe how some Ghanaians in the United States foolishly "worship" their non-Black bosses! We need to wake up from our slumber and embark on a long-term crusade to reject the white-is-better nonsense! To be successful, we must start the re-education of our children, letting them know that it is their of consumers achievements in this world, and their contributions to humanity, that matter the most, and not the color of their skin. After all, we have many examples to emulate: Kwame Nkrumah, Kofi Annan, and many other Ghanaians, dead and living, who had left, and continue to leave, indelible footprints in the sands of human achievement!

References

1. Amey-Obeng Grace. Social Activism Through Skincare *www.youbeauty.com/skin/african-akin-lightening-education*

2. BBC News Africa. 24 January 2013. The Ghanaian woman who made millions fighting skin-bleaching *http://www.bbc.com/news/world-africa-21173196*

3. Juliana Azumah-Mensah, Minister of Women and Children's Affairs (MOWAC), Ghanaians cautioned about skin bleaching *http://vibeghana.com/2012/02/17/ghanaians-cautioned-about-skin-ble...*
4. Pryce Daniel K. Skin-bleaching among Ghanaians: exposing the dangers. Feature Article. 25 April 2008. *http://www.qhanaweb.com/ghanHomePage/features/Skin-bleaching-*
5. Kuffour RA, Emmanuel Dartey, Wellington Owasu and Philip M. Dabouh Level of awareness of effects of the use of cosmetic bleaching products among women : A case Study of Bolgatanga Municipality of Ghana *Research on tlumaruties and Social Science.* 2014; 4(11): 57-62.
6. Source: Ghana | Myjoyonline.com | Naa Sakwaba Akwa | faustine.akwa@myjoyonline.com
Date: 27-08-2015 Time: 01:08:08:pm - See more at: http://www.myjoyonline.com/news/2015/August-27th/fda-to-ban-skin-bleaching-products-in-2016.php#sthash.uZQjuyiP.dpuf
7. Osei Kwame. Ghanaian women and skin bleaching— did God make a mistake? *Women's health special features: Ghanaian women and skin bleaching…* 14 July 2010 http://www.modernghana.com/news/284437/womens-health-specia...
8. Sylvia Arthur. Dying to be White. Clutch Magazine. *http://www.clutchmagonline.com/2008/01/dying-to-be-white.*
9. Ama K Abebrese's campaign against bleaching *LOVE YOUR NATURAL SKINTONE. SAY NO TO SKIN BLEACHING AND SKIN TONING.* The Ama K Abebrese Foundation. *http://infoboxdaily.com/your-world/ghana/item1723-ghana-skinbleaching.*
10. Gogo Gorden. Tinny, Kan-I against skin bleaching. *News Ghana. http://www.newsghana.com.gh/tinnykan-skin-bleaching/*
11. Abdul-Karim Mohammed A. Skin Bleaching: The Silent Killer. *http://www.modernghana.com/news/488197/1/skin-bleachin-the-silent...*
12. Jessica Edmond. PROJECT. Skin Bleaching in Ghana: Media and Cultural impact. *http:pulitzercenter.org/reporting/africa-ghana-skin-bleaching-women-…*
13. Sena Quashe. Should bleaching products be banned in Ghana too? http://pulse.com.gh/filla/morning-teaser-should-bleaching-products-be...
14. The Ama K. Abebrese Foundation partners Ghana Girl Guides Association to fight skin bleaching.*http://www.zionfelix.com/ama-k-abebrese-foundation-partners-ghana-girl-guides-association-fight-skin-bleaching/*
15. Tom Dorkenoo. In: "Dying to be white" by Sylvia Arthur. *http://www.clutchmagonline.com/2008/01/dying-to-be-white*
16. Mire Amina. Skin-Bleaching: Poison, Beauty, Power, and the Politics of the Colour Line. *Resources for feminist Research.* 2001; 28: (3-4):13.
17. de Souza M. The concept of skin bleaching in Africa and its devastating health implications. *Clinics in Dermatology* 2008; 26: 27-9.

Analysis of the contents of some skin lightening creams in Ghana

Doreen Amponsah *et al* [1] in a study, analyzed the levels of mercury and hydroquinone in 50 samples of skin-lightening creams and their potential risk to the health in Ghana. The concentration of mercury in the creams ranged from below 0.001 to 0.549µg/g and that of hydroquinone ranged from below 0.0001 to 3.45%. Amponsah *et al* conclude that all the creams sampled for mercury had concentrations less than the US Food and Drug Administration's acceptable limit of 1µg/g. **"The low concentrations of mercury detected in the cream samples analyzed therefore do not pose any potential risk to consumers".** Amponsah *et al* further state: Eight percent (8%) of cream samples analyzed contained hydroquinone levels higher than the recommended WHO limit of two percent (2%). The use of such creams may lead to health hazards. Therefore, it is recommended that all skin-lightening creams should be checked for hydroquinone levels before marketing.

Voegborlo *et al*[2] examined the total mercury content of skin toning creams and the potential risk to the health of women in Ghana. In the study, sixty nine (69) samples of skin lightening creams were analyzed for total mercury. The concentration of mercury in the creams ranged from below 0.001 to 0.311 µg g^{-1}. All the creams sampled had concentrations less than the US Food and Drug Administration's acceptable limit of 1µg g^{-1}. **The low concentrations of mercury detected in the cream samples analyzed therefore do not pose any potential mercury related health risk to the population particularly women."**

Comments on the above "conclusions"

Factors that determine adverse health effects of mercury and severity

It has been clearly stated that as regards mercury the factors that determine whether health effects occur and their severity include:

— The type of mercury concerned;
— The dose
— The age or developmental stage of the person exposed (the foetus is most susceptible)
— The duration of exposure
— The route of exposure (inhalation, injection or dermal contact).

See the sections on "MERCURY" and "HYDROQUINONE"

Reports from Ghana[3,4] revealed that mothers are now engaging in the practice of using skin lightening products for their babies. Mercury is also known to be more toxic to infants. Furthermore the skin of babies is known to be more vulnerable than adults to percutaneous absorption of chemicals.[5,6,7] Worse still, once initiated into the bleaching culture, these babies are more likely to grow up into childhood and adulthood as lifelong skin bleachers.

The **method of use** of bleaching products in the USA is completely different from the method of use in Africa. (See the Section on "**Body Works**"). Furthermore are infants being bleached in the USA as is done in Ghana?

US FDA permissible level of mercury in cosmetics *not* safe in Africa

The spas in Nigeria, and possibly other African countries, have designed a **unique** method of applying the skin-lightening products called "The body works"/Exfoliation which maximally amplifies the percutaneous absorption of the skin lightening chemicals (including mercury) through the *total body surface* of the skin. Is the US FDA permissible level of mercury in cosmetics of 1μg/g really relevant to Africa? The method of application of the mercury containing cosmetics in Africa is *completely different* from the USA. Furthermore the innovation of using the skin-lightening products on babies with immature cutaneous barrier function, and thirdly, the pervasive non-compliance by manufacturers to even the stipulated US FDA permissible level, since many product were found to contain chemicals at concentrations above the permissible limit, the recommendation is that only ***Zero level*** of mercury in cosmetics is acceptable for Africa. See the chapter on the ADVERSE HEALTH EFFECTS OF MERCURY ON THE BABY AND CHILDREN in chapter 13.

It is noteworthy that the above studies in Ghana[1,2] that resulted in **dangerous** conclusions that the products analyzed "did not pose any potential mercury related risk to the population particularly women" were probably made by basic (physical) scientists (detached from clinical reality), and are not **biological** scientists – physicians e.g dermatologists, pediatricians and gynaecologists who are on a daily basis exposed to the reality on ground – seeing and managing the adverse health consequences of bleaching products on mothers and children.

As regards the safety of "2 percent" hydroquinone, read the chapter on HYDROQUINONE: **"The fallacy about the safety of "2 percent" hydroquinone,"** and Amina Mire's research publication entitled- "Skin-Bleaching: Poison, Beauty, Power, and the Politics of the Colour Line."[8] Even at 2 percent concentration, hydroquinone causes skin damage. In addition, Schulz *et al*[9] have argued that skin damage resulting from hydroquinone poisoning depends on the **amount of hydroquinone absorbed by the skin** which, in turn, depends on the **frequency** and **duration** of application and not on the concentration of hydroquinone. See the section on **History of skin bleaching in South Africa.** In 1982, when the Black Consciousness (BC) activists succeeded in limiting the maximum concentration of hydroquinone allowed in cosmetics to two percent, bringing South African regulations into accord with US guidelines, this did not end the agitation by the activists who argued that despite thetwo percent regulation, skin lighteners **continued** to cause problems because the U.S regulations were inadequate for South Africa where black consumers experienced more intense exposure to ultra-violet rays and applied skin lighteners more heavily, more frequently, and for longer durations than their American counterparts, BC and medical activists jointly urged the government to **ban hydroquinone completely from cosmetics.** It becomes clear that Ghana, with perennial high intensity of sunshine **cannot** be regarded as a country where hydroquinone at any concentration can be tolerated as safe for its citizens. Furthermore, the use of hydroquinone in medications for skin blemishes is for a limited area of the skin and for a very short duration. See Chapter 21 on COSMECEUTICALS.

References

1. Amponsah Doreen, Sebiawu GE, Voegborlo R. Determination of Amount of Mercury in Some selected Skin-Lightening creams sold in the Ghanaians Market. *International Journal of Engineering Research & Technology (IJERT)* 2014; 3(6): 344-50.
2. Voegborlo RB, Agorku SE, Buabeng-Acheampong B and Zogli E. Toatl mercury content of skin toning creams and the potential risk to the health of women in Ghana. *Journal of Science and Technology.* 200; 28(1): 88-96.
3. Sylvia Arthur. The New Skin Bleaching Phenomenon. *http://www.ghanaweb.com/GhanaHomePage/NewsArchive/artikel.php?ID=22240*
4. Dorkenoo T. Skin Bleaching. "The Pandemic is Here" Weekly *Spectator* 1998; vol 572 p2
5. Rutter N. Clinical consequences of an immature barrier. *Semin Neonatol* 2000a 5:281-7
6. Rutter N. *Physiology of the newborn skin.* Oxford: Blackwell Science 2000b.
7. Harpin VA, Rutter N. Barrier properties of the newborn infant's skin: *J Pedi*atr 1983; 102:419-25.
8. Mire Amina. Skin-Bleaching: Poison, Beauty, Power, and the politics of the Colour Line. *Resources for Feminist Research.* 2001; 28(3-4):13.
9. Schulz EJ and Sher MA. Rescinding of legislation to ban hydroquinone containing creams. *South African Medical Journal.* 1990; 77:372. Reprinted in *The British Medical Journal* 1992; 305: 903-4.

GAMBIA

Gambia government enacted the Skin Bleaching Decree in 1995, and the law was extended in 2002. Under the Law people caught bleaching their skins are fined. Indeed the government went further and instructed security forces and police to arrest and detain anyone found with such products. As repressive as the law appears, however, this control remains extremely difficult with the **bribe** culture in Gambia.[1]

A document in response to the government's ban is reproduced below, unedited:

President Jammeh's ban on skin bleaching

By A Concerned Gambian[2]

"Dear Pa,

I am writing in support of President Jammeh's ban on skin bleaching. However, I kindly ask him not to fire these women from their jobs because most households in the Gambia are headed by women, and their families (mostly children and the elders) depend on these incomes for day-to-day sustenance. I would suggest that he (President Jammeh) gives them a warning and allows them two to three months to stop bleaching for good.

With that in mind, I clearly understand why President Jammeh wants to put a stop to skin bleaching. Skin bleaching is not good. It is not sustainable. Period. There are many problems associated with skin bleaching, amongst which are: psychological, economical, physical, emotional and medical/health. I will elaborate on these implications another time. For now, I will keep this article short to give people time to read and digest its content.

The most troubling factors that should be of concern to all of us are the medical/health problems associated with skin bleaching. I was informed by a Board Certified Dermatologist (Skin doctor) that bleaching creams/lotions, especially those manufactured in Africa, cause permanent skin damage, skin cancer (s), discoloration (inconsistent color distributions to the skin, e.g., lighter face, dark feet, dark lower extremities, etc, etc.); excessive breakouts of the face and neck areas (big fat dark pimples) and even diabetes (due to the chemicals and other additives/ingredients that are used in these products). The doctor did not say skin bleaching is the main cause of diabetes, but it does contribute to developing diabetes. In its totality, skin bleaching contributes greatly to the decline of women's health in Africa.

Let me reaffirm and validate that African women are absolutely beautiful in all our hues and we must do all we can to uphold, celebrate and cherish our gorgeous God given blackness and be proud of it.

Lastly, we need to examine our African men's obsession with "white skin" or "light skin" women, and how their attitudes and behaviors toward our dark skin women drive our women to bleach their skin. We need African men to support dark skin women by embracing our blackness.

Thank you.

Anonymous.

Bleaching: not a solution to flawless skin[3]

There has also been an excellent article to strengthen the people that there is absolutely no need to lighten the skin colour with chemicals. The article by Halimotou Ceesay is reproduced below:

"Hello and a warm welcome to yet another edition of She-she-she, your weekly column that deals with issues of women and girls within the country and beyond.

Every woman's dream is to have a good skin tone that will be the centre of attraction for that 'Lucky Man'.

Every woman wants to have good looking skin that is smooth, spot-free and flawless but does this mean that to get such a skin one needs to bleach by using chemicals? A good number of women are into skin bleaching. Some are into it with the hope of getting more beautiful than they were before, while others are into it due to peer pressure. No matter the case, either of these women knows the dangers attached to skin bleaching while others tend to ignore the dangers attached to it. Some women are also addicted to it so much so that when they are out of pocket to buy the chemicals at the market, they go in for local chemicals at home level that are cheap but dangerous.

The global issue of skin bleaching or lightening has become a public health crisis of epic proportions. Many people of color purchase and use skin bleaching products that later cause skin discolouration, skin cancer and other medical problems. Due to the depth of this phenomenon, we will devote a two part series to this issue in order to explore the ethical and public health challenges involved in skin bleaching, especially involving people of colour.

The issue of skin bleaching is more dangerous and deadly for people of colour throughout the world because the practice also affects psychological and physical faculties. The psychological impact for many people of colour to lighten one's skin in order to fit within the larger society's definition of beauty is now more widespread than ever. **Skin bleaching also symbolizes more complex psychological issues such as self-perception and self-esteem that have plagued people of colour.** Although many African women may not view their actions as medically dangerous, numerous medical studies have already indicated that excessive usage of these skin whitening products can have an adverse effect that may cause skin cancer. Some African nations have even considered limiting the sale of skin whitening products due to the mass and, sometimes, excessive usage of these products by African women.

When interviewed by news outlets, many African women have expressed that media images portraying white women as beautiful greatly influenced their decision to whiten their own skin. Furthermore, these women have added that although skin whitening products may have harmful effects, they would still use these products to look and feel more beautiful. One has to wonder whether such a mass consumption of these products will eventually cause a self-induced public health crisis within a segment of the larger global population. The reality is that without the conscious awareness of the negative impact of some coercive measures and a strengthening of one's individual identity, those who are faced with similar issues will not be able to overcome similar challenges. **The ethical issue involved in skin bleaching is that many skin bleaching products cause great harm to customers due to high levels of mercury.** Thus, many customers who buy these products are endangering the health of their skin, while skin care product companies continue to benefit financially from selling these products. In many instances, customers are uninformed about the medical risks involved in consuming excess amounts of skin lightening creams such as Artra. This product, in particular, is globally advertised to encourage women of colour to purchase it in order to have lighter and more beautiful skin, according to popular standards of beauty.

Skin bleaching can be a good option to get rid of the black spots or any other type of spots on skin. But skin whitening options have become very complicated these days and there are plenty of options available in the market leaving the customers confused. Although skin bleaching or whitening could be a good option for getting rid of dark spots or skin discolouration, the process is not free from side effects.

Some of the products are rather very harmful and cause skin cancer too. Therefore, it is very important you find out the side effects of skin bleaching before you opt for the whitening of your skin.

Harmful effects of skin whitening or bleaching[3]

Dark grey spots, skin cancer, acne, swelling of the skin, thinning of the skin, cataracts, setting down of fat on face, chest, upper back and stomach, increase in appetite and weight gain, osteoporosis, neurological and kidney damage due to high level of mercury used in the creams, psychiatric disorders, severe birth defects, asthma, and liver damage. Some of these side effects could be seen almost immediately while some are seen after prolonged use of skin whitening creams.

Natural ways of skin bleaching

Here are some of the natural ways for getting flawless and fair skin without using skin bleaches. Diet—Diet is the most important part that you should take care of if you want a flawless skin. Take away all refined food products and replace them with healthy and nutritious ones. Water—Increase your intake of water. This helps keep skin free of dehydration and so the look is healthy and unblemished. It also gives you lighter skin and flushes toxins out of your body system. It also gives you increased energy and better concentration. Remember, the body is 70 per cent water, so take a lot of water every day. Cleansing—Take proper care of cleaning your skin. Choose the product that is natural and effective. Pay attention to exfoliating your skin from time to time so that you get rid of the dead skin. Limes and Lemons—Citric acid is natural bleach and will help you have a lighter skin tone without any side effect. You can make a face mask with lime juice, few drops of glycerin and flour to make a paste. Apply this on your face and leave for 20-30 minutes. Wash with normal water. These methods are harmless and even cost you nothing extra.

Women should not forget that there is nothing more beautiful than having and nurturing the Black skin that God has given them. Black is beautiful and it costs you nothing but skin bleaching costs you more than you can afford in a lifetime because the more you use it, the more addicted you are to it and the poorer you become. Stop bleaching today, save money and guard your skin jealously against cancer.

Dont Carry Skin Bleaching Products

A message from the Trip Advisor staff, Jammeh[4,5]

"Be very careful if you bring any steroid creams or any other products that can be used to bleach skin into TG. You must have a GP's letter confirming your need."

Jammeh is apparently on a crusade against the rising number of young girls trying to lighten their skin

Some of the products used to bleach the skin are Omic Gel, Top Extra Gel, Topsone Gel, Neoprosone Gel, Regge Lemon Gel, Prosone Gel, Lemonvate Cream, Betnovate, Movate Cream, MGC Cream, Mekako Cream, Ambi Cream, Simba, Lexus, Fair and White Gel, Fair and Lovely Cream and Pro Beta-Zone. There is also Madonna Cream, Bu-Tone, and Glo-Tone (Chisolm 2002; Daily Gleaner 1999; Karamagi, Owino & Kata-bira 2001; Mills 2001; Star 2002). Some bleachers use household products like curry power, household bleach, cornmeal, milk powder and tooth paste to bleach their skin[6]

References

1. Gambia Extends Ban on Bleaching of Skin. BANJUL, Gambia—Military authorities in the West African state of Gambia have decreed a total ban on skin bleaching. News.google.com/newspapers?nid=1350&dat…id…
2. Anonymous. (A concerned Gambian) President Jammeh's ban on skin bleaching. *Freedom Newspaper Online.* Nov 30, 2013. http://www.freedomnewspaper.com/Homepage/tabid/36/newsid367/9...
3. Halimotou Ceesay. Bleaching: not a solution to flawless skin *THE POINT, Newspaper, Banjul.* Sept 04, 2014 *http://thepoint.gm/africa/gambia/article/bleaching-not-a-solution-to-fla...*
4. Jammeh. Don't carry skin bleaching products. *Tripadvisor* Gambia Travel Forum-*TripAdvisor.* *hhtp://www.tripadvisor.com/showTopic-g293794-i9249-k6218686-do…* March 2014
5. To review the TripAdvisor Forums Posting Guidelines, please follow this link: May 12, 2009. *http://www.tripadvisor.com/pages/forums_posting_guidelines.html*
6. Andrews MA. In. Skin bleaching and the deconstruction of blackness C. Charles *IDEAZ* 2003; 2(1): 43-53.

IVORY COAST

Ivory coast has banned skin-whitening creams because of the health concerns, the health ministry says.[1] He says "cosmetic lightening and hygiene creams that depigment the skin are now forbidden. The ban affects whitening creams and lotions containing mercury and its derivatives, cortisone, vitamin A and more than two percent hydroquinone—a lightening agent that is used to develop photographs.

Christian Doudouko[2], a member of Ivory Coast's pharmaceutical authority says "The number of the people with side effects caused by these medicines is really high, warning that they could cause skin cancer. Elidje Ekra,[2] a dermatologist at the Treichville university hospital in Abidjan says "lightening products can also lead to hypertension and diabetes.

"In our culture, some people think women with light skin are the most beautiful. This beauty standard push many girls to de-pigment their skin," Ekra said, What we see in the media is the lighter ones skin is, the better one's life " he added, referring to advertisements that fill the streets of Abidjan, Ivory Coast's biggest city, showing models with lighter than average skin. While the craze is most widespread among women, some men use the cream too, Ekra said.

However, analysts say the ban may not stop people buying the products. They are still used in the Gambia despite a ban. South Africa has the world's toughest laws against skin lighteners, having prohibited the most active ingredient-hydroquinone, but a University of Cape Town study found that more than a third of South African women still buy them.

British consultant dermatologist, Justine Kluk, told the BBC the major concern was over unregulated products, which may contain ingredients such as mercury or excessive amount of steroids, "if one thinks about steroids being present in these products, they're often present in much higher quantities than we would prescribe." She said the creams can cause a variety of health issues, such as "acne" thinning of the skin, glaucoma or cataracts if applied near the eyes," or if applied liberally to the whole body, they can cause high blood pressure, diabetes, osteoporosis, weight gain, mood disturbances due to absorption of large amount of steroids" she said.

In fact, organizers in Ivory Cost have gone so far as to create a new and controversial beauty pageant called, "Miss Authentica." The Miss Authentica pageant was designed to speak back to the white beauty regime, raise awareness about the dangers of skin bleaching, and highlight "natural" African beauty[4]. The important criterion for participation in this pageant is natural, non- bleaching skin. Although this pageant has taken a creative approach to revaluing African aesthetics, it has not eliminated the premise that women should be valued for their bodies and their physical beauty. White beauty is a discourse of white supremacy and patriarchy. So, while efforts like

"Miss Authentica" are an important critique of racial beauty regimes, their reliance on the beauty discourse limits their ability for social transformation.

References

1. Ivory Coast bans skin %whitening creams. 7 May, 2015. *BBC News. Africa. http://www.bbc.com/news/world-africa-32628240*

2. Standard Digital News%Kenya; Ivory Coast bans skin whitening creams. *http://www.standardmedia.co.ke/article/2000161357/ivory-coast-ban*

3. No More Vera Sidikas in Ivory Coast As The Country Bans 'Bleaching'! mpasho. Latest News Lifestyle May 8, 2015 *http://mpasho.co.ke/2015/05/no-vera-sidikas-ivory-coast-country-ba...*

4. James I. In pictures: Natural African beauty. BBC News. July 20 2009. Retrieved from *http://news.bbc.co.uk/2/hi/africa/8148719.stm*

MALI

In Mali, the term **"tcha-tcho"** is used to describe the practice of skin bleaching[1]·. In Mali, the cosmetic use of bleaching agents by black people has become a social phenomenon. Mehé *et al* conducted a survey in Bamako, Mali[2] among women aged from 15 to 45 years in order to evaluate the prevalence of this practice and its socio-economic factors. Two-hundred and ten women were questioned during the cluster survey. Among these, 53% used bleaching agents which were topical cortico-steroids (37%), hydroquinone-containing products (21%), mercury derivatives (11%) and products of unknown composition (16%). Dermatological side-effects were observed, but they did not hinder the use of these agents. Bleaching was particularly frequent in unmarried women (39%), literate women (34%) and female students (45%).

The use of bleaching creams to lighten complexions seems to have reached epidemic proportions in Mali, despite widespread education campaigns. Joan Baxter[3] in an article titled 'The heavy cost of light skin' describes how women who refuse to bleach are discriminated against and ostracized in Mali. Women who refuse to bleach often find themselves regarded as second class citizens. A woman who did not bleach her skin said she is often not offered a chair at baptisms, and is asked to make herself scarce when group photographs are taken at marriages. A quick survey shows there are more than 100 bleaching products available on the market in the capital, Bamako. Sold under brand names such as Marie-Claire or Diana, the products come from Morocco, Nigeria, the United States or Saudi Arabia.

Dermatologists estimate that more than half the women in Mali are now using these creams to bleach their skin—and this is a real problem because if people who are leaders of opinion bleach themselves, you can imagine how deep the problem is." Many of the women who use these products say they do so because Malian men prefer women with bleached skin. But male musician Al Hassan Soumali disagrees. "I don't think Malian men like bleached women," he says. "It's better for Malian women to change their minds." lighten their skin. These products are costly and often cause pain and blemishes. So why are so many women in Mali using them? The answer is simple, according to one Malian woman singer: The creams make her white, and impart a certain charm. But Malian physician, Dr Ali Gindo, finds bleached skin anything but charming. "They are just burning themselves," he says. "It's painful and it's awful." Dr Gindo says bleaching can cause skin cancer and the poorest people are the most at risk, because the cheaper the product, the more dangerous it is. But he says it is not just the poor women who are bleaching their skin.

Dr Gindo says:
"We have also people who are well educated like lawyers, writers or professors, or people on the TV who bleach their skin—and this is a real problem because if people who are leaders of opinion bleach themselves, you can imagine how deep the problem is." Many of the women who use these products say they do so because Malian men prefer women with bleached skin. But male musician Al Hassan Soumali disagrees. "I don't think Malian men like bleached women," he says. "It's better for Malian women to change their minds."

References

1. Léocadie Kamagaju, Renato Morandini, Françoise Gahongayire *et al.* Survey on skin-lightening practices and cosmetics in Kigali, Rwanda. *Int J Dermatol* 2016; 55: 45-51.

2. Mahé A, Blanc L, Halna JM, Kéita S, Sanogo T, Bobin P. An epidemiologic survey on the cosmetic use of bleaching agents by the women of Bamako (Mali). *Ann Dermatol Venereol* 1993; 120(12): 870-3.

3. Joan Baxter. The heavy cost of light skin. *BBC News.* 18 April, 2000. *http://news.bbc.co.uk/2/hi/africa/718359.st*

SENEGAL

The first report from West Africa

The first report from West Africa about skin bleaching was by Marchand *et al*, in 1975, in a study in Senegal;[1] other reports soon followed. "Xessal is the term used by the Senegalese population to define the various techniques and preparations used to bleach the skin.

Prevalence from different studies

Pascal del Guidice and Pinnier Yves[2] conducted a study in Dakar from 1992 to 1993 among six hundred and eighty five Senegalese women. 26% of the women were using skin lightening creams at the time of the study; and 36% had used skin lightening creams at some time before. There were some limitations as 93% agreed to answer the questionnaire, but many of them may not have given real and complete response. Indeed, a proportion of women may have denied the use of "xessal" because this practice is usually hidden. Despite these limitations, the study provides data confirming the extensive and uncontroled use of bleaching agents in the female Senegalese population. Among the female adult population, the use of "xessal" was higher among married women and in those with higher cultural level, possibly due to economic uncontrolled use of bleaching agents in the female Senegalese population. Among the female adult population, the use of "xessal" was higher among married women and in those with higher cultural level, possibly due to economic reasons. Dr Pierre-Andre Aka[3] says that in predominantly Muslim Senegal, where polygamy is prevalent, rival wives lighten their skin to compete for their husbands favour.

Another study in two areas in Dakar[4] on the use of skin bleaching cosmetics, describes the prevalence according to the following variables: age, matrimonial situation, level and/or type of instruction, job, and type of agent used. For that purpose, the researchers conducted a transverse derivatives (61%), topical corticosteroids (37%) and agents from unknown origin (2%). The use of skin bleaching cosmetic was more prevalent among young women between 30 to 44 years (72.5%), married (72.2%), analphabets (75%), and working (77.6%).

Mahe *et al*[5] in a study at the maternity centre in Senegal demonstrated that 68.7% of selected women between 6 and 9 months gestation, attending a maternity centre in Senegal, Dakar, used skin lighteners for cosmetic purpose during their pregnancy. This included agents containing hydroquinone, highly potent corticosteroids and products of unknown composition. Interestingly, some of the women in this study reported starting or increasing their use of skin lighteners because of their pregnancy.

Bleaching Products used

Dermatologists say that many of the products include steroids corticosteroid and clobetasol propionate, a cream which should be used for the treatment of severe skin inflammation and prescribed by health professionals, and hydroquinone a potentially carcinogenic chemical which limits melanin production in the skin, and is banned in the EU. The most common products used were hydroquinone and corticosteroids e.g clobetasol.[2,4] Other products contained mercurials but 25% of women had used assorted concoctions containing e,g detergents, hypochloride of sodium, and creams of unknown composition. Soap seller, El Hadji Traore,[6] mixes together skin-lightening soaps that come from Ivory Coast, Mali and Ghana. This one is called 'three days before the wedding': It is too strong to use alone. You have to mix it with other products." Said Traore. "Women complain that products like this can sting their eyes or burn their skin. The harsh chemical can weaken the tissue, leading to stretch marks and infections, but still they don't stop."

Anne Look[6] reported that the products, even those claiming to have so-called "natural" components, can contain mercury, hydroquinone or caustic agents like sodium hydroxide. These are dangerous ingredients that can cause cancer and are potentially disfiguring. Some women in the capital city Dakar say the risks are simply the price of beauty. A beauty supply shop in Dakar, complete with a selection of skin-lightening creams and soaps: "This lotion, it is carrot based. It doesn't have hydroquinone. It will give you an amazing color," said shop clerk Adama Diagne. She said she uses a similar cream, and she tells clients to avoid the stronger ones that promise fast, dramatic results. Adama said "It's a personal choice. No one pressures me. Some women want to be black every day, but I prefer to be a shade of brown. It's better for me. I like it," she said.

Most products are easily available on the streets or in market places. They are sold without any medical prescription and control, and imported from neighboring countries.[7,8] The cheaper cost of such uncontrolled products is likely to be the main reason for their trade.

Critics[9] say that the cost of Khess Petch – at 1,000 CFA Francs a tube – less than £2—deliberately targets the products at women who are unaware of the risks.

"There are expensive face-lightening creams which are less dangerous, but products like Khess Petch are very cheap and very dangerous—they are deliberately targeted at women in the villages and the poor urban areas," said Deme. "Even when they discover the side-effects and want to stop using the creams, they find they cannot stop. It's only when you stop that the skin changes and begins to become completely burned."

"When women who use these creams stop, they look horrible," said Fall. "They actually start looking more black, all the side effects manifest at the same time, which they just can't. accept."

There is a law banning the sale of the products

Although Senegalese law includes controls over the creams, including a ban on creams with more than 2% hydroquinone, the laws are poorly enforced, with products with much higher levels freely available in stalls and market places in Dakar.

Adverse effects reported

In the study by del Guidice and Yves,[2] 75% of the women using such creams showed cutaneous adverse effects. Facial acne was the most common adverse effects. Table 1 shows the main cutaneous diseases in women using "xessal." The mean duration of use was 50.5 months; a few women had used "xessal" for longer periods, e.g 20 years.

Table 7.1 Main cutaneous diseases in women using "xessal"[2]

Cutaneous diseases	Frequency (%)
Facial acne	36
Facial hypertrichosis	19
Cutaneous atrophy	17
Stretch marks	17
Hyper-hypopigmentation	14
Intertrigo	10
Pyoderma	9
Tinea corporis	6
Purpura	3

Evidence of high mercury levels in the scalp hair of Senegalese women

Gras and Mondain[10] conducted an epidemiological study from twenty Senegalese women using mercurials cosmetics to determine the mercury levels in scalp hair. The mean value was 155.75 +/- 75.38ppm mercury in scalp hair while the normal level is less than 10ppm. This prompted an experimental study in monkeys (Papio papio) treated with a soap containing mercuric biiodide. After only three months of experimentation, there was a significant augmentation of mercury levels is all the organs and especially in the kidneys and the hair. This study corroborates the findings of Barr in Uganda.[11]

Motives for bleaching

Women in Senegal say they lighten their skin for the same reasons women the world over say they tweeze, squeeze or alter their bodies—in sometimes dangerous ways—to achieve a certain standard of beauty—to catch a husband, to stand out in the crowd, to smooth out imperfections, to get ready for a special event.[6]

The expected result of "xessal" in Senegal is to clear the skin to obtain the so-called "teint clair" which is supposed to "improve appearance" and is considered by women as a standard of elegance, beauty, and higher social level.

Responses and interventions

Dakar example[12,13,14]

In the West African nation of Senegal, the "I am black and proud" movement, "Nuul Kuuk" as it's known locally, is growing day by day.

The movement, says fashion designer show organizer and a key figure in the black fashion world, Adama Ndioye Paris, is inspiring more and more young women to stand tall and be proud of their black skin, and to believe that dark skin is beautiful. For someone like Paris, who has been fighting incessantly against skin lightening – especially among black models – it's a huge deal.

Adama, who started the annual Dakar Fashion Week in 2002, made headlines in 2013 when she banned models who use skin lightening creams from participating in the event. Dakar Fashion Week in Senegal has been showcasing beautiful African women and fashion since 2002 – but in 2013, the founder has something new in store. Senegalese fashion designer Adama Ndiaye reportedly said she banned models from the Dakar Fashion Week who lighten their skin, a process which she refers to as depigmentation. Ndiaye told FashionGhana.com that she's against the practice and doesn't find it pretty. "I'm trying to teach them to like themselves".

Oulimata Ba, who is Senegalese-American, said although she has never lightened her complexion, she knows family members who have. Ba was happy to hear what Ndiaye is now doing with Dakar Fashion Week. "I think it's a wonderful thing she's doing, but that action alone is not enough", she said. Ba added that the European standards of beauty are so deeply ingrained in the culture that this ban of skin-bleaching models cannot make a huge change. But she hopes it's a catalyst for more to come. Ba said, "It's funny because Senegalese women are very proud to be African, but it's a huge contradiction."

"I've been fighting the practice of skin lightening for some years, particularly among black models," Adama says. "Because I never take on models that use these products. I have seen that more and more black models are stopping using them, because they love fashion and because I have constantly repeated that I think their natural look is more beautiful.

That said, though, Paris believes there's still a lot of legwork needs to be done to reduce the practice of skin lightening, both in Senegal and elsewhere in Africa. Governments have a role to play, she says, in stopping what has become a serious public health issue. Advertisement that glorify skin-lightening creams as agents of beauty must be banned. Only then is there hope to change the prevailing mindset, that lighter skin is more beautiful than dark.

Senegalese filmmaker Khardiata Pouye Sall was so troubled by the trend, in particular among prominent female public figures in the media, that last year she made her international-award-winning documentary "This Color That Bothers Me." It aired nearly a dozen times on state television in Senegal.

"I used the most shocking images so that women would know what they are exposing themselves to," said Sall. "Many of them know the dangers, but don't think it will happen to them. It is hard to understand why a woman would tell herself that dark skin is not beautiful. It's in their heads. They want to please a man, to be loved. Or they want to please society, to succeed."

Sall said the government needs to better regulate the marketing and sale of these products, but also emphasized that educating women really is the only way to make skin-lightening go out of style.

Adverts for skin bleaching products in Senegal

Thomas Fessy[15] reports that an ad campaign for skin whitening cream that promises result in 15 days has ignited fierce debates on Senegalese social net works since September 2012. "Khess Petch"- loosely translated from the local Wolof as "All White" or "All Light" – printed on huge placards all around town portrays a woman "before" and "after" she'd used the cream – she is seen black and then fair white.

Nearly 2,000 people signed an online petition to bring the adverts down, and soon after, a counter-campaign "Nuul Kuuk" was set up defending Black skin pride. Doctors at the main dermatology hospital service in Dakar say they receive an average of 200 women per week in cases related to the use of skin-whitening products.

Reports have been broadcast on television about the risks of using whitening creams following the huge controversy. Many women with bad skin damage have sought to encourage others to stop using these products. "I bitterly regret having done that to myself," "But girls and women with fair skin would always seduce more men"- a 51 year-old woman said. Thomas Fessy reports that the woman wears a scarf to hide a long stain and spots that the products left on her skin. "It is ugly and it itches," she says.

The health minister eventually met with Nuul Kuuk activists who were told that current laws couldn't forbid ads campaign for these products, which are labeled as cosmetics. The ads for "khess Petch" are now down, but other creams have just started their own campaign. It is a familiar formula for persuading women to buy a new beauty product: plaster billboards of a beautiful model in the capital city, accompanied by a catchy slogan written in the language of the ordinary woman.[9]

But when new adverts for skin cream "Khess Petch" – a skin lightening cream whose name means "all white" – appeared in Senegal, they had the exact opposite effect. The ads, which boast extreme skin-whitening after 15 days, complete with dramatic before and after shots, provoked mass public outrage and calls for the government to introduce an industry-wide ban.

"We are used to seeing adverts for skin lightening, but when we first saw these adverts for Khess Petch we were really scandalized. We decided to act," said Aisha Deme, manager of an online events website in the Senegalese capital, Dakar.

"Society is constantly telling us that fair-skinned women are beautiful-in the media, on TV—and Senegalese women have started to believe it," Deme added. "So we want to show that dark-skinned women are really beautiful, and that natural black skin should be celebrated."

Deme[9] now co-ordinates a campaign called **Ñuul Kukk**- which means "pitch black" in local language Wolof – and has attracted thousands of supporters on Facebook and high-profile friends, including the actor Awa Sene Sarr and rapper Awadi.

Senegal's health minister, Eva Marie Coll seck,[9] has also met the group, and expressed her "outrage" about the advert, fuelled by the prevalence of fair-skinned images in films, magazines and advertising.

Pascal del Guidice and Pinier Yves conclude that the use of skin lightening creams in African countries, such as Senegal is ongoing despite information campaigns. The standard of beauty, "teint clair" (clear skin), promoted by African magazines will continue; therefore, we must be aware of such cosmetic practices in African women and provide safe products.

References

1. Marchand JP, N' daiye B, Arnold J, Sarrat H. Les accidents des pratiques dépigmentants cutanés cosmétiquechez la femme africaine. *Bull Soc Med Afr Noire Lque Frse* 1976; 21:190-9

2. Pascal del Guidice and Pirier Yves. The widespread use of skin lightening creams in Senegal: a persistent public health problem in West Africa. *The International Journal of Dermatology*. 2002; 41:69-72.

3. Aka Pierre-Andre. In Skin bleaching on rise in Africa. Penangnini Toure. Reuters News agency. *The Toronto Star*. March 10, 1977.

4. Wone I, Tal-Dia A, Diallo OF, Badian M, Toure K, Diallo I. Prevalence of the use of skin bleaching cosmetics in two areas in Dakar (Sénégal). *Dakar Med* 2000; 45 (2):157-7.

5. Mahé A, Perret JL, Ly F *et al.* the cosmetic use of skin-lightening products during pregnancy in Dakar, Senegal: a common and potentially hazardous practice. *Trans R Soc Trop Med Hyg*. 2007; 101: 183-7.

6. Anne Look. In Senegal, Skin-Lightening Remains popular despite health risks. http://www.voanes.com/content/in_senegal_skin_lightening_remaini...

7. Pitche P, Afonou A, Amanga Y, Tchangai-Walla K. Prévalence des accidents cutanés lies à l'utilisation decosmétiques dépigmentants chez les femmes à Lomé. *Cahiers Santé* 1997; 7:161-4.

8. Sylla R, Diouf A, Ndiaye B et al. Pratique de la dépigmentation artificielle de la peau chez les femmes à Dakar et étude analytique des products dits cosmétiques utilizes. *Dakar Méd* 1994; 39:223-6.
9. Afua Hirsch. Skin-lightening creams face West African backlash. *Guardian. Co.uk.* November 14, 2012 http://www.biyokulule.com/view_content.php?articleid=5534
10. Barr RD, Rees Ph, Cordly PE et al Nephrotic syndrome in adult Africans in Nairobi. *Br Med J* 1972 Apr 15:2 (5806): 131-4.
11. Grs G, Mondain J. The problémes poses par l'utilisation des cosmétics mercuriels au Sénégal. *Toxl Eur Res* 1981: 3(4):175-8.
12. Savita Iyer—Ahrestani. March 28th 2014 wwwyoubeauty.com/skin/African-skin-bleaching-history.
13. Models Who Bleach Skin Banned from Dakar Fashion Week/ Black P...
wwN.youbeauty.com/skin/adama-paris
http://www.blackpressusa.com/2013/08/models-who-bleach-skin-ba...
14. James J. In pictures: Natural African beauty. BBC News July 20; 2009
http://news.bbc.co.uk/2/hi/africa/8148719.stm
15. Thomas Fessy. Africa: Where black is not really beautiful. *BBC News, Dakar. http://www.bbc.com/news/world-africa-20444798*

TOGO

Motives for skin bleaching in Togo

A study was done by Lonzozou Kpanake *et al*[1] titled: "Skin Bleaching Among Togolese: A preliminary Inventary of Motives" published in *The Journal of Black Psychology.* Kpanake surveyed 219 women and 81 men from Togo (West Africa). Using the results, Kpanake gives seven main reasons as to why Togolese people bleach.

1. *Social Domination:* Lighter skinned people are seen as more important, affluent and civilized.
2. *Attraction and Seduction:* Light skin is seen as more beautiful, and men are more likely to love light-skinned women more than dark-skinned women.
3. *Fashion:* Whitening is what they saw top models in magazines, family members, and close friends practice.
4. *Strengthening the self:* They are dissatisfied with their current appearance and want to change it to feel better about themselves
5. *Success:* They will benefit economically and status- wise if they have lighter skin
6. *Compliance:* Respondents felt lighter skin will increase others' positive thoughts towards them.
7. *Pleasure and Sensuality:* They love and enjoy their light skin. Light skin is seen as "soft", blemish free and has the ability to make others jealous.

They did not practice skin bleaching as a demonstration of opposition to African culture.

Pitche *et al*[2] evaluated the occurrence of cutaneous complications among women who used bleaching cosmetics in Lomé,Togo. The prevalence rate of skin bleaching in Lomé, Togo is 60%. Of 536 women who used these cosmetics, 69.2% had at least one dermatological complication. The bleaching agents used were mercury derivatives (30.9%), hydroquinone (24%), topical corticosteroids (18.5%) and products of unknown composition (25.6%). The main dermatological side-effects were hypochromia (62.8%),hyperchromia (2.7%), melano-leucoderma (8.1%), acne (11.6%) and skin trophic disorders (14.8%). The occurrence of these complications was associated with the length of time for which the chemicals were used, the frequency and the simultaneous use of different classes of these cosmetics.

The researchers noted that the prevalence of complication was similar to the 70% in the series of Mahé in Bamako. They noted the limitations of their study design—they did not consider the skin infections (bacterial and fungal) which could complicate the use of skin bleaching products, nor did they search for the possible internal organ complications such as renal diseases, diabetes and corticosteroid-induced obesity/Cushion's syndrome. They concluded by emphasizing the need to sensitizing the users on the dangerous adverse health complications from the habitual use of skin bleaching product.

References

1. Kpanake L, Muñoz Sastre MT, Mullet E. Skin bleaching among Togolese: A systematic inventory of motives, *Journal of Black Psychology* 2010; 38: 350-68.

2. Pitche P, Afanou A, Amanga Y, Tchangai-Walla K. Prevalency of skin disorders associated with the use of Bleaching cosmetics by Lomé women. *Sante.* May-June 1997; 7(3): 161-4. *http://www.ncbi.nlm.nih.gov/pubmed/9296805*

3. Mahé A, Keita S, Bohin T, Complications dermatologiques de l' utilisation cosmétique des produits dépigmentants à Bamako (Mali). *Ann Dermatol Venereol* 1994; 121: 142-6.

4. Pabozi N, Santos A, La distribution des produits cosmétique et la protection des consomateurs au Togo. *Mémoire de maîtrise en droit. Faculty de droit Lomé. 1993; 160*

5. Mahé A, Blanck L. Halna JM. Keita S, Sanogo T, Bobin P. Enquéte épidémiologique sur l'utilisation cosmétique de produits dépigmentants par les femmes de Bamako (Mali). *Ann Dermatol Venereol* 1993; 120: 870–3

REPUBLIC OF BENIN

Atadokpédé *et al*[1] conducted a cross-sectional survey to evaluate the prevalence of skin bleaching in secondary schools in central Benin using a questionnaire. It was a descriptive and an analytical cross-sectional study on randomly sampled students in public and private Colleges of General Education (CEG) in Bohicon, a city in Central Benin. Students aged at least 15 years were included. 429 students were selected and 36.6% of the students engaged in skin lightening. 66.9% of the students practicing skin lightening were female and 31.1% male. The average age of the students who practiced VD was 18 years with a range of 18 to 27 years.

Products containing hydroquinone were the most used (42.0), followed by corticosteroids (22.7%), mercury compounds (19.7%); fruit acids (13.6%) and others (2.3%) The average duration of use was 20 months with a range of 1-98 months. The mean monthly cost of products was 2.6 US dollars with a range of 0.7 dollars to 10 dollars.

Parents supported and funded the cost of skin lightening in 70.1% of cases, and the choice of product used was made by parents in 52.2% of cases. The opposition of parents to skin lightening was noted in 10% of case in girls and 15.7% of boys. Motivations for skin bleaching was to treat skin defects 38.5% in males and 78.1 female; and aesthetic reason in 61.5% of males and 78.1% females. Products were applied all over the body twice a day in most students. Majority of them claimed they continued to bleach because they loved the light skin (76.2%), the products were effective and they did not want the skin to become black again.

The adverse skin disorders observed among the skin bleachers were dyschromia (32.3), stretch marks (20%), acne 18.5%, superficial mycosis (13.1%), skin atrophy (13.1%), and contact dermatitis (3%).

The researchers concluded that skin lightening is a real public health problem in central Benin. It also poses a problem of loss of core values in favour of artificial values. It is urgent that a true youth outreach program be set up to fight against the scourge, which could contribute to poor academic performance

Reference

Atadokpédé F, Adégbidi H, Koudoukpo C, Téclessou J, Aholoukpé C, Dedboé B, do Ango- Padonou F, and Yedomon H. Epidemiological and clinical aspects of skin bleaching in Secondary Schools in Bohicon, Benin. *Journal of cosmetics, Dermatological Sciences and Applications*. 2015; 5:1-6.

Chapter 8

Southern Africa

Story highlights I, II, III
South Africa
Zambia
Zimbabwe

Story highlights I

SOUTH AFRICA

- Colonialism and apartheid had a major impact on black and coloured women, since they suffered both racial and gender discrimination.
- **History of skin lightening in SA**

Commercial Skin lightening cosmetics has been sold in South Africa by the mid 1950s for decades, first mainly to whites and later to people of colour.

These cosmetics also appealed to black and ambiguously raced people, including Jews, who sought to navigate social hierarchies that privileged lightness, and to achieve aesthetic ideal rooted in both colonial and precolonial conceptions of beauty

The earliest evidence of skin lighteners being marketed to black South African women dates to the early 1930s. They surfaced through two different routes: one entailed the importation of products made by African American companies and the other, the distribution of products manufactured in South Africa. Under apartheid even more than prior forms of segregation, skin complexion could inform where one lived, one's school and work opportunities, whether one could vote, and whether one needed a government pass to move in and out of urban areas. In 1980, Findlay and De Beer drew attention to 'A

South African epidemic of Ochronosis of the face in black skinned individuals.'

- A study conducted twenty five years ago showed that seven out of ten patients in two hospitals in Pretoria practiced skin bleaching. However, in current times, prevalence rates variously stated as— one woman in three SA women, 38% of black African women; 27% of Indian women; 35.5% from a study of misuse of topical steroids among patrons of pharmacies in Pretoria.
- Expressed motives for skin bleaching—"to be white," "to be beautiful;" "Our men find lighter women very attractive;" "I just want to look smart and handsome."
- Determinants for skin lightening in SA
  i. Effect of Apartheid
  ii. Historical influence of colonialism and apartheid
  iii. Availability of cheap low-end bleaching products
  iv. Effect of celebrity skin bleachers
  v. Cultural issues
  vii. Ineffective legislation
  viii. The promotional effect of the media
  ix. The effect of institutionalized Black market, peer pressure, and ignorance about health risks.

- South Africans use the whole spectrum of products available on the market to lighten the skin colour. These are topical preparations (creams, serums, gels, soaps), pills, and injectable, and surgical methods already discussed in the relevant chapter.
- In 1992 South Africa passed the world's most restrictive regulations regarding skin lighteners; Government banned skin lightening ingredients including mercury and hydroquinone from cosmetics. Government also prohibited manufacturers from claiming in advertisements that their products can "lighten," "whiten," or "bleach."
- Although the sale of over-the-counter skin-bleaching creams containing hydroquinone was banned in South Africa, the products have continued to circulate on the black market. Recently, spice shops and newly opened India and Pakistani beauty parlours have been doing brisk business with "fairness" creams. Former beauty queen Sorisha Naidoo claims her products have sold out since picture of her "new fair self" appeared in newspapers.
- SA dermatologists and scientists are engaged in robust intervention strategies through health education programmes and research.

Story highlights II

ZAMBIA

- The derogatory name given to skin bleachers in Zambia is 'FBI'— Former Black Individuals.
- The prevalence of skin bleaching in Zambia is alarming though the exact prevalence is unknown.
- "Even the ones who should know better are doing it" We know a few artistes who are bleaching, some CEOs, some cabinet people and even some pastors."
- "The thing about bleaching is that no matter how decent or independent you are, you just end up looking like a desperate cheap person."
- There are women who bleach their children.
- Some hair salons have even resorted to applying corticosteroid creams on the scalps of their clients to enable hair to grow fast.
- Such is the pervasive culture of whitening the skin that only pale white face powders are available in the market, a cosmetic dealer says she no longer order for darker shades of powder because they don't sell fast as dark people are in extinction in Zambia.
- When skin bleachers are asked why they bleached these were the responses "Dark-skinned women nowadays are left with no choice but to use some skin-lightening lotions. This is necessary to deter men, in particular husbands, from leaving their dark skinned women or wives in search of light-skinned partners or wives; light-skinned women are more desirable by men!" **Helen**
- "Men are to blame for the increase in the number of women who are using skin lightening lotions because we fear that if we don't lighten our skins, our husbands will go after those who are light skinned. You will find that men leave their dark-skinned spouses in their homes and go after the light-skinned ones, so what are women expected to do?" **Lizzy**
- People' responses on social media were highly critical of the skin bleaching culture
- Some of the men have vehemently refuted the stories that they valorize light skinned women
- There is a high prevalence of skin bleaching among Zambia men
- The Zambian Pharmaceutical Regulatory Authority (PRA) has issued out warnings on the dangers of rampant abuse of skin lightening creams in Zambia and the unnecessary burden on the government, which will have to spend colossal sums of

money on treating patients with complications of skin bleaching

- The Public Health Forum (PHPE) has called on Government to ban the sale of skin bleaching creams in the country
- 5 responses to "skin bleaching in Zambia"
    (i) *"What's the point of bleaching your skin if God had a reason to make you black,,,if It's because you want to attract Mr or Miss right it's pointless because the one who truly loves you will love you for who you really are. Am black and I'am proud, if someone does not love me for my skin colour then I will know there and then that he is Mr wrong.....Zambians let us be proud of who we are, immitating the white man's skin will just put us in jeopardy when faced with the consequences of cancers in the future...".* Nelisa.

    (ii) *"I would be very uncomfortable to appear brown when am black in the actual sense. I am really proud of my colour and happy to be my beautiful black self because there is nothing as comforting as being yourself in life. I think people who bleach do not realise how much they alter their own natural beauty.."* Marita.

    (iii) *"I can't believe how bleaching is affecting me myself. I am proud to be black. Why would I want to look like white people. This is what happens when people are not proud of themselves even men"!* Gladys Mwamba.

    (iv) *"You are right my sister preach".* Mutale.
    (v) *"Yalya ama ten pin aleonaula mukushita ama chemicals. Uyu transport officer afwile ukushitilamo abana bakwe imichopo mulya muchibolya"!!!!* Willie.

Story highlights III

ZIMBABWE

- Skin lightening is highly prevalent in Zimbabwe
- Hip/bum enhancing is also highly prevalent
- Both men and women have taken to using skin bleaching products.
- In an article titled "*Beauty is in the eye of the skin bleacher,*" Robin Chaibva[1] says— "The definition of beauty is a tricky proposition.

> "For ages, debate on what beauty is has raged across the globe. Therefore, it comes as no surprise that some people have taken it upon themselves to change their looks after experiencing the bullying and discrimination of not "fitting in." **Robin**

"Women who use the creams are delusional to think that all men find light-skinned women attractive. Women who do not get **adequate** attention from men are the ones resorting to these **desperate** measures. Women need more self-confidence, and users of these products are "**short-term investors**" trying to swindle men." **Cliff**

"Enhancements were for women who saw themselves as mere sex objects.

"men who bleach their skin are most likely sexual deviants." **Anonymous**

- Finally, Robin asked: "Is beauty your personality, looks or how you present yourself? What people find attractive is always a personal preference from individual to individual and varies across geographical and social clusters. So what do we call beautiful in Zimbabwe?
- Mainini cautioned that most, if not all the skin lightening creams sold in the market, are a dangerous cocktail of compounds like steroids, hydroquinone, tretinoin and mercury. Hydroquinone and mercury are bleaching agents that are banned from use in cosmetics.
- Experts have warned that long term use of these products can lead to lethal health complications
- Mainini concludes that she has seen women who now cannot spend a minute in the sun because continued use of the skin lightening creams have damaged their skin, it cannot tolerate the sun anymore. She cautioned those who continue using it if it makes them feel happy but beware of the dangers.

SOUTH AFRICA

Apartheid

Apartheid[1] (Afrikaans pronunciation: [PÈpartf[it]; an Afrikaans[2] word meaning "separateness", or "the state of being apart", literally "apart-hood")[3,4] was a system of racial segregation in South Africa enforced through legislation by the National Party (NP), the governing party from 1948 to 1994. Under apartheid, the rights, associations, and movements of the majority black inhabitants and other ethnic groups were curtailed, and white minority rule was maintained. Apartheid was developed after World War II by the Afrikaner-dominated National Party and Broederbond organizations. The ideology was also enforced in South West Africa, which was administered by South Africa under a League of Nations mandate (revoked in 1966 via United Nations Resolution 2145),[5] until it gained independence as Namibia in 1990.[6] By extension, the term is currently used for forms of systematic segregation established by the state authority in a country against the social and civil rights of a certain group of citizens due to ethnic prejudices.[7]

Racial segregation in South Africa began in colonial times under the Dutch Empire, and continued when the British took over the Cape of Good Hope in 1795.[8] Apartheid as an officially structured policy was introduced after the general election of 1948. Legislation classified inhabitants into four racial groups—"black", "white", "coloured", and "Indian", the last two of which were divided into several sub-classifications[9]—and residential areas were segregated. From 1960 to 1983, 3.5 million non-white South Africans were removed from their homes, and forced into segregated neighbourhoods, in one of the largest mass removals in modern history.[10] Non-white political representation was abolished in 1970, and starting in that year black people were deprived of their citizenship, legally becoming citizens of one of 10 tribally based self-governing homelands called *bantustans*, four of which became nominally independent states. The government segregated education, medical care, beaches, and other public services, and provided black people with services that were inferior to those of white people.

Apartheid sparked significant internal resistance, violence, and a long arms and trade embargo against South Africa.[11] Starting in the 1950s, a series of popular uprisings and protests was met with the banning of opposition and imprisoning of anti-apartheid leaders. As unrest spread and became more effective and militarised, state organisations responded with repression and violence. Along with the sanctions placed on South Africa by the international community, this made it increasingly difficult for the government to maintain the regime. Apartheid reforms in the 1980s failed to quell the mounting opposition, and in 1990 President Frederik Willem de Klerk began negotiations to end apartheid,[12] culminating in multi-racial democratic elections in 1994, won by the African National Congress under Nelson Mandela. The vestiges of apartheid still shape South African politics and society. De Klerk began the process of dismantling apartheid with the release of Mandela's mentor and several other political prisoners in October 1989.[13] Although the official abolition of apartheid occurred in 1991 with repeal of the last of the remaining apartheid laws, nonwhites were not allowed to vote until 1993 and the end of apartheid is widely regarded as arising from the 1994 democratic general elections.

Colorism in South Africa

Coloured people consist of three mixed race populations in South Africa who were given more social privileges than other unmixed, indigenous African groups. During the **apartheid era**, in order to keep divisions and maintain a **race**-focused society, the government used the term *Coloured* to describe one of the four main racial groups identified by law: Blacks, Whites, Coloureds and Indians. (All four terms were capitalised in apartheid-era law). Many Griqua began to self-identify as "Coloureds" during the apartheid era. There were certain advantages in becoming classified as "Coloured". For example, Coloureds did not have to carry a ***dompas*** (an identity document designed to limit the movements of the non-white populace), while the Griqua, who were seen as another indigenous African group, did.

Women under apartheid

Colonialism and apartheid had a major impact on black and coloured women, since they suffered both racial and gender discrimination.[14,15] Jobs were often hard to find. Many black and coloured women worked as agricultural or domestic workers, but wages were extremely low, if existent.[16] Children suffered from diseases caused by malnutrition and sanitation problems, and mortality rates were therefore high. The controlled movement of black and coloured workers within the country through the Natives Urban Areas Act of 1923 and the pass laws separated family members from one another, because men usually worked in urban centres while women were forced to stay in rural areas. Marriage law and births[17] were also controlled by the government and the pro-apartheid Dutch Reformed Church, which tried to restrict black and coloured birth rates.

Asians during apartheid

Defining its Asian population, a minority that did not appear to belong to any of the initial three designated groups, was a constant dilemma for the apartheid government.

For political reasons, the classification of "honorary white" was granted to immigrants from Japan, Taiwan, and South Korea—

countries with which South Africa maintained diplomatic and economic relations[18]—and to their descendants.

Indian South Africans during apartheid were classified many ranges of categories from "Asian" to "Black" to "Coloured" and even the mono-ethnic category of "Indian", but never as White, having been considered "non-White" throughout South Africa's history. The group faced severe discrimination during the apartheid regime and were subject to numerous racialist policies.

Chinese South Africans—who were descendants of migrant workers who came to work in the gold mines around Johannesburg in the late 19th century—were initially either classified as "Coloured" or "Other Asian" and hence "non-white" and were subject to numerous forms of discrimination and restriction.[19] It was not until 1984 that South African Chinese, increased to about 10,000, were given the same official rights as the Japanese, to be treated as whites in terms of the Group Areas Act, although they still faced discrimination and did not receive all the benefits/rights of their newly obtained honorary white status such as voting.

Indonesians arrived at the Cape of Good Hope as slaves until the abolishment of slavery during the 1800s. They were predominantly Muslim, were allowed religious freedom and formed their own ethnic group/community known as Cape Malays. They were classified as part of the Coloured racial group.[20] This was the same for South Africans of Malaysian descent who were also classified as part of the Coloured race and thus considered "not-white".[21] South Africans of Filipino descent were classified as "black" due to historical outlook on Filipinos by White South Africans, and many of them lived in Bantustans.[21]

Presidency of F.W. de Klerk

Early in 1989, Botha suffered a stroke; he was prevailed upon to resign in February 1989.[22] He was succeeded as president later that year by F.W. de Klerk. Despite his initial reputation as a conservative, de Klerk moved decisively towards negotiations to end the political stalemate in the country. In his opening address to parliament on 2 February 1990, de Klerk announced that he would repeal discriminatory laws and lift the 30-year ban on leading anti-apartheid groups such as the African National Congress, the Pan Africanist Congress, the South African Communist Party (SACP) and the

United Democratic Front. The Land Act was brought to an end. De Klerk also made his first public commitment to release Nelson Mandela, to return to press freedom and to suspend the death penalty. Media restrictions were lifted and political prisoners not guilty of common-law crimes were released.
On 11 February 1990, Nelson Mandela was released from Victor Verster Prison after more than 27 years of confinement.

Having been instructed by the UN Security Council to end its long-standing involvement in South-West Africa / Namibia, and in the face of military stalemate in Southern Angola, and an escalation in the size and cost of the combat with the Cubans, the Angolans, and SWAPO forces and the growing cost of the border war, South Africa negotiated a change of control; Namibia became independent on 21 March 1990.

On 10 May 1994, Mandela was sworn in as South Africa's president. The Government of National Unity was established, its cabinet made up of 12 ANC representatives, six from the NP, and three from the IFP. Thabo Mbeki and de Klerk were made deputy presidents.

References

1. Colonialism. Wikipedia, the free encyclopedia. *http://en.wikipedia.org/wiki/Aparthied.*

2. *"Dictionary.com entry for 'apartheid'"*. Retrieved 11 August 2012.

3. Shore Megan. *Religion and Conflict Resolution: Christianity and South Africa's Truth and Reconciliation Commission*. Ashgate Publishing, 2009. p.36

4. Nancy L Clarkson & William H Worger. *South Africa: The Rise and Fall of*. Routledge, 2013. Chapter 3: The Basis of Apartheid.

5. *"Resolutions Adopted by the General Assembly during its 21st Session" (PDF)*. Retrieved 11 August 2012.

6. *Gallagher Michael. "The birth and death of apartheid". BBC News.* Retrieved 17 June 2002

7. Merriam-Webster. Merriam-Webster, n.d. Web. 23 Feb. 2015. <http://www.merriam-webster.com/dictionary/apartheid>

8. *Du Toit A, Giliomee HB. Afrikaner political thought: analysis and documents. University of California Press.* ISBN 0520043197.

9. Baldwin-Ragaven Laurel, London Lesley, du Gruchy Jeanelle. *An ambulance of the wrong colour: health professionals, human rights and ethics in South Africa.* Juta and Company Limited. 1999 p. 18.

10 *"South Africa – Overcoming Apartheid". African Studies Center of Michigan State University.* Retrieved 26 December 2013.

11. *Lodge Tom. Black Politics in South Africa Since 1945. New York: Longman.* 1993.

12. *"De Klerk dismantles apartheid in South Africa". BBC News. 2 February 1990. Archived from the original on 15 February 2009.* Retrieved 21 February 2009.

13. http://www.theguardian.com/world/2010/jan/31/nelson-mandela-de-klerk-apartheid

14. "Women's Charter, 17 April 1954 Johannesburg". *ANC.* Retrieved 15 January 2014.

consumers used skin lighteners for a variety of reasons which ranged from clearing blemishes to lightening tanned skin to brightening to look more 'modern' or sexy. Nonetheless, the broad 15. *Cotula Lorenzo. Gender and Law: Women's Rights in Agriculture. Rome: FAO. 2006. pp. 46–52.* ISBN 9789251055632.

16. *Lapchick Richard E, Stephanie Urdang. Oppression and Resistance: The Struggle of Women in Southern Africa. Greenwood Press. 1982. pp. 48, 52.*

17. *Bernstein Hilda. For their Triumphs and for their Tears: Women in Apartheid South Africa. International Defence and Aid Fund for Southern Africa.1985. p. 48.*

18. *"In South Africa, Chinese is the New Black". China Realtime Report. 19 June 2008.*

19. *Sze Szeming. World War II Memoirs, 1941-1945 (Digital ed.). Pittsburgh: University of Pittsburgh. 2014 p. 42.* Retrieved 7 November 2014.

20. Lemon Anthony. *"Overcoming the Apartheid Legacy in Cape Town Schools". Review.* 2009.

21. Patric Tariq Mellet *"Intro", Cape Slavery Heritage.* Retrieved 24 May 2011.

22. Roherty James Michael. *State security in South Africa: civil-military relations under P.W. Botha.* M.E. Sharpe. 1992. p. 23. ISBN 978-0-87332-877-7.

History of skin lightening in South Africa

Lynn Thomas,[1] the erudite Professor of History at the University of Washington, has researched extensively and written books on the history of skin lightening and skin lighteners in South Africa. Commercial Skin lightening cosmetics has been sold in South Africa by the mid 1950s for decades, first mainly to whites and later to people of colour.[1] During the nineteenth century, these preparations became popular and profitable commodities in Europe, the United State and various imperial outposts including South Africa. They appealed to white women and some men by playing on a bourgeois and racialized aesthetic that valued skin purged of evidence of outdoor labour and intimacy with dark-skinned 'others'. These cosmetics also appealed to black and ambiguously raced people, including Jews, who sought to navigate social hierarchies that privileged lightness, and to achieve aesthetic ideal rooted in both colonial and precolonial conceptions of beauty[2]

During the interwar period, skin lighteners fell out of favour with many white consumers, as pale skin became a sign of those confined to factory or office work, and tanned skin a symbol of having the leisure time and affluence to enjoy outdoor holidays and the health benefits of the sun's vitamin D. While skin lighteners decreased in popularity among white women, they continued to be heavily marketed to African Americans through the early 1960s.[3] And among black South Africans, skin-lightener sales did not peak until the 1970s

The earliest evidence of skin lighteners being marketed to black South African women dates to the early 1930s. They surfaced through two different routes: one entailed the importation of products made by African American companies and the other, the distribution of products manufactured in South Africa. By the 1920s, some of the largest and most profitable black-owned business in the United States, such as Madame CJ. Waker and Apex, sold cosmetics, including skin lighteners.[4] Soon after these U.S. products entered South Africa, some white pharmacists began advertising their own skin lighteners to black consumers.[3]

Local manufacture of skin lighteners took off after the Second World War as white businesses sought to cultivate black consumers and the right-wing National party's electoral victory in 1948 ensured that skin colour took greater significance and relevance. Under apartheid even more than prior forms of segregation, skin complexion could inform where one lived, one's school and work opportunities, whether one could vote, and whether one needed a government pass to move in and out of urban areas. Like the whites, black appeal of these products relied on the pernicious official and popular ideologies that linked lighter skin to power and beauty.[3]

Although little evidence suggests that blacks used skin lighteners specifically to obtain official reclassification within apartheid's four-tiered racial hierarchy (European', 'Asia', 'coloured' and 'African'), they were certainly thought to enhance prospects in social and work settings that privileged light skin. Some job advertisements invited only applicants who were 'light-skinned' or 'slightly coloured'.[4] Amid this pervasive racism and colorism, some companies undertook the mass production and aggressive marketing of skin lighteners. By the late 1960s, a remarkable sixty percent of urban African women reported using bleaching/lightening creams, making them the fourth most commonly used household product (after soap, tea and tinned or powdered milk).[5]

Since the market proved to be lucrative, Abraham and Solomon Krok, South African businessmen and twin brothers born to Jewish immigrant parents, began to manufacture SuperRose Freckle and Complexion Cream with ammoniated mercury. The Kroks marketed this new product by suggesting that it made women irresistibly attractive to men. By the mid 1960s, demand was so great that they moved production to a larger factory, employed ever 500 people, and reported sales totaling R3 million.[6] Dermatologists agreed that while ammoniated mercury might lighten skin in the short term, prolonged use at higher concentrations could result in patches of darker pigmentation as the mercury oxidized and deposited in the skin.[7] Such effects together with the concerns over kidney damage prompted the US. And South African governments eventually, in the 1970s to prohibit mercury from cosmetics.

By 1970s, in addition to SuperRose, the Kroks had developed other brands including He-Man, Hollywood 7, Super Scott, Kool Look, Aviva, Tanlite and Alco. The other notable manufacturer, Karroo went out of business because it still used ammoniated mercury.

By the mid 1970s African doctors had begun to warn of the visible complications of the effects of hydroquinone. Findlay documented how prolonged use of skin lighteners with hydroquinone (usually three years or longer), particularly at higher concentrations (above three percent), combined with the high levels of exposure to ultraviolet rays common in South Africa could produce a form of bluish-black hyperpigmentation known as exogenous ochronosis. Thirty percent of all black patients seen at a dermatology clinic in Pretoria sought treatment for hydroquinone-induced ochronosis. A follow-up study in 1980 showed that some of the products contained between 5.5 and 7.5 percent hydroquinone.[8]

Around the same time that the government banned mercury and doctors began expressing concern over hydroquinone, Black Consciousness activists started criticizing all skin lighteners on political and moral grounds. Influenced by African nationalism and the black Power movement in the United States, Black Consciousness (BC) attacked apartheid policies and advocated black pride and political self-reliance.

BC activists teamed up with medical allies to make opposition to skin lighteners into a progressive political issue. In 1982, they succeeded in limiting the maximum concentration of hydroquinone allowed in cosmetics to two percent bringing South African regulations into accord with U.S guidelines.[9] This did not end the agitation by the activists who argued that despite the two percent regulation, skin lighteners continued to cause problems because the U.S regulations were inadequate for South Africa where black consumers experienced more intense exposure to ultra-violet rays and applied skin lighteners more heavily, more frequently, and for longer durations than their

American counterparts.[10] BC and medical activists jointly urged the government to ban hydroquinone from cosmetics. Although their campaign did not immediately convince government officials, it did influence consumers: by the mid 1980s, skin-lightening sales began declining at an annual rate of ten percent.[11]

In the early 1980s, Jewish activists like Geoff Budlencler, a Jewish lawyer at the Legal Resources Centre (LRC) in Johannesburg and Marc Suttner, an activist from a Jewish family and founding editor of an adult literacy magazine **Learn and Teach**, played prominent roles in campaigning for a ban on hydroquinone.

Learn and Teach, articles emphasized the dangers of skin Lighteners, affirmed the Black Consciousness (BC) motto 'black is beautiful', and featured photographs of consumers whose faces had been disfigured.[12] Learn and Teach succeeded in pressurizing the popular magazine **Drum** to stop featuring skin-lightener adverts and forsake significant revenue.[13] By 1987, the national Black Consumer Union (NBCU) and the Dermatological Society of South Africa were leading the campaign to ban hydroquinone. The government finally responded to activists' demands by introducing a draft regulation banning hydroquinone from cosmetics. The South African parliament passed the regulation in December 1987, with an implementation date of 1 July 1988.[14] In August 1990, while the National Party government and the recently legalized African National Congress negotiated the country's transition from minority to majority rule, all cosmetics containing hydroquinone were prohibited. Furthermore, South Africa became the first and only country in the world to restrict cosmetics advertisements from claiming to bleach', 'lighten', or 'whiten'.[15] Hence, in forbidding the language of lightening from all cosmetics adverts as well as banning specific ingredients, South Africa's regulation bore the mark of the broad anti-racist. political movement from which it emerged.

However, since the early 1990s, a relatively robust illicit market in imported skin lighteners has existed despite the country's unique ban.[16] Nigerians and Congolese have been blamed for the illicit influx of skin lightening products into South Africa.[17]

Skin Lightener Timeline in South Africa in the 80's

From the manufacturers' point of view, skin care for the Black population can be divided into 'general purpose' and 'skin lighteners.'

In 1980 the combined yearly turnover, according to Creamer[1] was estimated at R25 million.[18] The market was described in Creamer's column as 'phenomenal,' 'ripe for the picking', 'a roaring trade', as indeed it must be to have produced such an epidemic of ochronosis.[19]

The advertisers of the skin lightening products also contributed to the patronage of the products.[20] For examples, the caption on an advertising picture for a bleaching cream reads 'Success people use…., the best skin lightening creams in the world.' One notices on the advert the calm, healthy and pale appearance of the two educated and successful characters (the doctor and nursing sister), while the patient is dark complexioned, presumably sick, unsuccessful, rather stupid and worried-looking. (See Figure 11.1 in Chapter 11).

The clients who bought these creams came from a generally under-educated and impressionable section of the population who were persuaded by shrewd advertising that all manner of social and economic success was associated with the lightening of the skin.

A pharmacist[21] also questioned the ethical standard for the pharmacist to exploit this sort of advertising and to sell a product which may well cause irreparable damage. Advertising revenue for bleaching creams was lucrative for those magazines aimed at the Black woman reader. However, the editor of one such journal[5] was distressed by the simple faith which her readers had in advertisers' claims, followed as it was by appeals in the 'agony' column from women who had used these skin lighteners. On the strength of this experience alone, the editor took the bold and costly step of refusing to place advertisements for bleaching creams.

In 1986, South Africa Law was passed to include less than 2% HQ in cosmetic formulations. 58 brands of skin lighteners were available across the continent.

In 1989, the SA cosmetic industry had grown to R390 million. 15% males and 42% females exhibited exogenous ochronosis. 69% of this cohort used skin lighteners.[3] there was an inverse relationship between ochronosis and education.

History of the observed ochronosis from hydroquinone in South Africa

In 1980, Findlay and De Beer[22] drew attention to 'A South African epidemic of Ochronosis of the face in black Skinned individuals.'

They reported that about 10 years ago a new skin disease affecting the face of Black women was seen in the Pretoria area. The skin over the sun-exposed aspects of the cheeks became darker, and scattered, fixed black papules containing a pigmented colloid were often present. Even the ear cartilage developed some darkening and degeneration on the outer surface. Such changes were encountered only among those who habitually used skin-lightening preparations. They had mostly been satisfied with the lightening effect for several years, but since the skin then became gradually darker instead of remaining light, this sometimes led to the frantic application of more cream. They observed an intense blackening of those parts more exposed to sunlight. Sometimes as many as 30% of patients who attended the dermatology outpatient clinic wanted treatment for ochronosis. The researchers found that women so affected had used these creams for an average of 3 years, after stronger hydroquinone creams were allegedly first marketed in 1966. Through hydroquinone assay of some of the products on the market, they also found that the safety of a preparation may not be ascertainable solely by the concentration found in the bottle, tube or jar. The amount, frequency, energy and overall time-span of application of hydroquinone-containing products may be far more significant. Furthermore, a warning on the package to stop using the products if untoward signs appear may lead a user to discard one brand in favour of another which contains the same harmful ingredient. Table 8.1 shows a sample of the products used at that time. The percentage of hydroquinone in the bleaching products assayed in 1980 ranged from 2.5-7.5%.[22]

The researchers concluded that "hydroquinone **judiciously** used is a valuable bleaching agent. Indeed, some well-formulated brands of the type of agent studied in South Africa have been useful for the removal of blemishes in Whites which may otherwise be difficult to treat. With due supervision, our patients have been astonished by the cheapness and excellence of such preparations when used with care and suitable adjuvant measures. By watching for contact dermatitis, using sunscreens as an adjunct, and restricting the application to a daily routine lasting only a few months, the results are indeed gratifying. It would certainly be unfortunate if their use for strictly medical purposes were prevented."

Table 8.1 Sample group of 13 popular brands of bleaching applications (Findlay GH and De Beer HA 1980)

Lotion

* 1. Hi-lite *Special (Cheseborough Ponds'* International)

‡ 2. Alco Lightening and Complexion Lotion (Lipworth)
‡* 3. Hollywood 7 New Look Lotion (Classique)
‡† 4. 3-Day Kool-Look (Dalway)
‡† 5. Super Rose Extra-X Skin Lightener - Super He-Man Lotion. (Twins)

Creams in tubes

‡*† 6. Hollywood 7-Day Extra Skin Lightening Cream (Classique)
*† 7. Clere Skin Lightening Cream (Amka)
† 8. Mister Artra Skin Lightening Cream (Artra)
* 9. Look of Nature (Toni)

Creams in jars

‡† 10. Super Rose Freckle and Complexion Cream (Twins)
† 11. Bu-Tone No. 3 Strong Complexion Cream (Adcock Ingram)
‡† 12. Alco Freckle and Complexion Cream (Lipworth)
† 13. Ambi Skin Lightening & Beauty Cream (Bima).

* Items acknowledged to contain hydroquinone on the package.
† Items claimed to be exceedingly rapid or powerful. A special suitability for men was a favourite way
of emphasizing how strong they were.
‡ These items appear to emanate from the same or neighbouring premises.

References

1. Thomas Lynn M. Skin Lighteners, Black Consumers and Jewish Entrepreneurs in South Africa. *History Workshop Journal.* February 2012; 73:259-83. Doi:1093/hwj/dbr017.

2. Noliwe Rooks. *Hair Raising: Beauty, Culture, and African American Women*, New Brunswick, 1996; Peiss, *Hope in a Jar*, chap. 7; Susannah Walker, *Style and Status: Selling Beauty to African American Women, 1920-1975*, Lexington, 2007, chap.1

3. Lynn M. Thomas, 'Skin Lighteners in South Africa: Transnational Entanglements and Technologies of the Self' in *Shades of Difference: Why Skin Color Matters ed*, Evelyn Nakano Glenn Palo Alto, 2009;

4. Farieda Khan, 'Creams that are Destroying Black Beauty', *Weekend Argus*, 25 August 1990

5. *The Urban Bantu Market: Understanding its Complexities and Developing its Potential Proceedings of a 2-Day Seminar held in February 1969, Durban, Natal,* National Development and Management Foundation, Johannesburg, 1969, p. 21.

6. Interviews with S. Krok, 8 and 12 Aug. 2008; 'Business Achievers of the Month', *Herald Times*, 31 July 1987, p. 6.

7. Nealon DF. 'Ammoniated Mercury and the Skin', *Drug and Cosmetic Industry* Denton and others, 'Inhibition of Melanin Formation' 1943; 52: 2

8. Findally GH, and De Beer HA. 'Chronic Hydroquinone Poisoning of Skin from Skin-Lightening Cosmetics: a South African Epidemic of Ochronosis of the Face in Dark-Skinned individuals.' *South African Medical Journal* Feb 1980; 57 (6):187

9. 'If the Health Department Keeps Its Promise . . . Say Goodbye to Skin Lightening Cream', *Learn and Teach* 2: 3, 1982; 'Regulations Governing the Sale of Cosmetics Containing Hydroquinone, Mercury, and Lead', *South African Government*

Gazette 210, 1982; 'Regulations Governing the Sale of Cosmetics Containing Hydroquinone, Mercury, and Lead', *South African Government Gazette* 219, 1983; interview with Dr Hilary Carman by author, 15 Aug. 2004, Johannesburg.
10.Findlay GH and De Beer HA, 'Chronic Hydroquinone Poisoning'; George H. Findlay, 'Ochronosis Following Skin Bleaching with Hydroquinone', *American Academy of Dermatology Journal* 1982; 6:6 Dr C. Isaacson, Department of Anatomical Pathology, University of Witwatersrand, to Dr Stevens, National Health and Population Development, Pretoria, 25 May 1987: Personal Papers of Dr Hilary Carman (hereafter PPHC).
11. 'Cosmetics: Skin Lightener Sales Still Strong', *Finance Week*, 6 April 1989.
12. 'If the Health Department Keeps Its Promise'; 'Skin Lightening Creams: a Big New Problem', *Learn and Teach* 1982; 2 (5):1-3
13. 'The Learn and Teach Challenge', *Learn and Teach* 2: 5, 1982; Martin Feinstein, 'Drum to Ban All Ads for Skin Lightening Creams', *Rand Daily Mail*, 8 Sept. 1982.
14. Government Gazette no. R2892; a draft of the regulation was introduced the previous May. McGibbon, 'Blooming Trade'; Press Statement by Dr E. Kuzwayo and Dr Hilary Carman, 'Ban of Hydroquinone and Other Harmful Ingredients in Skin Lighteners', 9 March 1988: PPHC; J. Tatham, Vice President, Housewives' League of South Africa to Director General, Foodstuffs, Cosmetics and Disinfectants Act, 'Banning of Skin Lighteners', 16 March 1988: PPHC.
15. Republic of South Africa, 'Government Notice No. R. 1227 of 24 June 1988', *Government*
Gazette, Pretoria, 1988; Republic of South Africa, 'Government Notice No. R. 1861 of 10 August 1990', *Government Gazette*, Pretoria, 1990; 'Venter Cracks Down on Skin-Lightening', *Daily Mail*, 14 Aug. 1990.
16. Babalwa Shota and Dina Seeger. 'Smugglers Cash In on an Illicit Market,' *Sunday Times*, 12 Dec. 1999; Sam Mathe, 'Curse of the Cosmetic Creams', *Drum*, 10 Feb. 2000.
17. Pumza Fihlani. Africa: Where black is not really beautiful. *BBC News Johannesburg*. 1 January 2013/Africa. http://www.bbc.com/news/world-africa-20444798
18. Creamer M. *Sunday Times (Business Times)*, Johannesburg. 22 October 1978; p4
19. Findlay GH, Morrison JGL, and Simson IW. Exogenous ochronosis and pigmented colloid milium from hydroquinone bleaching creams. *Brit J Dermatol.* 1975; 93:613.
20. White CL. *Women's Magazines 1693-1968;* London: Micheal Joseph. 1970; chap 6.
21. Cornewell L. *S Afri Pharm J.* 1978; 45:216.
22. Findaly GH, De Beer HA. Chronic Hydroquinone Poisoning of the Skin from Skin-Lightening Cosmetics. *S Afri Med. J.* 1980; 57:187-90

Prevalence of skin lightening practice in South Africa

Nonhlanhla Kumalo, a dermatologist in South Africa, says the real extent of skin lightening in South Africa is unknown, but research suggests that 35% of women use the products regularly.[1] A recent study by the University of Cape Town suggests that one woman in three in South Africa bleachers her skin. The reasons for this are as varied as the cultures in this country but most people say they use skin-lighteners because they want "white skin."[2] Malangu and Ogunbanjo studied the predictors of topical steroid misuse among patrons of pharmacies in Pretoria. The prevalence of the misuse of topical steroid products among the respondents was 35.5%.[3] According to a University of ZwaZulu-Natal (UKZN) study, the number is closer to 35 percent. This rate makes South African women the sixth-highest proportion of skin bleachers anywhere in the world. Nigeria has the highest in the world, with 77 percent of women using skin-lightening products. According to Dr Lester Davids, a molecular cell biologist at the University of Cape Town, the skin lightening trade has become so rampant and widespread that it is impossible for the government o regulate.[2] "They're certainly not doing a good job," agrees Dr Imraan Jhetam, a private dermatologist in Durban. Jhetam noted that the rise in international travel has increased smugglers' opportunities to respond to a voracious demand for skin lighteners. Mamy Pony, a marketer of skin-lightening products,[1] gets most of her creams from a shop up the street called Aegis, where a bus driver smuggles them in from the Democratic Republic of Congo.[1] But the illegal skin bleaching preparations are smuggled in by road, sea and air from all over the world.

A most recent study was conducted by Ncoza Dlova *et al*[4] to elucidate women's perceptions of the benefits and risks of skin-lightening creams in two large public hospitals in Durban SA. The study population consists of 579 African and Indian women aged 18-70 years. 292 were Africans and 287 were Indians. Of these 32.3% had used skin-lightening (38% of Africans and 27% of Indians). Most of those who had used skin lighteners (85% of Africans and 76% of Indians) claimed awareness of the adverse effects of the products, although this did not appear to inform knowledge of the products, how it is used, the decision to use the product. Most users (90%) expressed satisfaction with results achieved but 32% reported adverse events. Dlova *et al*[4] conclude that there is a poor understanding of the risks associated with the use of skin bleaching products. They recommended that public education campaigns are required to teach consumers about these risks and the importance of concomitant use of sunscreens with these products.

References

1. Susie Neilson. Why are women still dying to be white? http://www.iol.co.za/lifestyle/style/fashion/why-are-women-still-dying... 19 June 2014

2. Davids Lester and Kumalo N. When lightening strikes, it brings pale ailments *Mail & Guardian.* Oct 31, 2014. http://mg.co.za/article/2014-10-31-00-when-lightening-stikes-it-bring...

3. Malangu N, Ogunbanjo GA. Predictors of topical steroid misuse among patrons of pharmacies in Pretoria. *South Africa Fam Pract* 2006; 48 (1): 14a-14e.

4. Dlova Ncoza, Hamed Saja H, Tsoka-Gwegweni Joyce, Grobler Anneke, Hift Richard. Women's perceptions of the benefits and risks of skin-lightening creams in two South Africa communities. *Journal of Cosmetic Dermatology*. Sept 2014; 13 (3): 236-41. Article first published online: 6 Sept 2014. *DOI: 10.1111/jocd.12104.*

Demographic Characteristics of Skin bleachers in South Africa

South Africa is marketed to the world as Mandela's rainbow nation, where everyone is proud of their race and heritage. But for some black South Africans there is such a thing as being too black.

In a bustling African market in the centre of Yeoville in Johannesburg, it is skin lighteners galore. Many of the country's celebrities have resorted to lightening the skin[1]— some of these are former Kwaito star Mshaza, Sorisha Naidoo, former **Scandal**! actress, singer Kelly Khumalo, pop star Nicki Minaj. Psychologists say there are also underlying reasons why people bleach their skin—but low self-esteem and, to some degree self hate, are a common thread. The sale of over-the-counter skin-bleaching creams containing hydroquinone was banned in South Africa in 1992. However they have continued to circulate on the black market. Recently, spice shops and newly opened India and Pakistani beauty parlours have been doing brisk business with "fairness" creams. Former beauty queen Sorisha Naidoo claims her products have sold out since picture of her "new fair self" appeared in newspapers.

Writing under the title—**'The dark side of skin lightening'** in 2011, Niyanta Singh wrote that Durban-dark skinned people wanting skin lightening products are the basis of multi-billion-rand industries. Some products claim to be totally natural, while many contain potentially harmful ingredients that could scar and cause permanent damage to the skin.

Former Miss India South Africa, Sorisha Naidoo lightened her skin after feeling insecure about her complexion. According to India anthropologists, the desire to be lighter-skinned is ancient, carved into the culture by waves of light-skinned invaders, and is also linked to India's complex social hierarchy, or caste system. Those higher up the scale generally tend to have paler skins than people on the bottom rung. For those with naturally light skin, on the other hand, a tanned skin suggests exuberant health and beauty. Sonali Jairam, a sociologist said the infatuation with fair skin among India South Africa stemmed from India's history. "It's the legacy of a jumble of issues—colonialism, class, and a Hollywood culture that exports a white-skinned, blonde haired idea".

Malangu and Ogunbanjo studied the predictors of topical steroid misuse among patrons of pharmacies in Pretoria.[2] Of the 225 participants, 83% were female, 75.1% of the participants were black female Africans, 50.7% were 20-40 years old; 56% were employed, and 53.3% were married. 50.2% had high school education. The prevalence of topical steroids misuse for skin lightening was 35.5%. 64.5% participants claimed they used the topical steroids for therapeutic reasons, while 35.5% admitted they used them as skin lighteners. In terms of awareness of side effects only 19.1% of the participants was aware of the side-effects of prolonged use of corticosteroids. Participants mentioned the following side-effects: acne, moon face, and changes in skin pigmentation.

In 1989, Hardwick et al reported that 15% males and 42% females exhibited exogenous ochronosis[3] from the use of hydroquinone containing skin lightening products.

References

1. Pumza Filani. Africa: where black is not really beautiful. *BBC News, Johannesburg.* 1 January 2013 Africa. http://www.bbc.com/news/world-africa-20444798.

2. Malangu N and Ogunbanjo GA. Predictors of topical steroids misuse among patrons of pharmacies in Pretoria. *South Africa fam Prac* 2006; 48(1): 14a-14e.

3. Hardwick N, Van Gelder L, Van der merwe C, Vander Merwe M. Exogenous ochronosis: an epidemiologic study. *British Journal of Dermatology* 1989; 120(1): 229-38.

Motives for skin bleaching in South Africa

A recent study by the University of Cape Town suggests that one woman in three in South Africa bleaches her skin. The reasons for this are as varied as the cultures in this country but most people say they use skin-lighteners because they want "white skin".

▪ **Nomasoto "Mshoza" Mnisi**

BBC Africa recently posted on article by Pumza Fihlani entitled "*Africa: Where Black is not really Beautiful.*"[1] Highlighting the well publicized case of South African musician, ***Nomasonto "Mshaza" Mnisi,*** who openly (and unapologetically) acknowledges lightening her skin, the article positions skin bleaching the result of **"low self-esteem and, to some degree self-hatred."**

Local musician Nomasonto "Mshoza" Mnisi, now several shades lighter, says her new skin makes her feel more beautiful and confident.[2] She has been widely criticized in the local media and social networking sites for her appearance but the 30-year-old says skin-bleaching is a personal choice, no different from breast implants or a having nose job.

"I've been black and dark-skinned for many years; I wanted to see the other side. I wanted to see what it would be like to be white and I'm happy," she says candidly.

Over the past couple of years Ms Mnisi has had several treatments. Each session can cost around 5,000 rand (£360; $590), she tells the BBC. Unlike many in the country, she uses high-end products which are believed to be safer than the creams sold on the black market but they are by no means risk-free, doctors say.

Ms Mnisi says she does not understand the criticism about her new appearance.

"Yes, part of it is a self-esteem issue and I have addressed that and I am happy now. I'm not white inside, I'm not really fluent in English, I have black kids. I'm a township girl, I've just changed the way I look on the outside," she says.

▪ **Lucky Shesi**

At 49, ***Lucky Shezi*** believes that a change in his grooming habits **will help him in his long arduous search for love.**[3] Last year he started using a skin-lightening cream he had read about on the internet. "**I started using the cream because I just want to look smart and handsome**. It wasn't about me having a light skin; I naturally have chocolate skin. I am not so pitch black." He says that there hasn't been a drastic change in his skin colour. He is aware that there are problems linked to skin-lightening products, so he uses the cream sparingly. "But I can see an improvement when I look at myself in the mirror," he says with a self-assured nod. "I'm looking handsome."

And his female colleagues have noticed a change. "At some stage they kept asking me what I was using. They said I was changing …though they didn't say in as many words that I was handsome or anything. This means that my cream must be working."

Lester Davids, an Associate Professor in human biology at the University of Cape Town (UCT), says the main reason people like Shezi use skin-lightening products is their **desire to improve their appearance.**

Men like Shezi, who are willing to admit to using skin-lightening products, are an anomaly. But Davids, who has done extensive research into the use of skin-lightening creams among women, believes the number of men using the products will increase.

- **Special research studies**

However, a recent study conducted by Ncoza Dlova[4] and other dermatologists at an out patient clinic in the Durban area of South Africa found that 38% of black African women and 27% of Indian women (women of South Asian descent) reported using skin lighteners. In explaining their usage, 26% of these women cited the **desire to lighten their skin**, while 59% cited the **treatment of specific skin problems** including post inflammatory hyperpigmentation, melasma, and acne.

Bekezela Phakathi[5] writes that Nomazulu (not her real name) peruses shelves at a Grahamstown pharmacy on High Street for skin bleachers, lightening creams and salves. The young woman whose own complexion is a rich cocoa claims to have used skin lightening creams for over ten years. She doesn't see anything wrong with trying to enhance her beauty by making her complexion fairer. She says ***"Our men find lighter women very attractive."*** She also says skin lightening creams are popular among her friends as they want to brighten their skin. Her husband and other people even compliment her on her complexion now and again. "I rarely get the blemishes, but I am light most of the time, so I will not stop using these creams," she says.

Rhodes Politics department, Dr Louise Vincent says that in societies like South Africa where men and women's views of the world have been influenced by racism, to be beautiful is frequently confused with being white. Racist beauty!

"My research is replete with personal testimonies of young black girls growing up wanting long flowing hair, lighter skin and so on. The important point is not so much that they want to be white but that they want, like most young girls, to be beautiful."

Kumalo agrees that the image of black beauty is socially constructed. ***"It does not matter who you are or where you are from, how poor or rich you are,"*** she says. ***"What matters is what is inside of you."***

References

1. Pumza Fihlani. Africa: Where black is not really beautiful. *BBC News, Africa. Johannesburg.* January 2013. http://www.bbc.com/news/world-africa-20444798
2. A Skin Bleaching epidemic in Africa and Its Diaspora. http://atlantablackstar.com/2013/01/02/a-skin-bleaching-epidemic-in...
3. Ina Skosona. When lightening strikes, it brings pale ailments. http://mg.co.za/artcle/2014-10-31-00-when-lightening-strikes-it-brings...
4. Dlova Ncoza Hamed SH, Tsoka-Gwegweni Joyce, Grobler Anneke, Hift Richard. Women's perceptions of the benefits and risks of skin-lightening creams in two South African communities. *Journal of Cosmetic Dermatology.* Sept 2014; 13 (3): 236-41.
5. Bekezela Phakathi. Dark side to beautiful skin. *Grocott's Mail Online.* Tue, 27 Mar, 2007. http://www.grocotts.co.za/content/dark-side-beautiful-skin-27-03-2007.

Determinants of skin bleaching in South Africa

Effect of Apartheid

Pivotal to the understanding of the determinants of skin bleaching in South Africa is a brief review of Apartheid in South Africa.[1] **Coloured** people consist of three mixed race populations in South Africa who were given more social privilege than other unmixed, indigenous African groups. During the **apartheid era**, in order to keep divisions and maintain a **race**-focused society, the government used the term *Coloured* to describe one of the four main racial groups identified by law: Blacks, Whites, Coloureds and Indians. (All four terms were capitalized in apartheid-era law.) Many Griqua began to self-identify as "Coloureds" during the apartheid era. There were certain advantages in becoming classified as "Coloured". For example, Coloureds did not have to carry a ***dompas*** (an identity document designed to limit the movements of the non-white populace), while the Griqua, who were seen as another indigenous African group, did.

Historical influence of colonialism and apartheid

Nahomie Julien explores the historical influence of colonialism and apartheid on South Africa's skin bleachers; and the existence of gender disparity within South African skin bleachers.[2] Nahomie believes that skin bleaching in South Africa is one of the psychological scars of colonialism and apartheid. With the official dismantling of apartheid which promised equal human and civil rights for all its citizens, South Africa prides itself on being called "Mandela's Rainbow Nation" and its citizens are proud of their race and heritage. However, South Africans have not overcome many of the psychological scars of apartheid and colonialism, some of which are self-hatred and low self-esteem. These negative psychosomatic influence often push people to alter their physical appearance to feel better about themselves, and one of the most common methods of doing so is by bleaching the skin.

Nahomie Julien submits that South African women are more affected by the stigma left by colonialism and apartheid than men. During colonialism, black women were treated in a most dehumanizing way and were viewed as objects of the colony. During apartheid women were seen by their husbands as "submissive brainless creatures." They were always slaves or servants to their white counterparts during both periods, leading them to believe that only white was right. They were not treated as human beings during either era, which consequently left them with an inferiority complex and adesire to always others.

Owing to this negative emotional baggage, these women believe that their apparent unattractiveness is the cause of most of their predicaments in life. They therefore feel that in order to compete and to please their spouses, they needed to lighten their skin. For some of these women, the whiteness of their skin is associated with socioeconomic status[3,4]. The lighter a woman's complexion, the more likely she is to get a well-paying job, promotion, spouse, and/or to receive respect.[3,5] This conditioning and ingrained culture is unequivocally the reason women ignore all the health risks associated with skin bleaching and continue to use potentially dangerous chemicals to lighten their skin. Some people associate skin bleaching with the need to be beautiful; however, beneath the aesthetic reasons, there is the underlying issue of self-hatred and low self-esteem[4,6] Also see section on MOTIVES. above

Lynn Thomas[7] in one of her submissions noted that skin color prejudice has been forged through political institutions of slavery, colonialism, and segregation, but it has also been forged through the collateral movement of consumer capitalism and visual media. She says to understand colorism we need not only to grapple with the development of legal codes, labor systems, and acute economic inequality, but also with the rise of consumer culture, mass manufactured commodities, glossy photomagazines, films, light-skinned celebrities, and viral social media. Such modern formations and everyday technologies have been profoundly influential in circulating, visualizing and rein scribing skin color hierarchies.

Availability of cheap low-end bleaching products

Researchers pinpoint apartheid-era South Africa as a major driver in the quest for lighter skin in that country and across Africa.[8] Undoing the complex layers of history and social mores upon which the desire for lighter skin in based is no easy feat. For scientists like Lester Davids, usage is sky high in South Africa as well as in other parts of Africa. It is fueled by the widespread availability of a plethora of cheap, purported skin-whitening products. Many of these are homemade, Davids says; but others flood in across the borders from various African countries as well as from India and Japan. "It doesn't take long to copy a cream from a big cosmetics house that promises to remove dark sports, pigmentation, etc., and sell it at five or ten times cheaper for a much poorer market," Davids says. "The problem is that a lot of these creams have been tainted because of chemicals and compounds added in unscrupulously, without a scientific base. While the wealthier segments of African society can afford to buy better quality, properly regulated products, and can avail of dermatological guidance for their proper usage, the lack of education that prevails in many nations on that continent, couple with the over-arching goal of lightening the skin, results in a gross abuse of cheap creams, and the disastrous consequences of this, is one of the biggest problems Africa as a whole faces today.

Effect of celebrity skin bleachers

A recent study by the University of Cape Town[9] suggests that one woman in three in South Africa bleaches her skin. The reasons for this are as varied as the cultures in this country but most people say they use skin-lighteners because they want "white skin."

South African musician Nomasonto "Mshoza" Mnisi, now several shades lighter, says her new skin makes her feel more beautiful and confident. She has been widely criticized in the local media and social networking sites for her appearance but the 30-years-old says skin-bleaching is a personal choice, no different from breast implants or a having nose job. Psychologists say there are also underlying reasons why people bleach their skin—but low self-esteem and, to some degree self-hate, are a common thread. When women in the media and celebrities bleach their skin, it perpetuates the idea that whiter light-skinned people are more successful and desirable. See the chapter on CELEBRITY DISCOURSE—Chapter 6.

Cultural issues[9,10,11]

A study was conducted by Ncoza Dlova *et al*[9] to elucidate women's perceptions of the benefits and risks of skin-lightening creams in two large public hospitals in Durban SA. The study population consists of 292 Africans and 287 Indians. They found that skin-lightening products are used by a third of African and Indian women in South Africa and that Cultural and historical perceptions equating a fairer skin with social advantage are pervasive and strongly reinforced by the media.

Some Indian women are so concerned about pigmentation that during pregnancy they eat saffron, powdered gold and green grapes, and drink lots of milk, in the belief that this will make their babies lighter-skinned.[9] The sale of over-the-counter skin-bleaching creams containing hydroquinone was banned in South Africa in 1992. However, they have continued to circulate on the black market. Recently, spice shops and newly opened India and Pakistani beauty parlours have been doing brisk business with "fairness" creams.

Former beauty queen Sorisha Naidoo claims her products have sold out since pictures of her "new fair self" appeared in newspapers. Sonali Jairam, a sociologist, said the infatuation with fair skin among India South Africans stemmed from India's history. "It's the legacy of a jumble of issues—colonialism, class, and a Hollywood culture that exports a white-skinned, blonde-haired ideals," she said. Jairam said a distinct example revealed itself through marriage advertisements. India newspapers, the ethnic weeklies in the US, and South African marriage websites all contained adverts seeking light-skinned partners. Five advertisements on one South African website have skin-color designations ranging from "wheatish" to "very fair". Psychologist Sriddha Lutchman said Indian women's perception of how dark or fair they were affected their confidence. Lutchman conducted a study in which she asked participants to rate their likelihood of finding a marriage, given their skin tone. She found that the lighter the skin tone, or perceived skin tone of the person, the higher their self-esteem and belief in their eligibility. "This sense of being better because you are light-skinned has been ingrained from generation to generation. This does not bode well for a large sector of our population, as those who are darker begin to feel inferior. They feel that they are not worthy and that they cannot be beautiful. In their quest to be accepted they resort to dangerous measures, such as skin-lightening, without a second thought," said Lutchman. Sociologist Smitha Govender, who also conducted a study on the effects of skin-lightening, concurred. "Skin colour is still one of the fundamental characteristics taken into consideration before a women's education, professional status or personality. One of the ladies from the study said when people described her, they would still say she was of wheatish complexion, but thin. Only after that did they mention her educational qualification and profession", said Govender. She said the reality was that an "overwhelmingly brown nation looks down on those that are dark-skinned".

Personal insecurity

Naidoo, whose Pure Perfect skin-lightening creams are proving so profitable, said she'd decided to lighten her own skin because she was insecure about her colour. "A photo shoot in a bikini for FHM South Africa Magazine (SA version of the popular men's magazine) brought out my insecurities.[10,11,12] I really wanted to have beautiful skin and colour and began researching skin-lightening. I have no qualms about the fact that I lighten my skin, because I was unhappy with my original colour," she said. Spending almost R3 800 a month on skin-lightening products, just to maintain her colour, Naidoo said her skin had initially reacted to the products, as she abused them. "I made the mistake of using more in the hope of getting lighter quicker. You will only damage your skin. It will only lighten according to how your body will allow," she said. Naidoo insists her products are 100 percent Nyong'o read a letter from a fan. "Dear Lupita, I think you're really lucky to be this black but yet this successful in Hollywood overnight. I was just about natural and contain no banned substances that could cause long-term harm. She said her creams were successful because they combined all the natural skin-lightening ingredients available in one cream. At R1000 for a basic cream and R3 000 for a 113g jar, Naidoo's products are, however, not safety guaranteed none of her other family members use them. "My sister is quite pale and has no need for them. My husband (Vivian Reddy) will never use them, as I love him just the way he is. As for my children… I'm happy with their complexions and love them for who they are. If in the future they choose to use skin-lightening products, that will be their choice," she said.

Ineffective legislation

The sale of over-the counter skin bleaching creams containing hydroquinone was banned in South Africa in 1992. Yet they are still being sold by street vendors, like at the stall on the corner of President and Diagonal streets at Joburg. Mamy Pony is one of many hawkers in the Joburg city centre who sell the bleaching creams and oitments. She tells Susie Neilson[13] "This one comes from Italy, from a white country. White people make it better." Pony's friend Aniece adds, picking up an imported cream claiming to smell of lemon's "I am surviving because of this thing." Aniece, a refugee from the Democratic Republic of the Congo, supports several children with the profits she makes selling lighteners. Although she offers her first name proudly—" It's French"%she withholds her surname, fearful of being shut down. "You see people here, some of them eat out of the garbage. I don't want to eat out of garbage," she says, waving her hand at the rubbish-strewn hill across from the taxi rank. She points back at Pony's small, cluttered box of creams. "I am surviving because of this thing. You put this thing bad, the police will come."

South Africa has the toughest laws on skin lighteners of any country in the world, having banned its most common active ingredient—hydroquinone—as well as the words "bleach," "lighten" or "white" in cosmetics advertisements. Yet, apart from a few well-publicised raids by police or the Department of Health, the skin-lightening trade is robust and thriving on our streets. Also see the section on INEFFECTIVE AND INADEQUATE LEGISLATION, REGULATORY AGENCIES, AND POLICIES—Chapter 5.

The promotional effect of the media

Jhetam blames the media, noting that the West has exported its version of beauty all over the globe.[9,13] Social media erupt every now and then when black celebrities such as Beyonce, Halle Berry, Rihanna and Nicki Minaj are Photoshopped to look fairer than they are. Others stars are criticised for being bleached with cosmetics that are more expensive but no doubt much safer than those found on street corners. A flurry of black African celebrities have also embraced skin lightening treatments and other symbols of whiteness as part of their brand. Last year, Nigerian-Cameroonian pop star Dencia became the spokesmodel for Whitenicious lightening cream. Closer to home, Kwaito artist Nomasonto "Mshoza" Maswanganyi caused a stir in 2011 after appearing on the BBC to gush over her near-Michael Jackson-like transformation. Respected international beauty companies are cashing in on the hype with creams that purport to correct or even skin tone, promoted by black women bathed in light. The desire for a light complexion is so intense in Africa, Asia and the

Far East that women have started taking orally or by injection dodgy treatments that had previously been applied topically. If the biggest names in showbusiness can't resist the pressure to lighten up, it gives ordinary women the impression that you need to appear white to succeed or to be attractive.

Fortunately, there are a few notable holdouts. The rise to fame of actress Lupita Nyong'o has inspired women of colour around the world. Addressing the 7th annual Black Women in Hollywood Luncheon in February, Nyong'o revealed that as a teenager she had loathed her dark skin and had prayed every night for a fairer complexion. It was the appearance of dark-skinned role models like talk-show queen Oprah Winfrey and supermodel Alek Wek ("dark as night") who showed her that black could be beautiful. At the luncheon, to buy Dencia's Whitenicious cream to lighten my skin when you appeared on the world map and saved me." Said Nyong'o: "My heart bled a little when I read those words." For some, Nyong'o represents the beginning of a shift away from a Western beauty standard. But it's doubtful. After all, the appearance of Wek changed little. South African poet and actress Lebo Mashile says she was fortunate that she "rode a wave" to fame at a time when the country was shedding apartheid. "The county was in the throes of revolution, forming an identity. I was very lucky to find myself there." Today, she says, her "natural" look – her Afro, her plus-size body – would bar her from fame. "I could make a lot more money if I slapped on a wig. But I don't bat for team Yellowbone," she said, referring to a US slang term for lighter-skinned black women. "I think that's a load of s***." Jhetam says the best one can hope for is that one day there will be something safe and effective to lighten skin. But until then South Africa's black market skin-lightening industry "will thrive".

The effect of institutionalized Black market, Peer pressure, and ignorance

Melangu and Ogunbanjo in a study entitled "Predictors of topical steroid misuse among patrons of pharmacies in Pretoria." Identify some factors that drive the bleaching culture in South Africa.[14]

It is a matter of concern that some participants bought topical steroid products from flea markets and supermarkets, as these products should not be available by law at these outlets in terms of the Medicines and Related Substances Act No. 101of 1965 (as amended in May 2003).[15] This suggests that the demand for topical steroid products is probably fueling a black market.

Another interesting finding of this study is the influence of peer pressure, particularly from friends. It was shown both in the stratified and logistic analyses that initially being advised by a friend was associated significantly with misuse. This strong influence, coupled with a lack of awareness of the side effects, provides a foundation that sustains this type of practice.

Although cause and effect cannot be determined from the findings of this study, race and peer pressure on the one hand, and ignorance and gender on the other hand, seem to be related to the misuse of topical steroid products.

These findings have several important implications. Firstly, interventions to scale down misuse and preventive efforts need to focus on the black female African and her peers. These interventions should be multi-dimensional, involving educational, legal and managerial approaches.

Media and public education on topical steroid misuse is warranted, and the involvement of general practitioners, nurses and pharmacists is needed, with specific messages directed at rooting out ignorance of the danger of this practice being circulated widely among the targeted subgroups.[17]

Secondly, legal approaches should include the enforcement of the existing legislation related to the control of medicines, so that scheduled medicines cannot be sold from unauthorized outlets. These legal approaches should include measures aimed at strengthening the ethical responsibilities of pharmacists in advising patients on the safety of medicines bought over the counter.

Thirdly, the below-mentioned managerial approaches could be implemented at the primary care level. During anamnesis, female patients presenting with symptoms likely to be linked to topical steroid misuse should be questioned about these symptoms by their general practitioners and other primary health care workers. Measures and systems should be instituted to identify, advise andrehabilitate those identified as having the side effects.

References

1. Apartheid in South Africa. *http://simple.wikipedia.org/wiki/Aparthied_in_south_africa*

2. Julien Nahomie. Skin Bleaching in South Africa: A Result of Colonialism and Aparthied? *DISCOVERY: Georgia State Honors College Undergraduate Research Journal*: 2014; Vol 2, Article 4 http://scholarworks. gsu.edu/discovery/vol2/iss1/4

3. Hunter ML. Buying racial capital: Skin-bleaching and cosmetic surgery in a globalized world. *Journal of Pan African Studies*. 2011; 4 (4):142-64.
4. Hunter ML. 'If you're light you're alright': Light skin color as social capital for women of color. *Gender & Society*. 2002; 16 (2): 175-93.
5. Perry I. Buying white beauty. *Cardozo Journal of Law & Gender*. 2006; 12: 579 -607.
6. Charles CAD. Skin Bleaching, Self-Hate and Black Identity in Jamaica. *Journal of Black Studies*. 2003; (6):711.doi:10.2307/3180843.
7. Thomas Lynn M. "Colorism in Africa/ my research on skin lighteners" *Global Perspectives on Colorism. Washington University, Law School.* 2 April 2015.
8. Saviter lyer Ahrestani. The Social History of Skin Lightening in Africa. March 2 2014 www.youbeauty.com/skin/african-skin-bleaching-history
9. Dlova Ncoza, Hamed Saja H, Tsoka-Gwegweni Joyce, Grobler Anneke, Hift Richard. Women's perceptions of the benefits and risks of skin-lightening creams in two South Africa communities. *Journal of Cosmetic Dermatology*. Sept 2014; 13 (3): 236-41. Article first published online: 6 Sept 2014. *DOI: 10.1111/jocd.12104.*
10. Pumza Fihlani. Africa: Where black is not really beautiful *BBC News, Johannesburg. Africa.* January 2013. http://www.bbc.com/news/world-africa-20444798.
11. Ina Skosana when Lightening strikes, it brings pale ailments…mg.co.za/…/2014-10-31-00.when-lightening-strikes-it-… Mail & Guardian Oct 31, 2014.
12. Niyanta Singh. The dark side of skin lightening. Durban-Dark-skinned people want to be lighter. Light-skinned people want to be darker. http://www.iol.co.za/lifestyle/style/beauty/the-dark-side-of-skin-ligh...
13. Susie Neilson. Why are women still dying to be white? 19 June 2014. http://www.iol.co.za/lifestyle/style/fashion/why-are-women-still-dying...
14. Malangu N, Ogunbanjo GA. Predictors of topical steroid misuse among patrons of pharmacies in Pretoria. *South Africa Fam Pract* 2006; 48(1): 14a-14e.
15. National Department of health, Medicines and Related Substances Act (Act 101 of 1965, as amended in May 2003). Pretoria: National Department of Health; 2003.

Skin lightening products used in South Africa

South Africans use the whole spectrum of products available on the market to lighten the skin colour.[1] These are topical preparations (creams, serums, gels, soaps), pills, and injectables, and surgical methods already discussed in the relevant chapter.

As regards the topical preparations, a recent study was done by Ncoza Dlova *et al*[2] on the skin-lightening creams used in Durban, South Africa. Hydroquinone (HQ) was not found in the top 10 skin-bleaching products sold on the market–Table 8.2. Only one product contained HQ derivative. However, nearly 50% of the products contained mercury as an active ingredient, although there was no indication of this compound on the packaging label. The mercury containing products were manufactured in South Africa, United Kingdom and Taiwan, even though the export of mercury-containing cosmetics had been banned in the EU since 2003

Table 8.2. list of 10 creams analysed together with the active skin-lightening agents declared on the packaging labels and those found to be present (C. Dlova et al 2012)

Sample no	Products label	Country of manufacture	Company	declared active ingredients	Active ingredients found to be present
1	Lemon Lite – vanishing cream	South Africa	Adcock Ingram	–	Mercury
2	Movate Cream	Italy	Esapharma	Clobetasol propionate (0.05%)	Clobetasol propionate
3	Persivate	South Africa	Aspen	Betamethasone valerate	Betamethasone
4	Shirley	Taiwan	Shirley Chemical Corporation	Contains natural albumen and placenta base that have an effect on Lightening facial skin	Mercury
5	Bee-Co cream	—	Unknown	—	Resorcinol
6	Rico complexion Cream	UK	Rico Skin Care Ltd	—	Mercury
7	Eskamel – acne and pimple cream	South Africa	SmithKline Beecham	Resorcinol (2%)	Resorcinol
8	Ponds–vanishing cream	South Africa	The Elida Pond's Institute	—	
9	Cuticura	South Africa	Novartis	Phenol, 8-hydroxyquinoline	Mercury
10	Gentle Magic skincare cream	South Africa	Du Marc CC	—	HQ derivative

As part of the multidisciplinary study in University of Cape Town, a survey was conducted to identify popular skin-lightening brands.[3] Researchers identified 29 brands. The main ingredients that were found were hydroquinone and prescription-strength topical steroid. Another common ingredient is retinoid, a chemical compound related to Vitamin A. An unexpected finding of the laboratory tests conducted by Davids and Kumalo[4] on skin lightening creams was the frequent and high concentrations of mercury.

Lester Davids warns that the demand for skin-lightening products in South Africa has led to a surge in the availability of "unsolicited, untested" products on the market. "very often the good products are out of the price range of the majority, with the result that many people are going to be looking for cheaper products. These cheaper products are untested and have hit the market at a staggering rate and serious health risks are expected.

Davids says that not all skin-lightening products are illegal. The problem is the lack of effective regulation of cosmetic products in

South Africa. Before a drug is registered, the Medicines Control Council will request for a list of every ingredient that is in the drug and details of how it was tested before it is released into the market. Under the Cosmetics Act, this is not necessary. Hence, anyone can put any chemical in a container, label it elegantly without even listing the ingredients, and market it as a cosmetic over the counter. Hence, the consumers are at the mercy of the integrity and conscience of the manufacturers of the cosmetics products.

In South Africa hydroquinone is only allowed to be used if prescribed clinically and it cannot be used at more that 2% within a formulation.

In South Africa, potent topical steroids such as Clobetasol propionate and betamethasone dipropionate are prescription drugs. Yet they are easily purchased from street vendors at very low cost of R10 compared with the retail cost at pharmacies, which ranges between R100 and R150/unit. Furthermore the prescription drugs are readily available in the pharmacy shops without prescription.

It is noteworthy that an *Editorial* in the British Medical Journal[5] has recommended that cosmetic skin lightening products should rightly be regulated as a drug (not a cosmetic) because according to the scientific definition, a cosmetic should not alter the structure and function of the skin; but skin lightening products alter the structure and function by inhibiting melanogenesis.

References

1. Skin lightening Clinics in South Africa. http://www.whatclinic.com/beauty-salons/south-africa/skin-lightening
2. Ncoza C Dlova, Nicole E Hendricks, and Bice S Martincgh Skin-lightening creams used in Durban, South Africa. *International J Dermatol* 2012; 51 (Suppl 1):51-3.
3. Pumza Fihlani. Africa: Where black is not really beautiful. *BBC News, Africa Johannesburg*. January 2013. *http://www.bbc.com/news/world-africa-20444798.*
4. Davids Lester and Kumalo N. when Lightening strikes, it brings pale oitments...mg.co.za/.../2014-10-31-00.when-lightening-strikes-it-... Mail 7 Guardian Oct 31, 2014
5. Olumide YM. **Editorial:** Use of Skin Lightening creams. Lack of recognition and regulation is having serious medical consequences. *British Medical Journal* (BMJ). 2010; 341:c6102 doi:10.1136/bmj.c6102

Complications of skin lightening products in SA

As regards the skin complications of skin lightening products, exogenous ochronosis from hydroquinone used to be the commonest complication in the 1970s and 1980s.[1-3] Schulz reported in 1982[2] that dermatitis resulting from the use of bleaching creams was the third most common skin disorder in 324 black patients, 3% had acute contact dermatitis, and 15% had leukomelanoderma resulting from monobenzone containing creams; while 82% were found to have melanosis ochronosis or colloid millium from the use of hydroquinone containing creams. A survey of 5355 black people in Johannesburg in 2003,[3] where the first and largest number of ochronosis cases were reported by Findlay et al in 1975,[4] found that only 27 (0.5%) had ochronosis. However, in the most recent study in 2014,[1] ochronosis accounted for only 0.05% of the patients seen and they were all in the early and late sixties in age, implying that they are possibly survivors of the skin bleaching scourge of the 1970s and 1980s. A comparison of the prevalence data in five national surveys shows a dramatic decline in ochronosis from 10% in 1978 to 0.05% in 2014.[4] This decline is attributed to the success of the stricter South African government regulations regarding the sale and use of hydroquinone-containing skin lighteners.[5]

Dr Noora Moi-Joosub says he still continues to see patients who need help with treating their ochronosis.[6] Dlova[4] believers that these are possibly survivors of the skin bleaching scourge of the 1970s and 1980s because ochronosis accounted for only 0.05% of the patients currently in her clinic and they were all elderly people in their early and late sixties. In the most recent study by Dlova et al,[4] dyschromia constitute the third most common skin condition seen in a black population in Durban, SA in 2014 with a prevalence of 11.6%. Steroid-induced acne, steroid addiction syndrome and other steroid-induced cutaneous side effects were commonly seen in the clinic.

Dr Imraan Jhetam,[6] a dermatologist said "Products were not as sophisticated as they are today. People from the African community back then used products that contained hydroquinone and steroids. The results were that people had badly burnt and scarred skin, while those who used steroids have extremely thin skin." Many skin-lighteners have devastating health consequences for users. In some, acid removes older, darker skin to reveal lighter skin underneath. Others inhibit melanin production—the chemical that produces the colour in skin tone—and contain ingredients such as mulberry extract, kojic acid, arbutin and hydroquinone. Hydroquinone, a chemical used in photo processing and rubber production, can remove the entire outer layer of the skin.

Umhlanga dermatologist, Dr Ishaan Ramkisson, said creams with these chemicals caused itching, burning and blistering and eventually led to darker skin patches where the creams had been administered. "There is also evidence that the long-term effects of such creams may cause skin cancer. Creams containing hydroquinone should not be used at all. "We use hydroquinone to treat pigmentation, but under the strictest (control)," he said.

Dr Jetham said he received requests for skin-lightening on a daily basis. "Ethically we do not perform skin lightening to alter your God-given colouring. I do, however, treat pigmentation patches and other skin discolouration problems.[8]

The cost implications of the skin-lightening practice also needs to be addressed. Local musician Nomasonto "Mshoza" Mnisi, now several shades lighter, says her new skin makes her feel more beautiful and confident. Mnisi says over the past couple of years she has had several treatments. Each session can cost around 5,000 rand (£360; $590), she tells BBC. Unlike many in the country, she uses high end products which are believed to be safer than the creams sold on the black market but they are by no means risk free.

References

1. Dlova Ncoza, Mankahla Avumile, Madala Nomandla, Grobler Anneke, Tsoka-Gwegweni Joyce, Hift Richard. The spectrum of skin diseases in a black population in Durban, KwaZulu-Natal, South Africa. *International Journal of Dermatology*. 2015; 54:279-85.

2. Schulz EJ. Skin disorders in black South Africans. *S Afr Med J* 1982; 62:864-867.

3. Findlay GH, de Beer HA. Chronic hydroquinone poisoning of the skin from skin-lightening cosmetics. A South African epidemic of ochronosis of the face in dark-skinned indviduas. *South Afr Med J*. 1980; 57: 187-90.

4. Hartshorne S. Dermatological disorders in Johannesburg, South Africa. *Clin Exp Dermatol* 2003; 28:661-5

5. Regulations governing the sale of cosmetics containing hydroquinone, mercury, and lead. *S Afr Gov Gaz* 1983; 219:7-9

6. Pumza Fihlani. Africa: Where black is not really beautiful. *BBC News, Johannesburg*. January 2013. http://www.bbc.com/news/world-afrca-20444798

7. Findlay GH, Morrison JGL, and Simson IW. Exogenous Ochronosis and pigmented colloid milium from hydroquinone bleaching creams. *Brit J Dermatol.* 1975; 93:613

8. Niyanta Singh. The dark side of skin lightening. *IOL Lifestyle*. July 21, 2011. *http://www.iol.co.za/lifestyle/style/beauty/the-dark-side-of-skin-light...*

Some Recommendations and Interventions to help prevent and reduce the burden from skin-lightening practices in South Africa.

(i) Public education

Dlova *et al* conclude that there is a poor understanding of the risks associated with the use of skin bleaching products.[1] They recommend that public education campaigns are required to teach consumers about these risks and the importance of concomitant use of sunscreen with these products.

Dermatology researcher and consultant, Dr Nonhlanhla Khumalo,[2] says many black women are blissfully unaware of the dangers that some skin creams pose in the long run. "Some creams contain mercury, which is known to cause neurological and kidney damage, speech and hearing impairments, and can also lead to psychiatric disorders" Khumalo told a recent talk shop. "I would advise ladies never to attempt using skin lighteners as they are not good for your skin." Khumalo explained that some skin lighteners create a thick black pigmentation which is irreversible and can even make the skin darker. Look out for ingredients like hydroquinone, which can cause blue-black discolorations and also lead to neuropathy, a disease of the nervous system.

Local cosmetics clerk, Elizabeth Jacobs,[2] says she usually discourages her clients from using lighteners. "A person can use them for some time, but after a few years they will see the repercussions. You get pimples, rashes or black spots that turn into wounds and they hardly ever heal." Jacob says she encourages her clients to use moisturisers which revitalize and repair the skin.

Melangu and Ogunbanjo[3] studied predictors of topical steroid misuse among patrons of pharmacies in SA. They recommend that interventions to scale down misuse and preventive efforts need to focus on the black female African and her peers. These interventions should be multi-dimensional, involving educational, legal and managerial approaches. Media and **public education** on topical steroid misuse is warranted, and the involvement of general practitioners, nurses and pharmacists is needed, with specific messages directed at rooting out ignorance of the danger of this practice being circulated widely among the targeted subgroups.

(ii) Enforcement of existing legislation; Pharmacists addressing ethical issues

Melangu and Ogunbanjo also recommend that legal approaches should include the enforcement of the existing legislation related to the control of medicines, so that scheduled medicines cannot be sold from unauthorized outlets. These legal approaches should include measures aimed at strengthening the **ethical responsibilities of pharmacists** in advising patients on the safety of medicines bought over the counter.

The below-mentioned managerial approaches could be implemented at the primary care level. During anamnesis, female patients presenting with symptoms likely to be linked to topical steroid misuse should be questioned about these symptoms by their general practitioners and other primary health care providers. Measures and systems should be instituted to identify, advise and rehabilitate those identified as having the side effects.

Lester Davids *et al* decry lack of regulation for ensuring safe cosmetics manufacture

"Lack of effective regulation"[4]

Not all skin-lightening products are illegal in South Africa. Davids says the problem is the lack of effective regulation of cosmetic products in South Africa.

"If I wanted to sell a clinically or medically related drug, I would have to go through the Medicines Control Council, which will request [a list of] every ingredient that is in the drug and details on how it was tested. All this even before the drug actually comes on to the market. However "Under the Cosmetics Act, that is not necessary. So I can put a cream in a container, put a nice label on it and market it as a cosmetic and it will be available over the counter," says Davids. "It's not illegal, but the information regarding what is actually in that formulation is very scarce."

A 2010 *British Medical Journal* Editorial calls for the stricter regulation of skin-lightening products, particularly in Africa, because these creams "alter the chemical structure of the skin by inhibiting the synthesis of melanin and should therefore be regulated as drugs% not cosmetics".[5]

Davids says that in the absence of effective regulation it is up to the consumer to be informed about the long-term effects of these products.

Lester Davids *et al* teach on how to shop for safe cosmetic products[4]

"Don't forget, you are using the cream now, but you are only going to be seeing the consequences of the chronic and long-term use in about six to eight months' time," he warns. "Then you are going to be suffering the effects of a damaged skin and irreversible damage."

Many people are using low-end, unsafe skin-lightening creams because they are cheaper than products that have been tested. Lester Davids, a lead researcher in a multidisciplinary study at the University of Cape Town, warns that the exact ingredients of many cheaper skin-lightening creams are unknown and not usually listed on the packaging. Products that are safe "will be supplied with an insert that will have all the ingredients listed, and will have all of the bases of use and will have instructions on how to use them". "Those instructions [are not available] with the cheaper creams that you will get at a station market or that you can get in an unlabelled bottle or tube at any of the markets anywhere." Very often the problem lies in the distribution of these products. "By the time it actually hits the shops, the shop owner has absolutely no idea what is in the cream." Davids says that there are a few questions one should ask before buying a skin-lightening cream:

- *What is in this cream?*

"This seems like a very obvious question to ask but you'd be shocked and amazed at how few people actually ask it. "When I buy a cream for my skin in a shop, the first thing I look at is: What is actually in this cream? "Most of these creams don't even have an ingredient label on them."

- *Where is the cream from?*

"It is important to know who actually supplies the cream. For example, if you want to buy meat, you would want to know who supplies the meat to the shop that you go to, because that relates to the quality of the meat. "In the same way you have the right to ask where this [cream] is supplied from."

- *How long has the formulation been in this container?*

"Under normal circumstances, any tube that you buy that comes with a little insert will have an expiration date on it, and it will have a date of distribution on it. So you will be able to tell how long the cream has actually been around. "The longer a cream stands, the more oxidised it becomes and these polyphenolics, if there are any in the cream, become more toxic."

- *Have these formulations been properly tested?*

"I think this is the fundamental question because, when you market products under the Cosmetics Act, half of the stringency and the need for testing that is required for medical or clinical drugs goes out the window. "And so we are quite concerned about the fact that a lot of these creams are hitting the market without being scientifically tested."

(iii) SA Government passes very stringent regulations regarding skin lighteners

In 1990, in the waning months of the apartheid regime and in response to considerable pressure from the anti-apartheid movement, South Africa passed the world's most restrictive regulations regarding skin lighteners:

1. Government banned skin lightening ingredients including mercury and hydroquinone from cosmetics.

2.They also prohibited manufacturers from claiming in advertisements that their products can "lighten," "whiten," or "bleach."

> –The second restriction bears the mark of anti-racist movement from which the regulations emerged.

See the section on HISTORY OF SKIN LIGHTENING IN SOUTH AFRICA above.

(iv) Research needs

Cape Town gets world-first safety lab for hair and skin cosmetics[6,7]

On 29 May 2015, the University of Cape Town (UCT) and Groote Schuur Hospital (GSH) launched a unique Hair and Skin Research Laboratory (HSR Lab) that will focus on comprehensive hair testing and safety in cosmetic formulation. The HSR Lab, established with support from the National skills Fund for R8.6m, is the brainchild of Prof Nonhlanhla Khumalo, Head of the Division of Dermatology at the University of Cape Town and Groote Schuur Hospital.

Nonhlanhla Khumalo, and her team, are on a mission to get harmful beauty products off the streets of SA. The lab tests skin-lightening products bought from informal traders and from pharmacies in Cape Town. Her team checks them for substances such as mercury and hydroquinone. The lab offers opportunities for clinicians and scientists to collaborate in the effort to protect people from preventable harm," Khumalo said. The executive director of the Cosmetic Toiletry and Fragrance Association of SA, Sally Gnodde, welcomed the establishment of the lab. *"Dark skin tones are beautiful naturally and there is no need to use dangerous products to change your natural beauty."* Said Gnodde.

SA Dermatologists and Scientists consistent research on skin lightening practices

— The original reports and characterization of exogenous ochronosis were done by SA Dermatologists and Scientists.

— Most of the empirical researches on the Skin bleaching culture in Africa have been done by South African Dermatologists and Scientists.

— Currently, a trans-disciplinary and multi-disciplinary research group in the University of Cape Town is releasing evidence-based guidelines and recommendations for reducing the burden of the skin lightening culture in the continent of Africa.

— There are ongoing collaborations between national and internationally recognized scientists, governments and recognized scientific journalists. These collaborations have resulted in implementation and publishing of scientific, ethically sound studies in South Africa and Africa.

·— In March 2015, the University of Cape Town hosted a Skin Lightening Workshop sponsored by the Programme for the Enhancement of Research Capacity (PERC). The Workshop was a most successful one because of the diversity and quality of research presentations and discourse on the subject–skin bleaching. The workshop has helped to widen the scope for future studies and network-building.

Recommendations by Lester Davids and Nina Jablonski–Highlights[8]

- Education is the KEY!!
  — Popular Press
  — Seminars/Public Talks.

- Advertising agencies/Cosmetic companies need a **Watchdog** organization
- Change in "**Self-image**"
- Cosmetic ethics and legislature
- **LOVE THE SKIN YOU'RE IN!!... IT'S THE ONLY WE'VE GOT!!!**

References

1. Dlova Ncoza, Hamed Saja H, Tsoka-Gwegweni Joyce, Grobler Anneke, Hift Richard. Women's perceptions of the benefits and risks of skin-lightening creams in two South African communities. *Journal of Cosmetic Dermatology*. Sept 2014; 13 (3): 236-41. Article first published online: 6 Sept 2014. *DOI: 10.1111/jocd.12104*.
2. Bekezela Phakathi. Dark side to beautiful skin. *Gracott's mail Online*. Tue, 27 Mar, 2007. http://www.grocotts.co.za/content/dark-side-beautiful-skin-27-03-2007
3. Malangu N, Ogunbanjo GA. Predictors of topical steroid misuse among patrons of pharmacies in Pretoria. *South Africa Fam Pract* 2006; 48 (1): 14a-14e.
4. Pumza Fihlani. Africa: Where black is not really beautiful. *BBC News Johannesburg*. 1 January 2013/Africa. http://www.bbc.com/news/world-africa-20444798
5. Editorial. Use of skin lightening creams. Lack of recognition and regulation is having serious medical consequences. *BMJ* 2010; 341: c6102 doi: 10.1136/bmj.c6102.
6. Cape Town gets world-first safety lab for hair and skin cosmetics. 29 May 2015. http://ww.health24.com/Lifestyle/Live-allergy-free/Cape-Town-gets...
7. Nashiro Davids. Dark cloud over skin-lightening creams. Nonhlanhla Khumalo is on a mission to get harmful beauty products off our streets. 02 June, 2015. http://www.timeslive.co.za/thetimes/2015/06/02/Dark-cloud-over-skin-lightening- creams.
8. Davids Lester M and Jablonski Nina. Is Africa in the Dark About seeing the Light? Insights into Global Skin Lightener Use. http://www.ehrn.co.za/download/lecture_series_08.pdf

ZAMBIA

The derogatory name given to skin bleachers in Zambia is 'FBI'— Former Black Individuals. Hildah Lumba[1] wrote an interesting article on "Dangers associated with skin bleaching." Bleached people in Zambia are ridiculed and called 'FBIs' (Former Black Individuals). Hildah is so disgusted with mothers who bleach their babies that she cursed:

"As for the women who bleach their children: may you melt in the sun and have your nose fall off"

Hildah interviewed Dr Pierre Yassa, consultant dermatologist at the skin Clinic, University Teaching Hospital who elaborated on the adverse health effects of skin lightening chemicals, and the dangerous consequences from removing the melanin pigment which protects us from the carcinogenic effects of excessive exposure to ultraviolet rays in the sun. Hildah also clarified some of the toxic effects of mercury and hydroquinone which are regular ingredients in skin bleaching products. Some hair salons have even resorted to applying corticosteroid creams on the scalps of their clients to enable hair to grow fast. She adds

"the thing about bleaching is that no matter how decent or independent you are, you just end up looking like a desperate cheap person."

"Even the ones who should know better are doing it" We know a few artistes who are bleaching, some CEOs, some cabinet people and even some pastors."

"Last time I bumped into one of these Zambian players plying their trade at TP Mazembe looking bleach their skin but really, do our Zambian players have to morph into that syndrome as well?"

Should women bleach their skin?

Brighton Sinkala,[2] the Lusaka-based comedian, during Comedy Calabash show in Kitwe put women's beauty in three categories: **"*Extremely beautiful*"**—in all aspects, physical appearance, colour and general morphology; **"Where beauty is a matter of one's opinion;"** and **"where it depends on the beer-holder"**—where to approach one, one had to be drunk". Sinkala's categorization might not be appropriate but for many a woman, it appears beauty is all about being light skinned. It is not unusual to see many light-skinned women on the streets these days. And if Kitwe could be used as a yardstick for all the other towns in Zambia, one can safely predict that being dark skinned and natural is almost heading for 'extinction'. If what I heard the other day from two humble middle-aged women is true, then there is a lot of work that needs to be done to put issues of beauty and love in their right context because it is clear from these women's explanation that to them, beauty is all about being light skinned.

According to one of the women whose identity will be revealed later, dark-skinned women nowadays are left with no choice but to use some skin-lightening lotions. She says this is necessary to deter men, in particular husbands, from leaving their dark skinned women or wives in search of light-skinned partners or wives. In her view, light-skinned women are more desirable by men!

Helen Sibamba is a trader at Chisokone Market in Kitwe and shares her views about skin bleaching and the use of skin lightening lotions. A single mother of twins, Sibamba admits that her light complexion is aided by some skin lightening creams but she only does it for "beauty" and making her skin "smooth".She says that for women to look beautiful, they need to have smooth, light skins.Lizzy Chansa, also a trader at Chisokone market and a mother of six, explains why women use skin lightening creams and lotions. "Men are to blame for the increase in the number of women who are using skin lightening lotions because we fear that if we don't lighten our skins, our husbands will go after those who are light skinned," she says."You will find that men leave their dark-skinned spouses in their homes and go after the light-skinned ones, so what are women expected to do?" she asks. If Chansa's view is representative of the majority of women using skin lightening creams, questions like "What is love and how far can a woman go just to please her man?"; "Is it really true that light-skinned women are more beautiful and more attractive than their dark skinned counterparts?"

Should beauty or love really be a justification for someone's decision to bleach their skins?"

These questions remain for you to answer.

But not all women share Sibamba and Chansa's view.

Elizabeth Mfula, a member of the Zambia National Marketeers' Association (ZANAMA) discourages all forms of skin bleaching for whatever reason. Mfula says she would personally not allow her daughter to bleach her skin because this comes with serious consequences. She says although it is important for a woman to look beautiful, it is not true that this beauty would only be achieved with a light skin. Mfula says simply being neat and using creams that smoothen but not lighten skins is all one needs. She observes that a lot of women have lost their natural beauty and complexion because of bleaching.

A number of men spoken to disagree with the views that they indirectly encourage skin bleaching by going after light-skinned women. According to Farley, a businessman of Kitwe, most men hate skin bleaching. "There was one time my wife used a lotion that started lighten up her skin. I ordered her to stop using the lotion because I just like her being natural...I wonder what kind of husband would encourage his wife to bleach." Musonda says it was nonsense for women to believe that men could leave their wives if they were not bleaching. And Peter of Kitwe discloses that he quit a four-year relationship with his fiancé after she came back from University of Zambia with a lightened skin. "She went to the University of Zambia as a natural beauty but I was surprised that when she came back, she was looking like a Cape-Coloured, so I told her that 'it's either you quit this bleaching or there will be no marriage' and that was it," he said.

Peter observes that skin bleaching had devastating effects on one's skin whereby a woman's skin wrinkles very badly after they stop using the same soaps, creams and lotions. He describes women with bleached skins as unattractive more so that the light skin is not even. "I wonder what makes them feel attractive because how can somebody who looks very light on the face but are very dark when they undress attract you?" he asked. Peter also wonders why some men had joined the habit of bleaching or lightening their skins and urges medical practitioners to step in and help educate the masses on the effects of skin bleaching. One can only wonder if this obsession with being light skinned is all about beauty or an inferiority complex. It is very likely that we will hear more about this issue from a dermatologist's point of view soon.

Responses to the question by Mwila Chansa @gmail.com[3]

"Should beauty or Love really be a justification for women to bleach

- *Never in my life will I bleach my skin, I would rather not get married if one of the conditions is to bleach for a man to marry me. Black is beautiful; that's what I call myself.* Mofya Chisenga Mukunta
- *Black is beautiful* Terry Oreilly.
- ***I prefer unbleached woman. Bleaching women are inferior and usually not confident*.** Michael Chipande
- *I think each person has the rights on her body, because some men appreciate women with bleached skin and some don't!. it's just like smoking. Some appreciate husbands like that and other don't! that's my point of view anyway. I have'nt bleached my skin and I,m proud of myself!!* Haulie Temb
- *The Malakoz are dark. Natural women are the best, whether dark or light.* Obinna Chuma Onukogu
- *I can say, BEAUTY is what we all possess; confidence is all it takes to bring it (beauty) out. I,ve seen girls who still lack confidence even after having bleached their skin. I guess it is because they feel stange in some sort of a borrowed skin. Be proud of your natural beauty girls!!* Mwich grace Kangwa.

- *It really amazes me why women want to destroy their faces with these harsh creams. The government has also not done their part in ensuring that this skin bleaching is stopped.* Ella Mwinji Zkonde Zulu

References

1. Hildah Lumba. Dangers associated with skin bleaching. *TIMES OF ZAMBIA* March 1, 2014
2. Brighton Sinkola. Should women bleach their skin? *http://www.facebook.com/peralink.php?story-fbib=138030709574...*
3. Mwila, chansa@gmail.com. The Post Newspaper Zambia

Zambian Men with Bleaching Skin: New Trend

Black is beautiful, so goes the saying. But not for some people, so it seems. A colleague told me how one day, while he was in a beauty supply shop, he saw the shelf stockpiled with Deproson, Betazole, Demo Gel, Amira C, Top Lemon, Lemonvet, Extra Claire, Bio Claire, Carolite, Maxlight, Bu-tone et. He was having a conversation with the owner of the shop, a dark-skinned woman, when a man, thought to be in his late 20s, came-in and picked an assortment of skin bleaching products from the shelf. The guy did not look embarrassed at all, but he could notice a little of discomfort from the shop owner as the man downloaded the bleaching stuff on the counter ready to purchase. After he had left, she explained to my friend that make-up and bleaching creams are increasingly becoming popular among men. And she can't be mistaken; it is easy nowadays to come across Zambian men with make-up as well as those using bleaching creams in the name of keeping with trendy world of fashion. This is unlike in the past when men were associated with moderate, comfortable and conservative outlooks. In fact, in the past, and please no offence intended, any man with a bleached skin was thought to be from Congo, specifically, a Kasai. The easiest way to identify a Kasai was through their skin appearance.

Early in 2010 the widely respected New York Times reported finding many of these creams on the shelves of ethnic beauty stores in Brooklyn, New York. Since the harmful chemicals are often not listed, or listed under many different names,buying bleaching creams in stores not monitored by a corporate structure could mean you are buying counterfeits. No prizes for correctly saying whether any of our shops are under supervision whatsoever.

I strongly think that it does not matter what color your skin is, as long as you feel confident in the one you have.

Admittedly, for many people skin bleaching is a way to achieve brighter, clearer skin, and to remove dark patches on many areas of the body. Often used during this process are chemical peels, whitening creams and even lasers to lighten and even your skin tone. Creams, which can be purchased at many shops without a prescription, are the most commonly used.

Most of these products can provide long-lasting results when used correctly, according to the marketers of these products. But we know that there are many risks and complications associated with use bleaching products. For a start, there is the is the issue of toxic ingredients. A doctor friend says some topical skin bleachers may use ingredients that can be harmful to both one's skin and indeed the overall health.

For instance, he says hydroquinone, which is also used in film development, is a primary active ingredients in many skin whitening creams. It is a known carcinogen, and has been linked with other complications such as adrenal dysfunction. He says if used continuously, hydroquinone can cause black and blue skin discoloration, a condition known as "ochronosis". A quick check on the internet reveals that many countries including Europe, Japan, and Australia have banned it sale as a skin lightener although the U.S retains it for this particular purpose.

Another toxic ingredient is mercury, a potentially risky element which has been linked to many illnesses, including Alzheimers and neurological dysfunctions.

This, according to medical experts, is known to have serious effects on the central nervous system, as well. It is easily absorbed through the skin, and is not readily expelled by the body. This means that, over time, you could build up a mercury level that could lead to toxicity. Now, with all these risks, it is difficult to understand why Zambian men, would embrace skin bleaching. A bit of make-up for purpose of photo shots or television camera is understanding, but skin bleaching is certainly out of our system as black Zambian men. The argument of going with the fashion trends does not even hold water. If anything the argument of discussion about dark skin and light skin is actually dumb. A lot of people do not like dark skinned people because they think they are ugly while mistakenly thinking that light-skinned people are prettier. I strongly believe that it does not matter what colour your skin is, as long as you feel confident in the one you have.

Reference

Daimone Siulapwa. Zambian men bleach skins: New trend? December 23rd , 2010. *http://ukzambians.co.uk/home/2010/10/31/zambian-men-bleached-skins-trend/*

Ban Sale of skin-bleaching creams-PHPF

The Public Health Partnership Forum (PHPF) in Zambia has called on Government to ban the sale of skin-bleaching creams in the country[1], arguing that indiscriminate use is harmful to the body. The PHPF publicity secretary, Enock Kaputula, said Zambia has become a dumping ground for such products. He said that the indiscriminate use of the creams can cause many health problems such as skin cancer, pigmentation disorders, speech and hearing impairment and kidney problems. He noted that the prevalence of women who were using high dose of steroids, hydroquinone and mercury to bleach has reached alarming level. He regretted that the creams are sold in many places including supermarkets, beauty and hair salons and drug stores. He observed that some hair salons have even resorted to applying steroid creams on the scalps of their clients to stop skin inflammation and to enable hair to grow fast. He described skin bleaching as a "disease" in the general definition of health because skin bleaching is caused by "genetic and socio-economic factors and the root cause is the need by users to overcome perceived suffering from social norms. He concluded that since skin bleaching is a psycho- social and health problem, it needs to be addressed with interventions aimed at changing the user's perceptions of themselves and educating people on its consequences.

The Zambian Pharmaceutical Regulatory Authority (PRA) has issued out warnings on the dangers of rampant abuse of skin lightening creams by Zambian women and men. PRA has expressed worry about the high number of cases of cancer, compromised immune system and diabetes among people abusing corticosteroid such as diprosone "medicines meant to treat and cure skin ailment such as eczema" as skin lighteners. The PRA said that at the Zambia International Trade Fair in Ndola, it was clear that there had been increase in the number of people abusing prescribed medicines. harmful to human health. He said abuse of steroids compromised the immune system leading to cancer and diabetes,among other diseases. He said 'using these creams just for the sake of transforming one's skin from a 'dark' to a 'light' complexion is outright reckless. It is like taking a course of anti-malaria drug such as coaterm or quinine when you are not suffering from malaria, just because it makes you feel good. It is surprising that educated people, who should know better the dangers of misusing chemicals, have been consistently applying the creams, and paid dearly for the 'sin' in many cases. Besides endangering their own health, the abusers of these creams should realize that they are also placing an unnecessary burden on the government, which will have to spend colossal sums of money on their treatment and care once they are afflicted with one or more diseases associated with skin bleaching creams.

Some outlets, especially in Lusaka, have even put up tantalizing billboards and posters inviting unsuspecting members of the public, especially women, to go for skin bleaching which they do not actually need.

There is even more alarming information that may not have reached the PRA, that some women have been mixing diprosone, epidermo, eggs and medicated soap into a concoction they are using as a skin lightener. Something must really be done about this, and urgently.

References

1. Enock Kaputula. Ban sale of skin-bleaching creams–PHPF Zambia Daily Mail. *www://lusakatimes.com/2010/03/31/ban-sale-skinbleaching.*

2. Rampant abuse of skin lightening creams by Zambian women. July 7, 2011 *http://ukzambians.co.uk/home/2011/07/07/rampant-abuse-of-skin-lightening-creams-by-zambian-women/*

Comments from Zambians to the call to ban skin-bleaching products

There is a general pervasive resentment in Zambia against skin lightening, end indeed the majority of the comments from bloggers are in favor of banning the sale skin lightening products including steroids like 'diprosone'. Some other comments include:

"If you women don't accept yourselves the way God has made you it is one way of saying you don't appreciate God for you to be black, don't blame God. You should learn to accept your skin color"

"This is good news, (ban) the nonsense should be stopped or these women will soon look like zombies. It seems they lack self esteem."

"I went to a chemist the other day looking for face powder and all I could find were these pale white powders. I asked the sales lady why they didn't have darker shades and she told me it was because they sell fast as she and I were the only dark people left in Lusala. It's a terrible inferiority complex"

"Hey it's not only women who use these things. However, the even strang argument is that when the mercury in the lightening creams and soaps destroy their liver they are likely to pass such defects to the rest of society. Jaribu cream/soap is especially known for doing so. You are right, it's not only women that use these bleaches, many men use them including Chiluba".

"Yes ban all other sources of evil, ban beers, ban polygamy, ban adultery, ban women doing the cooking alone in homes, ban wife grabbing, ban marrying women fit to be a grandchildren, haha the list is long. Look those women who use skin lightening creams know why they are doing that. In addition it is their own business. If they get ill well it is themselves to blame and no one else. Beer drinking causes lever problems that lead to deaths, smoking causes cancer that leads to deaths. Why hasn't the Govt. banned all this crap? I know many Zambian women here in Denmark who have been using skin lightening cream and the end results are there for all to see, however it is no one's business what others are using. Just let them be and one day they will find out when they start turning black again".

"Congolese men are the culprits in using these creams. But with our Zambian ladies who use these creams"

"Growing up, I use to think a couple of Zed women nurses were from South Africa because their skin tone was fair, little did I know that the nurses I thought where naturally fair skin toned South Africans where local Zedian nurses who use to steal skin medication creams like betnovate with side effects of bleaching skin to use as 'beauty products" when the hospitals ran out of medication which was either stolen and sold out as bleaching cream. One woman I met years later tried to hide from me because her skin color had changed to charcoal black, from that of a fake light brown one".

"For young people reading this article, your way out is EDUCATION and looking after your HEALTH. Forget about attracting rich husbands or other get- rich-quick schemes".

"Diproson should be banned, we don't need FBI'S(former black individuals)"

"Please ban the products – am tired of seeing orange, ashy, burnt faces – its like you are in the Twilight. I remember when I was growing up the only people using these creams and soaps where bar maids and sex for hire technicians".

"Those that have used the creams in the past and are regretful for doing it must go to schools and educate the young ones on the dangers of using such creams".

"Those who are saying leave them to bleach their skins are being ignorant. The fact is that it might affect you or your family if not now later. The skin lighteners are

usually toxic and cause harm to the reproductive system, brain or liver. If one of your kids marries a user of these bleaches the offspring may have problems which include gingivitis, tremors psychological changes and spontaneous abortions. Since you men love these FBIs you are bound to leave behind offspring that are deformed because you slept with a mercury infested woman and the other way round".

"You keep referring to Caucasians tanning to be darker. Newsflash,—the tanning creams don't have harmful ingredients like mercury as skin lightening creams"

"I would rather go for a woman with stretch marks than one with a bleached face… very disgusting. They should start arresting them now".

"You are saying skin creams cause damage to the reproductive system,:- and so does alcohol and other substance people take in but know are harmful to their health but has there been a time when they said ban alcohol or cigarettes? People should learn to mind their own business. And yes white women too put tan on their bodies to make their complexion darker".

"The original MEKAKO brand, MADE IN ITALY only has pink/purple/orange packages.
Blue/Green ones made in India/Africa/China are potentially unsafe and dangerous (might contain mercury or hydroquinone). Original soaps and creams don't. Avoid them and only trust the originals from mekako. Italy or mekako.france" (only official websites)"

5 Responses to "Skin bleaching in Zambia"

1. *"What's the point of bleaching your skin if God had a reason to make you black,,,if It's because you want to attract Mr or Miss right it's pointless because the one who truly loves you will love you for who you really are. Am black and I'am proud, if someone does not love me for my skin colour then I 'am will know there and then that he is Mr wrong…..Zambians let us be proud of who we are, immitating the white man's skin will just put us in jeopardy when faced with the consequences of cancers in the future…".* Nelisa Jan 31. 2011.
2. *"I would be very uncomfortable to appear brown when am black in the actual sense. I am really proud of my colour and happy to be my beautiful black self because there is nothing as comforting as being yourself in life. I think people who bleach do not realise how much they alter their own natural beauty.."* Marita Dec 16, 2010.
3. *"I can't believe how bleaching is affecting me myself. I am proud to be black. Why would I want to look like white people. This is what happens when*

people are not proud of themselves even men"! Gladys Mwamba Dec 12, 2010.

4. *"You are right my sister preach".* Mutale Dec 12, 2010
5. *"Yalya ama ten pin aleonaula mukushita ama chemicals. Uyu transport officer afwile ukushitilamo abana bakwe imichopo mulya muchibolya"!!!!*

Willie Dec 18, 2010.

Reference

http://ukzambians.co.uk/home/2010/10/30/skin-bleaching-zambia/

ZIMBABWE

In an article titled "*Beauty is in the eye of the skin bleacher,*" Robin Chaibva[1] says— "The definition of beauty is a tricky proposition. For ages, debate on what beauty is has raged across the globe. Therefore, it comes as no surprise that some people have taken it upon themselves to change their looks after experiencing the bullying and discrimination of not "fitting in."

One of the most talked about issues is skin bleaching and hips/bum enhancing. In Zimbabwe, men and women who use skin bleaching and hip enhancing products are hardely aware of the deadly and dangerous side-effects. Beyond the streets, some users of such products end up being suppliers to others who want to join the movement. Aside from knowing the unwanted side effects, users also undergo the risk of not getting the desired result from using these drugs. For example, a drug advertised to give curvy hips and a rounded bottom, may end up causing uneven fat deposits. Some skin bleaches may work in certain portions and leave other areas darkened. In May 2015, Cote d'voire banned the sale of skin bleaching products. In Zimbabwe, though, their use remains prevalent, it appears that medical authorities can ban the sale of these drugs from registered pharmacies but they cannot completely ban their use as the demand is very high on the black market. Instead of discussing the side effects and dangers— users are ignoring the message and continuing anyway.

The historian Burke notes that women's consumption of skin whiteners in modern Zimbabwe was considered as a sign of (re)colonization and "selling-out" to the white regime.[2]

Robin decided to find out some of the "social" side effects by asking the general public their thoughts about skin bleachers or people that use drugs to enhance their hips.

Farai, a 35 year old Harare man, thinks that women who use the creams are delusional to think that all men find light-skinned women attractive; while Cliff, a 32 year old, also from Harare, thinks that women who do not get "adequate" attention from men are the ones resorting to these "desperate" measures. Cliff believes women need more self-confidence, and users of these products are "short-term investors" trying to swindle men. Another older women who spoke to this publication on condition of anonymity, concurred with Cliff, saying enhancements were for women who saw themselves as mere sex objects. She also thinks men who bleach their skin are most likely sexual deviants. A social media survey by Robin revealed that people who seek to modify themselves in one way or another have insecurity issues, low self-esteem or identity crises. James Nyamhini, a pharmacist, said while measures would be taken to ban registration of these drugs, managing illegal vendors and sellers is where the major issue was.

There are, however, safer and more moderate ways to solve skin imperfections, available from registered pharmacies and cosmetic retailers. The use of specific exercises and wearing body shaping undergarments are some of the ways to enhance one's body shape too.

Finally, Robin asked: "Is beauty your personality, looks or how you present yourself? What people find attractive is always a personal preference from individual to individual and varies across geographical and social clusters. So what do we call beautiful in Zimbabwe?

Zimbabwean model Angeline Mandaba bleached her skin to vampire white.

Mainini Beatrice[4] expressed disgust at the whole idea of men bleaching their skin particularly after seeing a man who claimed to be "Reverend"—"Obadiah guy," bleach his skin. Beatrice says "I used to think this was only reserved for women only. Well, at least here in Zimbabwe I thought it was a preserve for the women. You see, in the 70s, when I was in my late teens, it was common for young urban women like me and the older ones too, to use skin lighteners. Even rural women too, vaiyuzawo! What it meant was that we were using skin lightening creams like Ambi, and Butone, the hot brands then. All those efforts were in search of the elusive beauty. Women searching for beauty! WOMEN! Both men and women have taken to using skin bleaching products. A colleague later told me it was common to find men in Zambia, the Democratic Republic of Congo, the other Congo (Brazzaville) and Tanzania who use skin lightening creams. What are these brothers trying to do? Change their skin colour? Do they hate themselves that much, that they want to become like them? Chiiko? I wonder what they tell their children, if they have them anyway"

Mainini continues: "Even though in my mind I will tolerate a woman who uses skin lighteners, this does not make it right. I really do not know why people try to change their skin colour. Some people have said these are the results of colonialism; that the colonized eventually aim to look like their colonizers. After all, the colonizers have hammered it in the colonized, that all lighter skins are better looking than darker ones. And by the way, this lighter-skin-better-attitude is not only confined to Africans (the most pitch dark skinned people on this earth). You go to India, and you find their caste system is also based on the tone of the skin. The lighter your skin colour is, the better caste you are in and the more societal benefits you enjoy. Just for being light skinned!"

Mainini cautioned that most, if not all the skin lightening creams sold in the market, are a dangerous cocktail of compounds like steroids, hydroquinone, tretinoin and mercury. Hydroquinone and mercury are bleaching agents that are banned from use in cosmetics.

Experts have warned that long term use of these products can lead to lethal health complications like permanent pigmentation, skin cancer, liver damage, mercury poisoning and a host of others. According to the UK's National Health Service (NHS) website, a cream that you buy over the counter is not necessarily medically approved and could permanently damage your skin. Yet locally in Zimbabwe, these creams are available all over the place. Kumupedzamhamo, in flea markets, people's homes. Everywhere! Most of them come with user instructions that are written in mostly strange Chinese or Arabic languages. Most of these creams are banned products, but you find them readily available. Who is responsible for their distribution and who should monitor their entrance in Zimbabwe? Where is the Medicines Control Authority of Zimbabwe? Do we have adequate legislation to deal with the proliferation of these creams? I doubt!

Information on the NHS website also says although steroids can be useful in treating some skin diseases, such as psoriasis and eczema, this must take place under the supervision of a skin specialist. These skin lightening creams, according to the NHS website can cause: permanent skin bleaching, thinning of skin, uneven colour loss, leading to a blotchy appearance, redness and intense irritation.

Mainini concludes that she has seen women who now cannot spend a minute in the sun because continued use of the skin lightening creams have damaged their skin, it cannot tolerate the sun anymore. She cautioned those who continue using it if it makes them feel happy but beware of the dangers

References

1. Robin Chaibva. *Beauty is in the eye of the skin bleacher The Sunday Mail.* Sunday Jun 28, 2015. *http://www.sundaymail.co.zw/?p=37974*
2. Burke Timothy. Lifebuoy Men, Lux Women: Commodification, Consumption, and Cleanliness in Modern Zimbabwe. Durham, NC: Duke University Press. 1996.
3. Muchadeyi E, Thompson S, Baker N. A survey of the constituents, availability and the use of skin lightening creams in Zimbabwe *Central Afr J Med* 1983; 29:225-7.
4. Mainini Beatrice. Reverends now skin-bleaching? *The Sunday Mail* Zimbabwe. 11 May, 2014. *http://www.sundaymail.co.zw/?p=3945.*

Chapter 9

East Africa

Story highlights
Kenya
Tanzania
Uganda
Sudan

Story highlights I

Kenya

- Skin bleaching products are called "mafuta" in Kenya.
- Skin lightening in East Africa has more to do with globalization of European ideals than with colonization.
- Skin lightening has been a part of Kenyan culture since the 60s
- The exact prevalence of skin lightening in Kenya is not known, but the practice is undeniably on the rise, especially amongst the young in urban areas.
- Skin lightening products were banned in 1999 but the products and the practice have continued to thrive unabated due to institutionalized corruption in Kenya's security forces
- Kenya women say they bleach to be (i) more beautiful (ii) more successful (iii) to satisfy the expectation of the opposite sex because Kenyan men prefer light complexioned women; hence to facilitate getting married quicker and prevent losing their husbands to other light complexioned women, Kenyan women find it expedient to bleach their skin.
- Media advertising enhances the stereotypes that light skinned people are advantaged socially and romantically.

- Unregulated clinics offering backstreet skin-bleaching injections have become increasingly popular with Kenyan women. Nairobi's River Road, a bustling area with a reputation for prostitution, black market goods and crime, has become a hub for illicit beauticians that provide these injections.
- Skin lightening creams containing mercury are used as injectables by the wealthy Nairobi women at US$ 70 per shot. The shots contain alpha hydroxy acids and mercury-containing creams
- Shop assistants with no knowledge of the products mix the gels, creams and ointments themselves
- Owing to the nature and medical and legal unacceptability of the practice, a lot of secrecy shrouds the production and sale of the merchandise.
- Counterfeit and misbranded products abound.
- Strict prescription products are readily given out by pharmacies on demand without prescription and sold in back streets
- Some physicians are known to give out concoctions with no known formula of contained ingredients
- Those with ill effects of bleaching products shy away from medical attention due to guilt complex or deny use of the products even when they consult physicians.
- Analysis of substances and products for content of ingredients is costly and often an impossibility
- A clinical investigation of Kenyan women with damaged kidneys revealed that they suffered from a high incidence of nephrotic syndrome which was attributed to the use of skin lightening products containing mercury.
- Badly administered injections of unregulated substances could also result in HIV, Hepatitis C, TB, permanent disfigurement and nerve paralysis.
- In Kenya more than half the population lives on less than US $ 1 a day yet some women spend up to KSH 10,000 per month on the pills and US$ 70 for a shot of mercury containing injection. Some women sell sex to sustain the skin bleaching practice.

- Story highlights II

  Tanzania
- Concocted skin bleaching products are called "mkorongo" in East Africa.

- Tanzania, the largest geographic East African country, is the main hub where empirical research has taken place on the skin lightening practice
- Tanzanians have high internalized Eurocentric standards of beauty as well as political affiliations with the Civic United Front party (CUF)—a nationally based liberal political party that is heavily represented by Zanzibaris of mixed ancestry.
- The tourist industry and increased access to mercury from gold and copper-lead mines help to drive the skin-bleaching culture
- The estimated prevalence rate of skin bleaching in Tanzania is about 30%.
- Tanzania was one of the first countries that banned the manufacture, importation and marketing of skin bleaching products early in 1968, but skin bleaching is still rife in Tanzania
- Tanzania women concoct affordable skin bleaching products by mixing dangerous caustic agents to lighten their skin
- Researchers found that artisanal gold mining with mercury amalgamation and the use of mercury containing imported creams and soaps touted as "antiseptics" have caused renal damage among Tanzanians and Kenyan's
- What would make a Tanzanian women say she "started bleaching to be beautiful and to look like Arabians or Europeans and attractive to people, especially men"?
- What would make Tanzanian women say they "lightened their skin to enhance opportunities in life (especially job opportunities), and to reduce the experience of negative stereotypes that are applied to dark skinned people?
- Why should "dark" skinned people be envious of those with lighter skin and attempt to achieve the same status by engaging in skin-lightening practices
- In addition to educating the people as recommended by researchers, what governmental action is required in Tanzania as regards skin bleaching?

- Story highlights III
  Uganda
- Uganda is one of the first countries to ban the skin bleaching products in 1972, yet skin bleaching has continued to thrive in the country.
- The products are easily accessible anywhere in Uganda as over-the-counter products in pharmacyshops, roadside or by hawkers,

and vendors Cross border smuggling from neighboring countries is big business in Uganda

- Both men and women use the products in Uganda not only on the visible parts but also on the genitalia and perineal area.
- The Uganda National Bureau of standards and National Drugs Authority has tried to crack down on bleaching cosmetics, but their efforts have not been successful. The trend is actually going up though still 'hush hush' among the public. Ugandan celebrities have been known to bleach their skins from way back. The bleaching trend has actually shot up over the years as homemade cosmetic and dermatological products have become easily accessible. Inspite of a ban on bleaching products, they are continuously being smuggled in.
- Adverse effects from the products have been reported by doctors of Makerere University Medical School. The adverse effects reported are both physical and psychological due to disfigurement of the face.
- Some doctors believe that skin bleaching is common among the uneducated and that those who bleach have low self esteem
- Kidney damage (nephrotic syndrome) and nerve damage (neuropathy) from the use of skin lightening chemicals have been reported in Uganda.
- Some Ugandan people believe that skin bleaching in Uganda is due to Ugandans internalizing Eurocentric ideals and failure to bring up their children to love their look and skin colour and to value themselves and others by their personalities and not by how they look.
- Some others believe that the effect of the media in promoting Eurocentric values like Botox and cosmetic facial and body reconstructive surgeries is a major driving force that fuels the skin bleaching practice

- **Story highlights IV**

Sudan

- A popular phrase in Sudan is *al-Husnu ahmar* (beauty is red). Whiteness is the ideal color in most Arab societies
- This debate over the right skin colour to have to be South Sudanese is a tiny part of the wider tensions created by east African returnees, ex-Khartoum residents, and the broader tensions between the 'browner' Equatorians and 'black' Nilotic-

origin people; women continue to reflect—painfully—the cultural and political narratives of national identity.

- War caused displacement that sent waves of people to urban areas where they were introduced to new colours and new standards of beauty that Sudanese had to live up.
- In Sudan, lighter skin is considered prettier and a sign of being enlightened.
- In the Sudanese culture if you want to remain natural and love your skin you are seen as a radical women instead of a woman who is proud of whom she is.
- Women have been told from early age, in folktales, that women, have to be beautiful. The standards of beauty now are light-skin and long hair. They want to get married because they are born to think that this is their traditional role; to be wives and mothers.
- In the Sudanese society, a woman is anything more than a pretty face. A woman is a "girl" until she is married and marriage has become so incumbent on looks. The women carry a heavy burden.
- A Sudanese professor says: "The level of beauty has gone down, i.e. most of them (Sudanese women) are ugly, very much so… using skin bleaching creams. An ugly woman creates distress in a person… it makes me feverish, I suffer a lot. All the big poets used to write about the beauty of women. But now, you can't find a girl worth writing poetry about." This comment generated a great controversy among women in Sudan.
- A man in Godele divorced his wife because of her habitual skin bleaching and says
- "I will not accept my wife again in my home as house wife, because she broke both my order and culture". The wife said when she visited Khartoum, she found all her former school mates who went to Khartoum have changed their color from black to brown, and then she was forced to do the same to win the love from her husband.
- In 2012 female students were suspended at Juba day Secondary and Comboni Secondary School for skin bleaching.
- Sudanese began grasping the dangers of this trend when a popular male musician died of kidney failure a few years ago reportedly, after applying a bleaching cream.

KENYA

History of skin bleaching in East Africa

Skin lightening in east Africa has more to do with globalization of European ideals than with colonialism.[1] The 60s, as Kenya gained Independence and Pan- Africanism was all the rage, saw the initial surge of East African women using skin lightening products – an era that also saw the rise of television and American media, where the practice of preferential treatment for light-skinned black Americans was well established, and the black stars exported were Chuck Berry, Diana Ross and Jimi Hendrix. But as this idea grew, so did the forces against it, with postcolonial African politicians deeming it racial betrayal. On the insistence of medical professionals, who were also opposed to skin lightening, Tanzania became the first country to ban the practice in 1968, followed by Uganda in 1972. While Kenya never enacted a total ban, it prohibited ads for Ambi soap, one of the most popular products at the time, on the basis that it insinuated that modern, post-colonial Africans were light skinned.

However, it wasn't a clear-cut case of racial pride versus globalisation, as the many social revolutions occurring during that time also included feminism. Audrey Wipper, a Canadian sociologist who was living in Kenya in 1972, criticised the range of bans in East Africa, arguing that "prohibition of Western fashions and beauty aids were efforts by postcolonial male politicians to use urban African women as scapegoats for the nation's problems." Skin lightening and, beyond the practice itself, the desire for light skin, had become contentious issues in the country, and women who used the products did so discreetly. Fifty-five-year-old Eunice who was a form two high school student in 1974, said "I remember Ambi and Snowfire as products we used to use. The creams were cheap, and most high school-going girls who felt that they weren't light-skinned enough could easily buy either from their neighbourhood shop. I was partial to Snowfire because my skin became lighter and smoother faster than my friends who'd been using Ambi."

While the Kenya Bureau of Standards (KEBS) came down hard on cosmetic products that were deemed unsafe in 1999, banning more than 100 lightening agents that used hydroquinone, mercury and steroids, by then the practice had essentially reached critical mass – enough women were lightening their skin that it was no longer something to keep hidden. While you're not likely to see women boldly proclaiming their use of the products today, asked point blank they're honest about whether or not they lighten their skin – and why

Perspective, Determinants and Expressed Motives in Kenya

An investigating journalist Josephine Mojiti asks Winnie why she bleaches her skin, and this was the response: "My skin gets me noticed," "I started lightening my skin after high school with body cream, and I love my colour now," she tells Josephine Mojiti earnestly. Progressing next to pills that were nearly KSH 10,000 (US $98.10) per month and now using injections that are even more expensive, Winnie has invested in her colour. "I know I might sound vain, but to me light skin is more beautiful than dark." Winnie, a bank teller and chronic skin bleacher, justifies the benefits of skin bleaching by drawing attention to the duration it took the modelling industry to accept dark skinned models like Alek Wek and Ajuma on their runways? Winnie adds—"Light skin is more appealing, it is a sign of purity, it makes you stand out of the crowd. It gives you preferential treatment, gives an easier time finding a job, makes one prettier, more attractive, and facilitates getting married quicker."

This perception, as well as the idea that lighter skin will make them more successful, plays a key role amongst Kenyan women who make the bold step to change their complexions. And it's true that a light skinned person in Kenya, be it male or female, will stand out in a crowd.

Nineteen-year-old Rita Irungu in Kenya says for years when she was at school she bought creams not knowing what they contained. She now has a weekly session with a beautician because of her bodly damaged skin. Dermatologists in Kenya fear that young African women who think lighter skin is beautiful are harming themselves by using skin lightening creams. Dermatologists in Kenya are now calling for skin creams to be labeled better.

Rita says "it was peer pressure, especially the expectations of the opposite sex, that persuaded her that light skin was better. You would really like this boy but he would go for the lighter girl." Boys would say to her. "Okay, you look good but I think you would look better if you were light."

Skin lightening has been a part of the Kenyan culture since the 60s. The exact prevalence in Kenya is not known but the practice is undeniably on the rise, especially amongst the young in urban areas. Skin-lightening in Kenya does not look like a practice that would stop any time soon but is most likely here to stay! Josephine Mogiti[1] explores this trend and its potential side effects, both for the women using these products and society as a whole, as the effects are not always what is expected.

She received reports from chronic bleachers like Mose who claimed she once enjoyed a beautiful, spotless, smooth face until "her youth finally caught up with her", and she started using the skin bleaching products. She eventually developed "red and blue black patches that looked burnt" on her upper back, nape and earlobes which she was then compelled to hide with a weave-on. Mose further admits "I can't stand heat of any kind. I can't walk under direct sunlight either, as my skin becomes taut starts cracking and bleeding." Dr Melanie Miyanji-de Souza, a dermatologist at the Aga Khan university Hospital, has stood behind the ban of certain skin lightening products since becoming familiar with the issue in 2001. Miyanji-de Souza says "We [the dermatologists] have had a lot of conferences on the matter because this thing has to be squashed, and we've come a long way. People who have been bleaching their skin come crying to me to help them, because the damage is not only on the skin but in the brain, kidneys, and liver."

Another chronic bleacher, Ann, says her curiosity got the better of her when a close friend divulged that she lightened her skin. "I was a little hesitant at first, but eventually started lightening mine since my friend's skin looked really good." Ann states.

This perception, as well as the idea that lighter skin will make them more successful, plays a key role amongst Kenyan women who make the bold step to change their complexions. And it is true that a light skinned person in Kenya, be it male or female, will stand out in a crowd.

The opinions of most Kenyan's on skin lightening is best described as ambivalent. There are Kenyan's who would like to see the country, as a whole, grow out of this 'phase' of considering dark skin to be somehow inferior.

"Why would you expose yourself to diseases all in the name of attracting the opposite sex?" asks Memusi Tira, an administrator at Film Aid. "I think it's a matter of self confidence – if you have an issue with your colour, check yourself rather than your colour!"

Mogiti says: it's easy to dismiss those who use the products as vain or having low self-esteem, but the truth of the matter is that light skin has been proven to have some benefits globally. In America, a study on prison inmates found that black prisoners with light skin typically received lighter sentences than darker skinned men who committed similar crimes. Meanwhile, in India parents looking to arrange marriages for their sons specifically search out light-skinned women, as do Afro-Arab families living in the Middle East.

The general preference for light is well established internationally right or wrong, but what makes it interesting in Kenya is that this is a country where the majority of the population is black, and there is still the idea of striving towards what is, essentially, whiteness.

Light skinned or dark skinned, Kenyans dissect every aspect of a woman's beauty routine; if she's in a weave, she is too Westernised, if her hair is kinky or nappy, she is not paying enough attention to her looks. From head to toe, from her make up to her choice in shoes, the Kenyan woman is always under scrutiny for how she balances Kenyan-ness and the Western beauty ideals that are being adopted here. And this is not going to change. Skin lightening has been a part of the Kenyan culture since the 60s, and it's most likely here to stay. What we have to decide is whether or not women should have to use chemical treatments to be able to look in the mirror to like what they see.

Media advertising greatly enhance the stereotypes that light skinned people are advantaged socially and romantically. An article on the web site **www.africana.com** said: "One Kenyan TV ad features a young woman staring lovingly at her boyfriend in a college cafeteria. Another pretty woman with slightly lighter skin walks by, upon which the man jokingly asks the girlfriend how he can tell the woman that she is the "most beautiful girl I have ever seen." Devastated, the young woman responds to a voiceover advising her to use "Fair and Lovely", a skin cream promising "special fairness vitamins" and guaranteed to lighten her complexion in just six weeks. The young woman uses the cream and, sure enough, keeps her man."

Market research in Kenya: Keny's backstreet# Bleachedbeauty trade

Unregulated clinics offering backstreet skin-bleaching injections have become increasingly popular with Kenyan women - a trend that health professionals find alarming.

Nairobi's River Road, a bustling area with a reputation for prostitution, black market goods and crime, has become a hub for illicit beauticians that provide these injections - often sitting outside their shops or booths hissing at passing women to attract customers.

- **Availability of banned items in Kenya**

River Road is a dusty, dingy business hub in Nairobi's downtown Central Business District (CBD). The street is busy and littered with plastic bags. This area is home to a number of products that are not necessarily legal, skin lighteners among them. Similar to an open-air market, shop owners call out to potential consumers, yelling **"Customer mafuta,"** referring to skin bleaching oils, creams and lotions that are available. To entice the passers-by even more, some of the models on the packages include celebrities like Beyoncé and Tamar Braxton. Amidst all the confusion and chaos that characterises the area, the stalls here specialise in body creams and lotions, and the shelves are fully stacked with rows and rows of the products, many of them, like the Clere labels that stare down from shelf after shelf, on the list of KEBS-banned products.

Shops elsewhere in Nairobi's CBD are no different, with the same illegal products being 'prescribed' by shop attendants. "Depending on the product, some may take a fortnight to a month for one to see results," says Wamuyu, one of these street experts. There are bleaching products that tone as well as lighten the skin, and everything she recommends claims to have sunscreen to protect users from UV rays. Interestingly, Wamuyu is insistent that I don't see a dermatologist. "You have flawless skin," she says, looking me [Josephine Mogiti] over. "So there is no need for seeking a dermatologist's opinion. You would only do so if you have problems like acne. Otherwise, you will just be throwing your money away for nothing." says Wamuyu.

- **The art of 'mixing' the skin lightening products and other observations.**

This art of **mixing** is important because of its relationship to the release of **Dioxane**— a veritable breast carcinogen. (See chapter 22).

Josephine Mogiti explores the scenes "Behind the Products." She writes:

Cindy, one of the stalls' attendants who looks to be in her late 20s, shows me how to **mix** the gels, creams and ointments that she says would be ideal for my skin type. She looks at me earnestly throughout her unhurried explanation, and when the step-by-step becomes overwhelming, she writes it down like a prescription. This is the norm on River Road. Shop assistants, having learnt the trade on the job, are not only billboards for their products – almost all of them using lighteners themselves – they also have an answer for everything, passing down conventional wisdom without any professional background or knowledge to base it on.

- **A dermatologist who is in the art of skin bleaching**

One of Nairobi's most reputable skin specialists, Dr. Pranav Pancholi of the Avane Cosmetic Clinic told the investigative journalist, "Products with safe agents like Morus Alba are a little bit pricey, but they are actually good, they are not going to cause problems with your skin," he says, adding that the price ranges between KSH 4,000 and KSH 15,000 (US $ 40-150). He's got a range of options on offer, including pills, injections and organics, but stresses the idea of 'good products', as all of these agents can be dangerous if used incorrectly or without the guidance of an actual professional.

- **Why the ban on products has been largely ineffective in Kenya**

On River Road the skin bleaching specialists hawk their goods sitting on stools in the street or standing in the doorways of their shops, some of which are just wooden booths rammed full of small colored boxes and creams. The more ramshackle beauty salons have gaudy hand painted signs, and sit sandwiched between seedy bars, DVD sellers, and starkly lit brothels. Others are slightly more upmarket, with large glass windows and neon signs. The sellers are all women and know how to hustle. They can be brash and aggressive, often standing outside and whispering and hissing at women who pass by to entice them into their shop.

When I first went to River Road and started to talk to people about taking photographs the sellers harassed me, asking me what I wanted, and even pushing me into a room where they could quiz me about what I was doing. They demanded over $500 to tell their story then kicked me out onto the street with dirty looks when I refused to pay it. Skin bleaching is a sensitive topic in a conservative and religious country like Kenya, and operating unlicensed salons that offer injections is against the law. It only survives though institutionalized bribery and if any of the skin bleachers get into trouble it's likely they'll need to make a hefty payout to avoid jail.[3]

Though medical professionals have serious concerns about the increasing popularity of the skin-bleaching injections, institutionalized corruption in Kenya's security forces means police are reluctant to intervene to stop the practice. Pancholi says skin bleachers operating on River Road make regular payments to the police, and a crackdown on their businesses is unlikely. "It is illegal for a non-medic to inject a client, but bribery allows the trade to continue,"[4,5]

- **Skin lightening creams used as injectables in Kenya**[1,3]

A worrying skin-lightening practice has emerged in Kenya and possibly some other African countries. There is a booming black market where creams that are intended for topical use are used as injectables by the wealthy Nairobi women for quicker action to lighten the skin because Kenyan men like women with whiter skin. The $70 (seventy US Dollars) treatment is so 'strong', it is said to be capable of turning a user into an 'albino.' The shots contain alpha hydroxy acids and mercury-containing creams.

Operating a small booth in the River Road area, Rose has worked in the skin-lightening business for more than five years. A range of skin-bleaching creams is displayed outside the booth. Rose also offers inside injections, but only to clients she trusts. She says injecting is considered taboo, but the process could lead to more effective results than other techniques.

"If you want an even colour and fast results, injecting is much better than a cream," says Rose, who gave only her first name fearing police arrest. "Some girls go back to their village and tell them the water of Nairobi made them lighter. There is great shame for wanting to change what God gave you."

Beauticians claim "the injections can make customers look six years younger and their skin a shocking ten shades lighter; and they are gaining particular popularity on Nairobi's River Road— a busy marked place notorious for its black market commerce and bribed law enforcement. Rose, a beautician, who does the injecting says "The injection lightens you from inside. It makes women clean." She says most of her clients are wealthy and some are national celebrities. Many are Somali or Indians. But, those ones never come to my shop. They send a driver with a photo of their skin color and I supply what they need:"

'Big money to make'[6,7]
Many of the products injected into River Road clients come from unregulated and imported materials from countries such as the Democratic Republic of Congo and China. Some list dangerous chemicals among their ingredients, including alpha hydroxyl acid (AHAs), a type of corrosive compound used in chemical peels.

"They promise the injection is safe, but it is not," say Dr Pranav Pancholi, a Harvard-trained dermatologist who works at Kenya's Shah Hospital. "The products are packaged and marketed to look attractive, but anything could be inside. Injecting products containing AHAs is abnormal. It can kill body tissue and serious infection."

Dr Adam Friedmann, a dermatologist at London's Harley Street dermatology Clinic, agrees that the increasing popularity of the injections is a worrying trend. "With bleaching creams from places like China and Africa there is no quality control. Bleaching creams contain dozens of chemicals, most of which are not labeled. Unregulated creams could–and often do–contain powerful steroids. They can cause thinning and skin damage." Friedmann says badly administered injections of unregulated substances could also result in HIV, Hepatitis C, TB, permanent disfigurement, inflammation or critical infection–but those seeking whiter skin continue to purchase them if they hear of short-term positive results by word of month. "People will take anything they think works," Friedman says. "In the beauty industry, you can only go by anecdotal evidence. The effectiveness of such products is often subjective… If people report positive results then the product sells. There is big money to be made if people are injecting such creams."

Is skin bleaching worth the cost in Kenya?
For most Kenyans their budget to pursue whiter skin is much lower than Sidika's, but spending on illicit backstreet treatments can still represent a serious investment in a country where UNICEF says more than half the population lives on less than $1 a day. It has been found that some of them sell sex to be able to purchase the products.

Rose charges $70 per shot and says the treatment can require a number of visits before results begin to show. The promise of whiter skin is worth the investment, according to one of Rose's clients, a woman in her mid-20s who also sells skin creams and gave her name as Mercy. She says she has been using lightening creams for a number of years and is trying the injections in an attempt to get more dramatic results. "My husband prefers half-caste woman to darker girls, and he is proud to be mine when we go to the club," she says. "I get far more male attention now I am lighter." Mercy cries cut out when the needle pricks her skin but after the injection she seems pleased that she went through with it. Grinning she gives shrug and says, "Nairobi is very competitive and Kenya men like women with whiter skin."

Research needs

The systemic effects of **injecting** Alpha hydroxy acid cosmetic products are unknown. There is need for animal studies to identify the possible adverse health effects of (i) injectable alpha hydroxy acid and (ii) injecting a mixture of glycolic acid mixed with mercury containing creams.

Some notable interventions in Kenya

What dermatologists have done in Kenya

Melanie Miyanji de Souza[8] a dermatologist in Nairobi Kenya, documented her experience in Kenya.

Dermatologist Dr Melanie Miyanji treats dozens of women of all ages who have abused skin lightening creams, and are now suffering the very visible consequences. She says the adverts are still giving the wrong message to Kenyan women. "The message that goes round is not right because when they talk of blemish-free skin they usually link it to lighter skin, or at least that's the way people look at it, so everyone tries to go for something lighter." The salient points are as follows:

Owing to the nature and medical and legal unacceptability of the practice, a lot of secrecy shrouds the production and sale of the merchandise.

Counterfeit and misbranded products abound.

Strict prescription products are readily given out by pharmacies on demand without prescription and sold in back streets

Some physicians are known to give out concoctions with no known formula of contained ingredients

Those with ill effects of bleaching products shy away from medical attention due to guilt complex or deny use of the products even when they consult physicians.

Analysis of substances and products for content of ingredients is costly and often an impossibility

Adverse health effects depend on the chemicals in the products used, the extent of use—localized or generalized—but most users use the products all ever the entire skin surface. Her guess is that products containing hydroquinone and corticosteroids are the most used.

Skin lightening is a time-consuming exercise because it is a daily ritual. She also listed the possible complications from chemical skin lightening

Melanie Miyanji de Souza concludes thus:
"After several years of grappling with this issue, against all odds, by educating the public and health workers, using the local and foreign media and trying to alert government authorities, we (dermatologists) have made headway. In May 2001, skin bleaching products were banned in Kenya. Other neighboring countries followed, and some are in the process of doing so. Some African countries impose fine and penalties for those found marketing or even using such products. Although this practice continues, it is to a much less extent. The good news is that many consumers are aware of what they purchase and use. Some who were victims of such a practice have visited physicians for help. This is a first important step for consumer safety. Law enforcement—proper surveillance and continued information to the consumer—is necessary to wipe out this scourge. The responsibility and challenge lies with dermatologists and other health workers.

Government ban of skin lightening product[1]

The Kenya Bureau of Standards banned several lotions, gels and soaps used for skin lightening that contained hydroquinone. Other African countries have done the same. This however does not necessarily stem the practice. The list of products is featured in APPENDIX. 12

Some other interventions against the skin lightening culture in Kenya

Campaigners want regulations to be tightened so that creams containing harmful substances already banned in the West do not appear in places like Kenya. Policing what is on sale in a market like Kenya's is a main problem. If a woman wants to lighten her skin, she could probably get what she needs

It is hoped that a group of girls taking part in the M-Net Face of Africa competition, who each dream of a career strutting the catwalks of Paris or Milan, will become the role models who could change attitudes. To win the competition, they need perfect skin. If they had been tempted to change their colour, they would probably not have been able to participate.

Intervention by Kenyan's film maker

WATCH: " Yellow Fever" by Ng'endo Mukii[9]

In this short thesis film, Kenyan filmmaker and recent graduate of the Royal College of Art, ***Ng'endo Mukii*** explores the globalization of beauty ideals and its impact on African women's self image. The trailer is only a little over one minute long, but the imagery and animation are immediately captivating and intensely beautiful. An observer said 'I have lived this scene too many times to count, and without even watching the film in its entirety, I understand exactly what Mukii describes as the "almost schizophrenicself-visualization" that she and many others have grown up with.'

Vera Sidika[10]

Vera Sidika, the supermodel dubbed "Kenya's Kim Kardashian", recently sparked a national debate when she unapologetically spoke out on national television about undergoing expensive skin-whitening treatment in the UK—saying she spent the equivalent of $170,000 on the transformation, which started the viral hashtag #BleachedBeauty on Twitter.

Vera has joined the long list of Celebs being criticized for using lightening cream— the likes of Cameroonian singer, Dencia, Cameroonian actress, Thelina O'khaz, Ghanaian actress, Yvonne Nelson and Nigeria bleaching expert, Pela Tonye. Vera sidika is sometimes dubbed "Kenya's Kim Kardashian, as-like Kardashian-she is famed for posting photos of her voluptuous backside on social media.

She gave an interview on Kenya TV in which she spoke openly about the skin lightening treatment she has recently undergone. "Looking good is my business." "My body is my business, nobody else's but mine. Change is good—if you do it the right way." She says she's already seen an increase in demand for her services. The response on Kenyan social media was huge. The interviewer—Larry Madodo, told BBC "I was accused of promoting or endorsing a white-centred view of beauty for African girls by interviewing her." She then decided to run a follow-up programme to discuss skin lightening, and encouraged people to share their thoughts using **#Bleaching beauty**. More than 4,000 people responded, and many of the comments have been damning. "# Bleacher Beauty is fake. Only those with low self-esteem would do that," (tweeted one). "# Bleached beauty ladies will soon begin bleaching their brains so they come up with bright ideas," (tweeted another). But others commenting on You Tube came to

Sidika's defense, praising her "openness and honesty" in speaking about the issue.

Larry Modowo describes the reaction on social media as "Fascinating," "astounding" and "hypocritical." Many men in Kenya do indeed prefer light-skinned women, he says — referring to them affectionately as "yellow, yellow." Dark-skinned women are sometimes derogatively called "tinted."

A little over two months since Vera over bleached, the effects have started being felt. Vera has since been in hiding because of shame as she now looks **ugly** and close to an Albino in skin tone. She has stopped posting update pictures of herself on Instagram, Facebook and Twitter but we were able (as usual) to get exclusive pictures of how Vera now looks:

Unlike in India where skin lightening creams are very common, in Kenya, skin lightening remains quite hush-hush, and is generally done in small backstreet venues. Experts believe it's on the rise, and warn of the dangers of unregulated black market treatments.

Orie Rogo Manduli, a former Miss Kenya and an advocate for women's rights, named Sidika "the most despicable woman we have ever had in this country," and called for media blackout on her activities to "protect our young girls from her bad influence and misguided ways." Sidika responded by saying she should be respected as a self-made woman from a poor background. "It is the society that is promoting the skin lightening or bleaching." She says. "When you… walk into modeling agencies, the girls there who get picked up for jobs are usually fair skinned." She also scorned the backstreet treatments offered on River Road, saying the practitioners there were offering low quality "skin bleaching" that could harm."

See the story of Vera Sidika under "CELEBRITY DISCOURSE."– Chapter 6.

References

1. Josephine Mogiti. SKIN DEEP. Destination Magazine. *http://www.eadestination.com/investigative-journalism/467-skin-deep 6/3/2015*

2.Banned Skin Bleaching/Skin Whitening products. *http://www.whiterskin.com/banned-skin-bleaching.html*

3. Annabel Fenwick Elliot. Kenyan men like women with whiter skin: The rise of wealthy Nairobi women illegally injecting themselves with skin-lightening creams. *http://www.dailymail.co.uk/femail/article-2650766/kenyan-men-like-women-whiter-skin-The-rise-wealthy-Nairobi-women-illegal-INJECTING-skin-lightening-creams.html*

4. Celeste Hibbert and Wil crips. Rich Kenyns are injecting themselves with black market creams to become white. *http://www.vice.com/read/rich-kenyans-bleach-their-skin-whiter*

5. Celeste Hibbert/AI Jazzera. Kenya's backstreet# BleachedBeauty trade. Nairobi has become a haven for toxic skin-lightening treatments such as those used by model Vera Sidika. *http.www/Aljazeera.com/indepth/features/2014/06/Kenya-backstreet-bleachedbeauty-trade-20146231346838141 7.html.*

6. Catty Jenkins Fighting against skin lightening. *BBC News AFRICAN/* Friday, 12 January, 2001. *http://news.bbc.co.uk/2/hi/africa/114088.stm*

7. Kay Motano. The fairest of them all: Dija Ayodele on the culture of skin-bleaching. *THANDIEKAY http://thandiekay.com/2014/07/31/the-fairest-of-them-all-dija-ayodele*

8. de Souza Miyanji Melanie. The concept of skin bleaching Africa and its devastating health implications. *Clinic in Dermatology*. 2008; 26:27-29

9. Ng'endo Mukii WATCH: "*Yellow Fever*" *by Ng'endo Mukii. http://yabablay.com/yellow-fever-by-ngendo-mulkii/*

10. BBC Trending #BBCtrending: Is Kenya's Vera Sidika a # Bleached Beauty? 10 June 2014. http://www.bbc.com/news/blogs-trending-27768032

TANZANIA

Concocted skin bleaching products are called "mkorongo" in East Africa.Tanzania, the largest geographic East African country—is the main hub where empirical research has taken place on the skin bleaching culture. Harada *et al* identified high mercury levels in head hair from a total of 14 subjects who resided around Lake Victoria, Tanzania. The researchers attributed this finding to the habitual use of toilet soap containing considerable amounts of mercury.[1,2] Lewis Kelley et al[3] examined the historical and cultural influence of skin bleaching in Tanzania. The authors acknowledge that the bleaching culture is problematic because users, especially women combine dangerous caustic agents (automotive battery acid, washing powder, toothpaste, cloth bleaching agents) with common bleaching products that are high in mercury and lead; together these increase the risk for severe health problems, such as irreversible skin damage, skin cancer, leukemia, and liver or kidney failure. Despite these great risks, skin bleaching is prevalent in Africa, with estimated rates nearing 30% in East Africa.

Little research has examined how the historical legacies of slavery, colonization, and westernization in East Africa may have shaped internalized dominant cultural ideals, resulting in the dangerous practice of skin bleaching. The authors took an exploratory look at the institutions of slavery, colonization, westernization, and neocolonialism in East Africa and argue that these institutions may have placed Tanzanians in a colour-conscious society. This also may have fueled potent skin-color ideals that have resulted in efforts to assimilate to dominating groups.

In their attempt to understand the demography of skin bleachers in Tanzania, Lewis et al[4] found several common characteristics among users. Findings suggest users are typically older (20+ years), higher income earners, married, and from the southwest region of Tanzania (a higher income-earning region due to tourism, and with increased access to manufactured mercury skin-bleaching products due to gold and copper-lead mines. Lewis et al also found that skin bleachers in Tanzania have higher internalized Eurocentric standards of beauty as well as political affiliations with the Civic United Front party (CUF) – a nationally based liberal political party that is heavily represented by Zanzibaris of mixed ancestry. Lewis et al argue that individuals possessing these common characteristics, likely have greater access to resources such as higher quantities of more potent skin-bleaching creams and possess more widespread idealized beliefs that lighter skin is better than darker skin, possibly due to influences of westernization and neocolonialism on subordinate groups.

In one Tanzanian study[5] women claimed Tanzania men preferred white, soft-skinned girls. Thus, skin-lightening was of utmost importance in attracting men. And once you've got a guy, you want to hang on to him. Another woman in the study explained that she used skin-lightening products to prevent her husband from being attracted to other girls, while yet another, a 25 years old, reported that she "started bleaching to be beautiful and to look like Arabians or Europeans and attractive to people, especially men. We are all competing for mates, and we do whatever we can to give ourselves an advantage over the next person. Men would probably be content to live in caves if they didn't have to acquire the trappings necessary to compete for the most desirable woman, and there would be less incentive for women to lighten their skin if men didn't keep valuing lighter skinned sisters over darker skinned ones."

The women in the study also said they lightened their skin to enhance opportunities in life (especially job opportunities), and to reduce the experience of negative stereotypes that are applied to dark skinned people. The negative stereotypes call to mind the associations with skin colour drawn out from black American kids by black American film maker Kiri Davis when she recreated the 1940's "doll experiment" a few years ago in ***A Girl Like Me***. In the Tanzania study many participants felt that their lighter skinned peers have higher status, income, education, job opportunities, as well as more friends. These women are not deluded; misguided, definitely, but not deluded. They see the evidence around them. It is not surprising then that some "darker" skinned people are often envious of those with lighter skin and attempt to achieve the same status by engaging in skin-lightening practices.

Lewis et al found that there are six key motivations behind why Tanzanians bleach their skin: (1) to remove pimples, rashes, and skin diseases; (2) to have a soft skin (3) to be white, "beautiful," and look more Europeans; (4) to remove the adverse affects of extended skin bleaching use on the body; (5) to satisfy one's partner or attract male mates; and (6) enhance job opportunities, status and income.

The few interventions implemented to prevent skin bleaching in Tanzania show marginal success in decreasing these numbers.[6] A study was conducted which took steps to identify the most effective means of prevention for a Tanzanian community where skin bleaching practices are prevalent. A team of 20 Tanzanians worked toward this goal using participatory research techniques. Results yielded components for the structure of an ideal intervention program, including (a) didactic education, (b) governmental action, and (c) educational media.[7]

References

1. Harada Masazumi, Nakachi Shigeharu, Cheu Taketo *et al.* Monitoring of mercury pollution in Tanzania: relation between head hair mercury and health. *Science of the Total Environment.* March 9, 1999; 227 (2-3)

2. Glahder CM, Appel PWU, Asmund G. *Mercury in Soap in Tanzania.* Copenhagen, Ministry of Environment and Energy. National Environment Research Institute (NERI) Denmark Technical Repot No 306; 1999, p19. http://www.2.dm.dk/1_viden/2_publicationer/3_fgrapporter/rapporter/fr306.pdf)

3. Lewis KM, Harris S, Camp C, Kalala W *et al.* The historical and cultural influences of skin bleaching in Tanzania. In: The Melanin Millennium: Skin Color as 21st Century International Discourse. Publisher Springer Netherlands 2013 pp 19-38

4. Lewis KM, Younge S, Njoku LC, Andrews E & Young L. The case of skin bleaching in Tanzania: who does it? *International Journal of Africana studies* 2010; 15(2):1-18

5. Lewis KM, Robkin N, Gaska K, Njoku L. Investigating motivations for women's skin bleaching in Tanzania. *Psychology of women Quarterly* 2011; 35 (1):29-37.

6. Lewis KM, Robkin N, Gaska K, Njoku LC, Andrews E and Jetha K. The Tanzania reponse to dangerous skin bleaching products and the gendered politics

involved: A critical analysis. *Jenda: Journal of Culture and Africa Women Studies.* 2009; 10, 18-35.
7. Lewis KM. The need for interventions to prevent skin bleaching. A look at Tanzania. http://jbs.sagepub.com/content/43/7/786.abstract

UK made mercury containing soaps and creams. Studies in Tanzania and Kenya

During a pilot project in Tanzania,[1] financed by RUF under the Danish Ministry of Foreign Affairs, the Danish participants discovered that mercury-bearing soaps and creams manufactured in the United Kingdom were illegally smuggled into the country and sold on the markets in towns and villages. These products are claimed to be antiseptic, but the real purpose of using them is to obtain paler skin and hair. At the market in Mpanda in western Tanzania on 27 September, 1999, three different brands of soap were bought and two types of cream were bought for analysis. The trade names and producers, as well as the country in which the products are manufactured, are listed in Table 1. All the products were analysed for mercury at NERI, Dept of Arctic Environment.

Table 9.1. Soaps and creams purchased at the Tanzanian market.

Product	Trade name	Declaration	Producer	Country
Soap 1	Rico	2% Hg iodide	Rico Skin Care Ltd.	United Kingdom
Soap 2	Jaribu	2% Hg iodide	Anglo Fabrics (Bolton) Ltd.	United Kingdom
Soap 3	Jambo	2% Hg iodide	Jambo	United Kingdom
Cream 4	Movate	Hydroquinone	Pramil srl Melzo (Milano)	Italy
Cream 5	Dear Heart	Hydroquinone	Cosmetic Expression Ltd.	United Kingdom

In Tanzania, import of these products is forbidden.[2,3] In spite of these restrictions, soap and cream containing mercury is manufactured in European countries, mainly the UK, and sold as antiseptic soap to Third World countries. These products are also sold in areas of Europe that have a substantial black population, such as London and Brussels. This indicates that the UK-produced soap containing mercury is exported to Third World countries, and then re-imported to the UK and Belgium. WHO[4] reports that these soaps contain in the order of 1 to 3% mercury iodide. Creams meant for bleaching the skin often contain 1 to 10% mercuryammonium. The soap and cream is meant to be applied to the skin, then left to dry and left on overnight.

Mercury in users of soaps and creams

Mercury from soap and cream enter the body through the skin and via inhalation. The following studies are derived from WHO.[4] A group of 60 women from Kenya, who had used cream containing 5 to 10% ammoniated mercury, had an average of 0.1 mg mercury per litre of urine, and 26 of these women had an average of 0.15 mg mercury per litre of urine. The latter group had developed the nephrotic syndrome (renal diseases). Another study showed that a group of 6 women, who had used cream with 1 to 3 % ammoniated mercury had 0.03 to 0.6 mg mercury per litre of urine.

A study carried out in Tanzania amongst gold miners and people not employed in gold mining or amalgamation showed that some women, who were not active in gold mining or amalgamation, had up to 0.1 mg mercury per litre of urine, and it was concluded that the mercury was derived from soap and cream containing mercury.

The mercury levels in human bodies can be measured by analyzing samples of hair. Kahatano *et al.*[3] found that 5 out of 9 women had an average of 244 mg mercury per kg hair (range 20 to 490 mg per kg), whereas the remaining 21 persons in the study had on average 2.3 mg mercury per kg hair. The very high mercury contents were ascribed to usage of soap and cream containing mercury.

Reports of renal problems due to mercury in skin bleaching products in Nairobi

The use of skin lightening products has been associated with serious complications such as renal disease in Nairobi.[5] Barr *et al* reported that adult nephrotic syndrome in Nairobi is predominantly encountered in young sophisticated African women, most of whom began to use skin-lightening creams containing mercury before the symptomatic onset of their illness. The particular form of mercury involved is well known to cause the nephrotic syndrome in other circumstances—for example, when applied to the skin in the treatment of psoriasis.

Harada et al[6] studied the mercury levels in head hair of residents around lake Victoria, Tanzania. They found high levels of mercury in the head hair. They speculated that this might be attributable to the habitual use of toilet soap containing considerable amounts of mercury. A similar study was replicated in Kenya among residents around Lake Victoria. A total of nine goldminers, 44 fishermen and their families, and 12 residents of Kisumu city, Kenya, volunteered for the study. Fourteen types of toilet soap were collected in Kisumu. The total mercury levels in the soaps ranged from 0.41-6.2%. All the subjects with high hair mercury level (>36.1ppm) had habitually used the mercury containing soaps. They also had various manifestations of mercury poisoning such as lassitude, vertigo, neurasthenia and black and white blots.

Now that Kenya women have started to **inject** themselves with mercury containing creams, one can only imagine what is happening to the kidneys of Kenya women. (See the section on KENYA above).

Conclusion and recommendations

Several studies have shown that women using soap and cream containing mercury attain mercury concentrations in their urine from 0.03 to 0.15 mg per litre. At these concentrations, there is a major risk of negative effects on their central nervous system and kidneys, since such effects have been demonstrated at concentrations from 0.02 to 0.5 mg per litre. In one study, women with an average urine mercury concentration of 0.15 mg per litre had developed kidney diseases. In a study of mercury in hair, five women had average mercury contents exceeding the threshold for an acute risk of poisoning, which is 50 mg mercury per kg hair (Appendix 13). The high mercury contents in their hair were ascribed to their use of soaps and creams with mercury.

The remainder of the mercury in the soap and cream goes with the waste water into the environment where it enters the food chain and returns in methylated form via fish to humans. Methylmercury therefore is efficiently transferred to unborn babies, and affects their mental abilities.

There are, therefore, many reasons for banning mercury-containing soaps and creams, which are manufactured and sold under the presumption of being antiseptic, although the real purpose is to bleach human hair and skin. In spite of this ban, these products can be bought in Tanzania, other African countries and some countries in Europe. In Tanzania, import of these products is forbidden. However, it is very difficult to prevent illegal import, and large amounts of soaps and creams are apparently smuggled into Tanzania. The most efficient way to restrict the use of these soaps and creams is to control their manufacture, most of which are located in Europe, and especially in the UK. In EEC the use of mercury in cosmetics is legal only in eye makeup cleansing products containing max. 0.07 % phenylmercury salts, whereas the manufacture of mercury-containing soaps and creams is not illegal. Inorganic mercury compounds are listed in the PIC (Prior Informed Consent) Convention (UNEP/FAO) for certain hazardous chemicals in international trade, but refers to pesticide use only (Danish Environmental Protection Agency, pers. comm.). Despite the fact that the manufacture of mercury-containing products is not illegal in EEC, we find it immoral that companies within the EEC exploit Third World countries by producing and exporting these products, which pose serious health hazards to mankind and are very toxic to the environment.

References

1. Glahder C, Asmund G. preliminary results from a pilot project on artisanal gold mining in Tanzania in 1999. *National Environmental Research Institute/Geological Survey of Denmark and Greenland.* 1999.

2. Glahder Christian M, Appel Peter Will and Asmund Gert. Mercury in Soap in Tanzania. *NERI Technical Report No* 306. 1999. *http://www2.dmu.dk/1_viden/2_publikationer/3_fagrapporter/rapporter/fr306.pdf*

3. Kahatano, JMJ, Mnali, SR, and Akagi H. A Study of Mercury Levels in Fish and Humans in Mwakitolyo Mine and Mwanza Town in the Lake Victoria Goldfields, Tanzania. - In: Lars Landner (ed.): Small–Scale Mining in African Countries. *Proceedings of an International Conference/Workshop* 29th September – 1st October. 1997 Dar es Salaam, Tanzania. 1998

4. WHO. Environmental Health Criteria 118. Inorganic Mercury. – World Health Organisation, Geneva. 1998

5. Barr RD, Rees PH, Cord PE, Kungu A, Woodger BA, Cameron HM. Neprorotic syndrome in adult Africans in Nairobi. *Brit Med J.* 1972; Apr 15: (5806): 131-4

6. Harada M, Nakachi S, Tasaka K *et al.* Wide use of skin-lightening soap may cause mercury poisoning in Kenya. *The science of the Total Environment* 2001, 269: 183-7

UGANDA

Halimah Kisule[1], a journalist in northern Uganda gave a most valuable insight into the skin bleaching culture in Uganda. Scores of Ugandans continue to bleach their skin despite a government ban on the sale of several lotions, creams, gels and soaps which are largely used to whiten and even tone the skin. Due to ineffective enforcement of the ban, these dangerous cosmetics are easily accessible anywhere in Uganda; whether sold over the counter, along the roadside or by hawkers, vendors move the skin lighteners easily due to high demand. Such is the popularity that skin-whitening products have gained today in Uganda. In Uganda, the practice of skin bleaching is common among adults with dark skin, especially women, but men also do it with little regard for the dangers posed to their bodies. Some people even use the products for anal bleaching to reduce naturally darker pigmentation of the genital and perineal area.

The Uganda National Bureau of standards and National Drugs Authority has tried to crack down on bleaching cosmetics, but their efforts have not been successful. The trend is actually going up though still 'hush hush' among the public. Ugandan celebrities have been known to bleach their skins from way back. The bleaching trend has actually shot up over the years as homemade cosmetic and dermatological products have become easily accessible. In spite of a ban on bleaching products, they are continuously being smuggled in.

Observed adverse effects.

Consumers of bleaching cosmetics claim that they want to enhance their beauty. One woman who declined to be named, explains, "One has to look good, by having fair, lighter skin."

Unfortunately, her skin is now multi-colored from bleaching. She has red skin on her face, yellow on her arms and dark skin on her back. The skin on her knees, toes and finger joints failed to lighten and remain black.

For this woman, the condition of her skin has only brought her shame; she now tries to cover most parts of her body in an attempt to conceal the damage done by the products she thought would enhance her beauty. Those in the medical profession explain that this condition occurs from allergic dermatitis or irritant dermatitis (abnormal, extensive and often local inflammation of the skin).

"I have cases where people get severe skin burns. Says Dr. Misaki Wayengera of Makerere University Medical School. He explains that the skin of the people using these bleaching products get inflamed, turns red, enlarges and begins to loose function as the cells fail to produce melanin. Wayengera says that bleaching can be achieved medically using low dosage hydroquinone, recommended at 2%. He advises that it should be used only in the areas of the skin that need to be lightened. He also advised consumers to always read the contents of cosmetics because those that bleach cause health problems like skin cancer, leukemia, thyroid disorders and delay or prevent the ability to diagnose leprosy. Mercury is the most toxic of these ingredients and leads to liver and kidney problems.

Prolonged use of bleaching cosmetics can indeed be disastrous both psychologically and physically. Halimah Kisule encountered one lady on the street who declined to be named nor talk about her skin. Her dry, pale face showed no happiness. She had wrinkles too - not from old age, but from the effects of starting and then stopping the use of these cosmetics. Halimah Kisule could easily read the disappointment in her face when she asked her to talk about her skin. Her response is a clear testimony to the negative effects of bleaching cosmetics and hint at the lengths some will go to for beauty. Her unhappiness is the other side of beauty that we rarely see, but one that can easily be avoided.

Barr et al[2] described Nephrotic syndrome in adult Africans in Nairobi who had used mercury-containing skin-lightening creams. Among the patients studied, skin lightening creams seemed to be particularly associated with a minimal-change (light-negative") renal glomerular lesian present in half of the patients using the cream. The prognosis in this group of patients seems remarkably good, with 50% entering remission, 77% of these doing so spontaneously on discontinuing the use of the creams. This finding corroborates the finding of the experimental studies of Gras in Senegal[3]. Karamagi et al[4] reported a case of hydroquinone neuropathy in Uganda following use of skin bleaching creams.

Though the East African Custom Management Act of 2006 banned the import of all soaps containing mercury, products like Mekako soaps are readily available in the country having been smuggled in before being re-exported to neighboring Kenya, Tanzania and Rwanda. "They are smuggled in jerricans disguised as water while others come in through ordinary containers but are declared as cosmetics, when [in reality] they are drugs that fall under the NDA mandate," says Gyavira Musoke, Head of Imports Inspection at Uganda's National Bureau of Standards (UNBS).

UNBS says that Kenya is blaming Uganda for failing to stop the importation of this toxic cosmetic despite the existence of the law. This is just one of the 400 prohibited cosmetic ingredients (that are defined as drugs under the Uganda National Drug Authority (NDA) regulations) that are on the open market. Products containing hydroquinone are still for sale after traders asked the Ministry of Tourism to give them some time to sell off their stock.

Ready markets for these highly valued cosmetics suggest that smuggling won't stop any time soon, but demand alone does not explain why one would continue to use these dangerous products. "Such a person lacks self-esteem, has low self-efficacy and a perception that she or he looks ugly," says Mr Robert Wandera, Coordinator of the Psychology Department at Makerere University. "It is common among women who are not educated," he adds. Wandera's colleague, Mr Calistas, says that it is very dangerous to have low self-esteem because severe cases can lead to suicide. He urges, "Do something positive to counter [your low self-esteem]. Take advantage of the good parts of your body or talents."

Responses

- *Nancy Vining Van Ness* says: Halimah, your article revealed to me a new area of concern for women, and some men, who are affected by unreal standards of beauty. I did not realize that the need to conform to unnatural standards was such a pleaque in Africa, but I ought to have guessed. It isn't only uneducated women who are the most susceptible to things that will make them look like the unreal standard that is put before them. Highly educated women in the US spend billions of dollars on cosmetics and surgery to make themselves conform to the look that the global corporate media tell us is desirable.
- *Aralena Leroy* says: It is a shame that women around the world continue to put their health at risk to meet someone else's standard of beauty. The media bombards us from day one with the message that we will never be good enough until we've applied their anti-wrinkle cream, gone under the knife, been jabbed with Botox needles, starved ourselves weak, and spent half of our income on their—largely useless products. It's a great way to get our minds off politics and the economy, though, isn't it? With women dedicating so much time to eliminating cellulite, they won't have time to worry about where their tax dollars are being invested… Aralena leroy astutely points out the seduction of the media as it relates to our collective self-worth. Ironically, many women of European descent have invested their money in cultivating African features (full lips, large hips, round ass, voluptuous breasts, i.e.) once considered savage yet now are deemed 'popular' in the lucrative fashion industry.

Marcus garvey once said, "people who don't know their history are doomed to repeat it." Beauty is not in the eye of the beholder; beauty is a biological inheritance – yet women of African descent must learn to affirm the divine within. Loving ourselves and each other in our own image is a good place to start.

- *Mjtlove* says: the truth is dark-skinned men and women of African descent continue to suffer the legacy of white world supremacy. The desire to bleach one's skin is similar to the obsession to lose weight: a racist society devalues women of african descent and market women of European descent as beautiful, intelligent and powerful.

- *Suad Hamada* says: The upbringing of children is important in enhancing the confidence of individuals, as children should be raised to love their look and color of their skin by teaching them to love themselves and others by their personalities and not how they look.
- *Yakinican* says: I'm white, I don't like my skin tone, I love to tan and make it darker. If I like to make my skin darker I have no problem with black people trying to make their skin lighter. To me its' just personal preference. Its' just like some of the thousands and thousands of people who do plastic sugery to have breast implants or facial restructures they want to look the way they want to and if its' what makes them happy I am happy for them as well.

References

1. Kisule Halima Abdallah. Skin bleaching thrives despite Ugandan government Ban on dangerous cosmetics. August 12, 2008. THE WIP. http://thewipeinent/2008/08/12/skin-bleaching-thrives-despite-ugandan-...
2. Barr RD, Rees PH, Cordy PE et al. Nephrotic syndrome in adult Africans is Nairobi *Br Med J* 1972; 2:131- 4
3. Gras G, Mondain J. The problem of the use of mercurials cosmetics in Senegal. *Toxicol Eur Res* 1981 July, 3(4) :175- 8.
4. Karamagi C, Owino E and Katabira ET. Hydroquinone Neuropathy following use of skin bleaching creams: case report *East Africa Medical Journal.* 2001; 78(4): 223-4

SUDAN

The identity of Southern Sudan

Deng Aling[1] says: It's hard to claim that South Sudanese culture is Arab or African in a globalized world where it is very difficult to claim cultural uniqueness as a group, let alone a group such as South Sudan which blended with the North for more than a decade. Speaking about culture, many claimed that Sudan is an Arabo-Islamic country, thus the culture is associated with the Arabs. Southern writers refuted these claims, calling for the Africanization of Sudan. Affiliation to Islam and speaking in Arabic doesn't change a person's identity and does not necessarily mean being Arab. Dr Dhieu Wol[2] thinks that the Southern identity is certainly African; being part of Sudan and speaking Arabic does not mean the Southerners are Arabs.

The history of Arabization and Islamization of Sudan remains a complex process of local interactions and external links with Egypt. The South was not spared from these intimate interactions of Arabo-Islamic cultures with African ones. The identity discussion on whether Sudan was Arab or African came to an end after the secession of the south. The Southern identity resistance began in Sudan before the

Egyptian—British colonialism when the South was a hotbed of slave trade. The resistance continued on during the colonial period, regardless of Gordon's futile efforts to ban the trade.

Although communication between the North and South has continued until today, many writers propose that Southern Sudanese culture has now become purely African after separation from North. Today's world is moving towards acculturation, where cultures blend together freely. This is what Jürgen Habermas calls the "inclusion of the others,"[3] where we build relations with another which is completely different than us, but the result of this relationship is valuable. Thus, it becomes difficult to refer to the Southern culture as definitely Arab or wholeheartedly African. The culture of South Sudan isn't purely Arab, or purely African, it is a humanistic culture that absorbed values from cultures to its East and West.

References

1. Deng Aling. Exploring the identity of Sudanese culture. Is it Arabic or African? *THIS IS AFRICA. http://thisisafrica.me/1613-2/* February 16, 2016.

2. Dhieu Wol. *Politics of Ethnic Discrimination in Sudan: A Justification for the Secession of South Sudan.* LAP LAMBERT Academic Publishing (December 14, 2010) ISBN-10: 3843369305, ISBN-13: 978-3843369305.

3. Jürgen Habermas *The Inclusion of the Other.* Studies in Political Theory. Edited by Ciaran P. Cronin and Pablo De Greiff 1988.

Colorism in Sudan

A popular phrase in Sudan is *al-Husnu ahmar* (beauty is red). Whiteness is the ideal color in most Arab societies. The second ranking is *asmar* (light tan), followed by *dhahabi* (golden), *Gamhi* (wheatish), *Khamri* (the color of wine), *akhdar* (light black/green). *Akhdhar* is used as a polite alternative to 'black' in describing the color of a dark-skinned Arab. Last and least is *azraq*, Literally "blue', used interchangeable with aswad to mean "black" – although in the past it referred to whiteness or light skin[1].

Motives for bleaching in Sudan

Nyabouy Gatbet[2] writes about skin bleaching and the south Sudanese community. Nyabouy is a south Sudanese Ethiopian-Canadian, poet, model, human right activist, and a university student in Canada. She writes: "There is a huge epidemic of skin bleaching in South Sudan, and that it seems the women are so insecure to go as far as using chemicals to abolish any trace of south Sudanese in them." She admits that everyone is entitled to their own life path and choices. She is compelled to comment on the matter because she has people in her community who are using skin lightening excessively without knowing the hazards associated with skin bleaching. She is saddened because of the negative message the bleachers are sending to the young women like the writer, because the bleachers are basically saying without lighter skin you are worth nothing. The subliminal message is with lighter skin you'll have a better life

Nyabouy says **"Some women bleach for beauty'** – If you are bleaching because you want to attract a better husband or boy friend you need to evaluate yourself. A man that is in love with your complexion and not your real you the relationship is doomed. A man that can easily be attracted by your beauty and stay because of your beauty is not a real man in my opinion. A man should love and be with you because of your brain and substantial character. Any man that supports his woman skin bleaching has some inner inferiority complex he needs to deal with. Because your partner is a reflection of who you are; and your partner mirrors everything you are. It is wrong for a person to bleach for love. The only love you can attract with fake skin is conditional love because those men aren't there because they care for you. If they truly care for you they make you stop bleaching because the long term effect of skin bleaching is cancer. It's common sense you are using chemicals to kill the natural melanin and pigmentation to achieve a man-made skin.

Some women bleaching for acceptance – Most of the south Sudanese women are skin bleaching because they want to be accepted by everyone in the society. They see lighter skinned women get all the attention while they are abandoned. They become color struck and envious of their lighter skinned female counterparts because they perceived them as having an easier life compared to them. These women's lives are based on their skin tones. They make limitations based on the color of their skin. They understand that with certain skin tones comes certain attention. Most of these women never received any male attention or any attention from people prior to skin bleaching. With their man-made skin they become who they always aspire to be—a lighter skinned version of themselves. As if they have transitioned from darkness to light. Now they live in the spot light

She then listed the symptoms of mercury toxicity as irritability, headaches, difficulty concentrating, forgetfulness, memory loss, numbness, tingling in the hands, feet or around the lips, insomnia depression and weight loss. Furthermore, mercury can have serious health consequences. It can damage the kidneys, and the nervous system, and interfere with the development of the brain in unborn children and very young children, as stated by Dr Charles Lee. Nyabouy also listed the side effects of the corticosteroid. The most serious is Cushing's syndrome—a malfunction of the adrenal glands leading to an over production of cortisol. Other side effects include increased appetite and weight gain, deposits of fat in chest, face, upper back, and stomach, swelling, slow healing of wounds, osteoporosis, cataracts, acne, muscle weakness and thinning of the skin.

She cautioned "To avoid unknowingly using harmful skin care products, never use unmarked products, including unmarked products that are given to you by friends, family or acquaintances or purchased at flea markets, swap meets or small unofficial beauty stores. If the product does not have an ingredient list, don't use it. If you have used any products that fit this description, it is important to know the signs of mercury toxicity

As you see bleaching your skin presents more risks than advantages. The sad thing in this culture is when you want to remain natural and love your skin you are seen as a radical woman instead of a woman who is proud of whom she is. To be happy with whom God made you to be seem so odd to this generation. If it is rebellious to maintain my dignity and a sense of myself so let it be. I won't let society pick at my wounds or through salt to benefit at my expense. To be proud of who you are is a rare thing, yet a very rebellious thing in a society where people behave like sheep waiting on their shepherd to tell them what to do. If you are the type of person who follows your own path—congratulations! You are a rare gem in a world full of stones. If you are a type of person who loves to be true to themselves, stay true to yourself because that's all you have in a world that tries to dictate everything.

Reem Abbas[3] published an article titled **"In search of beauty: Sudanese women throwing caution to the winds"**. In Sudan, lighter skin is considered prettier and a sign of being enlightened. To keep men interested, most women will do anything, even when the dangers are obvious. Skin lightening creams, some of which have had corrosive effects on many skins, often become their option. The costs are not very friendly to all, but due to their demand, skin lighteners are well stocked in different sizes for the different market segments.

"We have been told from an early age, in our folktales, that as women, we have to be beautiful," says Hadia Hasaballah, a Gender and Women's Studies professor at Ahfad University for Women. "The standards of beauty now are light-skin and long hair." Sudan is a country divided between a number of dominant ethnic groups, a few of whom have a lighter-complexion. For a long time, the dominant groups have looked to the lighter north, that is Egypt and the rest of North Africa for beauty inspiration. With that comes the colour complex. On the streets of Khartoum, women are busy. There is a crowded shop on street 40 in the capital that understands women and their skin complexes. Here, they can buy a spoon or a jar full of skin-lightening creams depending on their financial ability. And this in not a new trend because skin-lightening is an age-old tradition for Sudanese women, but the methods used have now shifted from natural to chemical. For years, Sudanese women resorted to scrubs made out of orange, yoghurt and natural products to change their skin. Now, with the media setting the standards for beauty by portraying light-skin presenters as hot, Sudanese women are opting for instant options. The marginalized groups of Western Sudan and the new south, on the other hand, look up to the image of the lighter-skin Sudanese.

It is not so simple, says Hasaballah who has carried out research on skin-lightening creams. "War caused displacement that sent waves of people to urban areas where they were introduced to new colours and new standards of beauty that Sudanese had to live up," she says, but adds that even the educated middle-class girls bleach their skins excessively. "***They want to get married because they are born to think that this is their traditional role; to be wives and mothers***," she says.

Chemicals used and health implications

Sudanese began grasping the dangers of this trend when a popular male musician died of kidney failure a few years ago, reportedly after applying a bleaching cream. Gadoora's death sparked a lot of debates, but not enough to ban creams containing harmful chemicals like mercury and hydroquinone. "Mercury causes kidney problems and hydroquinone causes diabetes, hyper-tension and high blood pressure if used in large doses," explains Maha El-Taher, a dermatologist. A spot-check around Khartoum confirmed fears that many shops sell skin-bleaching creams without knowledge of the chemicals they contain. "In some case, they know that they are selling chemicals that are illegal," added Dr El-Taher who has been advising her patients to avoid applying the creams. One of the most commonly used creams in Sudan are Rose and Diana, which have been blacklisted elsewhere because they contain mercury. Products containing the chemical have been banned in many countries after Europe did it in 1976. A pharmacist who worked in East Sudan, Doha Atta says that most girls look for low-quality creams. "Most girls ask for the pills. They act faster," says Atta. "Some of my friends have suffered many skin damages because of using such creams, I strongly advised them to stop," says Esam, a beauty conscious lady based in Khartoum.

Skin bleaching, women, morality and national character in Juba

Skin bleachers are "internally displaced"[4]. Anyone who has looked closely at non-European skin products knows that skin bleaching is a serious industry in Sudan. The international issues of race, racism and beauty standards must be addressed in any discussion of skin lightening and aspirations to white skin. It is hard to buy a soap, face cream or anti-acne product here in Juba that does not contain skin lightening agents.

The skin lightening trend in Juba is catching on, particularly among young women, and public opinion has been hot to condemn these girls for their vanity and apparent self-destruction. In October, 24 2012, female students were suspended at Juba Day Secondary for skin bleaching – some of whom said that they didn't realize the acne creams they were using were skin lighteners. Another 7 female students were suspended from Comboni Secondary School at the same time. More recently, a man in Godele was reported to have divorced his wife because of her habitual skin bleaching. "I will not accept [my wife] again in my home as housewife, because she broke both my order and culture." But, the wife said when she visited Khartoum, she found all her former school mates who went to Khartoum have changed their color from black to brown, and then she was forced to do the same to win the love from her husband.

However, what is frustrating—although interesting—is that the local discussion of this, in newspapers and on the radio, has centred around two targets: the usual condemnation of women's sexuality and vanity, and more interestingly, the idea of this practice undermining national culture and character. Skin bleaching is not part of South Sudanese culture, according to all the commentators; women here are supposed to be black. How black, though, is at issue. In the recent beauty pageants here (Miss Malaika and Miss South Sudan, working in competition), there were the usual Equatoria-Nilotic tensions that centred repeatedly around the preferred skin tones of the female contestants; many Equatorians felt that a Dinka or Nuer woman would win because extremely black skin is seen as 'properly' South Sudanese. However, lighter skin tones are more popularly understood as 'better', particularly among those returning from Khartoum and East Africa.

This debate over the right skin colour to have to be South Sudanese is a tiny part of the wider tensions created by East African returnees, ex-Khartoum residents, and the broader tension between the 'browner' Equatorians and 'black' Nilotic-origin people; women continue to reflect – painfully – the cultural and political narratives of national identity.

Sara Elhassan[5], writing under the title "**Women in Sudan: What the 'ugly' debate tells us about society"** describes how her response to a TV program created a storm which clearly depicts women in Sudanese culture as people to be seen but not heard.

She said it all began when she saw a video clip from a program aired on Blue Nile TV, a Sudanese satellite channel. A man identified as a Sudanese professor talked about the changes he noticed on returning to Sudan after 25years living abroad.

"The level of beauty has gone down, i.e. most of them (Sudanese women) are ugly, very much so An ugly woman creates distress in a person, I mean me personally, it makes me feverish, I suffer a lot" he said.

The professor went on to compare today's young Sudanese women to those of his generation. He said today's young Sudanese women were unattractive to him: using skin bleaching creams and "this kind of thing. According to the professor "all the big poets used to write about the beauty of women. But now, you can't find a girl worth writing poetry about".

Sara admitted that what the professor said was not that shocking, the words were not new or unfamiliar. These conversations happen daily, and the opinions expressed so widely that it is practically considered the norm. Sudanese people are consumed by appearance, the reigning look is light skinned women with long (straight) hair. The people are caught in a vicious cycle of pressure to conform to an image which for many, if not most, is far removed from what they were born with. What angered Sara and made her respond to the professor was the need to confront a society not interested in women as anything more than a pretty face. A woman is a "girl" until she is married and marriage has become so incumbent on looks. Women carry a heavy burden

Sara shared her response to the professor's remarks on YouTube and, within 24hours, over 20,000 views have been shared. It had gone viral on facebook, Twitter, and WhatsApp. The reactions were overwhelming shows of support from both men and women, But, as expected, some reacted negatively with comments questioning her audacity confronting the professor, that portrays a woman in Sudan as someone to be seen but not heard.

Anita Fabos[6] wrote about how in Sudan, a Muslim cultural discourse of 'propriety' has influenced Muslim Arab Sudanese ethnic identity in two locations and time periods in an expanding diaspora. Focusing in particular on women and their embodied practices of whitening and propriety in Egypt in the nineties and the United Kingdom a decade later, she argued that the recent turn towards Muslim expressions of Sudaneseness is a form of resistance to a racial labelling. While Sudanese have rejected being labeled 'black' in Egypt and in the UK, their renegotiation of a Muslim religious identity in the diaspora nevertheless confirms a racialized Sudanese ethnicity. Her study contributes to the rethinking of ethnicity in a transnational space where ethnic nationalism and globalized Islamic discourse intersect with local histories and hierarchies of race and gender[7]

References

1.Discrimination based on skin colour. http://en.wikipedia.org/wiki/Descrimination-based_based_on_skin_color#cite_note_22

2. Nyabouy Gatbet. Skin bleaching and the South Sudananes Community. February 10 2014. *http:www.nyabouygatbeleng.com/blog/skin-bleaching-and-the-south-sudanese-community.*

3. Reem Abbas in Khartoum. In search of beauty: Sudanese women throwing caution to the winds. *AFRICA REVIEW* June 15 2012. *http://www.africaview.com/Special-Reports?On-a-lighter-skin/-/a...*

4. Internally displaced. Skin bleaching, women, morality and national character in Juba. December 25, 2012. *http://internallydisplaced.wordpress.com/2012/12/25/skin-bleaching...*

5. Sara Elhassan. Women in Sudan: what the 'ugly' debate tells us about society. *The guardian* 10 December 2014. *http:www.theguardian.com/world/2014/dec/10/-sp-sudan-ugly-wo…*

6. Anita Fabos. Resisting 'Blackness', embracing Rightn How Muslim Arab Sudanese Women Negotiate Cultural Space in the Diaspora. *Ethnic and Racial Studies* 2011, pp 1 – 19.

7. Al-Baqr al-Affif Mukhtar. *The crisis of Identity in Northern Sudan: The Dilemma of a Black people with a white culture.* In Fluehr-Lobban and Rhodes, Race and Identity in the Nile Valley. Pp 213 – 24.

Chapter 10

Central and North Africa

Story Highlights I-IV
Democratic Republic of Congo
Rwanda
Jordan
Saudi Arabia

Story highlights I

Democratic Repulic of Congo

- Skin bleaching is called ***"maquillage"*** in the Democratic Republic of the Congo
- Almost everyone—men and women—including doctors, bleach in the Democratic republic of Congo.
- Congo was a Belgian colony and the Belgians were really colorist and favored the light skinned Congolese with Anglo features.
- Congolese engage in heavy cross border smuggling of bleaching products to neighboring countries.
- The skin bleaching problem among the Congolese both at home and in the diaspora is sensitive, complex and difficult to deal with since it involves issues strongly burdened with emotions such as one's ethnic and personal identity. The practice has an addictive dimension.
- Both the health risks and the social and symbolic aspects of the practice must be tackled to stem the tide of skin bleaching.

Story highlights II

Rwanda

- Skin bleaching is called "kwitukuza" in Rwanda.

- About 35% of Rwandese bleach their skin.
- In Rwanda, foreigners from Congo were the ones who often bleached themselves. But the trend is fast catching up with the Rwandans.
- Bleaching products have been banned in Rwanda but they are smuggled into the country.
- There is a notion that most Rwandan men prefer light skinned women, but Rwandan men deny this.
- Those who can afford it buy expensive creams and pills. Those who cannot resort to harsh and cheaper means of lightening their skins.
- *Rwanda Today* is informed that there is a mixture of creams, soaps, and Jik known as "*mkorogo*" that is used by women who cannot afford to buy the expensive creams.
- Only administrative penalties e.g warning, seizing the goods or closing of the business are used against defaulters
- A doctor teaches the people on some of the complications of skin bleaching.
- Those who bleach admit they are aware of the adverse effects of bleaching the skin.
- Those who do not bleach are restricted by family, religion and Rwandese culture.
- "Safer" products for bleaching are recommended.

Story highlights III

Jordan

- 60.7% of Jordanian women bleach their skin.
- Skin bleaching cuts across all demographic groups and skin complexions.
- The main reasons for bleaching are (i) belief that those with lighter skin tone are more beautiful; (ii) lighter skin tone contributes to a better employment opportunity; (iii) lighter skin tone increases a woman's chances of getting married as men perceive lighter skinned women as more attractive; (iv) for therapeutic reasons e.g to treat hyperpigmentation like melasma on the face.
- TV advertisements contribute to the practice as it presents models with light skin tone as being more attractive and the symbol of success.

- Interestingly the prevalence of usage among women from the lowest (less than 200JD) and the highest economic status (more than 600JD) are almost equal (69.2% vs 71.4%). (1 Jordanian Dinar is equivalent to 1.41 US Dollar). Further, although the prevalence of usage increases as the skin tone becomes darker, the percentage of users in the light skin tone population is considered high (44.1%).
- The skin lightening products contain hydroquinone or corticosteroids.
- All brands regardless of their composition are available without prescription from pharmacies.
- User's awareness of the active ingredients in the products and their adverse side effects appear to be lacking.
- Key issue to address is to educate Arab women to start to change their beauty perception and value their natural skin tone.

Story highlights IV

Saudi Arabia

- Although the skin colour among Saudi Arabia women is relatively light (skin type IV-V), 38.9% of the women use skin lightening products. Women of all sociodemographic variables use the products.
- In Saudi markets a wide variety of different brands of skin-lightening creams are available, either imported from overseas or manufactured locally by traditional herbalists.
- The products are sold by street vendors and at herbal shops
- The main reasons for using the products are:
    - i. to make them more beautiful
    - ii. to make them more confident
    - iii. for therapeutic reasons to treat hyperpigmentation
- 30% used more than 100g of bleaching creams monthly
  64.6% applied the products on their faces
  7.3% use the products all over the body
  10.3% continued to used it in pregnancy
  20.8% continued to use it during lactation
  Others use them on their necks or as hand creams
  16.7% reported they spent more than US$53.4 a month on bleaching products
- Various dermatological complications are reported by the users
- There is need for a nationwide health-education campaign to tackle this issue

- Bleaching products are legal in Saudi Arabia; the government has not banned any of the bleaching products suspected to be harmful
- Health regulators must focus on limiting the herbal preparations that have unknown or harmful components.
- Detailed pharmacological examination of the components of these bleaching agents needs to be conducted.

DEMOCRATIC REPUBLIC OF CONGO

Skin bleaching is called ***"maquillage*"** in the Democratic Republic of the Congo (DRC)[1]. Rhiannon speculated on why the Congolese like to bleach their skin[2]. She says "I live in Zambia which boarders Congo and I guess it's a part of their culture. Congo was a Belgian colony and the Belgians were really colorist and favoured the light skinned Congolese with thin noses just like they did in Rwanda. Skin bleaching is illegal in Zambia because of how badly it affects the skin but there are still loads of Congolese people in Zambia who smuggle in bleaching creams from Congo. Skin bleaching is common throughout other African countries but it is just more common in Congo. In Zambia it's more common with uneducated girls but in Congo it's **everyone.** My neighbour was a Congolese, the woman was a trained doctor but she still bleached her skin, but yeah I think it's something that has stayed on since Colonialism". Sonia says: "It's called colonialism!"

Giovanni Vassailo[3] reported a research on the use of skin whitening products among African people. The study was conducted in Italy and the Congo. The study was on the social and economic repercussions of the issue. He interpreted the study as an attempt to investigate these aspects, which implicate the social building of beauty as a concept and its representation in a globalized world. The data was collected in Italy and the Congo RDC by means of inspections carried out in Italian ethno-cosmetics shops, and Congolese markets, and by interviewing immigrant women and men in Italy who make use of skin whitening products in the Congo.

Giovanni concludes that the problem is sensitive, complex and difficult to deal with, since it involves issues strongly burdened with emotions such as one's ethnic and personal identity. The practice has an addictive dimension. Both the health risks and the social and symbolic aspects of the practice must be highlighted in order to stem the tide of skin bleaching. The speculative and marked factors carried along in the ensuing marketing and distribution of the products cannot be disregarded.

References

1.Léocadie Kamagaju, Renato Morandini, Françoise Gahongayire *et al.* Survey on skin-lightening practices and cosmetics in Kigali, Rwanda. *Int J Dermatol* 2016; 55: 45-51.

2.Why DR Congolese like to bleach their skin. 20 April, 2014. *https://imanafricaninny.wordpress.com/2007/04/11/why-dr-congolese-like-to-bleach-their-skin/*

3. Giovanni Vassallo. The use of skin whitening products among African people: Research in Italy and the Congo. *JENdA. A Journal of Culture and African Women Studies.* 2009; 14.

RWANDA

In Rwanda, skin bleaching is called ***"kwitukuza"***, which literally means rendering his/her skin red.[1] In Rwanda, skin lightening (SL) is a confidential practice as in many other African countries,[2] and is highlighted by the common saying: "we do SL, but we don't speak about it."

Very few data are available on depigmenting practices in Rwanda. Published findings derived from a 1987 report by Scarpa and Guerci, discussed the beginning of skin-whitening products importation by students.[3] According to a survey of traditional practitioners,[4] in the past, people tended to use natural products from traditional medicine (plant extracts). However, since the SL effect of these products are slow to appear, most people now turn to chemically defined depigmentation products.

Studies and surveys from Central Africa indicate that skin lightening (SL) is practiced mostly by females.[2,5] A poll in Brazaville, however, showed that more than a quarter of men aged 15-24 years regularly use SL products. This proportion may be as high as 45% if occasional users are included.[6]

Léocadie Kamagaju *et al*[1] conducted a survey on skin-lightening practices and cosmetics in Kigali the capital city of Rwanda. The aims of the study was to evaluate the extent of the practice of skin-lightening in Kigali, the capital city of Rwanda, the motivations behind this practice and the complexity of the adverse effects observed.

Because of the secrecy of the practice, the researchers used several approaches for the study (i) an inventory of the creams and ointments available on the Kigali markets; (ii) a questionnaire to evaluate the proportion of cosmetics actually bought and used in Kigali city by random selection of people (students, motorcycle/taxi drivers, executives, traders, cultivators, and jobless people; (iii) questionnaire interview of dermatologists and general practitioners (GP) and (iv) sociological profiles of male and female adolescents (aged 15-20) in two secondary schools and two centers for street youths and orphans and their motivations for practicing SL.

Prevalence

35% of the surveyed population (120 women) were found to use products with skin-bleaching properties, but only 27% admitted that they used the products specifically for their depigmenting properties. Of the 30 men surveyed, 23% practiced SL. They claimed they simply used their wives' creams or those considered by their wives to be good for the skin.

However, these figures were regarded as under-estimation because from the design of the questionnaire and method of survey. Only about half of the hydroquinone preparations marketed and none of the corticosteroids products were cited as being cosmetically used. The researchers could not ascertain whether the products containing the most active depigmenting agents: (i) really were not used by the study population; (ii) were used but not reported because they were not considered to be cosmetic products; (iii) were used but concealed by the interviewees who were fully aware of their real use; or (iv) were used only as prescription drugs.

Products used

It is noteworthy that Rwanda Bureau of Standards legislation (RBS 66:2005) does not approve any amount of hydroquinone in cosmetics. Products containing hydroquinone are reserved for medical purposes and given only with a physician's prescription[7]

The Bureau observed that most of the cosmetic products containing hydroquinone entering the Rwanda markets came from the Democratic republic of Congo (DRC). Since December 2009, inspections have been carried out regularly for a series of cosmetics containing hydroquinone at La Corniche Border (between Goma and Rubavu) and in nearby markets and shops. The products include Skin Light, La Crème Éclaircissante Traitante, Caro Light lightening oil, Caro Light lightening beauty lotion, Caro Light lightening cream, Elegance Lemon Plus lotion, Sivoclair Lait Éclaircissant, Maxi Claire cream, Clairmen and Elegance RICO, Crème Éclaircissante.[7] Most of these products were, however, largely available in Kigali during the time of survey. During the survey, it was found that the most common products **used** were the hydroquinone-containing Caro Light and Peau Claire.

Motives for bleaching

When specifically asked why they bleach, expressed motives were a wish for perceived overall beauty, a desire to attract men and/or a craving for a desirable, smooth, beautiful, finer, and unblemished skin. However, the majority of Rwandan men involved in the survey (57%) claimed that they preferred women with a black or "intermediate" skin complexion.

When arriving in the city, Rwandese people tend to lighten their skin to disguise their rural origins. Rural activities effectively expose people to the sun, which darkens their skin, much more than most urban activities. The same observation applies to people born in Kigali whose work requires them to spend most of their time under the sun, such as sellers in the small uncovered markets, 42% of whom were found to practice skin lightening. This motive is akin to that reported by Petit in France[8] who reported that African women living in Paris have been found to begin the practice of SL as soon as they arrive in France. Hence the practice of SL may reflect a desire for change that can be interpreted as the wish to conceal a type of background and a consequence of increase income—upward mobility.

As regards female adolescents around the age 15 years, the motivations for practicing SL can be divided into three components: (1) esthetic concern; (ii) a desire to do as others do—peer pressure; and (iii) need for social recognition (light skin is associated with higher social class). Those who did not practice SL said they were aware of the practice but were restricted by family, religion, and Rwandese culture. Other reasons for the non-practice of SL were described as not having access to the creams, cost, fear of side effects, having no interest in doing it ('feel good like this').

The researchers concluded that although many people acknowledge that there are possible adverse effects of using preparations commonly used in SL, the practice is generally continued. While it is important to question the rationale behind the practice of SL, it is equally important to develop and propose safer products.

Women resort to cheap 'mixtures' as skin lighteners

The quest for fair skin by African women has become a battle of the titans. People doing this are, however, not aware of the health risks they are putting themselves into.

Those who can afford buy expensive creams and pills. Those who cannot resort to harsh and cheaper means of lightening their skins. Unfortunately, there is a notion that most African men prefer light skinned women.[9] But African women are not alone here. Men are increasingly becoming culprits of bleaching with the Congolese men leading the pack. Koffi Olomide, Madilu System and General Defao are on the list of Congolese men who are known to have bleached themselves.

In Rwanda, foreigners from Congo were the ones who often bleached themselves. But the trend is fast catching up with the Rwandans. Not long ago products known to contain bleaching agents were banned in the country. Some of the skin lightening products available in shops assure the buyer of a new and improved image. Nzaire Philip, the director for Quality Assurance at the Rwanda Bureau of Standards, says that his office conducts market surveys every few months. And that these products do not pass through the normal channels. "The penalties for selling such products range from warnings, seizing of the goods to closing of the business, all these are administrative penalties" he said.

Rwanda Today is informed that there is a mixture of creams, soaps, and Jik known as "*mkorogo*" that is used by women who cannot afford to buy the expensive creams. Sophia sells "*Mkorogo*" on Biashara Street known as *cartier matteus* in Kigali. She sells her "*mkorogo*" between Rw35,000 to Rwf50,000 depending on the products used in the concoctions. But at any given time she uses more than 10 creams to come up with a concoction. One of the four dermatologists in the country, Kayitesi Kayitenkore, who runs Kigali Dermatology clinic, lists three main chemicals in the skin lightening products — corticosteroids, hydroquinone and mercury. According to Kayitesi Kayitenkore.[10] Hydroquinone stops skin pigmentation and blocks the amount of melanin which makes the body more vulnerable to UV rays. This pigment is the skin's own protector from the harmful ultraviolet rays of the sun. Corticosteroids make the skin thinner and prone to infections and difficulty in healing when you get wounds. Stretch marks, wrinkles and loss of water making the skin dry are among the effects of using bleaching products containing corticosteroids, Dr Kayitenkore says, with continued use of bleach, the skin thins out losing its elasticity and collagen. There are some studies that have shown people who use bleaching creams extensively can poison their bodies through such chemicals thus developing kidney failure, hypertension and diabetes. Doctors avoid surgical procedures on people who have used bleaching creams extensively. Because the mechanisms of skin repair will not work normally. In extreme cases, patients have been known to die on operating tables, because stitching cannot hold the skin for it has lost its elasticity.

Dr Kayitenkore says cancer of the skin in black people was known to be rare, because of the natural pigmentation that protects the black skin. But black people are known to suffer from cancer of the palm and the soles because these are white areas that can develop malignant melanoma. The common features for people who bleach are black knuckles and elbows and discoloration of the nails. In some cases, we have seen women with "moustaches", as an adverse effect of using these creams. Dr Kayitenkore advises people to seek professional advice.

Mama Papi is a Congolese business woman; she sells jewellery on the streets of Kigali. Her facial skin is burnt and has red patches. She tries to look for a shade where she can protect her already burnt face, but due to her nature of business she cannot afford to stand in one place for long. She says she has used bleaching creams for 20 years. She started using bleaching creams in her native Democratic Republic of Congo while still in school.

The use of bleaching creams became common because women with darker skins were shunned by men, while those with lighter skins were always favoured; hence the rise in the use of bleaching creams.

References

1. Léocadie Kamagaju, Renato Morandini, Françoise Gahongayire *et al.* Survey on skin-lightening practices and cosmetics in Kigali, Rwanda. *Int J Dermatol* 2016; 55: 45-51.

2. Morand JJ, Ly F, Lightburn E *et al.* Complications of cosmetic skin bleaching in Africa. *Med Trop* 2007; 67:627-34.

3. Scarpa A, Guerci A. Depigmenting procedures and drugs employed by melanoderm populations. *J Ethnopharmacol* 1987; 19:17-66.

4. Kamagaju L, Morandini R, Bizuru E *et al.* Tyrosinase modulation by five Rwandese herbal medicines traditionally used for skin treatment. *J Ethnopharmacol* 2013; 146: 824-34.

5. Rwandan Bureau of Standards. *Campaign Against Hydroquinone.* Rwanda Bureau of Standards Newsletter, 2010.*http://eacquality.net/fileadmin/rwanda/user_documents/RBS_Newsletter_issue_7_ED.pdf* [Accessed April 10, 2013]

6.Bonniol JL. Beauté et couleur de la peau. *Communications* 1995; 60:185-204
7.Mbemba-Ndoumba G. *Ces Noirs qui se Blanchissent la Peau. La Practique du "Maquillage" Chez les Congolais.* Paris; Editions L Harmattan, 2004: 124
8.Petit A. La depigmentation volontaire. Réalités, interprétations, résistances. Mémoire de Maîtrise 2007; University of Paris 13. *http://www.clinique-transculturelle.org/pdf/memoire_du_petit.pdf.* [Accessed May 12, 2013]
9.The East African. Women resort to cheap "mixtures" as skin lighteners. *http://www.theeastafrican.co.ke/Rwanda/Lifestyle/Women-resort-to-...*
10.Risks of 'skin deep' beauty
URL:http://wwww.theeastafrican.co.ke/magaz1.URL:http://wwww.theeastafrican.co.ke/magazine/-/434746/852812/-/14hhkgmz/-/index.html

JORDAN

Saja Hamed *et al* [1] explored the skin-lightening practice among women living in Jordan. The researchers investigate the determinants, the prevalence and users awareness associated with the use and misuse of skin-lightening products among women living in Jordan. Since this publication is described as the first report on skin lightening practice in Jordan as well as an Arab community, it is being reproduced in details.

The study population are female patrons of pharmacies in Jordan who were randomly asked to complete a questionnaire. 60.7% of the 318 respondents reported the use of skin-lightening products. The level of skin tone of the respondents are 'light' (32%), 'Light brown' (39.6%), 'Dark brown' (14.5%), and Black (13.2%). However, the researchers did not clarify if these skin tones were '*before*' or '*after*' the use of skin bleaching products.

The respondents cut across all socio-demographic groups.

Determinants

As regards women's perception of lighter skin tone, the questions asked were structured as follows:

i. Lighter skin tone is more beautiful
ii. Lighter skin tone provides women with higher self-esteem
iii. Lighter skin tone gives female a younger looking
iv. Lighter skin tone implies that a woman belongs to a high social class
v. Lighter skin tone helps a woman get a better job opportunity
vi. Lighter skin tone increases a woman's chance of getting married
vii. Men consider lighter skin tone more beautiful
viii. The way skin lightening products are advertised on TV has influence on a woman's preference of lighter skin tone.

The answers to the questions were graded as "strongly agree", "agree", "disagree", "strongly disagree", and "no answer".

The majority of the participants (62.3%) believe that lighter skin tone is considered more beautiful regardless of their skin tone and age group. This belief appears to be an important contributing factor to the prevalence of this practice as it is higher among skin lightening products users (72%) compared with nonusers (47.2%).

On the influence of lighter skin tone on women's perception of self-esteem and age, the majority of the women in the study population disagree with the notion that lighter skin tone contributes to the perception of higher self-esteem and youth (52.3%) and 59.6%, respectively. However, the percentage of women who associate lighter skin tone with self- esteem and youth is highly significant among skin lightening products users compared with nonusers. On the other hand, the social classification does not appear to be a determinant of the practice of using skin-lightening agents as the majority of user's and nonuser's (69.9% and 76%, respectively) do not associate lighter skin tone with being from a higher social class.

The respondents were almost equally divided on the issue of the influence of having a lighter skin tone on getting a better job opportunity. However, a statistically significant higher percentage of users (55.4%) believe that a lighter skin tone contributes to a better employment opportunity compared to non users (35.5%). The position of the respondents on this issue was clearly affected by their skin tone where 59.5% of women with dark skin tone believe in the influence of lighter skin tone in getting a better job opportunity compared to 43.6% of women with light skin tone. This points out job opportunities and employment as a significant factor promoting this practice. It is worth noting that as the level of education increases the perception of the importance of this factor decreases significantly.

The role of lighter skin tone in mate selection and the potential perception by men that a lighter skin tone is more attractive are two important reinforcing factors for the use of skin-lightening products. The majority of respondents believe that lighter skin tone is perceived by men as being more attractive and increases a woman's chances of getting married (62.6% and 63.4%, respectively), these beliefs are, as expected, more common among skin lightening products users (71.5% and 70.5%).

TV advertisement contribute to the practice of using skin-lightening products by presenting models with light skin tone as being more attractive and more likely to achieve success in their **life** (i.e. employment opportunity and mate selection). This is evident from the higher percentage of respondents (77.4%) who believe that the way TV advertises skin-lightening products influences women to prefer lighter skin tone regardless of the their level of education.

Socio-demographic data of skin bleachers

Users of skin-lightening products are distributed among women from all age groups, economic levels, and marital status. Interestingly the prevalence of usage among women from the lowest (less than 200 JD) and the highest economic status (more than 600 JD) are almost equal (69.2% vs 71.4%). (1 Jordanian Dinar is equivalent to 1.41 US Dollar). Further, although the prevalence of usage increases as the skin tone becomes darker, the percentages of users in the light skin tone population is considered high (44.1%).

Motives for skin bleaching

With regard to the objective of using such products, 29.3%, 29.3% and 20.7% of the users used skin-lightening products to lighten their darker skin tone, to treat hyperpigmentary disorders on their faces such as melasma, and for both reasons, respectively.Women with light skin tone use the skin-lightening products mainly to treat hyperpigmentary disorders (50%) rather than to lighten their skin tone (9.1%). As the skin tone becomes darker the driver for usage is mainly the women's preference of lighter skin tone rather than the need to treat hyperpigmentary disorders.

In addition, women with low educational level appear to use the skin-lightening products mainly because of their preference of a lighter skin tone (66.7%) compared with women with higher educational level (Tertiary education); only 13.5% of them use these products solely because they prefer lighter skin tone, 33.8% use it to treat hyperpigmentary disorders, and 27% use it for both reasons.

Further, women with higher income levels (more than 600 JD) are more driven by the therapeutic application of skin-lightening products (80%) rather than using them solely to lighten their skin tone (20%), compared with women with low income level whom only 24.6% of them use these products to treat hyperpigmentary problems.

Skin lightening products used

Regardless of the accuracy of their knowledge, 22.6% and 1.9% of skin lightening products users reported that they use products containing hydroquinone or corticosteroids as the active ingredients, respectively. Most users obtain their skin lightening products from either pharmacy (52.6%) or from small make up and skin care products stores (31.8%). This points a spotlight on the role of pharmacists in recommending skin-lightening products and instructing the customers on their use. Most skin lightening products users (54.7%) reported duration of use of more than 1 year and products were applied mostly on the face (81.9%). The monthly cost of these products for most users was equal to or less than 20 JD/month (~28 US $/month) regardless of the respondent's monthly income. A total of 48 different brands of skin-lightening products were reported. Twenty two of the reported products do not contain ingredient label, seven products contain hydroquinone, one product contains corticosteroid, and seven products are sunscreens. All brands can be bought from make-up and skin care stores with the exception of steroid- and hydroquinone-containing creams having a pharmaceutical presentation which can be obtained only from a pharmacy. However, all brands regardless of their composition can be obtained without any medical prescription from pharmacies.

User knowledge and awareness

In regard to the products knowledge, most users (72.5%) reported that they do not know the active ingredients in the product they use. This takes on a special importance considering the potential side effects of some of these ingredients. This observation emphasizes the importance of user education by the pharmacist and the sales persons in the locations in which the products are sold.

A total of 63.5% of users believe in the importance of using sunscreen over the skin-lightening products when going out during the day compared with 27.1% of users who do not believe in that. User's awareness of possible side effects associated with the use of skin-lightening products appears to be lacking as 37.5% of users do not believe that skin-lightening products may cause undesired cutaneous adverse effects. The underestimation of the risk associated with this practice is a key issue in developing interventions to change it.

With regard to the level of users' satisfaction with the performance of skin-lightening products, 70.9% of users are satisfied with the efficacy of the products they used.

Conclusion

Saja Hamed *et al* conclude that the study is the first report on the issue of using skin lightening agents in Jordan as well as an Arab community. The study takes a special importance as a result of possible adverse effects associated with the chronic use or misuse of these products and their impact on health care services. The results show that the use of skin-lightening products is a common practice among women living in Jordan. This practice is reinforced by a number of perceived benefits associated with having a lighter skin tone including perceptions of beauty, personal and professional success (i.e. job opportunity and marriage). Regarding the objective of usage, one-third of the respondents used such products solely to lighten their darker skin tone and one-third of respondents used it solely to treat hyperpigmentary disorders on their faces. Hence, skin-lightening practice is a double-edged sword. These products are considered an important step in ameliorating melasma and postinflammatory disorders but at the same time, they can be misused while trying to achieve a light skin complexion that is valued by a number of cultural beliefs. Thus, these findings show the importance of developing realistic interventions to educate women in Jordan, in particular, and other countries on the proper use of skin lightening products. The safety of these products and the potential hazards associated with their misuse (e.g. products that contain hydroquinone, corticosteroids, or ones adulterated with mercury) are key issues to address in educating Arab women to start to change their beauty perception and to value their natural blemish-free even-toned skin since individuals of color have recently gained a greater presence in leadership positions and in the media worldwide. Even for women who use the skin-lightening products for the treatment of pigmentary disorders, there is a need for increasing awareness on the proper use, factors that may hinder the efficacy of the used products, and how to avoid the use of misbranded or adulterated skin-lightening products.

Reference

Hamed Saja H, Tayyem Reema, Nimer Nisreen, and AlKhatib Hatim S. Skin-lightening practice among women living in Jordan: prevalence, determinants, and user's awareness. *International Journal of dermatology* 2010, 49; 414-20.

SAUDI ARABIA

Al-Saleh *et al*[1] states that Saudi markets a wide variety of different brands of skin-lightening creams are available either being imported from overseas or being manufactured locally by traditional herbalists. They conclude that this high supply indicates that there may be a high demand for such skin-lightening products in Saudi Arabia. AlGhamdi[2] conducted a study to estimate the prevalence of the use of bleaching agents among women in Saudi Arabia, to assess the knowledge and practice of bleaching and to examine attitudes towards skin bleaching. The study was through a self administered questionnaire. The questionnaire was distributed to 620 women but 509 (82%) of the women aged between 10-59 years responded. The mean age was 29 + 9 years.

The constitutional skin colour among Saudi Arabia women is relatively light (skin type IV-V). Of the participants, 38.9% were current users of bleaching agents. Only 26.7% of the respondents used bleaching agents for medical purposes to treat localized abnormal skin hyperpigmentation. Of the respondents 30% used more than 100g of bleaching creams monthly. These products were applied to the whole body in 7.3% of the cases. While 10.3% continued to apply the bleaching products during pregnancy, 20.8% did so during lactation. No associations could be found between the various sociodemographic variable and differences in the attitude towards the practice of using bleaching creams.

Of the participants, 56.8% believed that lighter skin colour made them more beautiful, whereas only 15.9% believed that lighter skin colour made them more self-confident. Non-medical preparations sold by street vendors and at herbal shops were considered by 15.3% as safe to use. 20.8% stated that they would use bleaching creams that gave fast results even if the components were unknown. The products were applied to the whole body in 7.3% of the cases, 64.6% applied the products on their faces; 26.7% used them on their necks and 17.1 used them on their hands. The age of the participants when they first started to use bleaching creams varied from 10-57 years; and the duration of usage varied from 1-150 months. 18.6% had used the cream for more than 6 months.

The complications reported by the skin bleachers were “skin becomes darker than before” (10%); “skin returns to its normal color” (24.40%); Rash (11.20%); skin dryness (16.10%). 30% reported they obtained the bleaching products from herbal shops. The monthly cost of the bleaching products varied from 5 to 3000 Saudi Riyals (SR). 16.7% reported they spent more than 200 SR per month on bleaching products (US $ 53.4).

Bleaching products are legal in Saudi Arabia; the government has not banned any of the bleaching products suspected to be harmful.

Conclusion

The researchers concluded that future research should investigate the prevalence and type of cutaneous and systemic complications of bleaching agents in Saudi Arabia. Furthermore, detailed pharmacological examination of the components of these bleaching agents needs to be conducted. Education of the public on the risks of bleaching product use is clearly imperative and would mitigate the side-effects of their use. Health education programmes should target women through various media options including leaflets, television and radio. Within hospitals, the researchers suggest that education programmes about the dangers of misuse and overuse of topical bleaching agents be integrated into existing health education programmes. Health regulators must focus on limiting the herbal preparations that have unknown or harmful components. The sales and marketing of bleaching products must be controlled, which could be done by imposing fines and penalties on the marketers of such products. There is a need for a nationwide health-education campaign to tackle this issue.

References

1. Al-Saleh I, Al-Doush I. Mercury content in skin-lightening creams and potential hazards to the health of Saudi women. *J Toxicol Environ Health.* 1997; 51:123-30.

2. Al Ghamdi KM. The use of topical bleaching agents among women: a cross-sectional study of knowledge, attitude and practices *European Academy of Dermatology and Venereology* 2010; *JEADY* DOI:10.1111/j1468-

Chapter 11

Colorism in Sub-Saharan Africa

Story Highlights
Skin-color preference in Sub-Saharan Africa
Colorism in sub-Saharan Africa: Nigeria as a case study
General public comments on colorism and skin bleaching in Africa retrieved from social media

Story highlights

- It has long been noted that black men prefer lighter-skinned women in sub-Saharan Africa. Several extracts from ethnographic literature corroborate this cross cultural preference for lighter skin in women.
- In Africa 'yellow girls' / lighter "brown" girls are usually considered to be more beautiful than 'black' girls. A bright, clear complexion held social significance in pre-colonial Nigerian society.
- The more successful commercial sex workers are invariably light-skinned and skin bleaching was traditionally associated with women in the sex trade.
- Colorism refers to prejudice based on skin tone, which is typically practiced *within* races, as opposed to racism *between* races. Colorism creates a hierarchical relationship that privileges lighter complexions.
- In Nigeria skin whitening is perceived as a route towards achieving a range of social and economic benefits. In addition to enticing men romantically, skin bleachers expect that light complexion would enable them to "enter into connection with high calibers, attain high social standard, become more successful in life, look

fashionable, express positive self-concept and be able to compete well with their male counterparts. Whether real or imagined, the perceived benefits of fair skin expand far beyond one's appearance.

- In Nigeria and Ghana, colorism is reflected in the over representation of light-complexioned models, actresses, and beauty pageant winners.
- There is shame around skin lightening in some cultures "either because one should 'naturally' have light skin not chemically derived light skin, or because some believe that lightening the skin implies a shame of one's race or ethnic identity."
- Marriage prospects carry a host of socioeconomic implications for women and their families, such that beauty can produce tangible economic payoffs.
- Advertisements in print media are unlike other forms of media in that they almost exclusively sell idealized images of life, rather than reality. With this enhanced picture comes an image of perfected appearances for consumers to aspire to. Additionally, print media can employ Photoshop technology to sell an unrealistic or even impossible image of beauty.
- Interestingly, like television programming and films, Nigerian print media often reflects some of the same colorist rhetoric present in Western media.
- The vast majority of celebrities and models are the same race as the country's consumers, yet their phenotypes are typically more in line with Eurocentric ideals than the average woman of each country.
- Unlike most local media, Western media typically embodies the image of global modernity and progress, an idea that seems to be increasingly appealing to women in the developing world who want to claim membership in a transnational, cosmopolitan culture.

> **"Colonialism and Westernization can be understood as intersecting rather than as distinct, unrelated phenomena. In its aftermath, colonialism left a region vulnerable to Western influences, including media images that portrayed lighter-skinned individuals as valuable and more powerful. Western media images reinforced the earlier racial hierarchies that were in place."**
>
> **Regardless of the impetus for colorism in Nigeria, the real propeller of the preference for**

lighter skin is the "global association of light skin with power."

What is the character of this "power"?

Love—**security,** value—**self-worth,** and purpose—**significance!**

- The general comments on social media can best be described as ambivalent but the overwhelming majority of views is against the skin bleaching culture in sub-Saharan Africa.

SKIN-COLOR PREFERENCE IN SUB-SAHARAN AFRICA (SSA)

Men valorize lighter-skinned women

Peter Frost extensively reviews the literature on studies done as regards skin color preference in Sub-Saharan Africa.[1]

It has long been noted that black men prefer lighter-skinned women, both in sub-Saharan Africa and in the black diaspora. For the United States, we can quote several writers. "A fair Negro woman … has such superior marriage chances that this fact is generally recognized as the major explanation of why passable women do not seem to pass out of the Negro caste as often as do passable men".[2] "The frequency with which Negro men choose women fairer than they are attests at least in part to the connection in the mind of the black man between fair skin and beauty".[3] "Several research projects conducted in the last few years suggest that African-American men are more attracted to women who are lighter than they are, and that African-American women believe light skin makes them, or would make them, more appealing"[4]

In sub-Saharan Africa, women often use skin-bleaching products, usually hydroquinone but also mercury, topical steroids, and Javel water.[5] Cites prevalence rates of 25% in Bamako, Mali, up to 52% in Dakar, Senegal, up to 35% in Pretoria, South Africa, and up to 77% in Lagos, Nigeria. He adds, "the majority of black men prefer light-skinned women as partners, girlfriends or wives. Several authors have stated that these light-skinned women are perceived as attractive, intelligent, moral, sexually more desirable, even chaste; whereas dark-skinned are regarded as mean, evil, stupid, even as not trust-worthy."

This preference is often put down to European influence. Myrdal[2] for instance, felt that African-Americans were internalizing Euro-American color prejudice. Others, like Layng[4], simply see an adoption of dominant norms of beauty: "it was the Europeans and their descendants who were both numerically and economically dominant. so it is not surprising that, over time, a greater number of African-Americans, especially those who were upwardly mobile, adopted the prevailing views on physical attractiveness."

There is evidence, however, that this aesthetic preference for light skin is native to Africa. Ardener[6] found it to be widespread among the Ibo of Nigeria, including generations born before the colonial period. In a survey of the *Human Relations Area Files*, van den Berghe and Frost[7] noted a **consistent** cross-cultural preference for lighter skin in women but not in men. Sub-Saharan Africa is no exception. Peter Frost featured several extracts from ethnographic literature to corroborate this cross cultural preference for lighter skin in women.

Studies done in Mali,[8] Tellensi (Ghana),[9] Hausa (Nigeria),[10] Ibo (Nigeria)[6], Azande (Sudan)[11], Berti (Sudan)[12], Somali (Somalia)[13], Masai (Kenya, Tanzania)[14], Rundi (Rwanda, Burundi)[15], Granda (Uganda)[16], Nairobi (Kenya)[17], Ila, Lunda, Luvale, and Chokwe (Zambia)[18], Ngoni (Malawi)[19], Kgatla (Botswana)[20], **consistently** showed that black men prefer lighter-skinned women. Among the Ibo of Nigeria, in the choice of a wife, yellow-skinned girls are regarded as beauties, and, other things being equal, they command higher bride prices. In Kenya, the lighter "brown" girls are usually considered to be more beautiful than "black" girls–and the more successful prostitutes are invariably "brown"[17]

The preference for light skinned women has remained prevalent over time in all cultures: Asia, European, African, Caribbean and American. However, there are exceptions like the maasai in Kenya who associate light complexions with being cursed or witchcraft.[20] One study on men of the Bikosso tribe in Cameroon found no preference for attractiveness of females based on lighter skin colour, bringing into question the universality of earlier studies that had exclusively focused on skin colour preference among non-Africa populations[21]

References

1. Frost Peter. Skin-color preference in Sub-Saharan Africa. December 2006. The Unz Review: *An Alternative Media Selection.* December 21, 2006. *http://www.unz.com/pfrost/skin-color-preference-in-sub-saharan/*
2. Myrdal G. *An American Dilemma.* New York: Harper & Row. 1944
3. Grier WH and PM Cobbs. *Black Rage.* New York: Basic. 1968.
4. Layng A. Color Counts: "… it is evident that differing color holds considerable importance within the black community and is measurably influencing self-esteem, prestige, and marital status." *USA Today* (Society for the Advancement of Education), March, 2006. *http://findarticles.com/p/articles/mi_m1272/is_2730_134/ai_n16108105*
5. Ntambwe M. 'Mirror mirror on the wall, who is the FAIREST of them all?' *Science in Africa* March, 2004. *http://www.scienceinafrica.co.za/2004/march/skinlightening.htm*
6. Ardener EW. Some Ibo attitudes to skin pigmentation, *Man1954;* 54:71-3.
7. Van den Berghe PL and Frost P. Skin color preference, sexual dimorphism, and sexual selection: A case of gene-culture co-evolution? *Ethnic and Racial Studies* 1986: 87-113.
8. Henry J. *L'âme d'un peuple africain.* Münster: Aschendorff. 1910.
9. Fortes M. *The Dynamics of Clanship among the Tallensi.* London: Oxford University Press. 1945.
10. Smith MF. *Baba of Karo: A Woman of the Muslim Hausa.* London: Faber & Faber.1965.
11. Evans-Pritchard EE. *Witchcraft, Oracles, and Magic among the Azande.* Oxford: Clarendon Press.1937.
12. Holy L. Gender and ritual in an Islamic society: The Berti of Darfur, *Man* 1988; 23:469-87.
13. Lewis IM. *Marriage and the Family in Northern Somaliland.* Kampala: East African Institute of Social Research.1962.
14. Merker M. *Die Masai.* Berlin: Reimer. 1910.
15. Albert E. Women of Burundi, in D. Paulme (Ed.), *Women of Tropical Africa.* London: Routledge & Kegan Paul.1963.
16. Lugira AM. *Ganda Art.* Kampala: Osasa pub. 1970.
17. McVicar KG. *Twilight of an East African Slum.* Ann Arbor, University Microfilms (UCLA Dissertation 1968). 1969.
18. White CMM. Correspondence, *Man 1954;* 54:147.
19. Barnes JA. *Marriage in a Changing Society.* Cape Town: Oxford University Press. 1951.
20. Skin bleaching/African Science Heroes. *https://afrisciheroes.wordpress.com/tag/skin-bleaching*
21. Dixson BJ, Dixson AF, Morgan B, Anderson MJ. Human physique and sexual attractiveness: Sexual preferences of men and women in Bakossiland, Cameroon. *Archieves of Sexual Behaviour.* 2007; 36: 369-75.

Aesthetic preference different from mate preference/mate choice in Africa

Among the traditional rural Africans e.g. traditional Zulu, physical beauty was not regarded a first primary or even an important qualification in a wife.[1] people formerly looked for strength rather than beauty and tended to marry black girls because it is claimed that black people had greater powers of endurance. Mc Vicar[2] makes a similar observation among Kenyan women when contrasting 'black' and 'brown' African women. He says "among these tribes black girls are usually regarded as had workers, possible because many consider themselves fortunate enough to be married," Among subsistence farmers in Bakossiland, Cameroon, no consistent[3] preference of skin color of a potential female partner was identified. Sub–Saharan Africa, together with New Guinea differs from most cultures because of its high level of polygamy and correspondingly low level of paternal investment in child care.[4-7] To maximize their reproductive potential, African men seek self-reliant women who can raise children largely on their own. This traditionally meant being able to produce enough food through hoe farming–outdoors and in the sun. There was thus a premium on darker women.

Today, hoe farming is disappearing. As agriculture becomes mechanized and as people move off the land, Africa is entering a new social environment where men no longer choose wives for their ability to work hard in the sun. Increasingly, African women are supporting themselves and their children through work in the service economy–with its emphasis on charm and visual presentation. The circumstances of life are now promoting rather than hindering the aesthetic preference for lighter-skinned women.

References

1. Vilakazi A. *Zulu Transformations.* Pietermaritzburg: University of Natal Press. 1962

2. Mc Vicar KG. *Twilight of an East African Slum.* Ann Arbor, University Microfilms (UCLA Dissertation) 1968.

3. Dixson BJ, Dixson AF, Morgan B, Anderson MJ. Human physical and sexual attractiveness: Sexual preferences of men and women in Bakossiland, Cameroon. *Arch Sex Behav* 2006.

4. Bourguignon E and Greenbaum. *Diversity and Homogeneity in World Societies.* HRAF Press 1973.

5. Goody J. Polygyny, Economy and the Role of Women, in J Goody (Ed). *The Character of Kinship* Cambridge: Cambridge University Press 1973; pp 175-90.

6.Pebley AR and Mbugua W. Polygyny and Fertility in Sub-Saharan Africa. In RJ Lesthaeghe (Ed). *Reproduction and Social Organization in Sub-Saharan Africa,* Berkeley: University of Califonia Press. 1989, pp 338-64.

7. Welch CF and Glick PC. The incidence of polygamy in contemporary Africa: A research note. *Journal of marriage and the Family*. 1981; 43: 191-3.

COLORISM IN SUB SAHARAN AFRICA: NIGERIA AS A CASE STUDY

Colorism refers to prejudice based on skin tone, which is typically practiced *within* races, as opposed to racism *between* races. Colorism creates a hierarchical relationship that privileges lighter complexions. (See Chapter 17 on COLORISM).

Imani Franklin,[1] in a well researched dissertation titled "living in a Barbie World: skin Bleaching and the Preference for Fair Skin in India, Nigeria and Thailand," eminently dissected the 'determinants' for skin lightening in two countries that were previously colonized (India and Nigeria) and one that had no history of colonization (Thailand). Nigeria, the most populous country in Africa with the highest use of skin lightening products in the world, is used as the case study for black African countries which is the subject of this discourse.

Some people have adopted a simplistic approach to the phenomenon of skin bleaching in Africa by arguing that women lighten their skin not because of rational social and financial incentives, but because of perverse, irrational psychologies. Proponents of the psychological argument assert that women of color who practice bleaching have subconsciously internalized white supremacist ideologies and suffer from low self-esteem and self-hatred. One 2010 study of 97 Shona women in Masvingo, Tanzania, finds that "68% (28 out of 41) of skin bleachers saw dark skin as "embarrassing and humiliating" and therefore participate in their own "self-destruction."[2] Proponents of this idea argue that, because skin bleaching is "based on racist assumptions rather than reasoned analysis," women must just be taught to love themselves and embrace their racial identities.[2] The fallacy in this thinking stems from the fact that women's decisions to bleach are often based in reasoned analysis. For example, Dr Robert Wandara, Coordinator of the Psychology Department of Makerere says "such a person lacks self-esteem, has low self-efficacy and a perception that she or he looks ugly." He also says that skin bleaching "is common among women who are not educated." Mr Calista, Wandara's colleague, says that it is very dangerous to have low self-esteem because severe cases can lead to suicide. He urges skin bleachers – "Do something positive to counter your low self esteem.

Take advantage of the good parts of your body or talents." (See chapter 9 on UGANDA)

However, observations in all the nations where skin lightening is practiced show that this is a phenomenon that cuts across ***all*** socioeconomic strata– from the analphabetic to the most learned preofessionals– academics, legal luminaries, even "men of God," doctors and nurses! (See the sections on SOCIO-DEMOGRAPHIC CHARACTERISTICS in the various countries in Africa)

As Margaret Hunter describes, many female bleachers observe the acute correlation between race and socioeconomic class and want to improve their opportunities in the local employment and marriage markets, as well as adopt a cosmopolitan, modern identity.[3] It would be both unfair and inaccurate to assume that such women are simply hoodwinked, drowning in their own self-hatred. Blay found that women in Ghana who used bleaching products were trying to attain beauty vis a vis light skin. She argues that light skin and beauty were the vehicles through which women attempted to gain "social capital."[4]

Race historian Lynn Thomas notes that the psychological and financial explanations of skin bleaching cannot be completely separated into distinct categories as the two have become highly entangled. It is hard to imagine that one could be consistently economically and socially devalued in a society because of her skin tone without some negative psychological repercussion.[5] In their work on skin bleaching in Sub Saharan African (SSA), a group of Georgia State University professors aptly summarizes, "As a function of living in a color-conscious society where people of darker skin tones are systemically and socially regarded as less desirable, individuals who fall within this group may begin to develop feelings of inferiority and internalize negative beliefs about themselves, come to value lighter skin tones, and reject aspects of themselves."[6] The very real social and economic disadvantages attached to dark skin around the world feed into a compromised psychological sense of self. Disrupting this psychological damage requires addressing the larger system by which dark skin comes to symbolize a lack of life opportunity. Given that the power attached to white skin globally has deep historical roots and is reiterated by contemporary popular media, this is not an easy paradigm to shift. It would be naïve to expect women of color in the developing world to simply embrace their dark skin in the name of self-love and abandon skin-lightening practices. A sustainable solution for countering the fundamental motivation behind skin bleaching requires disrupting the perceived link between disproportionately high life opportunity and fair skin ***Colorism!***

The reality is that many nations and regions outside of Europe have significant populations of European ancestry. Examples of such nations are South Africa, Namibia, Zimbabwe, Kenya, Algeria, Mauritius, Ivory Coast, Canary Islands, Seychelles and Somalia. Hence colorism may be a significant issue in such communities. However, Nigeria does ***not*** belong to such group of nations with a significant subset of populations of European ancestry. Hence post-colonization Nigeria is eminently suitable as a **Case Study** of what colorism looks like in Sub-Saharan Africa

So that unnecessary repetitions can be avoided in this chapter, see the relevant chapters on

(i) NIGERIA: History of skin bleaching
Chapter 4 Motives for skin bleaching
Perspectives on skin bleaching
Skin bleaching: A cry for help.
(ii) DETERMINANTS FOR SKIN BLEACHING I and II—Chapters 5,6.
(iii)COLORISM; BEAUTY; PHYSICAL ATTRACTIVENESS; SEXUAL ATTRACTIVENESS; SOCIAL IMPORTANCE OF BLEACHING FOR WOMEN—Chapter 17
(iv) EPIDEMIOLOGY —Chapter 3
(v) GHANA —Chapter 7

Case study: NIGERIA

Nigeria, the world's 7th most populous country, is home to 170 million people and 50% of its total population lives in urban areas.[9] Nigeria exhibits the highest use of skin lightening products in the world, with an estimated 77% of women in Nigeria using some form of skin lightening product, according to the World Health Organization.[10] It is important to understand Nigeria's unsettlingly high demand for skin-lightening products, partly because the country serves as a primary port for these creams to travel to other African nations that have stricter regulations of such products. Sociologist Margaret Hunter observes, "Many skin-whitening products with dangerous chemical ingredients are manufactured in Europe or the United States, sent to Nigeria, and then distributed throughout Africa in both formal and informal markets."[11] The centrality of Nigeria in Africa's skin bleaching market renders it an important case study for research. Nigeria's GDP per capita is $2,600, putting it in the World Bank's lower-middle income bracket.

Several studies have been done on the subject in Nigeria. Those that assessed prevalence rates have ***consistently*** recorded high rates%77.3%,[12] 62.4%[13] 92%[14] and 64.9%[15]. A study among market traders in Lagos yielded 77.3%,[12] another study at the Enugu State University of Science and Technology (ESUT) yielded 62.4%[13], yet another study at the Lagos State University Teaching hospital recorded 92% of female patients had used the bleaching products in the past, but at the time of study, the figure had dropped to 40% because of unacceptable adverse effects, disapproval by family and peers, pregnancy and inability to sustain the habit due to financial constraints.[14] Another study among undergraduate students at the University of Benin in Benin City showed that 64.9% of the respondents used skin bleaching products.[15] Latest snap poll[16] results released by NOI polls have revealed that 64% of Nigerians are of the opinion that skin bleaching has become highly predominant in the country, especially amongst Nigerian females (97%). This finding supports the claim by the World Health Organization (WHO) that Nigeria has the highest number of women that use skin-lightening products in the world. The poll further revealed that despite the negative effects of skin bleaching affirmed by 83% of respondents; the top reasons why people still engage in the practice of skin bleaching are the need to look beautiful" (35%) and to "look attractive to the opposite sex" (32%). Skin bleaching was also reported as being most predominant amongst Nigerians within the age groups of 18-25 years (48%) and 26-40 years (43%). NOI polls is the No1 for country-specific polling services in the West African region, in technical partnership with Gallup (USA) to develop opinion research in Nigeria. Jide Ojo a journalist in Nigeria, has described Nigeria as the "world capital of skin bleaching"[17] and Dija Ayodele described Nigeria as "the skin-lightening hothouse of the world".[18]

Colorism in Nigeria

What does colorism look like in a country where the overwhelming majority of women bleach their skin? Education researcher Irene Durosaro, cites the 1940s as the beginning of the formal use of skin lightening products in Nigeria.[19] On a regional level, Sub-Saharan Africa (SSA) experienced an escalation in the use of skin bleach products throughout the second half of the 20th century. South Africa's Drum magazine expanded throughout much of SSA, including Nigeria, and, by the 1950s, became the most influential vehicle for marketing skin lightening products to African women.[20] By the 1970s, "skin lighteners were common commodities in most of southern Africa" and the industry was effectively in motion on the continent.[20] Advertisements for skin bleaching in SSA have adopted less overtly racist marketing strategies over time, yet the message remains the same:"lighter is better." The early 1900s saw classic colonial-era advertisements for Pears Soap depicting benevolent white people cleaning dirty and savage black Africans.[21] Figure 11.1 shows a classical advert for commodity racism. Figure 11.2 shows "***PERFECT WHITE"*** bill board – one of the current numerous adverts for skin bleaching products on the streets of Lagos. Note the white-skinned Asian used to advertise it. In Figure 11.1, the light-skinned doctor and the nurse are portrayed as successful because they use Ambi skin lightener. The apprehensive dark-skinned patient looks wretched and needs to "emulate" the successful light-skinned medical personnel.

In Nigeria, Ghana and several African countries, the songs some of the musicians compose contain lyrics that are always glorifying light skinned ladies. Read about the role of legendary Victor Olaiya in promoting the valorization of light skin-color in Nigeria women. In Ghana, a lady who has been bleaching for the past 37 years has this to say

"When we were growing up most men of our time preferred fair-colored women to those who are black. Even just listen to some of the songs our musicians compose; they are always glorifying fair ladies so I decided to change my colour" Madam Bimpong[22]

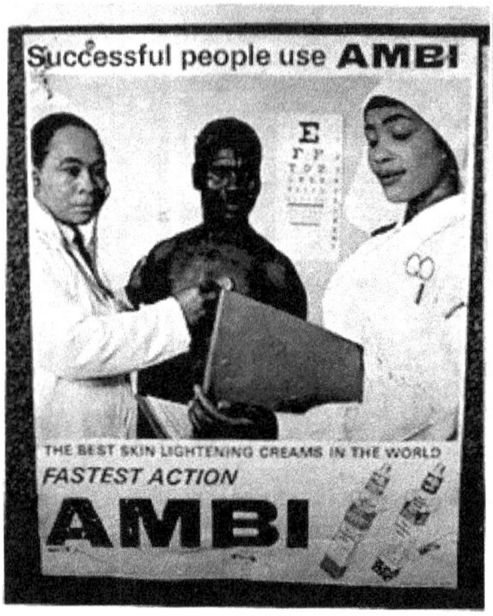

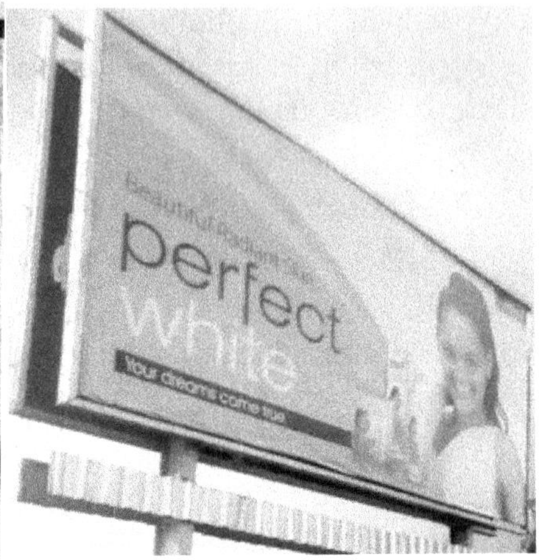

Figure 11.1 Skin lightening cream Advert Figure 11.2 "Perfect white" bill borad in Nigeria

Today, Nigeria serves as a port for harmful skin bleaches to enter SSA. Though Nigeria has some level of legal regulation limiting the entrance of dangerous skin bleaches, the country's lack of state control over informal markets renders such regulations ineffective. Given this state of inefficacy, "many skin-whitening products with dangerous chemical ingredients are manufactured abroad, sent to Nigeria, and then distributed throughout Africa in both formal and informal markets."[23] Skin lightening products are manufactured in many countries, for example, consumer protection agencies in the European Union and the United State of America have identified mercury-containing products in China, the Dominican republic, Lebanon, Mexico, Pakistan, the Philippines, Thailand, UK and the USA.[24,25] as manufacturers and exporters of mercury containing products. Nigeria's central role in the distribution of skin lightening products to other markets of SSA may contribute to its unparalleled rate of bleaching among women, and among female traders in particular. (See the relevant chapters on REDUCING THE GLOBAL BURDEN OF SKIN BLEACHING; WHY THE VARIOUS BANS HAVE BEEN INEFFECTIVE; WHERE ARE THE PRODUCTS MANUFACTURED?; WHERE CAN THE PRODUCTS BE PURCHASED?—Chapters 19, 20, 3 respectively).

The practice of skin bleaching has evolved over the years from simply maintaining one's natural complexion to complete, full-body bleaching, sometimes including the bleaching of genitalia and anus.[26] (See the section on INTIMATE BLEACHING—Chapter 13). Many have internalized the idea that fair skin brings enhanced social capital and material wealth, an association that is also highly gendered. In a recent survey at one skin clinic in Lagos, Nigeria, 92% of female patients had used skin lightening creams, compared to only 5% of male patients.[14] What privileges does fair skin afford Nigeria women in particular? In a study of female secondary school students in Ibadan, Nigerian, Durosaro found that the girls perceived skin whitening as a route towards achieving a range of social and economic benefits. In addition to enticing men romantically, they believed bleached skin products would enable them to "enter into connection with high calibers, attain high social standard, become more successful in life, look fashionable, express positive self-concept and be able to compete well with their male counterparts."[19] Whether real or imagined, the perceived benefits of fair skin expand far beyond one's appearance. (See the section on THE SOCIAL IMPORTANCE OF SKIN BLEACHING FOR WOMEN—Chapter 17).

In Nigeria and Ghana[27], colorism is reflected in the over representation of light-complexioned models, actresses, and beauty pageant winners that Nigerians are exposed to. One does not need to look far to see that "women with lighter complexions are more often used to advertise a wide range of products including alcoholic beverages, detergents, cars, toiletries, cosmetics, textiles and telephone handsets etc."[28] "Siji Jabbar writes: "**Skin lightening ads, Kumasi, Ghana…..** *we take in these images and mimic the practice of colorism in our own ads and magazines. We see which black women are considered beautiful by the mass media, we see that the black models and singers who are making it are mostly lighter-skinned–Rihanna, Beyoncé, etc. We see which actresses get to play love–interest roles and which ones get relegated to bit parts, and we see which ones make in on to those Top 100 list." "When you look at the Nigerian film industry (the largest of its kind in Africa), you find that its lead characters tend to be light-skinned. Fela's condemnation of the practice in* ***Yellow Fever*** *(1976) doesn't seem to have done much good. Check the Ghanaian film industry and you'll find the same."*

A young girl who went to audition for a new Ghanaian film was bluntly told by the film director
"We like to work with fair skinned women in our films. Now, if you can tone your skin, we can consider you for future films."[29]

Famous Nigerian models and celebrities include Munachi Abii, Tonto Dikeh, Susan Maxwell, and Omotola Jolade, all of whom have markedly lighter skin than average Nigerian women. Slightly darker celebrities such as Genevieve Nnaji, the face of Lux Soap, and singer

Tiwa Savage provide skin tone diversity in the circle of famous Nigerian women, yet all have straightened hair or weave extensions, reinforcing a Eurocentric image of African beauty.

Nigerian Nollywood actresses clearly admitted that one of the reasons for bleaching their skin was *"to increase their professional relevance"*

Nollywood actress, Susan Maxwell, who sells her own brand of skin bleaching products has this to say:
"Black is beautiful, but I have no qualms with enhancing your complexion. 80% of Nigerian men want their women to be fair. They want a lady that draws attention to them. I've worked with many married women who complain of their men staring at fair women and they say to me, "Susan, make me fair, I want to be attractive to my man!" Some women have said their sons want them to visit their schools because they want to show off their fair mother." (See the section on CELEBRITY DISCOURSE—Chapter 6).

There is tension between Nigeria's traditional beauty standard –full bosoms, wide hips, dark skin like ebony to contrast with the brightness of white eyes[30] –and the image of female beauty in the West. "There are some cultures that would regard long hair and slim figures as unusual. In Ghana, it is unusual to see a woman with a slim figure. When the models arrived to the fashion and design week, one woman compared them to aliens. Women in Ghana have no desire to be skinny as a lack of weight is associated with AIDS and poverty and body fat is associated with wealth."[31] Two of Nigeria's beauty pageants represent this contradiction. The Miss Nigeria pageant seeks a winner who represents traditional Nigerian culture and beauty, a winner who challenges conventional Western beauty ideals.[32] Conversely, The Most Beautiful Girl in Nigeria (MBGN) pageant, which feeds candidates into the Miss World and Miss Universe pageants, seeks a "Cosmo girl" who is trendy and fashion-forward. MBGN pageant directors must position their candidates as competitive in the context of international beauty pageants.[32] In other words, pageant winners must fit the basic conventions of international beauty –long hair, relatively light skin, slim figure–in order to be competitive alongside women from around the world. In 2001, Nigerian Agbani Darego became the first black African winner of the Miss World title. Darego's light caramel skin, straight hair, slim figure, and thin nose sparked debate in Nigeria regarding the possibility of national beauty standards being confronted with quite different international standards. Should Nigeria succumb to the West's international definition of beauty in the spirit of global integration, or work to ensure that the next generation continues to value Nigerian women's natural beauty?

Nigerians seem to display more timidity and subtlety surrounding their society's preference for fair skin compared with Indians. According to Imani Franklin "whereas the Indians openly admitted personal and societal preferences for fair skin, many Nigerian youth were hesitant to discuss Nigeria's colorism and skin-lightening practices. One insisted that she personally had no color preference and that Nigerian society shows no real preference to fair skin. However, she also stated that lighter-skinned women do receive social benefits and that she doesn't mind that fair skin is considered more beautiful, because she believes that, 9 times out of 10, lighter women genuinely are more attractive".[33] This contradiction of describing Nigeria's colorism yet asserting that colorism does not exist was common. There was also confusion among Nigerian interviewees regarding the prevalence of skin bleach use. One Nigerian student said "the use of skin lightening cream is not common," ostensibly unaware that Nigeria holds the highest rate of skin bleach use in the world.[34] Perhaps this lack of recognizing or admitting the extent of colorism in Nigeria is tied to the embarrassment around skin discrimination in many black communities around the world. Hunter writes that there is shame around skin lightening in some cultures "either because one should 'naturally' have light skin, not chemically derived light skin, or because some believe that lightening the skin implies a shame of one's race or ethnic identity."[35] The anti-colonial, anti-Jim Crow international Black Power movement in the mid 20th century struck a chord with blacks throughout much of SSA and the U.S. As a result, many who subconsciously or consciously pride fair skin experience a level of shame, believing they should "know better."[36] "It is surprising that educated people, who should know better the dangers of misusing chemicals, have been consistently applying the creams, and paid dearly for the 'sin' in many cases.[37,38] The shame attached to this internalized racism creates a complicated set of emotions for black Africans who, despise themselves, have bought into the notion that "white is right."

One factor common across societies is the fact that women seek lighter skin not only for the sake of beauty, but because they perceive fair skin as bestowing a range of social and economic benefits.[3, 4] Hunter explains that, for many women in developing nations with emerging global economies, they recognize their employment competition to be international and believe that lighter skin will give them a leg up in the job market. Additionally, marriage prospects carry a host of socioeconomic implications for women and their families, such that beauty can produce tangible economic payoffs. What has prompted such diverse cultures, all of which have predominately populations of color, to endow light skin with such economic and social privilege?

"In Mali, 53% of women in Bamako use bleaching agents. Women who refuse to bleach often find themselves regarded as second class citizens. A woman who did not bleach her skin said she is often not offered a chair at baptisms, and is asked to make herself scarce when group photographs are taken at marriages." (See the chapter on MALI—Chapter 7).

Imani Franklin, in her dissertation asks the following questions: What has led young women like one 19-year-old Zimbabwean to believe, "If I am to keep my boyfriend from being snatched away by other ladies, skin bleaching is the only solution?" "What force has been most influential in propelling the preference for lighter skin in Nigeria?" In answering these questions, four potential driving forces were assessed by Imani Franklin.

1. Traditional | Pre-modern Preferences
2. Colonization
3. Local | Domestic media
4. Contemporary Western media

Limiting the Scope of Media Analysis

The term "media" is an umbrella term that encompasses television, movies, newspapers, magazines, music, and various other forms of commercialized art including digital media e.g facebook, instagram, blogs, twitter etc.

Historically, American television programming and films have been the most popular forms of Western media internationally. Throughout much of the 20th century, Hollywood enjoyed relative dominance over the entertainment industry internationally and made great inroads in emerging market nations. However, the past few decades have seen the rise of highly competitive domestic entertainment industries. India's Bollywood film industry produces over twice as many films annually as Hollywood and its viewer base is growing at a rate of 15% each year, compared to Hollywood's viewer growth rate of 5-6%.[38] Nigeria's Nollywood is the third most successful film industry worldwide, after Hollywood and Bollywood, and generated $800 million between 2010 and 2012.[39]

Studies assessing the waning dominance of American movies and television programs have found that, "when given a choice, audiences prefer domestic and regional content to foreign programs."[40] In other words, communities prefer to watch stories that reflect lifestyles relevant to their own rather than Western lifestyles. Professor Chioma Ugochukwu refers to this idea as a "cultural discount" that diminishes the appeal of foreign cultural products. Such products present difficulty for viewers around the world in identifying with the "styles, beliefs, institutions, and behavioral patterns of the material in question."[41] Magazines and advertisements also face this cultural discount, but less so than movies and television programs. Print advertisements enjoy greater flexibility in adjusting to local cultures when necessary.

Television shows in Nigeria can communicate in the local language, incorporate recognizable cultural symbols, and remove content that is irrelevant to a given society. Additionally, a direct image that can be easily interpreted across cultures is less vulnerable to the cultural discount than a complete story that requires greater cultural context to understand. Thus, Western magazines and advertisements seem to hold long-term potential for international success than Hollywood films and American television shows, which are experiencing growing competition from emerging markets. Second, *advertisements in print media are unlike other forms of media in that they almost exclusively sell idealized images of life, rather than reality.* With this enhanced picture comes an image of perfected appearances for consumers to aspire to. Additionally, print media can employ Photoshop technology to sell an unrealistic or even impossible image of beauty. (See chapter 17 on BEAUTY). Thus, magazines and print advertisements provide the best text for analyzing Western standards of idealized beauty. The following section will describe how various forms of Western media, and print advertisements and magazines in particular, are marketed and consumed in Nigerian.

Western Media in Nigeria

The most populous country in Africa, is projected to become the fourth most populous country in the world by 2050. Given this population rate and the fact that Nigeria is one of Africa's more urbanized nations, this country presents a significant marketplace for international media consumption. In an effort to increase domestic revenue from this consumer base, Nigeria has built its media industry to compete with Western imported entertainment. For example, when Nigerian television programming was in its infancy in the 1960s, foreign programming dominated the country's airways. During a period of protectionist policies in the 1970s, foreign programming fell to 10% and has now stabilized to occupy around 18-23% of Nigerian television.[42] Western film consumption has also been challenged, with the rise of Nigeria's thriving film industry Nollywood after 1992. Nigeria has built a star system similar to that of the U.S., with THEMA awards to mirror the Oscars, as well as celebrity and film publicity magazines. Researchers of Nigeria's film industry. Jonathan Haynes and Onookome Okome write, "Nowhere else in Africa has a domestic market been captured so successfully."[40]

Print newspapers and magazines constitute a thriving media market in Nigeria, and most are privately owned and urban based.[43] Whereas in 1965, around 80% of Nigerians were uneducated and illiterate,[44] Nigeria's adult illiteracy rate today has fallen to 39%.[45] This increasing level of education among ordinary Nigerian citizens provides a ripe market for print media. However, though Western print media is occasionally consumed by the Nigerian elite, the majority of print media in Nigeria is domestically Nigerian rather than American|British. Interestingly, like television programming and films, Nigerian print media often reflects some of the same colorist rhetoric present in Western media. In his analysis of hundreds of advertisements in Nigeria, communications researcher Emmanuel Alozie found that there is a relatively even balance between appeals to what he calls "Nigerian values" and "Western values" in Nigerian advertisements.[46] Appeals to the values of family and savings are balanced with invocations of youth and individualism. After comparing advertisements from three SSA nations, marketing professor Adesegun Oyedele concludes that one advertisement appeal that seems not to be balanced with local cultural characteristics is beauty. Appeals to physical appearance are less localized to specific national standards, and span cultures more broadly than other appeals in popular SSA advertisements.[47] The extent to which domestic Nigerian media reinforces colorist preferences is discussed below.

Methodology and Findings

Imani Franklin examined the pre-modern cultural standards, colonization, local media, and contemporary Western media. Ultimately, she concludes that the various social and historical forces motivating colorist preferences in Nigeria as well as India and Thailand share one underlying reality: the positive correlation between fair skin and individual prosperity. The equation of whiteness with social and economic privilege is present in each hypothesis she assesses. It is this association that can be understood as the fundamental force driving the preference for fair skin and incentivizing millions of women across the Global South to practice skin bleaching. Her paper treats skin lightening as a proxy for colorist preferences. For Nigeria, she looks at the pre-colonial (pre-1900), colonial (1900-1960), and post-colonial/global mass media (1960s-present). Based on anthropological studies, historical accounts, and primary text reviews of print advertisements from each case study, she determines which time period seems to have been the first in which colorism became hugely salient as it is today. She then attaches that time period to an explanation for the source of colorism – (1) traditional, pre-modern culture (2) colonization (3) local media (4) Western/foreign media. No one hypothesis necessarily fits all case studies. Rather, there may be a different explanatory phenomenon for each country at hand.

Hypothesis 1: Traditional/Pre-Modern Preferences

See the earlier section on SKIN COLOR PREFERENCE IN SUB-SAHARAN AFRICA and NIGERIA: HISTORY OF SKIN BLEACHING—Chapter 4.

One pre-colonial theory for explaining colorism is the idea that histories of conquest and class stratification privileged fair skin in Nigeria and Ghana.[3,4] In Nigeria, and West Africa more broadly, there is evidence to suggest that notions of racial hierarchy existed long before European colonialism. Race historian Lynn Thomas describes the process of female initiation that was common in many traditional SSA communities. In preparation for marriage, young women would undergo periods of seclusion from the community.[48] Part of the logic behind this practice was the idea that girls would experience a small transformation in appearance through cleansing, exfoliation, and a lightening of the skin from being out of sun. This example suggests that a bright, clear complexion held social significance in pre-colonial Nigerian society. Additionally, historian Bruce Hall writes extensively of the history of race in Muslim West Africa. Particularly in the 17th century, he explains, Arabs from North Africa increasingly dominated culturally and militarily over blacks to the South, marking what he calls the "Arabization" of the Sahel. This Arab influence created a racialized differentiation between Arabs (who often considered themselves white), Berbers, and black Africans. Hall writes,

> "By entering even more fully into the world of Arab Islamic culture, and by constructing and elaborating on genealogical connections to important Arab Islamic ancestors, the elite stratum in Sahelian pastoralist societies increasingly defined itself as part of one world and distinct from another".[47]

The process of African elite in the Sahel defining themselves as culturally and racially distinct from the masses marked an increased ethnic stratification of society that predates colonization. Interestingly, in the period of Arabization, whiteness became less about actual skin color, and more about "genealogical connection to important people in the historical and religious pantheon of Arab Islam. Blackness, by contrast, was defined most fundamentally by the lack of such connections."[49] In "The Historical and Cultural Influences of Skin Bleaching in Tanzania," a group of Georgia State University professors writes of a similar dynamic in the region of east Africa today known as Tanzania. Trade between local Africans and northern Arabs created a hierarchical relationship, in which "dark-skinned Tanzanians were considered 'primitive' and inferior to lighter-skinned Arabs."[50] (Also see the chapter on TANZANIA; SUDAN—Chapter 9).

Hypothesis 2: Colonization

Though historical indications of colorism existed before the onset of colonialism in Nigeria, Ghana and some other African nations, racial hierarchies that were loosely forming beforehand were cemented during British rule. (See the sections on PRE-EUROPEAN CONTACT "COLORISM"; COLONIALISM; NIGERIA: History of skin bleaching—Chapters 17,18,4 respectively).

The colonialism hypothesis for colorism essentially argues that the success in marketing and selling skin lightening agents today is "predicated upon European (colonial) promotion of idealized whiteness."[51] It is colonization, this theory asserts, that decisively imbedded skin-tone hierarchies into indigenous societies from West Africa to South Asia. Regardless of class level, black Nigerians were residentially segregated from white colonizers, were denied quality jobs, and were regularly supervised by less-qualified whites.[52]

Nigerian elite indirectly helped cement a racial and cultural hierarchy that valorized the British. On the most basic level, this colonial phenomenon equated whiteness with power and desirability. For the first time, the material payoff of being or appearing white became omnipresent in everyday Nigerian life. If this race/culture-based power gradation were not enough to embed a bias towards fair skin into Nigerian society, the British also intangibly assigned morality to different skin colors. Blackness symbolized ugliness, evil, and the dark side of the soul, while whiteness signified goodness, beauty, and godliness.[53]

Hypothesis 3: Domestic Media

The hypothesis that domestic media drives colorism is a challenging one to evaluate. In particular, it is difficult to determine whether the roots of colorism in Nigeria, Ghana and other African nations sprang from Western influence or are homegrown. In the local media of Nigeria, the vast majority of celebrities and models are the same race as the country's consumers, yet their phenotypes are typically more in line with Eurocentric ideals than the average woman of each country.

Popular forms of media include the myriad of wedding magazines that flood Nigerian newsstands, hip-hop music videos, and of course, the Nollywood film industry –which gained momentum in the 1980s and has a net worth of roughly $200 million per year.[54] Early forms of Nigeria's fashion and lifestyle magazines began in the late 1940s. Today, an average magazine typically costs less than one American dollar.[55] The 1959 establishment of Western Nigerian Television (WNTV) marked the beginning of Nigeria's television industry.[56] Between 1959-1984, 34 stations were initiated at a rate of 1.5/year.[56] In the same time span, the share of imported programming dropped from 90% to 20%, suggesting a growing demand and capacity for local media production.[41] While many Nigerian actresses and magazine models are lighter-than-average, there is significantly more skin tone diversity in Nigerian media than that of India. Dark and medium skin tones are surprisingly represented in publications like Drum magazine's Nigeria edition and fashion magazines like Bella Naija marketed to Nigeria's middle class. However, while color diversity does exist, medium to light skin tones are still disproportionately represented in Nigerian media, particularly in music videos of popular rappers like P Square and D'Banj.

Nigeria's local media does not seem to be the primary force behind colorism. This is partly because the beauty image in Nigerian media is not that radically different than women's natural phenotypes in the area. Moreover, widespread consumption of popular media in Nigeria is relatively recent, whereas Nigeria's colorism proves to be a long-standing phenomenon.

Hypothesis 4: Western Media

Josephine Mogiti has this to say about the influence of the western media on skin bleaching in Kenya.[57] Skin lightening in East Africa has more to do with globalization of European ideals than with colonialism. The 60s, as Kenya gained Independence and Pan-Africanism was all the rage, saw the initial surge of East African women using skin lightening products – an era that also saw the rise of television and American media, where the practice of preferential treatment for light-skinned black Americans was well established, and the black stars exported were Chuck Berry, Diana Ross and Jimi Hendrix." But as this idea grew, so did the forces against it, with postcolonial African politicians deeming it racial betrayal. On the insistence of medical professionals, who were also opposed to skin lightening, Tanzania became the first country to ban the practice in 1968, followed by Uganda in 1972. While Kenya never enacted a total ban, it prohibited ads for Ambi soap, one of the most popular products at the time, on the basis that it insinuated that modern, post-colonial Africans were light skinned. However in 2001, Kenya banned a list of products listed at the end of this chapter.

However, it wasn't a clear-cut case of racial pride versus globalisation, however, as the many social revolutions occurring during that time also included feminism. Audrey Wipper, a Canadian sociologist who was living in Kenya in 1972, criticised the range of bans in East Africa, arguing that "prohibition of Western fashions and beauty aids were efforts by postcolonial male politicians to use urban African women as scapegoats for the nation's problems." Skin lightening and, beyond the practice itself, the desire for light skin, had become contentious issues in the country, and women who used the products did so discreetly. Fifty-five-year-old Eunice was a form two high school student in 1974. "I remember Ambi and Snowfire as products we used to use." The creams were cheap, and most high school-going girls who felt that they weren't light-skinned enough could easily buy either from their neighbourhood shop. "I was partial to Snowfire because my skin became lighter and smoother faster than my friends who'd been using Ambi."

> This recent rise in the use of skin lighteners cannot be seen as simply a legacy of colonialism but rather is a consequence of the penetration of multinational capital and Western consumer culture. The practice therefore is likely to continue to increase as the influence of these forces grows.[58]

Unlike colonialism, Western media promotes colorism in a subtler manner, such that consumers can feel they are voluntarily buying into the preference for fair skin. The increased moral legitimacy of soft imperialism over pre-modern imperialism may decrease local backlash against it, rendering consumers more receptive to its messages. Unlike most local media, Western media typically embodies the image of global modernity and progress, an idea that seems to be increasingly appealing to women in the developing world who want to claim membership in a transnational, cosmopolitan culture.

As Glenn concludes in her work, regardless of unique national histories, "the desire for lighter skin and the use of skin bleaches is accelerating in places where modernization and the influence of Western capitalism and culture are most prominent."[58] Whether it is creating or simply reinforcing colorism, global mass media is a hugely significant piece in the puzzle of how the world has come to prefer fair skin.

> "Colonialism and westernization can be understood as intersecting rather than as a distinct, unrelated phenomena. In its aftermath, colonialism left a region vulnerable to Western influences, including media images that portrayed lighter-skinned individuals as valuable and more powerful. Western media images reinforced the earlier racial hierarchies that were in place..."[59]

Imani Franklin concludes:
In short, pre-colonial histories, colonialism, and modern-day media have intersected to produce a widespread preference for fair skin that shows no signs of abating in the short-term.

Regardless of the impetus for colorism in each case study, the real propeller of the preference for lighter skin is the **"global association of light skin with power."**[59]

According to the 2007 World Distribution of Household Wealth survey, North America and Europe alone own 64% of global wealth and the developed Asia-Pacific countries (Japan, South Korea, Taiwan, Australia, and New Zealand) own 24%.[60] India holds .9% of global wealth, Thailand .2%, and all of Africa a shockingly low 1%.[60] For women in the developing world observing this regional distribution of global wealth, it is difficult to ignore the uncanny association of whiteness with class privilege.

Even after the end of slavery or colonialism, "...as the capacity of whiteness to deliver is arguably diminished by the elimination of rigid racial stratifications, whiteness continues to be perceived as materially significant."[61] These perceptions of the historical and current material benefits of whiteness largely drive the $10 billion skin lightening industry. It is important to note that "whiteness" as a construct is relative, such that, even by lightening one's skin just a couple of shades, an individual can theoretically gain relative advantage over others in the community.

What is this *'POWER'* as regards skin bleaching in SSA?

South Africa Kwaito star Mshoza proudly states that she started undergoing skin-lightening and plastic surgery because she was "tired of being ugly." 'Beauty' in some communities has been associated with fair and honey-hued skin for too long, so many have fallen into the trap of believing it. Even Oscar award-winning actress, Lupita Nyong'O, publicly stated she grew up hating her skin tone and wanted it to be lighter. She would pray to God at night to wake up few shades lighter. It wasn't until Oprah Winfrey called brilliantly-dark Sudanese supermodel Alex Wek 'beautiful,'Nyong'O says, that she was able to start accepting her own beauty. "That made it a fact," she proclaimed at Essenc's annual Black Women in Hollywood Luncheon.

Advancing the popular Ghanaian aphorism, *ahoofe kasa*, means literally **'beauty talks'**, Blay[4] explores the politics of beauty among women in Ghana, particularly those who currently use or at one time had used skin lightening agents. Although the participants interviewed indeed express that their use of skin lightening agents is fueled by their desire to be perceived as more noticeably beautiful, critical analysis of the data reveals that what they are seeking is not an arbitrary beauty, but one that is functional and materialized via light skin. In this way, beauty via light skin as gained through skin bleaching, allows participants access to social capital, and for many, their newfound light skin color becomes a battering tool negotiable for economic capital.

Blay further clarifies the meaning of "power", in her publication entitled **'Skin Bleaching and Global White Supremacy: By Way of Introduction.'**[61]

"Weber's definition of power is instructive to understanding the European/White nationalist agenda. Weber defines power as "the probability that one actor within a social relationship will be in a position to carry out his will despite resistance, regardless of the basis on which this probability rests." (Einsenstadt, 1968, 15)[62]

And what are the components of this **'Power'** as regards Sub Saharan Africans who bleach? Love—**security**, value—**self-worth**, and purpose **significance!**

See the chapters on (1) MOTIVES FOR SKIN BLEACHING AMONG BLACK AFRICANS and (2) SOCIAL IMPORTANCE OF BLEACHING FOR WOMEN—Chapters 5, 6,17.

References

1. Imani Franklin. Living in a Barbie World. Skin Bleaching and the preference for fair skin in India, Nigeria and Thailand. Senior Honors Thesis Standard University. May 14, 2013

2. Gwaravanda, Ephraim Taurai. "Shona Proverbial Implications on Skin Bleaching: Some Philosophical Insights." *The Journal of Pan African Studies*, June; 29(3): 114. *http://www.jpanafrican.com/docs/vol4no4/Shona-20Proverbial-20Im plications_on_Skin_Bleaching.pdfhttp://www.jpanafrican.com/docs/vol4no4/Shona_Proverbial_mplicatio ns-20on_Skin_*
Bleaching.pdf

3. Hunter Margaret. Personal Interview with Imani Franklin. Nov. 2012.

4. Blay YA. Ahoofe kasa!: skin bleaching and the function of beauty among Ghanaian women. *JENda: A Journal of Culture and African Women Studies* 2009b; 14: 1-10.

5. Thomas Lynn. Phone interview with Imani franklin March 15, 2013.

6. Lewis, Kelly et. al. "Investigating Motivations for Women's Skin Bleaching in Tanzania." *Psychology of Women Quarterly*, March 2011; 35 (1) *http://pwq.sagepub.com/content/35/1/29.full.pdf+html.*

7. Discrimination based on skin color.*http://en.wikipedia.org/wiki/Discrimination_based_on_skin_color#cite_note_22*

8. Pumza Fihlani: Where black is not really beautiful. *BBC NEWS, Johannesburg. Africa.* January 2013. *http://www.bbc.com/news/world-africa-20444798.*

9. CIA World Factbook: Nigeria. *https://www.cia.gov/library/publications/the-world-factbook/geos/ni.html.*

10. "Lighter Shades of Skin." Beauty in Nigeria. *The Economist.* Sep 28, 2012. *http://www.economist.com/blogs/baobab/2012/09/beauty-nigeria*

11. Hunter, Margaret. "The persistent Problem of Colorism: Skin Tone, Status, and Inequality." *Sociology Compass:* 2007: 239. *http://onlinelibrary.wiley.com/doi/10.1111/j.1751-9020.2007.00006.x/pdf*

12. Adebayo SB. An epidemiological survey of the use of cosmetic skin lightening cosmetics among traders in Lagos, Nigeria *West Afr J Med.* 2002; Jan-Mar: 21(1): 51-5.

13. Ofondu EO. Cosmetic use of bleaching creams in Enugu. National Postgraduate medical College of Nigeria Dissertation 2003.

14. Ajose OA. Consequences of skin bleaching in Nigeria men and women. *International Journal of Dermatology.* 2005; 44 (Suppl1): 41-3.

15. Ofili AN, Eze EU, and Onunu AN. *Nigerian Medical Practitioner* 2006; 49: 1(2): 24-7.

16. NO1 polls. Predominance of Skin Bleaching Linked to Search for Beauty and Attractiveness. *http://www.no1-polls.com/root/indexphp?pid=182aparential=14aptid=1*

17. Jide Ojo. Nigeria as the world capital of skin bleaching March 26, 2014. *http:www.punchase.com/opinion/Nigeria-as-theworld-capital-of-skin…*

18. Kay Montano. The fairest of them all: Dija Ayodele on the culture of skin-bleaching. *THANDIEKAY* 31 July 2014. *http://thandiekay.com/2014/07/31/the-fairest-of-them-all-dija-ayodele..*

19. Durosaro AI *et al.* "Perceptions of Skin Bleaching Among Female Secondary School Students in Ibadan Metropolis, Nigeria." Journal of Education and Practice, 2012; 3(7): 43 http://www.iiste.org/Journals/index.php/JEP/article/viewFile/1847/1802.

20. Thomas Lynn cited in Glenn, Shades of Difference: Why Skin Color Matters. Stanford CA: Stanford University Press, 2009, 201.

21.*The Advertising Archives. http;//www.advertisingarchives.co.uk*

22. Hadiza Nuhhu-Billa Quansah. Black to white to black; tales of "nan so eben.*"(/index.php/articles-and-opinions-section/item/2282-black-to-white-to-black-tales-of-na-nso-eben) http://www.myghanalinks.com/index.php/articles-and-opinions-sectio...*

23. Hunter Margaret. "Buying Racial Capital: Skin-Bleaching and Cosmetic Surgery in a Globalized World." *The Journal of Pan African Studies*, June 2011; 4(4): 149. http://www.mills.edu/academics/faculty/soc/mhunter/Hunter_Buying_20Racial_20Capital.pdf.

24. World Health Organization (WHO). Preventing Disease Through Healthy Environments. Mercury in Skin Lightening products.
http://www.who.int/ipcs/assessment/public_health/mercury_flyer.pdf

25. Antony Barett and Zoe Smith. Toxic creams for sale as thousands seek whiter skin. *The guardian UK* 16 October 2005.
http://www.theguardian.com/uk/2005/oct/16/health.healthandwellbeing

26. Sowunmi Olayemi, Abulude Samuel. Skin Bleaching: Showbiz Personality Most Guilty. *LEADERSHIP* Aug 11, 2014.

27. Siji Jabbar. Who taught you to hate your [dark] skin? This is Africa. February 27, 2014 *http://thisisafrica.me//who-taught-you-to-hate-your-dark-skin/*

28. Olumide Yetunde M. Editorial: Use of skin lightning creams. *British Medical Journal (BMJ).* 2010; 341:c6102(Published 23 November 2010).

29. Akua Djannie. Skin Bleaching is a sin against God. *Ghanaian Chronicle / All Africa Global Media.* September 18, 2007.

30. Lawal Qudus. Interview by Imani Franklin. In-person interview. Stanford, CA, April 2013.

31. Hirsch A. Trend for Slim Fashion Models Only Skin Deep in Ghana. *The Guardian [online]*. Available at: *http:www.guardian.co.uk/world/2012/oct/09/skinny-fashion-models-ghana* Accessed: 16 March 2013.

32. Balogun Oluwakemi. "Idealized Femininity and Embodied Nationalism in Nigerian Beauty Pageants." *Gender & Society*, June 2012; (3):369, http://gas.sagepub.com/content/26/3/357.full.pdf.

33. Okoh Emem. Interview by Imani franklin. Email interview. Dec 12, 2012

34. Lanre-Ladenegan, Anjola. Interview by Imani Franklin. Email interview. Dec 12, 2012.

35. Hunter Margaret. "Buying Racial Capital: Skin-Bleaching and Cosmetic Surgery in a Globalized World." *The Journal of Pan African Studies*, June 2011; 4(4): 149 *http://www.mills.edu/academics/faculty/soc/mhunter/Hunter_Buying_20Racial_20Capital.pdf.*

36. Hunter Margaret. Interview by Imani Franklin. In-person interview. Oakland, CA, Nov 27, 2012.

37. Enock Kaputula. Ban sale of skin-bleaching creams- PHPF Zambia daily mail. *www://lusakatimes.com/201/03/31/ban-sale-skinbleaching*

38. Mahmood Shabnam and Manjushri Mitra. "Bollywood Sets Sights on Wider Market." *BBC Asian Network*. June 24, 2011. http://www.bbc.co.uk/news/business-13894702

39. "Nigeria's Movie Industry Becomes Third Richest Globally." *Ventures Africa*. Oct 25, 2012. *http://www.ventures-africa.com/2012/10/nigerias-movie-industry-becomes-third- richest-globally/*.

40. Waisbord Silvio. "McTV: Understanding the Global Popularity of Television Formats." *Television & New Media*, Vol. Nov 2004; 5 (4): 362. http://tvn.sagepub.com/content/5/4/359.abstract

41. Ugochukwu Chioma. "Cultural Resistance and Resilience Amid Imported TV Programming in Nigeria." *Africa Today*, Fall 2008; 55(1): 37. http://www.jstor.org/stable/27666950.

42. Okome Onookome and Jonathan Haynes. "Evolving Popular Media: Nigerian Video 112 Films." *Research in African Literatures*, Fall 1998; 29(3): 114. *http://www.jstor.org/stable/3820623.*

43. "The Nigerian Media and Entertainment Industry: More Than Fun, There is Good Money to be Made." *Economic Note: BGL Research and Intelligence: 5. http://research.bglgroupng.com/Documents/EconomicNote/ECONOMIC_20NOTE_The_Nigerian_Entertainment_Industry.pdf*

44. Baker Raymond. "Marketing in Nigeria." *Journal of Marketing*, July1965; 29(3): 40. *http://www.jstor.org/stable/1248544.*

45. "At a Glance: Nigeria." *UNICEF. http://www.unicef.org/infobycountry/nigeria_statistics.html*

46. Alozie Emmanuel. "Critical Analysis of Cultural Values Found in Nigerian Mass Media Advertisements." *SIMILE: Studies in Media & Information Literacy Education*, Nov 2003; 3(4): http://utpjournals.metapress.com/content/028t617g544w13v6/fulltext.pdf.

47. Oyedele Adesegun and Michael Minor and Salma Ghanem. "Signals of Global Advertising Appeals in Emerging Markets." *International Marketing Review*, Vol.2009; 26 (4/5) *http://www.emeraldinsight.com/journals.htm?articleid=1806003*

48. Thomas Lynn. Interview by Imanni Franklin. Phone interview. March 15, 2013.

49. Hall Bruce. A History of Race in Muslim West Africa, 1600-1960. *Cambridge University Press*, 2011: 57. http://ebooks.cambridge.org/ebook.jsf?bid=CBO9780511976766

50. Lewis Kelly et. al. "Investigating Motivations for Women's Skin Bleaching in Tanzania." *Psychology of Women Quarterly*, March 2011; 35(1): 23. *http://pwq.sagepub.com/content/35/1/29.full.pdf+html*

51. Oloruntoba-Oju Taiwo. "Body Images, Beauty Culture and Language in the Nigeria, African Context." Africa Regional Sexuality Resource Centre, Sep 2007: 36. *http://www.arsrc.org/downloads/uhsss/oloruntoba-oju.pdf.*
52. Kristin Mann. Marrying Well: marriage, status and social change among the educated elite in colonial Lagos. African Studies Series, 47, Cambridge: Cambridge University Press, 1985.
53. Gwaravanda Ephraim Taurai. "Shona Proverbial Implications on Skin Bleaching: Some Philosophical Insights." *The Journal of Pan African Studies*, June 2011; 4(4): 201 http://www.jpanafrican.com/docs/vol4no4/Shona_Proverbial_Implications_on_20Skin *_Bleaching.pdfhttp://www.jpanafrican.com/docs/vol4no4/Shona_Proverbial_Implications_on_Skin_Bleaching.pdf*
54. Haynes Jonathan. "Video Boom: Nigeria and Ghana." Postcolonial Text, 2007; 3(2): 7. *http://www.postcolonial.org/index.php/pct/article/viewFile/522/422.*
55. Rubenstein Joseph. "On Nigerian Pop Culture." *Dialectical Anthropology*, Aug 1978; 3 (3): 262. http://www.jstor.org/stable/29789937.
56. Umeh Charles. "The Advent and Growth of Television Broadcasting in Nigeria: Its Political and Educational Overtones." *Africa Media Review* 1989 3 (2): 54. *http://archive.lib.msu.edu/DMC/African_20Journals/pdfs/africa_20media_20review/vol3no2/jamr003002006.pdf.*
57. Josephine Mogiti SKIN DEEP. DM. *Destination Magazine. http://www.eadestination.com/investigation-journalism/467-skin-deep*
58. Glenn Evelyn Nakano. "Yearning for Lightness: Transnational Circuits in the Marketing and Consumption of Skin Lighteners." *Gender & Society* June 2008, 22: 289. http://gas.sagepub.com/content/22/3/281.
59. Hall Ronald. "Skin Color as Post-Colonial Hierarchy: A Global Strategy for Conflict Resolution." *The Journal of Psychology*, 2003; 137 (1):41 http://www.tandfonline.com/doi/abs/10.1080/00223980309600598#preview
60. Harris Cheryl. "Whiteness as Property." Critical Race Theory and Legal Doctrine. *The New Press, New York*, 1995: 285. *http://homepages.gac.edu/~lwren/AmericanIdentititesArt_folder/AmericanIdentititesArt/WhitenessProperty.pdf.*
61. Blay Yaba A. Skin Bleaching and Global White Supremacy By Way of Introduction. *The Journal of Pan African Studies*. June 2011; 4(4): p38.
62. Eisenstadt SN (Ed). Max Weber on Charisma and institution Building. Chicago: *University of Chicago Press*. 1968

GENERAL COMMENTS ON COLORISM AND SKIN BLEACHING IN AFRICA RETRIEVED FROM SOCIAL MEDIA.

It's a lazy Sunday. I was reading up on two interrelated topics that have fascinated me for quite some time now...Especially since my most recent visit to Somalia two summers ago when I witnessed, firsthand, the sad practice of skin bleaching and the way it ruins the lives of so many African women. It's even gotten to the point where the practice is Reaching epidemic proportions in several **African nations.**

There are many bleaching creams/products available in abundance all over Africa. These products are relatively inexpensive (the cheaper the product, the more toxic it is) and they are, for the most part, very easy to obtain with or without prescription. In a number of the African countries effected, medical & government officials have acknowledged the bleaching of skin as a widespread affliction that needs to be dealt with immediately. In some countries, the government has enacted laws banning the importing of the creams but the practice continues to thrive & the demand for the products spreads.

So when I went over to Somalia, my first time back there as an adult, I was just...so freaked out. I felt sadness afterwards but my initial reaction was one of horror. It's not that I was oblivious to the existence of the practice but the extent of it's popularity is what shook me....Most heartbreaking. I can't describe it in any other way. I'd be sitting with girls/women and they'd just have this bleaching as part of their beauty routines. Stripping themselves of their clothing, I'd watch on as they'd lather on the cream and slip plastic bags onto their limbs to seal off the air— maximizing the chemical burn. We'd go to a corner shop to grab an item or two and the younger girls would sneak off with the creams, giggling, the women would be purchasing skin bleaching products alongside their groceries. Anyway, I should note that I am aware of skin bleaching not being limited to Africa. Generally, it's common knowledge amongst people of colour all around the world. So. Enough of me rambling on. When reading articles/opinions regarding this subject, I'm always interested in which side of the argument a writer/person takes when it comes to tackling this basic question:

Who is to blame for the continued existence of Post-Colonial Clorism

Comments retrieved from social media

Are blacks/people of colour largely to blame for the continued existence of post-colonial Colorism?

I have girls trying to convince me that the products were perfectly safe skin cleansers & that I should give them a try because I am a boring (read: medium-to-dark) shade of brown. Of course many of them never had any sort of real formal education so I'd try to explain but for those who've been using it for a while, it's unfortunately too late for them to stop because their skins have adapted to the chemicals (they get blemishes/scarring when they stop using the cream). They've destroyed themselves. The long-time users you see walking around cowering from the sun..visibly excruciating in pain. That actually breaks my heart a little bit. (**evilted** Sept. 12th, 2005).

What exactly do they think skin-bleaching is going to do for them...do they get treated better by their black peers. It's so stupid and very contrary to the way they would be treated here in America. They would be outcasts and ridiculed but I guess
it's like getting a tummy-tuck over there.
(malloryrenee Sept. 12, 2005)
Some of the products are used to actually help even out skin tone. My sister and I use some of them not because we are ashamed of our skin. We use them to even out dark areas of our already medium brown skin. I am NOT advocating skin bleaching at all, I think many Black people are being brainwashed into thinking that Black is ugly, which is annoying and upsetting.
iI was researching the skin bleaching epidemic in Africa, and Latin America, and I think that it is just wrong. I forget the name of the product, we only use it sparingly, it might even be Ambi...if it is, we will stop using it due to this propaganda. (**Miyaunna** Sept.12, 2005)
If you bought it in Wal-Mart, it is most likely Ambi. They also have soap, but I had to stop using their stuff because it was making my skin feel dry, and the cream did not do anything to even out my skin tone. A hairdresser later told me that Ambi is not that good anyway. I forgot what she recommended instead, other than to stop buying black beauty products that are only sold in Wal-Mart. (**thegirliscrazy** Sept 12th, 2005).

See it's odd because it's a social stigma...but the idea that white/light is better is just rubbish.

So the key is to be as discreet as possible about the bleaching so others can think you're a naturally light-skinned black person. Of course most of these people almost always end up getting exposed in some way or another. I even learned how to spot the bleachers when I was there. Their body hair(arms, legs) would be blonde, then of course the blemishes & scarring. Also areas closer to bone/with less padding of flesh you'd see their big blue veins popping out all over the place because the skin gets so thin & diseased. (**evilte**d Sept. 12th, 2005).

I'm African. The reason they bleach in Africa is the same reason we do anything else to make us "whiter"%colonialism. Yes, lighter blacks do get treated better, and in America, lighter skinned people get treated better. Let's look at destiny's child...Beyoncé vs. Kelly. The two sound exactly the same. But..hmm. I don't even need to explain, I'll just say, yeah. Destiny's child."They would be outcasts and ridiculed." Do you ridicule light skinned people? The thing is, these bleaching creams do work, so you don't know who is or isn't using them in most cases. So, yeah, it has little to do with wanting to be treated better by black peers, more by white folk (who are coming back in large numbers to Africa, pissing us off some more), for jobs and all that, the whitish you are the better you're treated. Just my little insight. (**ritahritahritah** Sept. 12th, 2005).

They thought they were more attractive, yes. But in a way you can't blame them. It's the society. They've got men and women praising light skin as the ultimate ideal/sign of beauty. The girls want to look beautiful. But more importantly, with so many being fairly uneducated & poverty stricken, THEY NEED A MAN to survive. Marriage = shelter, food etc. So they do their best to fit the ideal. (**evilted** Sept. 12th, 2005).

"What's more strange is that East Africans have more..er.. I guess Caucasoid/sharp features than the usual black person in Africa since we've racial mixing from the past. On average, most of us are not THAT dark anyway. Some of us even look straight-up Arab. You see it in families all the time. I've got 2 bros & a sister who are seriously light skinned. " I know, that's the part that always made me wonder in general and in history we HAVE been treated a bit better than West Africans, and many say its because of our Caucasoid features...AND its important to note that this skin bleaching thing is more prominent in Western and Southern Africa. "Whereas in other African nations it's more common for men to bleach too." Again, very prevalent in West Africa. There is this singer who had lots of people lash out against him cause he had only hire dancers who bleached their skin like him. (**ritahritahritah** Sept. 12th, 2005).

In my opinion?

Are blacks/people of colour largely to blame for the continued existence of post-colonial Colorism? No. That always strikes me as "blaming the victim." At least when it comes to stuff that didn't exist before white racism came into play. Now, if white people owned up to all their racism and fixed the problems they caused... Then I guess people could start legitimately turning their attention to people of color perpetuating these things. I'm not saying that other people of color are "innocent victims." But I put 90% or more of the blame on white racism/colonialism. (**i_dreamed_i_was** Sept. 12th, 2005)

In Zambia they were even banned for a while (skin creams). Kenneth Kaunda famously complained about women with "fanta faces and coca-cola bodies". They're back on the shelves now. This reminds me of how glad I am to have come from such a dark-positive family. As in light-skinned people in the family are encouraged to darken the line, not lighten it, and people in my family are happy that I'm darker than both of my parents — when I popped out, they were really worried that I would be light. My son, however, is a hat-person. that is, when he's wearing a hat, you cannot tell that he's black. with NO prompting from me, he constantly goes on about how he wishes he were darker. I think that it's because he's always had so many positive black male role models in his life that he wants to be like them. (I don't include myself in that, even though he seriously looks up to me. (**Lindito** Sep. 12th, 2005)

In that picture the nurses hand is considerably darker than her face. Just something I noticed. (**Lapetitediva** Sept 12th, 2005)

I swear I saw a couple African women over the weekend who bleached their skin. It was really obvious because their faces were so raw and scabbed over. The skin wasn't even a color found in nature. No one has a complexion like that in real life, not even white people, it was just so pinkish and weird looking. Who are you fooling looking like that? It's scary what internalized racism/colonization can do to us. And like someone above mentioned, there must be huge levels of denial and cognitive dissonance involved. It really is beyond heartbreaking. (**kittylarock** Sep. 12th, 2005)

That picture is sad. : Horrible.
I think it's too much to say we are to blame. White/European is the standard of beauty, and when you grow up with constant reminders that white men are successful and white women are beautiful ie the Prince Charmings and Sleeping Beauties and Cinderellas and what not that we are bombarded with upon arrival, then the media slamming us with so many negative images of being black or being dark, creates this monster, and it will take a long time for us to get it out of our system.

Although we know what makes us feel as though we should change our appearance, and that it is wrong, it takes a lot for one individual to decide to go against such a.... huge prominent social standard. I wear an afro, and I do find myself at times listlessly turning pages in magazines, seeing long silky straight styles like, perhaps I should be a bombshell this week.......flat iron my hair and I'm like that, what a lot of work to do something I don't do naturally. When all Jessica did was shake and go this morn knowing that her straight hair is all she needs to fit the standard.

Not to mention weaves, nose jobs, starving ourselves, bleaching ourselves. Just like any other behavior that has been drilled in our heads, and we take over from there. They say we can't learn and are stupid, we don't go to school and call being smart white. They say black and nappy is ugly, we have a panic attack if someone says we are dark, press, perm and burn the nap out our scalps. They say we are funny silly buffoons, we coon it up till we can't coon no more.

So is it our FAULT, No. Are we largely to BLAME? No. But do we actively participate and contribute? Yes sir. And we need to quit. By the way, Beyonce has been looking like my dream brown lately so I doubt she is bleaching herself. If you compare her skin from Survivor album, to her in that cocoa brown dress tanned to death, It's such a big difference. I dream of a golden tawny glow like that *sigh*. (**chiefwiggins** Sep. 12th, 2005)

Reference

Evilted. Blackfolks. Livejournal. Colorism & The Bleaching Of Skin Sept. 11th, 2005.. *http://blackfolk.livejournal.com/2563814.html*

Further Shade and the politics of Skin Bleaching in Africa
Lighter Shade and the Politics of Skin Bleaching in Africa

We seem to be a carbon copy, if not an unreasonable facsimile, of the land of the free and home of the brave. South African Kwaito artist Mshoza is only doing very publicly what a number of Africans have been doing to themselves for years under what they believed to be the veil of secrecy. Skin bleaching was once such a problem in South Africa that the government banned the bleaching agent hydroquinone, which makes you " light and bright.' In fact hydroquinone was linked as a possible carcinogen according to the U.S. Food and Drug Administration, which is also proposing a ban on any products containing the chemical.

In Dec 2011, Kwaito singer Mshoza, appeared on the popular South African talk show Motswako to declare her "passion to be white". The horrified interviewer, Penny Lebyane, later said "Yes I was angry, Yes I took it personal! Yes I even wanted to shake her so I can get to realize what she's doing to herself!"

Now with all the jibes, twitter rants, expressions of horror and solidarity with blackness etc, let's get real.

Fact is the light skin amongst many societies, not least black ones, have always been considered most desirable or, if attainable, a mark of not only beauty but upward mobility. Mshoza's declaration goes one step better than the king of pop ever did – she admits she wants to look more white. To her whiteness is something she intrinsically believes will make her happy. Is she really to blame? Or is it the society we live in? As one smart person put it: "our femininity and aesthetic, particularly as Black women is a highly politicized…"

What I find strange are the people wanting to attribute Mshoza's choices to anything but societal pressures. ***How are we educating our girls? What kind of self-esteem message are we giving them?*** I know that we do not love our girls enough if this is the kind of nonsense that they eventually will end up doing. For a myriad number of reasons, we are taught to hate ourselves from day one, even by people who love us. But is Mshoza alone in her desire to emulate a certain Eurocentric image of beauty? Perhaps many of us need to have that discussion, with our weaves, our fake nails, and fake eyelashes. Until white people get not only tans but African curly, bouncy, thick and tangly natural hair transplants and weaves, I'm never going to buy that 'enhancement' argument.

I've only ever worn a weave once in my life. I bought a straight-haired wig to hide my bald head during winter. I kept forgetting I had it. It's not about enhancement, it's about denouncement, a worldwide phenomenon with black women. If much of what's on our screens, in our music and out of our mouths is anything to go by, we are a deeply hurt people. Can we not candidly discuss Mshoza's decisions as they reflect our society' ills? Whether her personal inspiration is *Christina Aguilera*, *Micheal Jackson* or *Rihanna,* we know that women's images are constantly being manipulated to suit a certain agenda. When do we get to take back the conversation, and set a new agenda?

- "I tried bleaching in 2013 and it was a nice journey. But I stopped and I'm back to being dark skinned and feel good to undergo that transformation. It makes you realize how beautiful dark skin is". (**Katlego** 21 July 2014)

- "I quite like looking through a post that will make men and women think.Also, many thanks for allowing me to comment!

This woman has low self esteem. FULL STOP! (**Magnific** July 13, 2013)

"Mshoza. I also want to bleach myself; I already done my face fill up, breast lift. The thing is they don't do it in South Africa. The bleaching, still hoping I will be able to do shipping of the products. Mshoza you are looking good girl." (**Zipho** Dec. 30, 2012)

"She looks horrible". (**Sade Mcneal** Dec. 14,2012)

"The weaves are just as destructive as the bleaching because of the baldness (alopecia) caused by it and also constant straightening can be permanent. Both stem from the belief that being black is ugly. A lasting legacy of slavery and the continued portrayal of fair skinned 'Black' women with long straight hair by the media which is only getting worse. You hardly ever see a real black women proud of her heritage on TV, just imitation white women and it's sickening. The people who fought for our freedom would be turning in their graves if they could see what they had fought for us to become% shackles of colonial mentality." (**Pabzito** June 17,2012)

"In a way, I don't care what Mshoza is doing. What bothers me is that she is in the public eye and young African girls are taking in all sorts of messed up message about their skin and features. Also, with India I've only just heard of this recently and am yet to confirm, but prior to European colonization, they were colonized by the light-skinned Aryans. I have to read more on this topic but apparently this age old colourism did not exist before then."

"Hi just wanted to say thanks for actually sharing this video. The way she thinks is not real to some people. But the fact that she has actually researched it and knows the perceived "benefit" of her wanting to change I find interesting. I feel sad that someone can feel like this. Considering some African cultures still have misgiving about albino. But her reasons are her reasons and maybe giving her this platform means that we all have to deal with this way of thinking. Is it any different to what we do to our hair? Is it not similar in thought to it? This is a misconception about what an "African woman" should look like. Again thank you for allowing us to debate this issue, there are similar limitations people place on the idea of being "Africa". (**Pamela** Dec. 10,2011)

Do not be sorry for the long comment, not at all! I am glad you responded. And I might have my own long response for you. Clearly, a simple post on this outlet will not cover the breadth of the issue, and I appreciate you citing another source of information for us. My generalization 'always' is certainly akin to the all-encompassing 'since the dawn of time' – and I was certainly not there! So – what does a short history lesson tell us? That it is not possible that all pre-colonial societies considered light skin as desirable as many post-colonial ones. We do need to delve more into the past to get an understanding of what ideas of beauty were in those times. Having lived in Botswana and the US most of my life, and now being in South Africa, I see the issues played out in similar ways. I call the US problems with colorism the house and field mentality. There is a fascinating book that I highly recommend everyone to read called The Color Complex. http://www.amazon.com/Color-Complex-Politics-African-Americans/dp/0385471610

Similar issues can also be seen in India, but that is a country where centuries of empire-building, before European colonization, rendered the caste system a malignant form of stratification. Thankfully, people fight for their rights. The Dalit castes of India, who are usually the darkest, and poorest people, are at the forefront of tearing down these outdated system of society. the caste/colour system has been so strong that a marriage between a (light) North India and a (dark) South India is something unusual, but happening more often now. This is why I was saying many societies have practiced forms of colour prejudice, and it hasn't only been because of colonization. European colonization only entrenched already widely practiced notions. It is what she is, I like her before and present she is pretty good, good my sister its your life and do whatever you want to do mwa mwa." (**Luso** Dec. 9, 2011.)

The issue of skin lightening/bleaching vs wearing a weave/braids is a bit like comparing stew to a salad, both are mixed but of a totally different notion and basis. Yes they might hinge on insecurities somewhat relative to societal influenced definitions of beauty, but the skin bleaching phenomena has much more

> extreme psychological nuances. I consider getting rid of blotches or acne scars etc as a different issue, but suppressing your melanin at cellular level%now that's like superficial genetic modification%I wonder what her (Mshoza's) kids think; but with media bombarding us with paler Beyonces and our kids in SA only exposed to whitecentric dolls and figures, they probably think%mom's cute%now what next? (**Rural Dexa** Dec. 21, 2011)

> At present the notion is heavy that the lighter you are, the prettier you are, as far as women are concerned, and that to my mind is destructive, naïve and totally wrong notion.

I disagree with this completely. I took issues with the earlier sentence due to the kind of high attention I pay to history and culture. A long time ago when I posted a similar sentence on my blog it came across like dark-skin has never been viewed as beautiful or as something to be attained ever. I feel a lot of us Africans think we are exempt from issues like colourism because we are not African Americans. However we are taking in the same message from the media and most of the time the media is not kind to dark-skinned African women. There is a lot of work that needs to be done and to change this we have to change the way we think altogether. In Africa it isn't even as obvious as that. We do need to go back in time and, like I said before, investigate the notions of beauty among many different societies. At present the notion is heavy that the lighter you are, the prettier you are, as far as women are concerned, and that to my mind is a destructive, naïve and totally wrong notion. (**Eccentricyoruba** Dec. 10, 2011)

> While I agree with much of this post, especially with regards to the self-esteem of African and dark-skinned girls, I take issues with this sentence;
> ***Fact is the lighter skin amongst many societies, not least blacks ones, have always been considered most desirable or, if attainable, a mark of not only beauty but upward mobility.***
> I strongly disagree with this sentence. I don't believe that light skin has always been considered most desirable in many societies, even African ones. I am not denying that some societies have placed people with lighter skin on top, however in Africa these societies did not from the majority. From what I've read, a lot of societies that favored light skin have a history of colonization and rule by lighter skinned populations. To be honest, one of the few books

I've read that spoke this supposedly natural preference for light-skin in all societies, even African societies only mentioned one or two African tribes (The Curse of Ham: Race and Slavery in Early Christianity," "Judaism and Islam"). I don't get how this forms the majority. If we're talking about societal pressures to be light-skinned, then we should also be talking about historical realities, the effects of Western colonization on our thinking and philosophy as well.

Now it is a good thing that so many discussions on Mshoza's bleaching have been popping up on African forums. Speaking as a Nigerian, I think a lot of us have self-hating ideas in our heads what we accept as 'natural Negroid features' in a Nigerian classroom. Looking back, it is amazing how even dark-skinned African children knew it was okay to deride features that are supposedly typically African (a big nose, full lips etc). I've only ever worn a weave once, to conform with expectations for secondary school prom. As an adult I decide to keep my hair natural and I was told that 'no Nigerian woman keeps her hair like that'. Like that%meaning in twist or a short afro. It is really bewildering the way we seem to hate natural aesthetics. I do not believe this is natural but a product of mental colonization. We need to free our mind from nonsense and learn to accept ourselves. (**Eccentricyoruba** Dec. 8, 2011).

Reference

Kwaito Singer Mshoza's Lighter Shade and the Politics of Skin Bleaching. *http://afripopmag.com/2011/12/mshoza-skin-bleaching-micheal-jackson/*

Chapter 12

The Skin Color Discourse

Story Highlights
Melanin pigmentation of the skin
human skin color
Social status, colorism and racism

Story highlights

- Skin pigmentation is affected by many factors: various genes, nutrition, environmental factors and one of the most notable is the **melanin** pigment.
- Melanin is a brown-black pigment and is found in the skin, hair, iris of the eyes, the inner ear, some parts of the brain and the adrenal gland.
- Some of the different types of melanin are **Eumelanin, Pheomelanin** and **Neuromelanin.** Eumelanin provides the black and brown pigment to the hair, skin and eyes**. It absorbs the harmful untraviolet (UV) rays and protects the skin from the harmful-cancer inducing rays from the sun.** Pheomelanin provides the pink and red colors and is the main pigment found among red-haired individuals. It enhances the skin sensitivity to sun and aggravates the aging process. Neuromelanin is found in different areas of the brain and eye; loss of this melanin may cause several neurological disorders.
- The top skin layer is called epidermis and melanin is synthesized at the bottom of the epidermis which is called the basal layer. Melanocytes are the special cells which are present in the basal layer and which produce melanosomes, packets of melanin.

- Melanogenesis is the production pathway for melanin production. The base amino acid is tyrosine, and tyrosinase is an important enzyme in the process of melanogenesis. Tyrosinase both initiates the synthesis of the two melanin and is involved in the steps further down the process line. Three enzymes are successively involved in melanogenesis: tyrosinase, TRP-2 (tyrosinase-related protein-2) and TRP-1 (tyrosinase-related protein-1).
- There are different skin colours and it is the amount of **melanin** pigment present which decides the skin color. The factors which decide the skin color are:

—the ratio of eumelanin to pheomelanin, where the more eumelanin is present, the darker the tone of an individual

—The melanocortin 1 receptor (MCIR) gene is primarily responsible for determining whether pheomelanin and eumelanin is produced in the human body.

—the absolute amount and concentration of melanin in the skin; and

—the size of the packets that melanin travels in (melanosomes), the number of melanosomes, and how well spread the melanosomes are.

- Human skin colour is classified according Fitzpatrick scale: Types l-Vl
- In general, people living close to the equator are highly darkly pigmented, and those living near the poles are generally very lightly pigmented. The rest of humanity shows a high degree of skin colour variation between these two extremes, generally correlating with UV exposure.
- The main function of the melanin pigment is to protect human beings against the adverse effects of the sun rays—ultraviolet (UV) radiation The photoprotective properties of melanin are directly related to the absorption and scattering of incoming radiation.
- The preferred skin tone varies by culture and has varied over time.
- Colonization and slavery by European countries inspired colorism and racism.

MELANIN PIGMENTATION OF THE SKIN

Introduction

Skin complexion is a characteristic that is affected by many factors. Various genes, nutrition, and environmental factors can play a role in the color of skin. One of the most notable components of skin that contributes to complexion is a pigment known as **melanin.**

Humans come in all types and colors. While some are lighter colored others are dark skinned. So why do we have these different gradation in color of the skin. Colors are formed by pigments. The one pigment in humans that is responsible for the color is **Melanin**. We all have heard of **Melanin,** either in our science class or mostly in the commercials on the **television** and magazines. The advertisements keep reminding us how they protect our skin from ultra violet rays and reduce the darkening of **melanin** pigment of our skin. Nowadays, studies on **Melanin** have become more intense as man is trying hard to find out solutions to reverse the **aging** effect of sun rays on the skin.

What is Melanin pigment?

Melanin is a complex polymer synthesized by living organisms. A polymer is a large chemical compound often made up of hundreds of smaller chemical parts, monomers. A variety of melanin can be found through biology, most commonly being composed of derivatives of acetylene, a black monomer.

Melanin is found naturally in our body and is present in various locations, from **brain** to the skin and from eye to the ear. The chemical composition of **melanin** differs at every location and is bifurcated accordingly. Until now, scientists have not been able to find out the exact information regarding the pathways and structures of various **melanin**, some mechanisms are still being evaluated. Chemically, **melanin** is insoluble, amorphous and it cannot be studied as a crystal form or as a solution. In order to understand the **melanin** properties better, partial degradation process has finally been devised by the researchers so as to study each component of melanin structure separately.

Melanin is found in several areas of the human body including:

- Skin where it provides skin color
- Hair
- Pupils or irises of the eyes
- Stria vascularis of the inner ear
- Areas of the brain, the substantia nigra and locus coeruleus
- The medulla and zona reticularis of the adrenal gland

What are the different types of melanin?

Some of the different types of melanin include **eumelanin, pheomelanin** and **neuromelanin.**

Eumelanin is found in the hair, skin and dark areas around the nipples. It is particularly abundant among black populations and provides black and brown pigment to the hair, skin and eyes. Eumelanin is brown or black color pigment and protects the skin from absorbing the harmful UV rays. People with darker skin tones have more of Eumelanin.This is the reason melanin pigments are called as photo-protectants which means a substance that can provide protection from the harmful sun rays. When eumelanin is present only in small amounts, hair may be blonde.

Pheomelanin is also found in the hair and skin. This type of melanin provides pink and red colors and is the main pigment found among red-haired individuals. This type of melanin is not as protective against UV-radiation induced cancer as eumelanin. Pheomelanin is a reddish color pigment and is a very weak absorptive of UV radiation and it also acts as a photosensitizer which means sensitive to **light.** Females tend to have more of this pigment in their skin than men. When this pigment enhances the skin sensitivity towards sun, in turn aging process also aggravates.

Neuromelanin is a form of melanin found in different areas of the brain and loss of this melanin may cause several neurological disorders. It is found in the brain and eye. But it is still not fully known what function Neuromelanin executes. It is found in the retina and also in the fovea area of retina. This area does not grow properly if melanin pigment is absent in the retina at the developing stage. But the other areas do not get affected by the presence or absence of melanin during development. Due to the presence of this pigment in the iris, it is opaque to light.

What is the work structure of Melanin? Where is Melanin produced?

The works structure of melanin is shown below in Figure 12.1

The top skin layer is called epidermis and **melanin** is synthesized at the bottom of the epidermis which is known as basal layer. **Melanocytes** are the special cells which are present in the basal layer and which produce melanosomes, packets of **melanin**. This is known as melanogenesis and when the skin cell nuclei get damaged due to ultraviolet radiations, this process is initiated. Melanosomes are carried by dendrites during this process and are spread to various skin cells (keratinocytes) all over the epidermis. Dendrites are tentacle-like projections. When the melanosomes are at the tip of the projections, they are squeezed into keratinocytes. These melanin packets then spread all above the nucleus for protecting the DNA placed within the organelle from dangerous UVR. Afterwards, these skin cells rise to the top layer of the epidermis and die. Eventually they are desquamated— shed away. Most skin pigment melanins working in other **organs** have still not been fully understood.

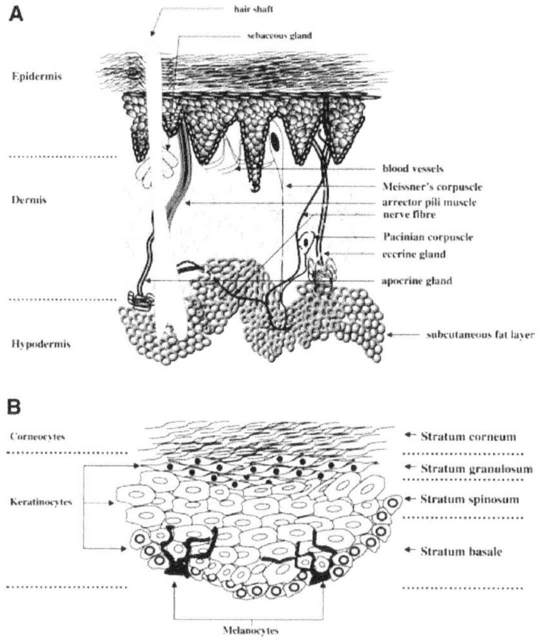

Figure 12.1. Structure of the skin. A*)* The different layers and components. Collagen, elastin, and other components of the extracellular matrix (ECM) of the dermis are not represented. B*)* Layers of the epidermis. The stratum lucidum usually present in thick epidermis such as palms and soles is not included; it is normally located between the stratum granulosum and stratum corneum and consists of flattened cells with no nuclei. Merkel cells (stratum basale) and Langerhans' cells (stratum spinosum) are not represented either.

Human skin pigmentation: melanocytes modulate skin color in response to stress

These melanocytes start producing melanin once damage occurs to the nuclei of cells in the skin, caused by ultraviolet radiation. This radiation can be either artificially (sunbeds) or naturally (sun) produced, and results in the biological release of alpha-melanocyte stimulating hormone (α-MSH). α-MSH binds itself to melanocyte cells, inducing the production of melanin within melanosomes. This overall process is termed melanogenesis. Once produced, melanin is transported to the upper levels of the skin through the outward growth of keratinocytes (skin cells). It has been found that the amount of melanocytes generally does not vary between people, but the number of melanosomes, and subsequently melanin, can vary dramatically.

What is melanogenesis?

The stages in melanogenesis are shown below in Figure 12. 2.

The production pathway of both eumelanin and pheomelanin is becoming better understood, it is known that the base amino acid is tyrosine, and tyrosinase is an important enzyme in the process of melanogenesis. Tyrosinase both initiates the synthesis of the two melanins, and is involved in steps further down the process line.

Skin and follicular/hair pigmentation is the result of the exposure of melanin at the surface of the skin and of the the hair follicle. Melanogenesis/synthesis of melanin is carried out specifically by the *melanocytes*, dendritic cells present in the basal layer of the epidermis, which put out branches for contact with the keratinocytes. The newly synthesized melanin is transferred from the melanocyte dendrites to the keratinocytes, which ultimately expose the melanin at the surface of the epidermis, thus providing uniform coloration of the epidermis.

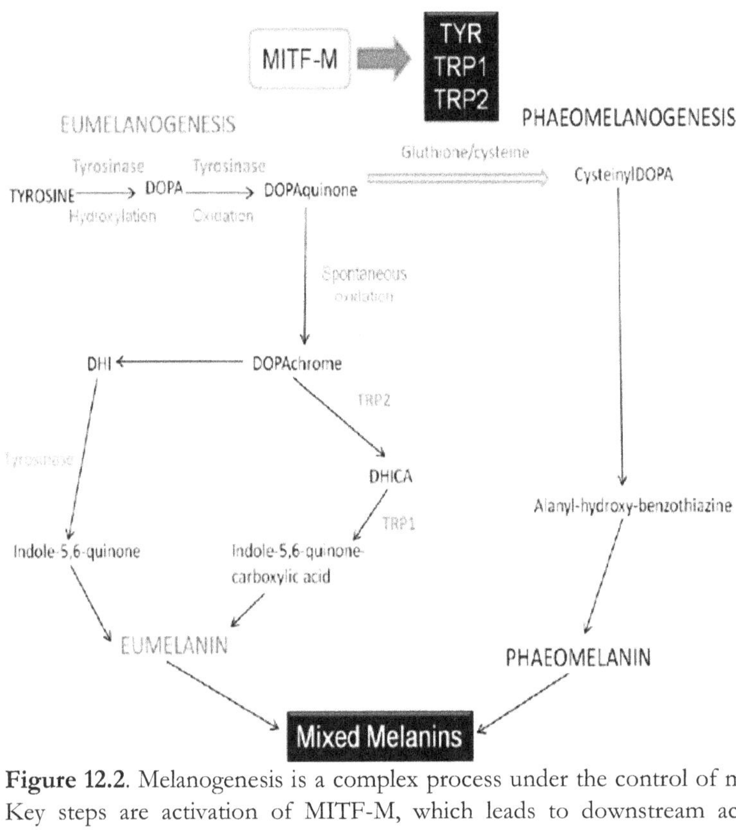

Figure 12.2. Melanogenesis is a complex process under the control of many genes. Key steps are activation of MITF-M, which leads to downstream activation of essential enzymes Tyrosinase, TRP1 and TRP2

The synthesis of melanins (pheomelanins, rich in sulfur, giving an orange color; eumelanins, conferring a brown color) is carried out in the melanosomes, which are melanocyte-specific lysosome-like organelles, by a complex enzymatic process. Three enzymes located on the internal face of the melanosomal membrane are successively involved in melanogenesis: tyrosinase, TRP-2 (tyrosinase-related protein-2) and TRP-1 (tyrosinase-related protein-1).

Melanin is a complex polymer derived from the amino acid tyrosine. Numerous steps are involved in the biosynthesis of melanin. The first step is catalysis of the chemical L-3,4-dihydroxyphenylalanine by tyrosinase. A lack of tyrosinase can lead to albinism. Tyrosinase is only found in specialized cells called melanocytes, inside which tiny granules of melanin pigment are contained in vesicles called melanosomes.

Tyrosine, a precursor for melanin synthesis, is hydroxylated to *Dopa* (dihydroxyphenylalanine) and then oxidized to *dopaquinone*, these two conversions being due to the action of tyrosinase. At this stage, the melanin synthesis can be oriented toward *pheomelanin* (orange-yellow melanin) which is encountered in blond individuals/ redheads, or toward *eumelanin* (darkbrown melanin) which is encountered in individuals with dark pigmentation.

Eumelanin results from the polymerization of dopaquinone so as to give leukodopachrome and then dopachrome. The latter is in turn converted either to 5,6-dihydroxyindole (DHI) or to 5,6-dihydroxyindole-2-carboxylic acid (DHICA) under the action of TRP-

2. At this level, the synthesis of eumelanin can be carried out according to two pathways. DHI is oxidized, under the action of tyrosinase or of a peroxidase, to indole-5,6-quinone, while DHICA, under the action of TRP-1, gives 5,6-dihydroindole-2-carboxylic acid. The indole-5,6-quinone and the 5,6-dihydroindole-2-carboxylic acid polymerize so as to form melanochromes and then eumelanin.

The synthesis of pheomelanin involves the formation of sulfur compounds (cysteinyl-DOPA) subsequent to the action on dopaquinone of glutathione and of cysteine. The cysteinyl-DOPA is converted to alanylhydroxybenzothiazine and then to pheomelanin.

Under the effect of solar radiation of UVB type, human keratinocytes produce and secrete endothelin peptide hormone which exerts a paracrine effect on the melanocytes. Endothelin activates a G protein-coupled membrane receptor (ETR) inducing melanocytes proliferation, and transcription of the genes encoding tyrosinase and the ETR. Similarly, in response to UV radiation, keratinocytes and melanocytes secrete the α-MSH peptide (melanocortin-stimulating hormone) which regulates melanocytes pigmentation activity. To do this, α-MSH binds to MC-R (melanocortin receptor), inducing activation of the cAMP/PKA transduction pathway, or even of the ser/thr kinase PKC, resulting in de novo synthesis of tyrosinase and in eumelanin synthesis. PKC-β appears to directly activate tyrosinase by phosphorylation of the cytoplasmic domain thereof. α-MSH also appears to facilitate the transfer of melanin to keratinocytes by stimulating melanocyte dendricity.

What factors determine the skin color?

Melanin is a pigment that is produced by cells known as **melanocytes** in the skin of most animals, including humans. This pigment comes in different shades, depending on the genetic make-up of the individual. Melanin comes in two basic forms, and can range from yellowish-red to dark brown. **Eumelanin** is the most common form of melanin, and is brownish in color. The other basic form is called **pheomelanin**, which produces reddish-brown color that is often associated with freckles and red hair. The production of melanin in the individual is determined by several factors.

Generally speaking, every individual on earth has approximately the same number of melanocytes. The difference, then, in the production of melanin is affected by:

i. Exposure to UV radiation. Melanin is produced as a response to UV radiation in order to prevent damage to the DNA in the integument. Individuals who are exposed to UV light, such as the sun, will produce more melanin for protection.
ii. Genetic make-up. Different ethnicities and cultures are genetically predisposed to producing particular shades and amounts of melanin due to inheritance. This is, essentially, one of the primary indicators used in determining race in the human population. (It is important to note that this is, and has historically been, a controversial form of human identification.)
iii. Size of melanocytes. Melanocyte size varies in different individuals, and may lead to a difference in the amount of melanin produced per cell.
iv. Disease conditions. Several diseases may affect melanin production, including **albinism** (a genetic inability to produce melanin) and **vitiligo** (a progressive loss of melanocytes).

These factors all play a role in the production and expression of melanin in the skin. While some factors are more prominent than others, ultimately, they are all important in the final complexion that is exhibited.

There are different skin colors and it is the amount of **melanin** pigment present which decides your skin color. The factors which decide the skin color are,

- The ratio of eumelanin to pheomelanin, where the more eumelanin is present, the darker the tone of an individual;
- The absolute amount and concentration of melanin in the skin; and
- The size of the packets that melanin travels in (melanosomes), the number of melanosomes, and how well spread the melanosomes are.

What is the function of Melanin as a pigment?

In the skin, melanin functions as an absorptive pigment. A pigment is a substance that, as a result of selective colour (wavelength) absorption, determines the colours of many plants and animals. In humans, the two types of melanin present in the skin (eumelanin and pheomelanin) are responsible for different skin tone (which is induced by ultraviolet radiation), and the constituent of freckles.

Eumelanin is a black or brown pigment, and is mainly concerned with the protection of the skin by absorbing incoming UV radiation. This protective ability warrants melanin to be termed a photoprotectant (a substance capable of providing protection against radiation from the sun). Pheomelanin is a reddish pigment, a very weak absorptive of UV radiation, further it also acts as a photosensitizer (makes your skin sensitive to light), where it increases sun sensitivity and skin ageing.

Melanin is able to protect the skin from UVR by several methods; it is able to scatter incoming UVR, absorb it, and can also absorb compounds produced by photochemical action which would be toxic or carcinogenic.

The amount of UV radiation that is absorbed or scattered is determined upon by a number of factors. The size, shape, and distribution of melanosomes, as well as the wavelength of the incident ray.

The photoprotective properties of melanin are directly related to the absorption and scattering of incoming radiation.

Once the energy is absorbed by melanin, electrons are raised to excited states and in turn, pass the energy on to the cell in which it is situated. Most (99%) of the energy absorbed is dissipated 'non-radiatively' within a nanosecond of excitation. The cell is then assumed to use this energy to regulate its conditions and drive chemical reactions, a role similar to that of chlorophyll in photosynthesis. It is widely supported that with increased melanin density in the skin, patients are less likely to encounter UV exposure related diseases. Aside from determining skin colour, the light absorbent melanin protects the DNA against UV radiation from the sun and it is considered a potential candidate in melanoma treatment.

References

1.Function of skin pigment. *Clinuvel Pharmaceuticals* http://www.clinuvel.com/en/skin-science/function-of-skin-pigment.

2. Meredith P and and Sarna T. The physical and chemical properties of eumelanin. *Pigment Cell Research.* 2006; 19:572-594.

3. Jablonski N and Chaplin G. The Evolution of human Skin Coloration. *Journal of Human Evolution* 2000; 39:57-106.

4. Chedekel, Zeise and Fitzpatrick, *Melanin: Its role in Human Photoprotection.* Valdenmar Publishing Company 1994.

5. John Williams. What is Melanin?— Definition, Production and Function. http://study.com/academy/lesson/what-is-melanin-definition-production...

6. What is the function of Melanin Pigment? http://www.innovateus.net/health/what-function-melanin-pigment

HUMAN SKIN COLOR

Human skin color ranges in variety from the darkest brown to the lightest pinkish-white hues. Human skin pigmentation is the result of natural selection. Skin pigmentation in human beings evolved primarily to regulate the amount of ultraviolet radiation penetrating the skin, controlling its biochemical effects.[1]

The actual skin color of different humans is affected by many substances, although the single most important substance is the pigment melanin. Melanin is produced within the skin in cells called melanocytes and it is the main determinant of the skin color of darker-skinned humans. The skin color of people with light skin is determined mainly by the bluish-white connective tissue under the dermis and by the hemoglobin circulating in the veins of the dermis. The red color underlying the skin becomes more visible, especially in the face, when, as consequence of physical exercise or the stimulation of the nervous system (anger, fear), arterioles dilate.[2]

There is a direct correlation between the geographic distribution of Ultraviolet (UV) radiation (UVR) and the distribution of indigenous skin pigmentation around the world. Areas that receive higher amounts of UVR, generally located closer to the equator, tend to have darker-skinned populations. Areas that are far from the tropics and closer to the poles have lower intensity of UVR, which is reflected in lighter-skinned populations.[3] Researchers suggest that human populations over the past 50,000 years have changed from dark-skinned to light-skinned and vice versa as they migrated to different UV zones,[4] and that such major changes in pigmentation may have happened in as little as 100 generations (~2,500 years) through selective sweeps.[4,5,6] Natural skin color can also darken as a result of tanning due to exposure to sunlight. The leading theory is that skin color adapts to intense sunlight irradiation to provide partial protection against the ultraviolet fraction that produces damage and thus mutations in the DNA of the skin cells.[7] In addition, it has been observed that adult human females on average are significantly lighter in skin pigmentation than males. Females need more calcium during pregnancy and lactation. The body synthesizes vitamin D from sunlight, which helps it absorb calcium. Females evolved to have lighter skin so their bodies absorb more calcium.[8]

The social significance of differences in skin color has varied across cultures and over time, as demonstrated with regard to social status and discrimination.

Melanin and genes

Melanin is produced by cells called melanocytes in a process called melanogenesis. Melanin is made within small membrane–bound packages called melanosomes. As they become full of melanin, they move into the slender arms of melanocytes, from where they are transferred to the keratinocytes. Under normal conditions, melanosomes cover the upper part of the keratinocytes and protect them from genetic damage. One melanocyte supplies melanin to thirty-six keratinocytes according to signals from the keratinocytes. They also regulate melanin production and replication of melanocytes.[6] People have different skin colors mainly because their melanocytes produce different amount and kinds of melanin. The genetic mechanism behind human skin color is mainly regulated by the enzyme tyrosinase, which creates the color of the skin, eyes, and hair shades.[9,10] Differences in skin color are also attributed to differences in size and distribution of melanosomes in the skin.[6] Melanocytes produce two types of melanin. The most common form of biological melanin is eumelanin, a brown-black polymer of dihydroxyindole carboxylic acids, and their reduced forms. Most are derived from the amino acid tyrosine. Eumelanin is found in hair, areola, and skin, and the hair colors grey, black, yellow, and brown. In humans, it is more abundant in people with dark skin. Pheomelanin, a pink to red hue is found in particularly large quantities in red hair,[11] the lips, nipples, glans of the penis, and vagina.[12]

Both the amount and type of melanin produced is controlled by a number of genes that operate under incomplete dominance.[13] One copy of each of the various genes is inherited from each parent. Each gene can come in several alleles, resulting in the great variety of human skin tones. Melanin controls the amount of ultraviolet (UV) radiation from the sun that penetrates the skin by absorption. While UV radiation can assist in the production of vitamin D, excessive exposure to UV can damage health.

MC1R

The melanocortin 1 receptor (MC1R) gene is primarily responsible for determining whether pheomelanin and eumelanin is produced in the human body.

Sexual dimorphism

The degree of differences between male and female anatomical traits is called sexual dimorphism. It has been observed that adult human females are consistently lighter in skin pigmentation than males in the same population.[8] This form of sexual dimorphism is due to the requirement in human females for high amounts of calcium during pregnancy and lactation. Breastfeeding newborns, whose skeletons are growing, require high amounts of calcium intake from the mother's milk (about 4 times more than during prenatal development),[14] part of which comes from reserves in the mother's skeleton. Adequate vitamin D resources are needed to absorb calcium from the diet, and it has been shown that deficiencies of vitamin D and calcium increase the likelihood of various birth defects such as spina bifida and rickets.

Natural selection has led to females with lighter skin than males in all indigenous populations because women must get enough vitamin D and calcium to support the development of fetus and nursing infant and to maintain their own health.[6]

The sexes also differ in how they change their skin color with age. Men and women are not born with different skin color, they begin to diverge during puberty with the influence of sex hormones. Women can also change pigmentation in certain parts of their body, such as the areola, during the menstrual cycle and pregnancy and between 50 and 70% of pregnant women will develop the "mask of pregnancy" (melasma or chloasma) in the cheeks, upper lips, forehead, and chin.[6] This is caused by increases in the female hormones estrogen and progesterone and it can develop in women who take birth control pills or participate in hormone replacement therapy.[15]

Disorders of skin pigmentation

Uneven pigmentation of some sort affects most people, regardless of bioethnic background or skin color. Skin may either appear lighter, or darker than normal, or lack pigmentation at all; there may be blotchy, uneven areas, patches of brown to gray discoloration or freckling. Apart from blood-related conditions such as jaundice, carotenosis, or argyria, skin pigmentation disorders generally occur because the body produces either too much or too little melanin.

Depigmentation

Various types of albinism are a result of genetic mutations affecting different parts of the melanin production pathway. In a person with albinism, melanocytes can be entirely absent, or fail to produce melanin, or melanosomes can fail to mature and be transferred to keranocytes. The ability to produce melanin in patches around the body is a condition known as vitiligo.

Hyperpigmentation

Increased melanin production, also known as hyperpigmentation, can be a few different phenomena

Melasma (formally called chloasma) describes the skin discolorations darkening of the skin caused by hormones. These hormonal changes are usually the result of pregnancy, birth control pills or estrogen replacement therapy.

Solar lentigo, also known as "liver spots" or "senile freckles" refers to darkened spots on the skin caused by aging and the sun. These spots are quite common in adults with a long history of unprotected sun exposure. The most typical cause of darkened areas of skin, brown spots or areas of discoloration is unprotected sun exposure. Once incorrectly referred to as liver spots, these pigment problems are not connected with the liver.

Aside from sun exposure and hormones, hyperpigmentation can be caused by skin damage, such as remnants of blemishes, wounds or rashes— post inflammatory hyperpigmentation. This is especially true for those with darker skin tones. On lighter to medium skin tones, solar lentigenes emerge as small- to medium-sized brown patches of freckling that can grow and accumulate over time on areas of the body that receive the most unprotected sun exposure, such as the back of the hands, forearms, chest, and face. For those with darker skin colors, these discolorations can appear as patches or areas of ashen-gray skin. Parts of the skin uncovered by clothing and maximally exposed to the sun are usually darker than the covered areas (Figure 12.3).

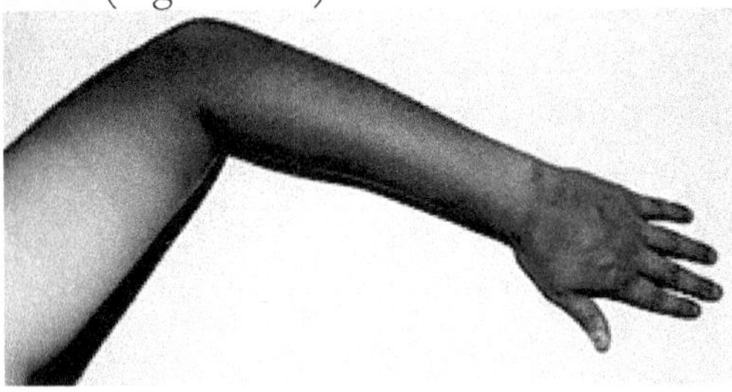

Fig 12:3. A suntanned arm showing darker skin where it has been exposed. This pattern of tanning is often called a farmer's tan.

Exposure of skin to solar radiation

Melanin in the skin protects the body by absorbing solar radiation. In general, the more melanin there is in the skin the more solar radiation can be absorbed. Excessive solar radiation causes direct and indirect DNA damage to the skin and the body naturally combats and seeks to repair the damage and protect the skin by creating and releasing further melanin into the skin's cells. With the production of the melanin, the skin color darkens, but can also cause sunburn. The tanning process can also be created by artificial UV radiation.

There are two different mechanisms involved. Firstly, the UVA-radiation creates oxidative stress, which in turn oxidizes existing melanin and leads to rapid darkening of the melanin, also known as IPD (immediate pigment darkening). Secondly, there is an increase in production of melanin known as melanogenesis.[16] Melanogenesis leads to delayed tanning and first becomes visible about 72 hours after exposure. The tan that is created by an increased melanogenesis lasts much longer than the one that is caused by oxidation of existing melanin. Tanning involves not just the increased melanin production in response to UV radiation but the thickening of the top layer of the epidermis, the stratum corneum.[6]

A person's natural skin color has an impact on their reaction to exposure to the sun. Generally, those who start out with darker skin color and more melanin have better abilities to tan. Individuals with very light skin and albinos have no ability to tan.[17] The biggest differences resulting from sun exposure are visible in individuals who start out with moderately pigmented brown skin: the change is dramatically visible as tan lines, where parts of the skin which tanned are delineated from unexposed skin.[6]

Modern lifestyles and mobility have created mismatch between skin color and environment for many individuals. Vitamin D deficiencies and UVR overexposure are concerns for many. It is important for these people individually to adjust their diet and lifestyle according to their skin color, the environment they live in, and the time of year. For practical purposes, such as exposure time for sun tanning, six skin types are distinguished following Fitzpatrick,[17] listed in order of decreasing lightness (Table 12.1). Figure 12.4 shows Von Luschan's chromatic scale.[18]

Table 12.1 Fitzpatrick scale

Type	Also called	sunburning	Tanning behaviour	Von Luschan's scale
I	Light, pale white	Often	Occasionally	1-5
II	White, fair	Usually	Sometimes	6-10
III	Medium, white to light brown	Rarely	Usually	11-15
IV	Olive, moderate brown	Rarely	Often	16-21
V	Brown, dark brown	Very raely	Sometimes darkens	22-28
VI	Very dark brown to black	Extremely rarely	Naturally black-brown skin	29-36

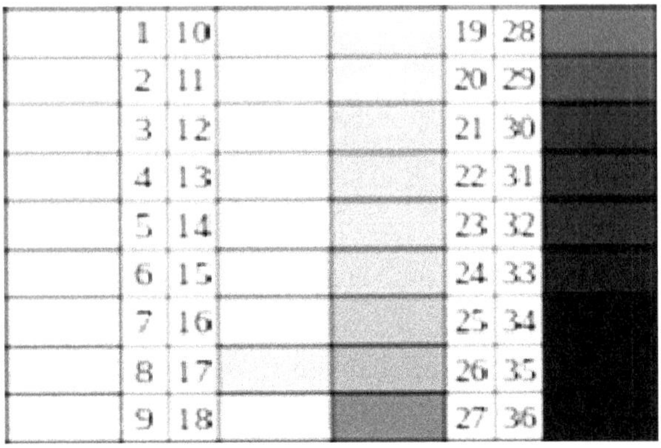

Fig 12.4 Skin colors according to von Luschan's chromatic scale

Dark skin with large concentrations of melanin protects against ultraviolet light and skin cancers; light-skinned people have about a tenfold greater risk of dying from skin cancer, compared with dark-skinned persons, under equal sunlight exposure. Furthermore, rays from sunlight are believed to interact with folic acid in ways that may damage health.[19] In a number of traditional societies the sun was avoided as much as possible, especially around noon when the ultraviolet radiation in sunlight is at its most intense. Midday was a time when people stayed in the shade and had the main meal followed by a nap,[20] a practice similar to the modern siesta.

In general, people living close to the equator are highly darkly pigmented, and those living near the poles are generally very lightly pigmented. The rest of humanity shows a high degree of skin color variation between these two extremes, generally correlating with UV exposure.

References

1. Muehlenbein Michael. *Human Evolutionary Biology*. Cambridge University Press. 2010; pp. 192–213.
2. Jablonski NG. *Skin: a Natural History*. Berkeley: University of California Press. 2006.
3. Webb AR."Who, what, where, and when: influences on cutaneous vitamin D synthesis". *Progress in Biophysics and Molecular Biology* . 2006; 92 (1): 17–25.
4. Jablonski Nina G. "Why Human Skin Comes in Colors". *AnthroNotes* Spring 2011; 32 (1).
5. "The Human Family Tree Facts". (http://channel.nationalgeographic.com/channel/a-night-of-exploration/articles/the-human-family-tree-facts/) *National Geographic*. Retrieved 2013-07-20.
6. Jablonski Nina. *Living Color*. Berkeley, Los Angeles, London: University of California Press. 2012; ISBN 978-0-520-25153-3.

7. Jablonski NG, Chaplin G. "Colloquium Paper: Human skin pigmentation as an adaptation to UV radiation". *Proceedings of the National Academy of Sciences.* 2010; 107: 8962–8.
8. Jablonski Nina, Chaplin George. "The evolution of human skin coloration." *Journal of Human Evolution.* 2000; 39 (1): 57–106.
9. Sturm RA. "A golden age of human pigmentation genetics". *Trends in Genetics* 2006; 22 (9): 464–9.
10. Sturm R A, Teasdale and Fox N F."Human pigmentation genes: Identification, structure and consequences of polymorphic variation". *Gene* 2001; 277 (1–2): 49–62.
11. Ito S, Wakamatsu K S, Wakamatsu K. "Diversity of human hair pigmentation as studied by chemical analysis of eumelanin and pheomelanin". *J Eur Acad Dermatol Venereol.* Dec 2011; 25 (12): 1369–80.
12.http://www.metacyc.org/META/NEW-IMAGE?type=COMPOUND&object=CPD-12380
13. Schneider Patricia. "The Genetics and Evolution of Skin Color: The Case of Desiree's Baby". *RACE – The Power Of An Illusion.* Public Broadcasting Service. 2003. Retrieved 14 April 2015.
14. Kovacs Christine. "Vitamin D pregnancy and lactation: maternal, fetal and neonatal outcomes from human and animal studies." *American Journal of Clinical Nutrition* 2008; 88 (2): 5205-85.
15. Costin and Hearing, Hearing VJ. "Human Skin pigmentation: Melanocytes modulate skin color in response to stress." *FASEB Journal* 2007; 21 (4): 976-94.
16. Agar Nita, Young Antony R. "Melanogenesis: a photoprotective response to DNA damage?" *Mutation Research/ Fundamental and Molecelar Mechanisms of Mutagenesis.* 2005; 571 (1-2): 121-32.
17. Fitzpatrick TB. "Normal skin color and general considerations of pigmentary disorder". *Fitzpatrick's Dermatology in General Medicine.* New York: McGraw-Hill. 2003; 819-25
18."Skin Tones/Tones chart" (http://www.fairandflawlessskin.com/skintonehtml). *Fair & Flawless.* Retrieved 2013-01-05.
19. Vorobey P, Steindal AE, Off MK, Vorobey A, Moan J. "Influence of human serum albumin on photodegradation of folic acid in solution." *Photochemistry and photobiology.* 2006; 82 (3): 817-22

Retrieved from *http://en/wikipedia.org/w/index.php?title=Human-skin_color&oldid=664640444*

SOCIAL STATUS, COLORISM AND RACISM

The preferred skin tone varies by culture and has varied over time. A number of indigenous African groups, such as the **Maasai,** associated pale skin with being cursed or caused by evil spirits associated with witchcraft. They would abandon their children born with conditions such as albinism and showed a sexual preference for darker skin.[1]

Many cultures have historically favored lighter skin for women. In Europe, before the Industrial Revolution, pale skin was preferred and was a sign of high social status. The poorer classes worked outdoors and got darker skin from exposure to the sun, while the upper class stayed indoors and had light skin. Hence, light skin became associated with wealth and high position.[2] Women would put lead-based cosmetics on their skin to whiten their skin tone artificially.[3] However, when not strictly monitored, these cosmetics caused lead poisoning. Achieving a light-skinned appearance was additionally brought about in various other ways, including the use of arsenic to whiten skin, and powders. Other methods included wearing full-length clothes when outdoors, including gloves and parasols.

Colonization and slavery by European countries inspired colorism and racism, led by the belief that people with dark skin were uncivilized, inferior, and should be subordinate to the lighter-skinned invaders. This has been perpetuated in modern times.[4] During slavery, lighter-skinned African-Americans were perceived as more intelligent, cooperative, and beautiful.[5] They were more likely to work as house slaves and were also given preferential treatment by plantation owners and the overseers. For example, they had a chance to get an education[6] while darker African-Americans worked in the fields and did not get an education.[7] The preference for fair skin remained prominent until the end of the Victorian era, but racial stereotypes about worth and beauty were still persistent in the last half of the 20th century and continue in the present day. African-American journalist Jill Nelson wrote that, "To be both prettiest and black was impossible,"[8] and elaborated:
"We learn as girls that in ways both subtle and obvious, personal and political, our value as females is largely determined by how we look. ... For black women, the domination of physical aspects of beauty in women's definition and value render us invisible, partially erased, or obsessed, sometimes for a lifetime, since most of us lack the major talismans of Western beauty. Black women find themselves involved in a lifelong effort to self-define in a culture that provides them no positive reflection."[8]

A preference for fair or lighter skin continues in some countries, including Latin American countries where whites are a minority.[9] A dark-skinned person is more likely to be discriminated against in Brazil.[10] Many actors and actresses in Latin America have European features—blond hair, blue eyes, and pale skin.[11,12] A light-skinned person is considered more privileged and has a higher social status;[12] a person with light skin is considered more beautiful[12] and it suggests that the person has more wealth.[12] Skin color is such an obsession in some countries that specific words describe distinct skin tones from "*jincha*", Puerto Rican slang for "glass of milk" to "*morena*", literally "brown".[12]

In India, pale skin is considered more attractive, while dark skin is associated with a lower class status, creating a massive market for skin whitening creams.[13] Fairer skin tones also correlate to higher caste status in the Hindu social order – although the system is not based on skin tone.[14] Actors and actresses in Indian cinema tend to have light skin tones, and Indian cinematographers have used graphics and intense lighting to achieve more desirable skin tones.[15] Fair skin tones are claimed to be an asset in Indian marketing.[16]

Skin whitening products have remained prominent over time, often due to historical beliefs and perceptions about fair skin. Sales of skin whitening products across the world grew from $40 billion to $43 billion in 2008.[17] In South and East Asian countries, light skin has traditionally been seen as more attractive, and a preference for lighter skin remains prevalent. In ancient China and Japan, for example, pale skin can be traced back to ancient drawings depicting women and goddesses with fair skin tones. In ancient China, Japan, and Southeast Asia, pale skin was seen as a sign of wealth. Thus, skin whitening cosmetic products are popular in East Asia.[18] 4 out of 10 women surveyed in Hong Kong, Malaysia, the Philippines and South Korea used a skin-whitening cream, and more than 60 companies globally compete for Asia's estimated $18 billion market.[19] Changes in regulations in the cosmetic industry led to skin care companies introducing high end skin lighteners. In Japan, the geisha are well known for their white painted faces, and the appeal of the *bihaku*, or "beautiful white", ideal leads many Japanese women to avoid any form of tanning.[20] There are exceptions to this, with Japanese fashion trends such as ganguro emphasizing almost black skin. Skin whitening is also not uncommon in Africa,[21,22] and several research projects have suggested a general preference for lighter skin in the African-American community.[23] In contrast, one study on men of the Bikosso tribe in Cameroon found no preference for attractiveness of females based on lighter skin color, bringing into question the universality of earlier studies that had exclusively focused on skin color preferences among non-African populations.[24]

Significant exceptions to a preference for lighter skin started to appear in Western culture mid-20th century.[25] Though sun-tanned skin was once associated with the sun-exposed manual labor of the lower class, the associations became dramatically reversed during this time — a change usually credited to the trendsetting Frenchwoman Coco Chanel making tanned skin seem fashionable, healthy, and luxurious.[26] Today, though an overall preference for lighter skin remains prevalent in the United States, many within the country regard tanned skin as both more attractive and healthier than pale skin.[27,28,29,30] Western mass media and popular culture continued to reinforce negative stereotypes about dark skin,[31] but in some circles pale skin has become associated with indoor office work while tanned skin has become associated with increased leisure time, sportiness and good health that comes with wealth and higher social status.[2] Studies have also emerged indicating that the degree of tanning is directly related to how attractive a young woman is.[32,33]

References

1. Africa: Dispelling Myths about Albinism, (http://allafrica.com/stories/2009091054.html), Pambazuka News, 10 September 2009

2. Kruszelnicki Karl "News in Science: Skin Colour 1". (March 1, 2001). http://www.abc.net.au/science/articles/2001/03/01/249992.htm?site=science/greatmomentsinscienceabc-net.au . Retrieved May 25, 2014.

3. Agredano YZ, Chan JL, Kimball RC, Kimball AB. "Accessibility to air travel correlates strongly with increasing melanoma incidence". *Melanoma Research* (February 2006). 16 (1) 77-81

4. Hall Ron. "The Psychogenesis of Color Based Racism: Implications of Projection for Dark-SkinnedPuertorriqueños"http://web.archive.org/web/20110106160600/http://www.jsri.msu.edu/RandS/research/irr/rr21.pdf

5."What Are "Good Looks"?". http://northbysouth.kenyon.edu/2000/Beauty/goodlooks.htm Kenyon College. Retrieved 2014-03-23.

6. "The Paper Bag Test".http://www.sptimes.com/2003/08/31/Columns/The_paper_bag_test.shtml St. Petersburg Times. 2003-08-31. Retrieved 2014-03-23.

7. "For Light-Skinned Only?". http://www.npr.org/blogs/newsandviews/2007/10/for_lightskinned_only.html 2007-08-16. Retrieved 2014-03-23.

8. Jill Nelson (1997). "Straight, No Chaser—How I Became a Grown-Up Black Woman— WHO'S THE FAIREST OF THEM ALL?" (http://comminfo.rutgers.edu/professional-

development/childlit/books/Straight.PDF). New York Times. Retrieved 2009-11-06.
9. "Documentary, Studies Renew Debate About Skin Color's Impact". http://www.post-gazette.com/lifestyle/2006/12/26/ Documentary-studies-renew-debate-about-skin-color-s-impact/stories/200612260092. *Pittsburg Post Gazette.* 2006-12-26. Retrieved 2014-03-23.
10. "Racism Takes Many Hues". http://www.miamiherald.com/multimedia/news /afrolatin/part5/index.html Miami Herald. 2007-08-24. Retrieved 2014-03-23.
11. Quinonez Ernesto. "Y Tu Black Mama Tambien". (2003-06-19). http://www.newsweek.com Retrieved 2008-05-02.
12. Jones Vanessa E. "Pride or Prejudice?". (2004-08-19). http://www.boston.com/news/globe/living/articles/2004/08/19/pride_or_prejudice/?page=2 Boston.com. Retrieved 2014-03-23.
13. Sidner Sara. "Skin whitener advertisements labeled racist". 9 September 2009. http://edition.cnn.com/2009/WORLD/asiapcf/09/09/india.skin/index.html. *CNN.com/asia* (CNN). Retrieved 2009-09-11.
14. Saxena Shobhan. "Caste: Racism in all but name?". http://articlestimesofindia.indiatimes.com/special-report/28005708_1_Caste-based-discrimination-caste-discrimination-dalit-human-rights). *New Delhi: Times of India.* 26 April 2009. Retrieved 2012-09-20.
15. Vaidyanathan Rajini. "Has skin whitening in India gone too far?". *London: BBC News.* 5 June 2012. Retrieved 2012-09-20.
16. Lakshmi Rama. "In India's Huge Marketplace, Advertisers Find Fair Skin Sells".(http://www.washingtonpost.com/wp-dyn/content/article/2008/01/26/AR2008012601057.html). *Washington DC: Washington Post.* 27 January 2008. Retrieved 2012-09-20.
17."Bleaching Creams: Fade to Beautiful?". http://news.medill.northwestern.edu/chicago/news.aspx?id=161243.html *Northwestern University.* 2010-03-10. Retrieved 2014-03-23.
18."Skin Deep: Dying to be White". (http://edition.cnn.com/2002/WORLD/asiapcf/east/05/13/asia.whitening/) *CNN.* 2002-05-15. Retrieved 2014-03-23.
19.Skin whitening big business in Asia. (http://www.pri.org/world/asia/skin-whitening-big-business-asia.html) Pri.Org. Retrieved 2011-02-27.
20.Mowbray Nicole. "Japanese girls choose whiter shade of pale". (http://www.guardian.co.uk/japan/story/0,7369,1185335,00html). *London: Guardian Unlimited.* 4 April 2004. Retrieved 2010-05-24.
21."The Heavy Cost of Light Skin". (http://news.bbc.co.uk/2/hi/africa/718359.stm). *BBC News.* 2000-04-18. Retrieved 2014-03-23.
22."Mirror mirror on the wall, who is the FAIREST of them all?" Skin lightening. (http://www.scienceinafrica.co.za/2004/march/skinlightening.htm) Scienceinafrica.co.za. Retrieved 2011-02-27.
23.Color Counts: "... it is evident that differing color holds considerable importance within the black community and is measurably influencing self-esteem, prestige, and marital status." | USA Today (Society for the Advancement of Education).

https://www.questia.com/library/1G1-143164170/color-counts-it-is-evident-that-differing-color questia.com. Retrieved 2012-09-25.
24. Dixson Barnaby. Human Physique and Sexual Attractiveness: Sexual Preferences of Men and Women in Bakossiland, Cameroon. (https://www.springerlink.com/content/b7414t360040220/fulltext.pdf.)
25. Singer Merrill, Hans Beyer. *Killer Commodities: Public Health and the Corporate Production of Harm.* 28 July 2008. (https://books.google.com./?id=64xpa-rhHLgC&pg=PA151&dq=sun+tan+lower+class&q=) AltaMira Press. p. 151. ISBN 0-7591-0979-6. Retrieved 2009-09-11.
26. Koskoff Sharon. *Art Deco of the Palm Beaches.* https://books.google.com.ng/books?id=RHdeo6uvlfYC&pg=PA2&lpg=PA2&dq=%22Coco +Chanel%22+%22Josephine+Baker%22+tan&q=%22Coco%20Chanel%22%20%22Josephine%20Baker%22%20tan 28 May 2007. Arcadia Publishing. p. 2. ISBN 0-7385-4415-9. Retrieved 2009-09-11.
27."Use of Sunscreen, Sunburning Rates, and Tanning Bed Use Among More Than 10 000 US Children and Adolescents". (http://pediatrics.aappublications.org/egi/content/full/109/6/1009.pediatrics.aappublications.org. 2002-06-06. pp. 1009–1014. Retrieved 2010-09-14. (PEDIATRICS Vol. 109 No. 6)
28. Broadstock Marita, Borland Ron, Gason Robyn. "Effects of Suntan on Judgements of Healthiness and Attractiveness by Adolescents". *Journal of Applied Social Psychology*. 2006-07-31; 22 (2): 157.
29. Leary Mark R, Jones Jody L. "The Social Psychology of Tanning and Sunscreen Use: Self-Presentational Motives as a Predictor of Health Risk". *Journal of Applied Social Psychology* 2006-07-31. 23 (17): 1390.
30. "Tan is 'In': Study Finds Light Brown More Attractive than Pale or Dark Skin".http://phys.org/news/2006-09-tan-brown-pale-dark-skin.html. Physorg.com. Retrieved 2012-08-18.
31.Balkaran Steven "Mass Media and Racism". 1999.(http://www.yale.edu/ypq/articles/oct99/oct99/oct99b.html).
32. Leary Mark R, Jones Jody L. "The Social Psychology of Tanning and Sunscreen Use: Self-Presentational Motives as a Predictor of Health Risk". *Journal of Applied Social Psychology* 1993; 23 (17): 1390–406.
33. Banerjee SC, Campo S, Greene K, Campo Greene. "Fact or wishful thinking? Biased expectations in "I think I look better when I'm tanned". *American Journal of Health Behavior* 2008; 32 (3): 243–52. (https://www.ethicshare.org/node/425236)

Chapter 13

Types Of Chemicals, Products Used In Skin Lightening and Some Adverse Health Effects

Story highlights I

Types of chemicals

- The products used in lightening the skin topically are available as creams, gels, serums and soaps. In African countries, hydroquinone, mercury and topical corticosteroids are the most common skin lightening agents, while worldwide, hydroquinone, magnesium-L-ascorbic L-2-phosphate (MAP), calcium ascorbate, L-ascorbic acid, mequinol, N-acetyl-4-S-cysteaminylphenol, arbutin, Kojic acid, Kojic acid dipalmitate, Azeleic acid, niacinamide, Bearberry, Kamana Egyptian milk, and natural home made products are the most widely used.
- Most skin lightening agents act by inhibiting the conversion of tyrosine to melanin through inhibition of tyrosinase enzyme
- Mechanisms by which steroids cause skin lightening have not been clearly elucidated. However, steroids were thought to initially cause vasoconstriction of skin, giving an apparent lightening of the skin, and later inhibition of epidermic melanogenesis by suppression of endogenous production of ACTH, a melanocortin which is one of the chemical/hormonal modulators of melanin synthesis.

Story highlights II

Mercury in skin lightening cosmetics

- Mercury is a very toxic natural occurring element and occurs largely in three forms (i) elemental mercury, (ii) inorganic mercury and (iii) organic mercury. The most toxic form is organic mercury — methylmercury
- Mercury in any form is poisonous, with mercury toxicity most commonly affecting the neurologic, gastrointestinal and renal organ systems.
- Poisoning can result from mercury vapor inhalation, mercury ingestion, mercury injection, and absorption of mercury through the skin.
- Once in the environment, mercury can be transformed by bacteria into methylmercury. Methylmercury then bioaccumulates in fish and shell fish. Bioaccumulation occurs when an organism contains higher concentrations of the substance than do the surroundings. Methylmercury also bio-magnifies. For example, large predatory fish are more likely to have high levels of mercury as a result of eating many smaller fish that have acquired mercury through ingestion of plankton. Exposure to mercury – even small amounts – may cause serious health problems, and is a threat to the development of the child ***in utero*** and early in life.
- Factors that determine whether health effects occur and their severity include:
  - the type of mercury concerned
  - the dose
  - the age or developmental stage of the person exposed (the foetus is most susceptible)
  - the duration of exposure
  - the route of exposure (inhalation, ingestion, injection, or dermal contact)

All the above factors are relevant to the use of cosmetic skin lightening products in Africa.

Methyl mercury is the type of mercury in the food chain to which the fetus is exposed. The vast majority of the mercury containing cosmetic products available on the market have mercury in excess of the US FDA maximum acceptable level. The method of application – "Body Works"—maximally amplifies the dose absorbed through percutaneous absorption. The duration of use is for decades—a life style. The route of exposure – mercury-containing skin lightening creams are now being used as *injectables.*

- Mercury is neurotoxic, nephrotoxic, teratogenic, carcinogenic, genotoxic, immunotoxic and has cardiovascular and reproductive toxicity.
- Mercury in skin bleaching products has public health implications to the baby, household contacts and the general public.

Story highlights III

Hydroquinone in skin lightening cosmetics

- The most common over-the-counter skin bleaching agent in the world, including North America and Europe, is hydroquinone (HQ). In human medicine, hydroquinone is used as a topical application in skin whitening to reduce the colour of the skin. This use is banned in some countries, including the member states of the European Union.
- Hydroquinone is known to competitively inhibit melanin production by inhibiting sulfhydryl groups and acting as a substrate for tyrosinase. HQ has cytotoxic (cell-killing or cell-damaging) activity on the melanocytes, as well as on many other cell types.
- It was once thought that concentrations of hydroquinone of 2% or less had negligible potential adverse effects. It is now known that this is not true, as the medical literature reports problems occurring with lesser concentrations.
- Most over-the-counter skin-bleaching chemicals available in the United States, Canada and Europe contain hydroquinone. In the United States, in 1990, $44 million of over-the-counter skin-bleaching products were purchased.
- Chronic use of hydroquinone containing products cause exogenous ochronosis and the "fish odour syndrome"
- Hydroquinone has been identified as both a potential clastogen and mutagen. A clastogen is a toxin that has the capability to cause breaks in chromosomes, cause sections of them to be destroyed, and to rearrange the sections and thus cause mutations which can lead to various types of cancer. A mutagen is a material that causes mutation and damage in DNA. When the DNA is altered, it can cause any number of chain reactions that can negatively impact the health, including cancerous growth of cells and cell division.
- HQ also weakens the immune system; it is toxic on the nervous system (neurotoxic). HQ also causes injury to the eyes leading to sensitivity to light, corneal ulcers, cataract and visual disturbances

- The world Health Organization states: "It is recommended that over-the-counter sales of creams containing hydroquinone be restricted. Health education programs should be developed to discourage the use of hydroquinone-containing creams".

Story highlights IV

Hydroquinone induced Exogenous Ochronosis

- Complications of hydroquinone use that have been reported are dermatitis, exogenous ochronosis, cataract, pigmented colloid milia, scleral and nail pigmentation and patchy depigmentation.
- Exogenous ochronosis is a diffuse pigmentation of the face; and blue black macular patches on the face and external ears and sun-exposed areas of the upper chest, upper back and extensor surfaces of the extremities following prolonged application of hydroquinone.
- Exogenous ochronosis is classified into three clinical stages: (a) erythema and mild hyperpigmentation; (b) hyper-pigmentation, pigmented colloid milium (i.e. caviar-like lesions) and scanty atrophy; and (c) papulonodular lesions.
- A more serious complication of exogenous ochronosis (EO) is loss of elasticity of the skin and impaired wound healing. After major abdominal surgeries like Caesarian section, myomectomy, hysterectomy etc, there may be catastrophic wound dehiscence, burst abdomen, and death from overwhelming infection.
- The chronic bleachers also exude an offensive fish odour in the sweat like the 'fish odour syndrome.' The 'fish odour syndrome,' also known as trimethylaminuria, is characterised by body odour of rotten fish. This is due to excretion of a chemical, trimethylamine in the breath, urine, sweat, saliva, and vaginal secretions.
- There is no known effective treatment for EO.
- A dip-stick method of testing for hydroquinone and mercury is necessary for use by consumers who may wish to verify the contents of a cosmetic product before use
- **Other names for Hydroquinone**

It is critical to note that, because the use of Hydroquinone in cosmetics has been banned in several countries, other names are often used on the ingredient labeling to camouflage the identity of the ingredient. Hence, other names for hydroquinone like Quinol, Tequinol, Benzene-1,4-diol, Idrochinone, 1-4 dihydroxy benzene, 1,4 hydroxy benzene, 1,4-Benzenediol, p-Diphenol, Hydrochinone, p-hydroxylphenol, Hydrochinonium, and Hydroquinol may be used

Story highlights V

Corticosteroids as skin lightening agents

- Topical corticosteroids TCs are subdivided according to strength (Class I–VII), with class I (i.e. clobetasol) being the most potent and class VII (i.e. hydrocortisone) the least potent. The strength of TCs is determined by the vasoconstriction assay, in which potency is associated with the degree of blood vessel blanching in the upper dermis. TCs have long been used for their skin lightening properties and are often the most commonly used skin lighteners in Africa. TCs are believed to bleach the skin through inhibiting pro-opiomelanocortin (POMC), the precursor protein for α-melanocyte-stimulating hormone (α-MSH), which is produced in the intermediate lobe of the pituitary to stimulate epidermal melanin production.
- Corticosteroids are *de facto* drugs, not cosmetic products.
- Some of the complications of topical corticosteroids are adrenal insufficiency, Cushing's syndrome, hypertension, diabetes, osteoporosis, cataract, glaucoma, myopathy, predisposition to bacterial, fungal and viral infections of the skin, acne, striae, hypertrichosis, skin atrophy, steroid addiction syndrome and contact eczema.

Story highlights VI

Intimate Area Skin Whitening and Tooth bleaching

- Intimate area skin whitening may be traced to commercial sex workers, but has now resurfaced as "Hollywood" trends.
- The private parts which may be bleached include the breasts, penis, vagina, anus, buttocks and the thighs.
- The ingredients may contain hydroquinone or Alpha Arbutin.
- Anal bleaching may result in scarring and strictures. Clients may also acquire herpes and bacterial infections from the spas.
- Dental **whitening** restores natural tooth colour and dental **bleaching** whitens beyond the natural color.
- Methods available for teeth whitening use bleaching strips, pen, gel and laser bleaching. The bleaching agents are carbamide peroxide and 6-phthalimido peroxy hexanoic acid (PAP).

Story highlights VII

Systemic skin whitening agents

- Systemic skin whitening agents are either pills or injections.
- The pills are glutathione

L-cysteine peptite
Tranexemic acid and other miscellaneous agents.

- None of the agents have been approved by the WHO nor FDA for use as a skin lightening agents.
- Some of the adverse effects are, internal physical stress, allergic reactions, liver damage and hormonal imbalance.
- Glutathione injection has caused anaphylaxis, Stevens-Johnson syndrome, Toxic epidermal necrolysis, kidney failure and thyroid dysfunction.

Story highlights VIII

Skin Whitening Injections

- The most commonly used systemic skin whitening agent is Glutathione (GSH) used alone or in various combinations, both as oral and intravenous formulations.
- **Side effects of Glutathione Injections**
  Hair loss
  White spots on the nails
  Numbness of extremities
  Shivers and shakes
  Depression and anxiety
- **Complications of Glutathione Injections**
  Allergy or Anaphylaxis (manifested by difficulty of breathing, tightness of chest, rashes, hives, and swollen skin)
  Systemic **Infection**
  Stevens–Johnson Syndrome
  Toxic Epidermal Necrolysis or Lyell's Syndrome
  Kidney Failure
  Thyroid Dysfunction
  Severe abdominal pain
- As already mentioned above, these agents are not FDA approved for skin whitening and no scientific evidence exists for their use. In addition, the injectable formulations are counterfeited and given by untrained people illegally and hence associated with the risk of sepsis, air embolism, transmission of human immunodeficiency virus, Hepatitis B, and use of non-sterile preparations that can lead to serious infections. According to the FDA, the US drug watchdog, side-effects of the injection range from skin rashes, disruption in thyroid function, kidney damage, Stevens-Johnson syndrome and toxic epidermal necrolysis. The last two life-threatening conditions

cause fever, severe rash, blisters and skin peeling. Affected people have to be treated in the hyper-sterile burns wards of hospitals.

Story highlights IX

Skin Lightening surgery and other techniques

- Laser surgery or cryosurgery is also used to whiten the skin by destroying the melanin cells
- Laser surgery is a very expensive procedure
- Other methods for lightening the skin are
    - Microdermabrasion
    - Chemical peels
    - Mesotherapy
    - Fraxel laser treatment
- The notable adverse effects that may arise from Laser surgery are heat injury, activation and dissemination of cold sores (herpes), scaring, infection and paradoxical darkening of the skin.

TYPES OF CHEMICALS AND PRODUCTS USED IN LIGHTENING THE SKIN AND ADVERSE EFFECTS

Types of chemicals and products

The products used in lightening the skin topically are available as creams, gels, serums and soaps. In African countries, hydroquinone, mercury and topical corticosteroids are the most common skin lightening agents,[1-4] while worldwide, hydroquinone, magnesium-L-ascorby L-2-phosphate (MAP), calcium ascorbate, L-ascorbic acid, mequinol, N-acetyl-4-S-cysteaminylphenol, arbutin, Kojic acid, Kojic acid dipalmitate, Azelaic acid, niacinamide, Bearberry, Kamana Egyptian milk, and natural home made products are the most widely used.[5-7] Use of combinations of skin lightening agents are very common and all ingredients are often not included in the labels.1,3,4. Skin lightening products containing hydroquinone and its mobenzyl ether and mercurial compounds are commonly used in Africa because they are cheaper and affordable to the low income people. However the middle and upper class use the expensive better regulated products. For example while a jar/tube of hydroquinone or mercury based product can cause as low of $2US, or a 500ml 0.6kg of Kanama Egyptian milk costs $400US.[8]

Mechanisms of Action of skin lightening agents[1-7]

Most skin lightening agents act by inhibiting the conversion of tyrosine to melanin by inhibition of tyrosinase enzyme[1,2]. Tyrosinase enzyme is the rate limiting enzyme in the melanogenesis which catalyse important steps in melanin formation: tyrosinase converts tyrosine to dihydroxy-phenylalanine (DOPA) and then to dopaquinone. All classes of topical steroids are commonly used as bleaching agents in African countries, and they are easily purchased in open markets. Mechanisms by which steroids cause skin lightening have not been clearly elucidated. However, steroids were thought to initially cause vasoconstriction of skin giving an apparent lightening of the skin, and later inhibition of epidermic melanogenesis by suppression of endogenous production of ACTH, a melanocortin which is one of the chemical/hormonal modulator of melanin synthesis[3,4,5] Table 13.1 shows the mechanisms of action of skin bleaching chemicals.

Table 13.1 Mechanisms of Action of skin lightening agents[1-7]

Mechanisms	Non plant extracts	Plant extracts
Competitive tyrosinase Inhibitors	a. Hydroquinone and its derivatives: 1. Hydroquinone (2-5%) 2. Mequinol (2%) (4-hydroxyanisol, monobenzyl ether of hydroquinone) 3. *N*-acetyl-4-5-cysteaminylphenol 4. Gentisic acid (methyl gentisate) b. Glutathione (thiol) c. Epicatechin gallates.	Azelaic acid (15-20%) (9-carbon dicarboxylic acid) Arbutin (3%) Alpha arbutin Deoxyarbutin Aloesin Kojic acid (2-4%) Flavonoids, flavones, flavonols, hesperidins Kuraninone Saponin Oregonin Yohimbin
Non-competitive tyrosinase inhibitors	Haginin A and *N*-acetyl glucosamine	Glabirdin (10-40%) (Licorice extracts); Hydroxystilbenes: (1) resveratol, (2) oxyresveratol, (3) ginetol, Piceatannol, Mulberry (mulberroside) and Polyphenols (procyanidins)
Newer tyrosinase inhibitors (require further *in vivo* and *in vitro* studies)	Hydroxyphenyl naphthol, Calycosin and Quinolines (chloroquine and quinine)	Diarylpropane
Reduces the transfer of melanosomes from melanocytes to keratinocytes or melanin transfer		Niacinamide (5%); Soy (soybean trypsin inhibitor)
Reduces tyrosine oxidation		P-coumaric acid
Copper chelation, anti-oxidant, and inhibits melanocyte proliferation		Ascorbic acid (5-10%) (Magnesium L-ascorbic acid-2- phosphate) and Ellagic acid.
Removes keratinocytes shortens the cell cycle and facilitates rapid pigment loss, interferes with pigment transfer and enhances penetration of other SLA	Alpha hydroxy acids: Glycolic acids (6-12%) and Retinoids: Tretinoin (Retinoic acid) (0.05 and 0.1%), adapalene (0.1%).	Liquirtin (Licorice extracts)

Mechanism of action of skin lightening cosmetics Morand JJ. LYF et al Med Trop. 2007; 67 (6): 627-34

References

1.Jombow K. Obata H, Pathak MA et al. Mechanism of Depigmentation by Hydroquinone. *J Invest Dermatol* 1974; 62:436.

2. Lerner AB, Fitz[atrick TB. Inhibition of melanin formation by chemical agents. *J. Invest Dermatol* 1952; 18:119-35

3. Kanthraj GR *Indian J Dermatol Venereol Leprol* 2010; 76:3-6

4. Policarpio B, Lui H Skin Lightening and Depigmentation Agents. *eMedicine Specialties > Dermatology > Cosmetics* 2009

5. Olumide YM, Akinkugbe AO et al Complications of chronic use of skin lightening cosmetics. *International Journal of Dermatology* 2008; 47:344-53

6. Tobin AM, Barragry J et al. *Ir Med J.* 2005; 98 (4): 118.

7. Komokshi R. Fairness via Formulations: a review of cosmetic skin-lightening ingredients. *J. Cosmet Sci* 2012. Jan-Feb; 63 (i): 43-54.

MERCURY IN SKIN LIGHTENING COSMETICS

Introduction

Mercury is a very toxic element but its use has been found in many areas including use for religious, cultural and ritualistic purposes. Mercury has also been used in some traditional medicines (such as certain Traditional Asian remedies), paints, jewelry as a preservative in some vaccines and other pharmaceuticals, and in skin-lightening (toning) creams and soap. The application of mercurial preparations to the skin has been practiced for centuries.[1,2] It is know from history that mercury was used in ointments by the Greeks and the Romans also used it for cosmetics.[3] Mercury-containing cosmetic preparations have been represented for many years as skin-bleaching agents or as preparations to remove or prevent freckles and/or brown spots.[4] Preparations intended for such use are regarded as drugs as well as cosmetics— Cosmeceuticals. In addition to such use as skin-bleaching agents mercury compounds have also been widely used as preservatives in hand and body creams and lotions; hair shampoos, hair sets and rinses, hair straighteners, hair colouring, and other preparations.

References

1. Cole HN, Schreiber N, and Sollman T. Mercurial ointment in the treatment of syphilis. *Arch dermatol* 1930; 21: 372-93

2.Turk JL and Baker H. Nephrotic syndrome due to ammoniated mercury. *Br J Dermatol* 1968; 80: 632¯4

3. Silverberg DS, McCall JT and Hunt JC. Nephrotic syndrome with the use of ammoniated mercury. *Arch Int Med* 1967; 120: 581¯6

4. Al- Saleh I and Al-Doush I. Mercury Content in Skin Lightening creams and potential hazards to the health of Saudi Women. *J Toxicol Environ Hlth* 1997; 51: 123-30.

Some facts about mercury

Mercury is a naturally occurring element that is found in air, water and soil. Mercury exists in various forms: elemental (or metallic); inorganic (to which people may be exposed through their occupation); and organic (e.g., methylmercury, to which people may be exposed through their diet). These forms of mercury differ in their degrees of toxicity and in their effects on the nervous, digestive and immune systems, and on lungs, kidneys, skin and eyes. Mercury is considered by WHO as one of the top ten chemicals or groups of chemicals of major public health concern.

Mercury occurs naturally in the earth's crust. It is released into the environment from volcanic activity, weathering of rocks and as a result of human activity. Human activity is the main cause of mercury releases, particularly coal-fired power stations, residential coal burning for heating and cooking, industrial processes, waste incinerators and as a result of mining for mercury, gold and other metals.

Once in the environment, mercury can be transformed by bacteria into methylmercury. Methylmercury then bioaccumulates (bioaccumulation occurs when an organism contains higher concentrations of the substance than do the surroundings) in fish and shell fish. Methylmercury also bio-magnifies. For example, large predatory fish are more likely to have high levels of mercury as a result of eating many smaller fish that have acquired mercury through ingestion of plankton. Exposure to mercury – even small amounts – may cause serious health problems, and is a threat to the development of the child ***in utero*** and early in life.

People may be exposed to mercury in any of its forms under different circumstances. However, exposure mainly occurs through consumption of fish and shellfish contaminated with methylmercury and through worker inhalation of elemental mercury vapours during industrial processes. Cooking does not eliminate mercury in food items.

Exposure to mercury

All humans are exposed to some level of mercury. Therefore there is a maximum permissible level of – "normal" range in blood or urine levels – below 10ppm. Most people are exposed to low levels of mercury, often through chronic exposure (continuous or intermittent long-term contact). Acute high level of exposure could occur, for example, due to an industrial accident.

Reference

WHO/Mercury and health. Fact Sheet N° 361.Updated September 2013. *http://www.who.int/mediacentre/factsheets/fs361/en/*

Mercury toxicokinetics

Mercury is considered one of the most toxic elements for plants and animals. Mercury is a highly volatile element with a long atmospheric half-life. As a result of these physical properties, it is ubiquitous in the environment and exposure is not an isolated concern but rather a global threat to human health. In recent years, research has revealed that even frequent exposure to very low concentrations of mercury has the ability to cause long-lasting neurological and kidney impairment. Human health risks from mercury exposure have been widely documented, and include neurological effects, impaired fetal and infant growth, and possible contributions to cardiovascular disease.

Mercury Compounds: Toxicokinetics

There are basically five chemical forms of mercury (Hg). Elemental mercury Hg^{o} (also known as metallic mercury), Mercuric Chloride ($HgCl_2$). Mercurous chloride (Hg_2Cl_2) (also known as calomel), Methylmercuric Chloride (CH_3HgCl) and Dimethylmercury (C_2H_6Hg). Methylmercuric Chloride is used experimentally to investigate the effects of methylmercury. Elemental mercury is only moderately water soluble but Mercuric Chloride is considerably more water soluble. In comparison, organic Hg such as methylmercury chloride, is much less water soluble. Dimethylmercury, a very toxic by-product of the chemical synthesis of MeHg also has a relatively low water solubility and is considered to be relatively lipid soluble. The solubility of the different forms of Hg might play a role in their differential toxicity. Table 13.3 shows toxicologically relevant mercury species.

Table 13.2 Summary Table Comparing Toxicologically Relevant Mercury Species

Methylmercury (CH_3Hg^+)	Elemental Mercury (Hg^0)	Mercuric Mercury (Hg^{2+})
• **Sources of Exposure**		
Fish, marine mammals, crustaceans, animals and poultry fed fish meal	Dental amalgams, occupational exposure, Caribbean religious ceremonies, fossil fuels, incinerators	Oxidation of elemental mercury or demethylation of MeHg; deliberate or accidental poisoning with $HgCl_2$
• **Biological Monitoring**		
Hair, blood, cord blood	Urine, blood	Urine, blood
• **Toxicokinetics**		
Absorption		
Inhalation: Vapors of MeHg absorbed	Inhalation: Approximately 80% of inhaled dose of Hg^o readily absorbed	Inhalation: Aerosols of $HgCl_2$ absorbed
Oral: Approximately 95% of MeHg in fish readily absorbed from GI tract	Oral: GI absorption of metallic Hg is poor; any released vapor in GI tract converted to	Oral; 7-15% of ingested dose of $HgCl_2$ absorbed from the GI tract; absorption proportional

	mercuric sulfide and excreted	to water solubility of mercuric salt; uptake by neonates greater than adults
Dermal: In guinea pigs, 3-5% of applied dose absorbed in 5 hr	Dermal: Average rate of absorption of Hg^0 through human skin, 0.024 ng/cm^2 for every 1 mg/m_3 in air	Dermal: In guinea pigs, 2-3% of applied dose of $HgCl_2$ absorbed
Distribution		
Distributed throughout body since lipophilic; approximately 1-10% of absorbed oral dose of MeHg distributed to blood; 90% of blood MeHg in RBCs MeHg-cysteine complex involved in transport of MeHg into cells	Rapidly distributed throughout the body since it is lipophilic	Highest accumulation in kidney; fraction of dose retained in kidney dose dependent
Half-life in blood, 50 d; 50% of dose found in liver; 10% in head.	Half-life in blood, 45 d (slow phase); half-life appears to increase with increasing dose	Half-life in blood, 19.7-65.6 d; 1st phase, 24 d, 2nd phase, 15-30 d
Readily crosses blood-brain and placental barriers	Readily crosses blood-brain placental barriers	Does not readily penetrate blood-brain or placental barriers In neonate, mercuric Hg not concentrated in kidneys; therefore, more widely distributed to other tissues In fetus and neonate, blood-brain barrier incompletely formed, so mercuric Hg brain concentrations higher than those in adults
Biotransformation		
MeHg slowly demethylated to mercuric Hg (Hg^{2+})	Hg^0 in tissue and blood oxidized to Hg^{2+} by catalase and hydrogen peroxide (H_2O_2); H_2O_2 production the rate-limiting step	Hg^0 vapor exhaled by rodents following oral administration of mercuric Hg
Tissue macrophages,		Mercuric Hg not

intestinal flora, and fetal liver are sites of tissue demethylation Mechanisms of demethylation unknown; free radicals demethylate MeHg in vitro; bacterial demethylation enzymes studied extensively, none has been characterized or identified in mammalian cells		methylated in body tissues but GI microorganisms can form MeHg
Does not bind or induce metallothionein		Binds and induces metallothionein
Excretion		
Daily excretion, 1% of body burden; major excretory route is bile and feces; 90% excreted in feces as Hg^{2+}; 10% excreted in urine as Hg^{2+} Lactation increases clearance from blood; 16% of Hg in breast milk is MeHg	Excreted as Hg^0 in exhaled air, sweat, and saliva, and as mercuric Hg in feces and urine	Excreted in urine and feces; also excreted in saliva, bile, sweat, exhaled air, and breast milk
Half-Life limination		
(Whole body) 70-80 d; dependent on species, dose, sex, and animal strain	58 d	1-2 mo
• **Toxicodynamics**		
Critical target organ		
Brain, adult and fetal	Brain and kidney	Kidney
Causes of Toxicity		
Demethylation of MeHg to Hg^{2+} and the intrinsic toxicity of MeHg	Oxidation of Hg^0 to Hg^{2+}	Hg^{2+} binding to thiols in critical enzyme (e.g., cysteine) and structural proteins
Latency period		
In Iraq, from weeks to month; in Japan, more than a year; differences suggested to be caused by Se in fish; no toxic signs during latency period		
• **Mobilization**		
DMPS, DMSA	After oxidation to Hg^{2+}: DMPS, DMSA	DMPS, DMSA

- **Possible Antagonists**

Selenium, garlic, zinc
MeHg-cysteine complex is structurally analogous to methionine.

Abbreviations: $HgCl_2$, mercuric chloride; DMPS, 2,3-dimercapto-1-propane sulfonate; DMSA, meso 2,3-dimercaptosuccinic acid; GI, gastrointestinal tract; RBC red blood cells.

Reference

Mercury: Chemistry, Exposure, Toxicokinetics and Toxicodynamics
http://www.nap.edu/read/9899/chapter/4

The rate of dermal absorption increases with the concentration of mercury and prior hydration of the skin. The degree of dermal absorption varies with the skin integrity and lipid solubility of the vehicle in the cosmetic products. Ingestion may occur after topical application around the mouth and hand-to-mouth contact. After absorption, inorganic mercury is distributed widely and elimination occurs primarily through the urine and feces. With long-term exposure, urinary excretion is the major route of elimination. The half-life is approximately 1-2 months.

Factors that determine whether health effects occur and their severity include:[1]

- The type of mercury concerned;
- The dose
- The age or developmental stage of the person exposed (the foetus is most susceptible)
- The duration of exposure;
- The route of exposure (inhalation, ingestion, injection, or dermal contact)

All the above factors are relevant to the use of cosmetic skin lightening products in Africa. Methyl mercury is the type of mercury in the food chain to which the fetus is exposed. The vast majority of the mercury containing cosmetic products available on the market have mercury in excess of the US FDA maximum acceptable level. The method of application–"Body Works"– maximally amplifies the dose absorbed through percutaneous absorption. The duration of use is for decades–a life style. (See the relevant section in chapter 4 on NIGERIA). The route of exposure –mercury-containing skin lightening creams are now being used as *injectables.* (See chapter 9 on KENYA).

Reference

1. Al-Saleh I, Shinwari N, EL-Doush I et al. Comparison of mercury levels in various tissues of albinos and pigmented mice treated with two different brands of mercury skin-lightening creams. *Biometals* 2004; 17:167-75
2. Mahe A, Ly F, Perret JL. Systemic complications of the cosmetic use of skin-bleaching products. *Int J Dermatol* 2005; 44 (Suppl 1):
3. Al-Saleh I, Khogali F, Al-Amodi M et al. Histopathological effects of mercury in skin lightening cream. J Environ Pathol Toxicol Oncol 2003; 22: 287-299.
4. El-Saleh I, El-Doush I, Shinwari N, et al. Does low mercury containing skin-lightening cream (fair & lovely) affect the kidney, liver, and brain of female mice? *Cutan Ocul Toxicol* 2005; 24:11-29
5. Al-Saleh I, El-Doush I. Mercury content in skin-lightening creams and potential hazards to the health of Saudi Women. *J Toxicol Environ Health* 1997; 51:123-30.
6. Mahe A, Ly F, Perrett JL. Systemic complications of the cosmetic use of skin-bleaching products. *Int J Dermatol* 2005; 44(Suppl 1): 38-8
7. Weldon MM, Smolinsku, Maroufi A, et al. Mercury poisoning associated with a Mexican beauty cream. *West J Med* 2000; 173:15-8.
8. Al-Saleh I, Shinwari N, Al-AModi M. Accumulation of mercury in ovaries of mice after the application of skin-lightening creams. *Bio Trace Elem Res* 2009; 131:43-54.

Mercury Toxicity[1]

Mercury in any form is poisonous, with mercury toxicity most commonly affecting the neurologic, gastrointestinal (GI) and renal organ systems. Poisoning can result from mercury vapor inhalation, mercury ingestion, mercury injection, and absorption of mercury through the skin.

Mercury has 3 forms: (1) elemental mercury, (2) inorganic salts, and (3) organic compounds. Perhaps the most deadly form of mercury is methylmercury. Only 2-10% of the ingested mercury is absorbed from the gut, and ingested elemental mercury is not absorbed at all; however, 90% of any methylmercury ingested is absorbed into the bloodstream from the GI tract. Organic mercury compounds, specifically methylmercury, are concentrated in the food chain.

Fish from contaminated waters are the most common culprits. Industrial mercury pollution is often in the inorganic form, but aquatic organisms and vegetation in waterways such as rivers, lakes, and bays convert it to deadly methylmercury. Fish eat contaminated vegetation, and the mercury becomes biomagnified in the fish. Fish protein binds more than 90% of the consumed methylmercury so tightly that even the most vigorous cooking methods (eg, deep-frying, boiling, baking, pan-frying) cannot remove it.

For centuries, mercury was an essential part of many different medicines, such as diuretics, antibacterial agents, antiseptics, and laxatives. In the late 18th century, antisyphilitic agents contained mercury. It was during the 1800s that the phrase "mad as a hatter" was coined, owing to the effects of chronic mercury exposure in the hat-making industry, where the metal was used in the manufacturing process.

In 1889, Charcot, in his *Clinical Lectures on Diseases of the Nervous System,* attributed some rapid oscillatory tremors to mercury exposure.[2] In Wilson's classic textbook of neurology, published in 1940, Wilson concurred with Charcot's attribution of tremors to mercury poisoning, but also described mercury-induced cognitive impairments, such as inattention, excitement, and hallucinosis.[3]

In 1961, researchers in Japan correlated elevated urinary mercury levels with the features of the previously mysterious Minamata disease. Before the etiology of Minamata disease was discovered, it plagued the residents around Minamata Bay in Japan with tremors, sensory loss, ataxia, and visual field constriction.[4] Minamata disease is an example of organic toxicity. In Minamata Bay, a factory discharged inorganic mercury into the water. The mercury was methylated by bacteria and subsequently ingested by fish. Local villagers ate the fish and began to exhibit signs of neurologic damage, such as visual loss, extremity numbness, hearing loss, and ataxia. Babies exposed to the methylmercury in utero were the most severely affected. Furthermore, because mercury was also discovered in the breast milk of the mothers, the babies' exposure continued after birth.[5]

References

1.Olson DA Mercury Toxicity. *http:emedicine.medscape.com/article/1175560-overview*

2. Charcot JM. Clinical lectures of diseases of the nervous system. *The Landmark Library of Neurology and Neurosurgery*. 1994; 186.

3. Wilson SAK. Neurology. *The Landmark Library of Neurology and Neurosurgery*. 1994; 739-40.

4. Harada M. Minamata disease: methlmercury poisoning in Japan caused by environment pollution. *Crit Rev Toxicol.* 1995; 25 (1): 1-24.

5. United Nations Programme: Minamata Convention on Mercury. Minamata on Mercury. Available at *http://www.mercuryconvention.org/convention.* Accessed October 18, 2014.

Young's Syndrome

Mercury toxicity can also cause Young's syndrome. Young's syndrome, also know as azoospermia, sinopulmonary infections, sinusitis-infertility syndrome and Barry-Perkins-Young syndrome, is a rare condition that encompasses a combination of syndromes such as brochiectasis, rhinosinusitis and reduced fertility.[1,2] In individuals with this syndrome, the functioning of the lungs is usually normal but the mucus is abnormally viscous. In Young's syndrome, there is low motility of sperm cells. The sperm cells are there, but they are not very motile; they can't move all the way to the tube from the vagina where they are deposited. By the time they get to the uterus, most of them are dead, because they are slow moving. The syndrome was named after Donald Young.[3] There have been several studies undertaken suggesting that contact with mercury might cause the syndrome.[4,5] The spouses of women who use mercury containing cosmetic products can inhale mercury from the vapour emanating from the woman and through this chronic exposure develop Young's syndrome.

References

1. Handelsman DJ, Conway AJ, Boylan LM, Turtle JR. "Young's syndrome. Obstructive azoospermia and chronic sinopulmonary infections." *N Engl. J Med.* January 1984; 310 (1): 3-9

2. Young's syndrome—General Practice Notebook. *http://www.gpnotebook.co.uk/simplepage.cfm?ID=-1214644174)*

3. Young M. "Obituary of Donald Herron Young". *BMJ* Janaury 2003; 326 (7382): 226.

4. Hendry WF, A'Hern RP, Cole PJ. "Was Young's syndrome caused by exposure to mercury in childhood? *BMJ* 1993; 307 (6919): 1579-82.

5. Lau KY, Lieberman J. "Young's syndrome. An association between male sterility and bronchiectasis." *West J Med* June 1986; 144 (6): 744-6.

Toxic effects of mercury

- **Neurodevelopmental toxicity.** Neurodevelopmental effects in the fetus are associated with maternal exposure.[1,2,3,4]
- **Nephrotoxicity** Inorganic mercury compounds are nephrotoxic and can cause kidney damage in children.[5]
- **Teratogenicity.** An agent that can cause maldevelopment of embryo in the first trimester of pregnancy (first 3 months)
- **Cardiovascular Toxicity.** Hearty function alteration has been described in children in association with methymercury exposure[6]

- **Carcinogenity** High exposure to methylmercury is associated with leukemia among adults.[7]
- **Genotoxicity, Mutagenesis** Causes genetic mutation—change in the genetic material of a person causing different physical characteristics to develop [8,9]
- **Reproductive Toxicity**. In the Minamata study there was an increase in the quality of male stillborn festuses,[10] abnormally low number of pregnancies.[11] Exposure of dental assistants to mercury vapor was associated with spontaneous abortions, stillbirths and congenital malformations[12] and male azoospermia in Young's syndrome
- **Immunotoxicity** Mercury is likely to be immunotoxic, as shown in animal models.[13,14] Studies of mercury exposure in the Amazonia region due to gold mining activities showed a positive association between mercury and malaria.[15]

References

1. Davidson PW, Myers GJ, Cox C, Axtell C, Shamlaye C, Sloane-Reeves J, et al. Effects of prenatal and postnatal methylmercury exposure from fish consumption on neurodevelopment: outcomes at 66 months of age in the Seychelles Child Development Study. *JAMA*. 1998; 280:701–7.
2. Myers GJ, Thurston SW, Pearson AT, Davidson PW, Cox C, Shamlaye CF, et al. Postnatal exposure to methyl mercury from fish consumption: a review and new data from the Seychelles Child Development Study. *Neurotoxicology*. 2009; 30:338–49. [PMC free article]
3. Myers GJ, Marsh DO, Davidson PW, Cox C, Shamlaye CF, Tanner M, et al. Main neurodevelopmental study of Seychellois children following in utero exposure to methylmercury from a maternal fish diet: outcome at six months. *Neurotoxicology*. 1995; 16:653–64.
4. Myers GJ, Davidson PW, Shamlaye CF, Axtell CD, Cernichiari E, Choisy O, et al. Effects of prenatal methylmercury exposure from a high fish diet on developmental milestones in the Seychelles Child Development Study. *Neurotoxicology*. 1997; 18:819–29.
5. Clarkson TW, Magos L. The toxicology of mercury and its chemical compounds. *Crit Rev Toxicol*. 2006; 36:609–62.
6. Grandjean P, Murata K, Budtz-Jorgensen E, Weihe P. Cardiac autonomic activity in methylmercury neurotoxicity: 14-year follow-up of a Faroese birth cohort. *J Pediatr*. 2004; 144:169–76.
7. Yorifuji T, Tsuda T, Kawakami N. Age standardized cancer mortality ratios in areas heavily exposed to methyl mercury. *Int Arch Occup Environ Health*. 2007;80:679–88.

8. Mergler D, Anderson HA, Chan LH, Mahaffey KR, Murray M, Sakamoto M, et al. Methylmercury exposure and health effects in humans: a worldwide concern. *Ambio.* 2007; 36:3–11.
9. Agency for Toxic Substances and Disease Registry . Toxicological Profile for Mercury. U.S. Department of Health and Human Service - Public Health Service - Agency for Toxic Substances and Disease Registry; Atlanta, Georgia: [cited 2009 August]. 1999. Available at: *http://www.atsdr.cdc.gov/toxprofiles/tp46.pdf.*
10. Sakamoto M, Nakano A, Akagi H. Declining Minamata male birth ratio associated with increased male fetal death due to heavy methylmercury pollution. *Environ Res.* 2001; 87:92–8.

11. Bakir F, Damluji SF, Amin-Zaki L, Murtadha M, Khalidi A, Al-Rawi NY, et al. Methylmercury poisoning in Iraq. *Science.* 1973; 181:230–41.
12. Sikorski R, Juszkiewicz T, Paszkowski T, Szprengier-Juszkiewicz T. Women in dental surgeries: reproductive hazards in occupational exposure to metallic mercury. Int *Arch Occup Environ Health.* 1987; 59:551–7.
13. Mergler D, Anderson HA, Chan LH, Mahaffey KR, Murray M, Sakamoto M, et al. Methylmercury exposure and health effects in humans: a worldwide concern. *Ambio.* 2007; 36:3–11.
14. World Health Organization Principles and methods for assessing autoimmunity associated with exposure to chemicals. *Environmental Health Criteria.* 2006; 236:1–333.
15. Silbergeld EK, Silva IA, Nyland JF. Mercury and autoimmunity: implications for occupational and environmental health. *Toxicol Appl Pharmacol.* 2005; 207:282–92.

Symptoms and signs of mercury poisoning

Minamata disease has devastating neurologic consequences as a primary outcome of methyl mercury intoxication; unfortunately, these are relatively resistant to treatment. Complications include the following:

- Acute perioral and facial paresthesias
- Visual-field constriction
- Respiratory distress and nonspecific dermatitis
- Extremity numbness eventually appears, along with headache, fatigue, and tremor
- Ataxia and dysarthria can also be observed

Severe poisoning eventually causes the patient to lie in a mute, semirigid posture that is broken only by episodes of crying or primitive reflexive movements. Babies exposed in utero are the most severely affected. They are affected by low birth weight, seizure disorders, profound developmental delay, incomplete visual loss (including tunnel vision) or total blindness, and hearing loss. Neurologic damage in the form of diffuse and widespread neuronal atrophy is most severe in patients exposed in utero. Long-term studies may indicate that even prenatal exposure at low concentrations can cause subtle, but detectable, decrements in the areas of motor function, language, and memory. Children so affected may have long-term stigmata, including motor impairment, visual loss, hearing loss, developmental delay, and seizure disorders.

Mercury in skin lightening cosmetics

Mercury is a common ingredient found in skin lightening soaps and creams. It is also found in other cosmetics, such as eye makeup cleansing products and mascara.[1-3] Skin lightening soaps and creams are commonly used in certain African and Asian nations.[1,4,5] They are also used among dark-skinned populations in Europe and North America.[2,6,7] Mercury salts inhibit the formation of melanin, resulting in a lighter skin tone.[8],

Mercury in cosmetics exists in two forms: inorganic and organic.[3,10,11] Inorganic mercury (e.g. ammoniated mercury) is used in skin lightening soaps and creams. Organic mercury compounds (thiomersal [ethyl mercury] and phenyl mercuric salts) are used as cosmetic preservatives in eye makeup cleansing products and mascara.[1-3,12]

Products, packaging and ingredients

- Skin lightening products come in different forms , including soaps and creams and lotions ; the soap is often sold as "antiseptic soap".[1,2] These products are supposed to be applied to the skin to dry overnight.[2] Women use the soap to wash their hair, arms or face or their entire body.[2] It is reported that some women use these products for as long as 20 years.[1]

- The soaps come in bar form and are sold individually in boxes.[6] The creams are generally packaged in tubes or jars.[6] The soaps contain approximately 1-3% mercury iodide, and the creams are composed of 1-10% mercury ammonium.[2] Some soap products tested contained mercury at concentrations up to 31 mg/kg, whereas cream products had mercury concentrations as high as 33 000 mg/kg.[13]
- A 2011 survey funded by the German Federal Ministry for the Environment, Nature Conservation and Nuclear Safety noted that

individuals from Brazil, Kyrgyzstan, Mexico and the Russian Federation believe that mercury-containing skin lightning products are easy to obtain.[14]

- Products with very high levels of mercury contamination look grey or cream coloured.[15]
- The amount or concentration of mercury in a product may be labelled on the packaging or in the ingredient list. Names to look for include mercury, Hg, mercuric iodide, mercurous chloride, ammoniated mercury, amide chloride of mercury, quicksilver, cinnabaris (mercury sulfide), hydrargyri oxydum rubrum (mercury oxide), mercury iodide or "poison"; directions to avoid contact with silver, gold, rubber, aluminium and jewellery may also indicate the presence of mercury.[1,6] However, companies selling products that contain mercury, do not always list it as an ingredient.

- **Effects of Using the Products:** Women who use mercury-containing skin lighteners often have elevated mercury levels in their hair, blood and urine. Several studies have found their hair mercury levels greater than 100 ppm in women using these products, compared with a "normal" range of below 10ppm.[2,16,17] Similarly far above normal levels of mercury have been measured in urine of women in Kenya[18] and Tanzania[17] who used mercury-containing skin lighteners, and users of these cosmetics in Hong Kong had elevated mercury levels in their blood and urine.[19]

Some manufacturers are no longer using mercury as a preservative in mascara and eye makeup cleansing products as a result of consumer pressure. However, most jurisdictions still allow the sale of makeup products containing mercury compounds.[25]

References

1. UNEP 2008. *Mercury in products and wastes.* Geneva, United Nations Environment Programme, Division of Technology, Industry and Economics, Chemicals Branch, 2008.
http://www.unep.org/chemicalsandwaste/Portals/9/Mercury/AwarenessPack/English/UNEP_Modl_UK_Web.pdf.

2. Glahder CM, Appel PWU, Asmund G *Mercury in soap in Tanzania.* Copenhagen Ministry of Environment and Energy, National Environmental Research Institute (NERI) Technical Report No. 306; 1999.
http://www2.dmu.dk/1_viden/2_publikationer/3_fagrapporter/rapporter/fr306.pdf).

3. Ladizinski B, Mistry N, Kundu RV. Widespread use of toxic skin lightening compounds: medical and psychosocial aspects. *Dermatologic Clinics*, 2011; 29:111-23.
4. WHO *Guidance for identifying populations at risk from mercury exposure*, Geneva, World Health Organization 2008.(http://www.who.int/entity/foodsafety/publications/chem/mercury/en/).
5. Lindsey K, Balagizi I, Hirt HM. *Be black and beautiful.* Winnenden, anamed international 2009.
6. New York City Department of Health and Mental Hygiene. *Mercury in soaps and creams.* New York, NY, Department of Health and Mental Hygiene. 2011.http://www.nyc.gov/html/doh/html/epi/mercury_sc.shtml.
7. McKelvey W, Jeffery N, Clark N, Kass D, Parsons PJ. Population-based inorganic mercury biomonitoring and the identification of skin care products as a source of exposure in New York City. *Environmental Health Perspective*, 2011; 119(2): 203-9.
8. Engler DE. Letter to the editor: Mercury "bleaching" creams. *Journal of the American Academy of Dermatology*, 2005; 52(6): 1113-4.
9. IPCS. *Elemental mercury and inorganic mercury compounds: human health aspects.* Geneva. World Health Organization, International Programme on Chemical Safety (Concise International Chemical Assessment Document 50; 2003. http://www.who.int/entity/ipcs/publications/cicad/en/cicad50.pdf).
10. ATSDR. *Toxicological profile for mercury.* Atlanta, GA, Agency for Toxic Substances & Disease Registry 1999. (http://www.atsdr.cdc.gov/toxprofiles/TP.asp?id=115&tid=24).
11. WHO. *Exposure to mercury: a major public health concern.* Geneva, World Health Organization (Preventing disease through healthy environment series; 2007. http://www.who.int/phe/news/Mercury-flyer.pdf).
12. Al-Saleh I, Al-Doush I. Mercury content in skin-lightening creams and potential hazards to the health of Saudi women, *Journal of Toxicology and Environmental Health*, 1997; 51(2): 123-30.
13. MDH. *Skin-lightening products found to contain mercury.* Minnesota Department of Health 2011 (http:///www.health.state.mn.us/topics/skin/).
14. Uram E, Bischofer BP, Hagemann S. Market analysis of some mercury-containing products and their mercury-free alternatives in selected regions. *Gesellschaft für Anlagenund Reaktorsicherheit (GRS) mbH*, March GRS-253;http://www.ipen.org/ipenweb/documents/ipen%20documents/grs253.pdf
15. Texas DSHS . *DSHS warns of mercury poisoning linked to Mexican beauty cream.* News release, 1 September 2011. Texas Department of State Health Services, 2011.(http://www.dshs.state.tx.us/news/releases/20110901.shtm).
16. Gras G and Mondai J. The problem of the use of mercurials cosmetics in Senegal (author's transl) [Article in French] *Recherche Eurpéene en Toxicologie* 1981; 3(4): 175-178.
17. Kahatano JMJ, Mnali, SR and Akagi H. A Study of Mercury Levels in Fish and Humans in Mwakitolyo Mine and Mwanza Town in the Lake Victoria Goldfields, Tanzania. – In: Lars Landner (ed.): Small-Scale Mining in African Countries. Proceedings of an International Conference/Workshop 29th September – 1st October, 1997 Dar es Salaam, Tanzania 1998.
18. World Health Organization. Environmental Health Criteria 118: Inorganic Mercury. Geneva, WHO 1991.

19.Sin KW and Tsang HF Large-scale mercury exposure due to a cream cosmetic: community-wide case series. Hong Kong Medical Journal 2003; 9:329-34; also see recent IPEN repot at: http:///.ipen.org/hgfree#grs.

Some reports of high mercury levels in cosmetics

The absorption of mercury from the skin and hence its toxic effects depends on the concentration of mercury in the products.

Skin-lighteners are sold as creams, lotions and soaps. Hundreds if not thousands of them are sold in the global market. Those that use mercury as an active ingredient often contain from 2 to 10 percent mercury by weight. Products tested in a variety of countries in Africa, Asia, Latin America and North America have contained from 660 to 57,000 parts per million (ppm) mercury[1]. Users of these cosmetics in Hong Kong had elevated levels in their blood and urine. Unfortunately, the most effective ingredients, which include mercury compounds and hydroquinone, are also the cheapest, and that induces many manufacturers to use them in products, despite their well documented toxic hazards.

Analysis of mercury levels in some locally manufactured Mexican Skin-lightening creams, using the cold vapor technique coupled with atomic absorption spectrometry (CV-AAS), showed a mercury content of the samples which varied between 875 and 36,000ppm, despite the fact that the US Food and Drug Administration (FDA) has determined that the limit for mercury in creams should be less than 1ppm. A total of 6 out of 16 randomly sampled skin lightening creams had measurable levels of mercury. No warning information was noted on the packaging.[2]

One study measured international skin-lightening products for their mercury content, focusing on products available to US consumers either online or in stores. The products were screened for mercury content using a portable x-ray fluorescence spectrometer. Of the 549 products tested, 6% contained mercury levels above 1000ppm, and 45% contained mercury levels that exceeded 10,000ppm. Of the skin lightening products purchased in the United States, 3.3% were found to contain mercury in excess of 1000ppm. According to the authors, the Food and Drug Administration (FDA) limits the amount of mercury in most cosmetic products to 1ppm.[3]

Despite national bans, however, recent tests show mercury-containing skin lighteners are still sold in developed countries like the US. In

New York City, the Department of Health and Mental Hygiene found five such products, one of which had caused a case of mercury poisoning.[4] The products had been imported from the Dominican Republic. An American newspaper, the Chicago **Tribune**, recently tested 50 skin-lightening products and found five, manufactured in China, Mexico, India, Lebanon, India, Pakistan, and Taiwan, that contained mercury levels ranging from 6,000 to 29,600ppm[5].

Another study in China on Minimal change disease caused by exposure to mercury-containing skin lightening cream showed that the cream contained very high mercury levels (7,420 – 30,000ppm). All the four cases studied were women. All the patients presented with nephrotic syndrome and heavy proteinuria (8.35 – 20.69g/d). The blood and urinary mercury levels were 26-129nmol/l and 316 – 2,521nmol/d respectively. Renal biopsy revealed minimal change disease (MCD) in all four patients. The duration of exposure to the mercury – containing skin lightening cream was for 2-6months.[6]

Skin lightening creams were randomly collected from local markets in Sultanate of Oman for analysis of mercury content. All the products collected were of low cost imported materials from different countries. Out of forty cream samples analysed, about one fourth of the samples contained higher levels of mercury which is more than the maximum mercury content of 1 microg/g permitted by the Food and Drug Administration (FDA regulation.. The mercury level in the analysed samples was found to be in the range from 0.02 to 25.7 microg/g[7].

Women who use mercury-containing skin lighteners often have elevated mercury levels in their hair, blood and urine. Several studies have found hair mercury levels greater than 100ppm in women using these products, compared with a "normal" range of below 10ppm.[8,9,10] Similarly, far above normal levels of mercury have been measured in urine of women in Kenya[11] and Tanzania[9]

References

1. Sin KW and Tsang HF Large-scale mercury exposure due to a cream cosmetic: community-wide case series. *Hong Kong Medical Journal* 2003; 9:329-34; also see recent IPEN report at: http://www.ipen.org/hg free#grs

2. Peregrino CP, Moreno MV, Miranda SV, Rubio AD, Leal LO: Mercury levels in locally manufactured Mexican skin-lightening creams. *Int J Environ Res Public Health;* 2011 Jun; 8(6): 2516-23.

3. Hamann CR, Boonchai W, Wen L, Sakanashi EN, Chu CY, Hamann K, et al. Spectrometric analysis of mercury content in 549 skin-lightening products: is mercury toxicity a hidden global health hazard? *J Am Acad Dermatol.* Feb 2014; 70 (2); 281-7. e3. [Medline]
4. New York City Department of Health and Mental Hygiene. NYC Health Dept. warns against use of "skin lightening" creams containing mercury or similar products which do not list ingredients. Press release, Jan 27 2005. http://www.nyc.gov/htm/doh/html/pr/pr008-05.shtml.
5. Gabler E and Roe S. Some skin whitening creams contain toxic mercury, testing finds. *Chicago* **Tribune**, May 18, 2010. http://articles.chicagotribune.com/2010-15-18/health/ct-met-mercury-skin-creams-20100518/skin-lightening-creams-mercury-testing.
6. Tang HL, Mak YF, Chu KH, Lee W, Fung SK, Chan TY, Tong KL: Minimal change disease caused by exposure to mercury – containing skin lightening cream: a report of 4 cases. *Clin Nephrol*; 2013 Apr; 79 (4): 326-9
7. Naser J, Kirm I: Mercury content in low cost skin lightening cream products. *J Environ Sci Eng.* 2012 April; 54(2): 245-8.
8. Gras G and Mondain J. The problem of the use of mercurials cosmetics in Senegal (author's trans) [Article in French] *Recherche Européene en Toxicologie.* 1981 3(4): 175-78.
9. Kahatano J M J, Mnali SR and Akagi H (1998) A Study of Mercury Levels in Fish and Humans in Mwakitolyo Mine and Mwanza Town in the Lake Victoria Gold fields, Tanzania – In: Lars Landner (ed): Small-scale Mining in African Countries. Proceedings of an International Conference/Workshop 29th Sept – 1st Oct, 1997 Dar es Salaam, Tanzania.
10. Glahder CM, Appel PWU and Asmund G Mercury in Soap In Tanzania. NERI Technical Report No. 306, 1999. National Environmental Research Institute, Ministry of Environment and Energy, Denmark.
11. World Health Organization. *Environmental Health Criteria* 118: Inorganic Mercury, Geneva, WHO. 1991.

Adverse health effects of mercury exposure to cosmetic products and clinical manifestations

Mercurials were popular as skin lightening agents until they were recognized as toxic. They have been shown to be nephrotoxic via the absorption of mercury through the skin following repeated use.[1,2] Although banned in many countries, some studies show that a number of marketed skin lightening products still contain mercury compounds.[3,4] As already documented these products are still being manufactured in China, Dominican Republic Lebanon, Mexico, Pakistan, the Philippines, Thailand and the USA (see chapter on Epidemiology). About 45% of commonly used skin-lightening creams in Saudi Arabia were shown to contain mercury above the FDA's acceptable limit of 1ppm[5]. Nephrological as well as neurological complications have been documented.[6,7] Experimental studies in mice have confirmed that mercury is toxic on the kidney, liver and brain.[4] In addition studies comparing mercury levels in various tissues brands of mercury skin lightening creams, found that mercury accumulated in the ovaries of treated mice. The clinical implication of this is that the use of mercury containing skin-lightening products may contribute to infertility and fetal damage (fetotoxicity).[8]

Elemental and methylmercury are toxic to the central and peripheral nervous systems. The inhalation of mercury vapour can produce harmful effects on the nervous, digestive and immune systems, lungs and kidneys, and may be fatal. The inorganic salts of mercury are corrosive to the skin, eyes and gastrointestinal tract, and may induce kidney toxicity if ingested, after inhalation, injection or dermal exposure of different mercury compounds.[1]

Mercury-based bleaching creams contain ammoniated mercury as a bleaching agent. Some of these creams may contain up to 2.5% mercury which can be harmful to our health, thus resulting in mercury poisoning, especially chronic mercury poisoning. Mercury use in cosmetic products can have adverse effects including skin rashes like dermatitis and acne venenata, and post inflammatory dyschromia. Long-term use of mercury-based skin lighteners often produces a characteristic "slate gray" skin color.[2] Hyperpigmentation is a common problem among African women, caused by mercury and/or hydroquinone in skin-lightening creams. Ammoniated mercury, used in some skin lightening creams can cause rashes and allergic reactions.[3] It can also reduce the skin's resistance to bacterial and mycotic disorders.[6,7] Gastro-intestinal symptoms include a metallic taste, gingivo-stomatitis, nausea and hypersalivation. Direct and prolonged exposure through the skin during repeated application can cause damage to the brain, nervous system and kidneys.

Neurological and behavioural disorders may be observed after inhalation, ingestion or dermal exposure of different mercury compounds.[4] Although inorganic mercury has poor lipid solubility and hence does not cross the brain barrier, in cases with chronic exposure to mercury, it has been seen to accumulate in the brain and cause neurological damage.

Mild subclinical signs of central nervous system toxicity can be seen in workers exposed to an elemental mercury level in the air of 20μg/m^3 or more for several years.

Symptoms and signs of mercury toxicity include neurotoxic problems such as ataxia, tremors, speech and hearing impairment, insomnia, neuromuscular effects, headaches and complaints like tingling, numbness, lassitude, vertigo, abdominal cramps, generalized aches and pains; mental problems such as irritability, fearfulness, depression and forgetfulness. All the classic signs of inorganic mercury poisoning that are seen with chronic mercury exposure may not be attributed to mercury exposure at all nor from skin bleaching products by the clinician. Mild, subclinical signs of central nervous system toxicity can be seen in workers exposed to an elemental mercury level in the air of 20μg/m^3 or more for several years. Kidney problems such as mercury-induced nephropathy and immunotoxicity may occur.

However, there are general characteristics associated with mercury poisoning, including a tight feeling of the chest, chills, diarrhea, metallic taste, nausea, vomiting, emotional instability, irritability, depression, forgetfulness, insomnia, muscular weakness, renal failure, and loss of teeth. depression, anxiety and paranoid delusion.

The kidneys are the major sites of inorganic mercury deposition; renal damage include reversible proteinuria, acute tubular necrosis and nephrotic syndrome. Kidney effects have been reported, ranging from increased protein in the urine to kidney failure. This is further discussed under a separate heading because of its importance. Mercury in skin lightening cosmetic products have raised serious public health concerns and also serious health issues as regards the fetus and early childhood. These shall be discussed under a separate heading because of their importance.

More disturbing reports have emerged of mercury-containing skin lightening creams being mixed with α-hydroxy acids and used as injectables for women who wish to lighten their skin quickly and effectively[3]. The potential serious adverse effects of this unorthodox method of administration of α-hydroxy acid and mercury are yet to be characterized

In addition, dermal exposure to skin-lightening creams containing mercury may contribute to infertility as a consequence of accumulation of mercury in the ovaries.[4] It may also cause foetal abnormalities.

References

1.Mercury/Toxicity WHO/ Mercury and health http://www.who.int/mediacentre/factsheets/fs36/en

2. Olumide Y.M, Odunowo BD, and Odiase AO. Regional dermatosis in the African. Part 1. Facial hypermelanosis. *International Journal of Dermatology* 1991; 30(3): 186-9.

3. Harada M et al. Wide use of skin-lightening soap may cause mercury poisoning in Kenya. *Science of the Total Environment* 2001; 269: 183-7.

4. Luderschdmidt C and Plewig G. Chronic mercury poisoning following topical application of skin bleachers. (author's translation) [Article in German] *Klinische Wochenschrift* 1979; 57 (6): 293-8.

5. Chan TY: Inorganic mercury poisoning associated with skin-lightening cosmetic products. *Clin Toxicol* (Phila); 2011 Dec; 49 (19): 886-91

6. 1. Annabel Fenwick Elliott. Kenya men like women with whiter skin: The rise of wealthy Nairobi women illegally injecting themselves with skin-lightening creams http://www.dailymail.co.uk/femail/article-265076/illegally-INJECTING-skin-lightening-creams-html

7. Al-Saleh I, Shinwari N, Al-Amodi M. Accumulation of mercury in ovaries of mice after the application of skin-lightening creams.*Biol Trace Elem Res* 2009; 131:43-54

8. Al-Saleh I, Shinwari N, Al Amodi M. Accumulation of mercury in ovaries of mice after the application of skin-lightening creams. *Bio Trace Elem Res* 2009; 131:43-54

Effects of mercury in skin lightening products on the kidneys

Mercury use in skin lightening products has resulted in the accumulation of mercury in the body after absorption through the skin especially in the kidney where it is mainly accumulated in the tubular region, giving rise to the occurrence of severe reactions.[1-5] The United States Food and Drugs Administration (US FDA) in 1992 established the maximum acceptable limit of mercury in cosmetic to be 1μg/g. A clinical investigation of Kenyan women with damaged kidneys revealed that they suffered from a higher incidence of nephrotic syndrome, which was attributed to the use of creams containing mercury.[3]

The kidneys are the major sites of inorganic mercury deposition; renal damage includes reversible proteinuria, acute tubular necrosis and nephrotic syndrome.

Inorganic mercury poisoning following the use of skin-lightening creams has been reported from Africa, Asia, Europe, Middle East,

USA, Latin America, Australia and Hong Kong.[6-15] Wherever there are dark-skinned people either as indigenes, immigrants or emigrants. Nephrotic syndrome, mainly due to minimal change or membranous nephropathy and neurotoxicity were the most common presenting features.

Kidney damage caused by long-term use of mercury-containing skin-lightening creams has been reported by investigators in China[7], Hong Kong[8] and the UK[9]. In those cases, once the source of mercury exposure was identified and the women stopped using the harmful products, their kidney function gradually returned to normal. Unfortunately, most women who use skin-lightening products are unlikely to be seen by a medical practitioner who could detect such kidney damage at an early stage and eliminate their mercury exposure before more serious disease develops. It has also been observed that most practising non dermatologist physicians are hardly aware of the cutaneous stigmatas of skin-lightening cosmetics and are most unlikely to associate the renal problem of the patient to the cosmetic use. In Nigeria, Ayobola Iyanda assessed the renal function of 23 skin-whitening users while 25 women served as controls. Serum urea and creatinine were significantly increased compared with the controls. This significant increase in the levels of renal indices show that these agents might be nephrotic after prolonged usage.[16]

There are no clear-cut guidelines regarding the urinary mercury levels at which chelation therapy is indicated. The chelating agents used for mercury poisoning are dimercaprol, DMSA (meso-2-3-dimercaptosuccinicacid) and DMPS (sodium 2,3-dimercapto-1 propanesulfonate). It is unclear whether the use of chelating agents will reverse the renal and neurological damage.[10]

References

1. Soo YO, Chow KM, Lam CW, Lai FM, Szeto CC, Chan MH, Li PK. A whitened face women with nephrotic syndrome. *Am J Kidney Di* 2003; 41:250-3.

2. Marzulli FN, Brown DWC. Potential systemic hazards of topically applied mercurials *J Soc Cosmet Chem* 1972; 23:875-86.

3. Barr RD, Woodger BM, Rees PH. Levels of mercury in urine correlated with the use of skin lightening creams. *Am J clin Pathol* 1973; 59: 36-40.

4. Berlin M. Mercury. In: F. Friberg GF Nordberg, and VL Vouk (Editors) Handbook in toxicology of metals. Amsterdam: Elsevier/North-Holland, 1979; 503-30.

5. Bourgeosis M, Dooms-Goossens A, Knockaert D, Sprenger D, Vsan Boven M, and Van tittelboom T. Mercury intoxication after topical application of a metallic mercury ointment. *Dermatologica* 1986; 1972: 48-51.
6. Chan, TY: Inorganic mercury poisoning associated with skin-lightening cosmetic products. Clin Toxicol (Phila); 2011 Dec; 49 (19): 886-91
7. Li SJ et al Mercury–induced membranous nephropathy: Clinical and pathological features. *Clinical Journal of the American Society of Nephrology* 2010; 5(3): 439-444.
8. Tang HL et al Minimal change disease following exposure to mercury–containing skin lightening cream. *Hong Kong Medical Journal* 2006; 12(4): 316 – 318.
9. Oliveira DB et al Membranous nephropathy caused by mercury–containing skin lightening cream. *Postgraduate Medical Journal* 1987; 63 (738): 303 – 304.
10. Risher JF, Amler SN, Mercury exposure: Evaluation and intervention the inappropriate use of chelating agents in the diagnosis and treatment of putative mercury poisoning. *Neurotoxicology* 2005; 26:691-9.
11. Chakera A, Lasserson D, Beck JR, Roberts ISD, Winearls QJM. Membranous nephropathy after use of UK-manufactured skin creams containing mercury 2010; doi: 1093/qjmed/hcq209
12. Bourgeois M; Dooms–Goossens A, Knockaert D, Sprenger D, Van Boven M and Van Tittelboom T. Mercury intoxication after topical application of a metallic mercury ointment. *Dermatologica* 1986; 172:48-51
13. Dorkenoo T. Skin Bleaching. "The Pandemic is Here" Weekly *Spectator* 1998; 572:2.
14. Glahder CM, Appel PWU and Asmund G. Mercury in Soap in Tanzania. *NERI Technical Report* No. 306 National Environmental Research Institute, Denmark 1999, p19.
15. Kibuhamusohe JW, Davies DR, Hutt MSR. Membranous nephropathy due to skin lightening cream. *Br Med J* 1974; 2:646-7.
16. Iyanda AA, Anetor John and Adeniyi FAA. Altered copper level and renal dysfunction in Nigerian women using skin-whitening agents. http://www.researchgate.net/profile/John_Anetor2

Public Health Concern: Mercury in skin-lightening products

Environmental impacts

These cosmetics containing mercury can harm not only the user, but also nonusers who come in contact with people using such products on a regular basis. Even though never having used the product themselves, contacts were also found to have high mercury levels.

Mercury from the soap and cream is transferred to the drainage system and thence into the environment. Here it enters the organisms either as inorganic mercury compounds, or is converted by bacterial action to organic mercury, e. g., methylmercury. Methylmercury is readily incorporated into the food chain and concentrated in fish and fish-eating birds. When fish are eaten by humans, the results can be fatal, for example, in Minamata in Japan. Elimination of methylmercury from fish and other aquatic organisms is slow.[1,2,3,4]

Mercury compounds are highly toxic to microorganisms even in concentrations as low as 0.005 mg inorganic mercury per litre. Organic mercury compounds are ten times more toxic to microorganisms. In aquatic environments, the organic compounds are generally more toxic than inorganic compounds. Aquatic plants are affected by concentrations as low as 1 mg inorganic mercury per litre, whereas organic compounds are toxic at much lower concentrations. Larvae of insects are generally more sensitive to mercury compounds than adults. Lethal concentrations (LC50-values) of inorganic mercury compounds to freshwater fish are in the range of 0.03 to 0.4 mg per litre, whereas sea-water fish seem to be more resistant. Low concentrations of mercury compounds have an impact on fish by reducing their reproduction. Terrestrial plants are generally unaffected by high mercury concentrations, whereas birds contaminated by mercury show a reduction in food intake, and consequent poor growth. These observations have been described in WHO [5,6]

Pregnant women who have eaten fish containing methylmercury transfer this mercury very efficiently to their foetuses. As a consequence their new-born babies have a much higher mercury contents in their blood than their mothers.[7] It has been demonstrated that even quite low mercury levels in mothers during pregnancy affect the ability of their children to solve mental problems, when these are presented to the seven year old children.[8]

The use of mercury-containing cosmetic products was also found to be of public health concern as it can contaminate the home. Mercury vapours from skin lightening cosmetics with high concentrations of mercury manufactured in Mexico and brought into USA by an immigrant was found to release measurable levels of mercury vapour. Close household contacts were also reported to have elevated urinary concentrations though they did not use the cream.[9,10] This phenomenon of inhalation of hazardous toxic mercury vapour is akin to non-tobacco smokers at risk due to inhalation of tobacco smoke from smokers. Male partners of the women can develop male infertility from inhalation of Mercury vapours. Mercury decreases both sperm count and sperm cell motility, which is the ability to move spontaneously and actively.[2,10,11]

In 2010 members of a Mexican-American family in California manifested symptoms of mercury exposure. California Department of Public Health (CDPH) investigated identified unlabeled skin-lightening creams with mercury content measured at 2.0%-5.7% by weight as the likely source of mercury exposure. Mercury vapor concentrations as high as 50μg/m^3 were measured in spot household locations.[12,13]

Estimation of the urine mercury concentration is the best marker of exposure of inorganic mercury and indicator of body burden. A 24-hour urine for measurement of mercury excretion is preferred; a spot urine mercury concentration should be corrected for creatinine output. Urine mercury levels greater than 25mg/L are considered as suggestive of poisoning and it is used as a diagnostic test for exposure to inorganic mercury[3].

A generation of women is being negatively affected by excessive usage of these products and in many instances the environment, including the water supply and food chain, is dramatically being affected in countries where people of color live and consume skin bleaching products. Therefore, it is reasonable to conclude that skin lightening products have caused a silent, but deadly epidemic in public health that needs to be addressed immediately. Although customers have the choice to purchase these products, the larger population is being affected healthwise. It is of utmost importance to protect the larger population than to protect individual rights to purchase skin bleaching products that contain mercury.

References

1. Kahatano J M J, Mnali SR and Akagi H A Study of Mercury Levels in Fish and Humans in Mwakitolyo Mine and Mwanza Town in the Lake Victoria Gold fields, Tanzania – IN: Lars Landner (ed): Small-scale Mining in African Countries. Proceedings of an International Conference/Workshop 29th Sept – 1st Oct, 1997 Dar es Salaam, Tanzania who used mercury-containing skin lighteners, and users of these cosmetics in Hong Kong had elevated levels in their blood and urine (1998).

2. Glahder CM, Appel PWU, Asmund G. *Mercury in soap in Tanzania*, Copenhagen, Ministry of Environment and Energy, National Environmental Research Institute (NERI) Technical Report No. 306; 1999.

3. Sin KW and Tsang HF. Large-scale mercury exposure due to a cream cosmetic: community-wide case series. *Hong Kong Medical Journal* 2003; 9:329-334; also see recent IPEN report at: http://www.ipen.org/hgfree#grs

4. Anekwe Obiora N. The Global Phenomenon of Skin Bleaching: A Crisis in Public Health (Part 1). Voices in Bioethics. Retrieved on October 12th, 2014, Restricted from
http://voicesinbioethics.org/2014/01/2014/01/29/theglobal-phenomenon-of-skin-bleaching-a-crisis-in-public-h&#8230

5. WHO Mercury and health Fact sheet No 361. September 2013. http://www.who.int.mediacentre/factsheets/fs361/en/
6. Zero Mercury Working Group Mercury in Fish: A global health hazard 2009. http://mercurypolicy.org/wp-content/uploads/2009/02 / MercuryInFishFullReportFinal021009.pdf
7. Hansen CT, Nielsen CO, Dietz R, Hansen MM. Zinc, cadmium, mercury and selenium in minke whales, belugas and narwhals from West Greenland. *Polar Biol.* 1990; 10:529-39.
8. Grandjean P, Budtz-Jorgensen E, Jorgensen PJ, Weihe P. Umbilical cord mercury concentration as biomarker of prenatal exposure to methylmercury. *Environ Health Perspect.* 2005; 113:905-8
9. 8 Common Causes of Infertility in men. *INFORMATION NIGERIA* http://www.informationng.com/2015/05/8-common-causes-of-infertility
10. Olson David A, Ramachandran Tarakad S. Mercury Toxicity http://emedicine.medscape.com/article/1175560-overview Updated Oct 20, 2014.
11. Male Infertility-Medscape Reference emedicine.medscape.com/article/436829-overview
12.Centers for Disease Control and Prevention (DCD). Mercury poisoning associated with beauty cream – Texas, Mexico, and California. 1995 – 1996. *MMWR Morb Mortal Wkly Rep* 1996; 45:400-3.
13.Gabler E and Roe S. Some skin whitening creams contain toxic mercury, testing finds. *Chicago Tribune,* May 18, 2010 See: *http://articles.chicagotribune.com/2010-15-18/health/ct-met-mercury-skin-creams-20100518/skin-lightening-creams-creams-mercury-testing*

The sources of mercury to mother, baby and children

Mercury in the mother is dangerous to the baby

The mother acquires mercury through

(1) Use of skin bleaching products containing mercury (before, during and after pregnancy)[1,2,3]
(2) Through consumption of contaminated fish with melthylmercury [4,5]
(3) Through mercury amalgamation (artisanal gold mining) [6,7,8,9] (See the section on TANZANIA)
(4) Through the use of Ayurvedic folk remedies and some ethnic and religious practices[10,11,12]
(5) If mothers eats any food contaminated with mercury e.g grains such as rice or maize treated with mercury containing fungicides.[13,14,15]

Sources of mercury to the baby

1. The fetus (unborn baby) acquires mercury from the mother through the placenta.[16,17]
2. After birth the baby acquires mercury through mothers breast milk,[18,19,20] through sucking the nipple coated with mercury skin

bleaching products, and through inhaling mercury fumes from the mother's skin.[21,22,23] (See the chapters on NIGERIA, GHANA, JAMAICA—4, 7 and 15).

3. Babies can directly absorb mercury through the skin when the mother uses mercury containing skin bleaching soaps and creams on the baby. The baby's skin is particularly vulnerable and permeable to chemicals in toiletries and cosmetics.[24] There was an epidemic of mercury toxicity among children in a refugee camp from widespread use of skin bleaching cosmetics creams and soaps on children.[25]
4. Babies acquire mercury from 'take home' sources if any member of the family is occupationally exposed to mercury e.g artisanal gold mining due to mercury amalgamation. The clothing and skin of such workers are coated with mercury, hence the home environment is contaminated with mercury fumes.[6,7,8,9]
5. There is a report of baby's diaper contaminated with mercury.[26]
6. Mercury containing teething powder have also caused mercury toxicity in babies
7. Adults, babies and older children can inhale mercury from latex paints.[27,28]

Sources of mercury to older children

1. Eating contaminated fish and shellfish and grains like the adults.
2. Child labor in artisanal gold mining%mercury amalgamation[9]
3. Inhalation of mercury fumes in a contaminated home environment [6,7,8,9]
4. The principal sources of exposure to mercury in schools is elemental mercury e.g broken thermometers, old barometers, electrical switches and liquid metal used in school laboratories.[29,30,31,32]

References

1. Al-Saleh I, Al-Doush I. Mercury content in skin-lightening creams and potential hazards to the health of Saudi women. *J Toxicol Environ Health.* 1997; 51:123–30.

2. Palmer RB, Godwin DA, McKinney PE. Transdermal kinetics of a mercurous chloride beauty cream: an in vitro human skin analysis. *J Toxicol Clin Toxicol.* 2000; 38:701–7.

3. Deleu D, Hanssens Y, Al-Salmy HS, Hastie I. Peripheral polyneuropathy due to chronic use of topical ammoniated mercury. *J Toxicol Clin Toxicol.* 1998; 36:233–7.

4. Aberg B, Ekman L, Falk R, Greitz U, Persson G, Snihs JO. Metabolism of methyl mercury (CH_3Hg) -compounds in man. *Arch Environ Health.* 1969; 19:478–84.

5. Miettinen JK, Rahola T, Hattula T, Rissanen K, Tillander M. Elimination of methylmercury in man. *Ann Clin Res.* 1971; 3:116–22.
6.United Nations Environment Programme%Chemicals. Global Mercury Assessment. Geneva: 2002. Available at: http://www.unep.org/gc/gc22/Document/UNEP-GC22-INF3.pdf.
7. Eisler R. Mercury hazards from gold mining to humans, plants, and animals. *Rev Environ Contam Toxicol.* 2004; 181:139–98.
8. International Labour Organization (ILO) International Programme on the Elimination of Child Labour (IPEC) http://www.ilo.org/ipecinfo/product/download.do?type=document&id=4146.
9. Bose-O'Reilly S, Lettmeier B, Gothe RM, Beinhoff C, Siebert U, Drasch G. Mercury as a serious health hazard for children in gold mining areas. *Environ Res.* 2008; 107:89–97.
10. Rai V, Kakkar P, Singh J, Misra C, Kumar S, Mehrotra S. Toxic metals and organochlorine pesticides residue in single herbal drugs used in important ayurvedic formulation—"Dashmoola" *Environ Monit Assess.* 2007; 143(1-3):273–7.
11. Saper RB, Kales SN, Paquin J, Burns MJ, Eisenberg DM, Davis RB, et al. Heavy metal content of ayurvedic herbal medicine products. *JAMA.* 2004; 292:2868–73.
12. Dargan PI, Gawarammana IB, Archer JRH, House IM, Shaw D, Wood DM. Heavy metal poisoning from ayurvedic traditional medicines: an emerging problem? *Int J Environ Healthc.* 2008; 2:463–74.
13. Cheng J, Yuan T, Wang W, Jia J, Lin X, Qu L, et al. Mercury pollution in two typical areas in Guizhou province, China and its neurotoxic effects in the brains of rats fed with local polluted rice. *Environ Geochem Health.* 2006; 28:499–507.
14. Feng X, Li P, Qiu G, Wang S, Li G, Shang L, et al. Human exposure to methylmercury through rice intake in mercury mining areas, Guizhou province, China. *Environ Sci Technol.* 2008; 42:326–32.
15. Bakir F, Damluji SF, Amin-Zaki L, Murtadha M, Khalidi A, Al-Rawi NY, et al. Methylmercury poisoning in Iraq. *Science.* 1973; 181:230–41.
16. Harada M. Minamata disease: methylmercury poisoning in Japan caused by environmental pollution. *Crit Rev Toxicol.* 1995; 25:1–24.
17. Akagi H, Grandjean P, Takizawa Y, Weihe P. Methylmercury dose estimation from umbilical cord concentrations in patients with Minamata disease. *Environ Res.* 1998; 77:98–103.
18. Grandjean P, Jorgensen PJ, Weihe P. Human milk as a source of methylmercury exposure in infants. *Environ Health Perspect.* 1994; 102:74–7. s
19. Vimy MJ, Hooper DE, King WW, Lorscheider FL. Mercury from maternal "silver" tooth fillings in sheep and human breast milk. A source of neonatal exposure. *Biol Trace Elem Res.* 1997; 56:143–52.
20.Yoshida M, Satoh H, Kishimoto T, Yamamura Y. Exposure to mercury via breast milk in suckling offspring of maternal Guinea pigs exposed to mercury vapor after parturition. *J Toxicol Environ Health.* 1992; 35:135–9.
21. Sandborgh-Englund G, Elinder CG, Johanson G, Lind B, Skare I, Ekstrand J. The absorption, blood levels, and excretion of mercury after a single dose of mercury vapor in humans. *Toxicol Appl Pharmacol.* 1998; 150:146–53.
22. Henriksson J, Tjalve H. Uptake of inorganic mercury in the olfactory bulbs via olfactory pathways in rats. *Environ Res.* 1998; 77:130–40.

23. Fang SC. Comparative study of uptake and tissue distribution of methylmercury in female rats by inhalation and oral routes of administration. *Bull Environ Contam Toxicol.* 1980; 24:65–72.
24. Weldon MM, Smolinski MS, Maroufi A, Hasty BW, Gilliss DL, Boulanger LL, et al. Mercury poisoning associated with a Mexican beauty cream. *West J Med.* 2000; 173:15–8. [Discussion, 19] [PMC free article]
25. Otto M, Ahlemeyer C, Tasche H, von Muhlendahl KE. Mercury exposure. *Nature.* 1994; 367:110.
26. Gotelli CA, Astolfi E, Cox C, Cernichiari E, Clarkson TW. Early biochemical effects of an organic mercury fungicide on infants: "dose makes the poison. *Science.* 1985; 227:638–40.
27. Agocs MM, Etzel RA, Parrish RG, Paschal DC, Campagna PR, Cohen DS, et al. Mercury exposure from interior latex paint. *N Engl J Med.* 1990; 323:1096–101.
28. Beusterien KM, Etzel RA, Agocs MM, Egeland GM, Socie EM, Rouse MA, et al. Indoor air mercury concentrations following application of interior latex paint. *Arch Environ Contam Toxicol.* 1991; 21:62–4.
29. Lee R, Middleton D, Caldwell K, Dearwent S, Jones S, Lewis B, et al. A review of events that expose children to elemental mercury in the United States. *Environ Health Perspect.* 2009; 117:871–8. [PMC free article]
30. Risher JF. The Concise International Chemical Assessment Document Series. World Health Organization; Geneva: 2003. Elemental Mercury and inorganic compounds: human health aspects. Available at: http://www.who.int/ipcs/publications/cicad/en/cicad50.pdf.
31. Zeitz P, Orr MF, Kaye WE. Public health consequences of mercury spills: hazardous substances emergency events surveillance system, 1993-98. *Environ Health Perspect.* 2002; 110:129–32. [PMC free article]
32.MacLehose R, Pitt G, Will S, Jones A, Duane L, Flaherty S, et al. Mercury contamination incident. *J Public Health Med.* 2001; 23:18–22.

Effect of mercury in skin bleaching products on the baby and children's health

Route of exposure

- *Transplacental*—through the placenta while still in the womb (prenatal exposure).[1,2]
- *Ingestion (orally)*— from mothers breast milk and from sucking the nipple skin coated with bleaching cream [3,4,5]
- *Inhalation*— by inhaling mercury vapour on the skin of the mother coated with mercury containing skin bleaching creams or contaminated air [6,7,8]
- *Transdermal*— absorption through the skin when the mother applies bleaching creams on the baby or bathes the baby with mercury containing soaps. The parents may also bring home mercury vapour on their body from work e.g artisanal gold mining.[9,10,11]

Clinical manifestation by the baby: symptoms and signs

- Baby can be affected even when the mother shows no signs nor symptoms[1]
- Signs of mercury toxicity in the newborn are muscular spasms, stiffness and high muscle tone. A foetus exposed to high levels of mercury may even be born without kidneys. A woman working at a mercury containing cosmetic product factory at W & E Products in UK gave birth to a baby with no kidneys, who died at three month.[12]
- Lauwerys *et al*[13] reported a case of slight renal tubular dysfunction associated with cataract and anemia in a 3-month-old black boy in Belgium. High levels of mercury were found in blood and urine of the child. They argued that the renal, ocular and haematological defects may have resulted from exposure to mercury during foetal life and the one month lactation period due to the extensive use of inorganic mercury containing cosmetics by the mother.
- Babies are born severely damaged with microcephaly (small underdeveloped brain and head); cerebral palsy (brain damage causing paralysis or muscle weakness); severe mental retardation, seizure disorders (epilepsy), blindness, deafness, and other malformations, delayed developmental milestones, language disorders, problems with memory.[1,2]
- The newest findings with long-term studies are increased incidence of high blood pressure and decreased heart rate.[14,15]
- Some other symptoms are delayed e.g **tremor** (regular involuntary rhythmic oscillation of a part of the body); **dysdiadochokinesia** (impairment of the power to perform alternating movements in rapid, smooth, and rhythmic succession%clumsy child); **ataxia** uncoordinated and unbalanced movement); increased **salivation**, **stupor** (a state of being unable to think or hear clearly etc, a state of depressed consciousness in which mental and physical activity are reduced to a minimum); **cachexia** (severe generalized weakness, malnutrition, and emaciation); **ptosis** (dooping of the upper eyelid); and **incontinence** (inability to control the natural evacuations of feces or urine).[14,15]

- Full expression can be delayed and deficits are irreversible; no effective treatment is possible.

Symptoms and signs of mercury vapor inhalation
Inhalation of elemental mercury vapor can cause acute and chronic intoxication. Depending on the dose and time, several symptoms can be observed.[16]

- Airway symptoms e.g **cough**, **dyspnea** (difficult or labored breathing) fever, ill-being, h**eadaches**, **central nervous system problems** (tremor, ataxia, coordination disturbances); **gingivitis** (inflammation of the gums), **stomatitis** (inflammation of the soft tissues of the mouth, mercurial **erethism** (excitability, loss of memory, insomnia, extreme shyness); **neurocognitive disorders** (impaired thoughts, perceptions, understanding and reasoning); **kidney problem** (protein in urine); and **skin symptoms** (acrodynia with painful, swelling of extremities, pinkish discoloration, peeling of skin.

Chronic Mercury Exposure and Skin Reactions
Mercury compounds, including inorganic and organic forms, can induce dermatotoxic reactions ranging from a chronic dermatitis to acrodynia. Acrodynia, Pink's disease, and Morbus Feer are synonyms used for a specific clinical picture of mercury intoxication. Acrodynia is a toxic reaction to elemental or inorganic mercury exposure that occurs mainly in young children, rarely in adults.[17-20] A special susceptibility may be present, because the symptoms can occur at low levels of mercury exposure. Among 32 published cases the urinary mercury concentrations were below 50 μg/L and in 4 children even below 10 μg/L.[17]

It is characterized by pinkish discoloration and desquamation of hands and feet, morbiliform, rubeoliform or scarlatiniform exanthems, (measles-like rash) erythema (redness of the skin), symmetrical, mainly hands, feet, and nose, predominantly distal, volar (palms and soles), especially in cold surroundings (Pink's disease), bluish, cold, wet extremities, itchiness, pain in the extremities, loss of hair, loose teeth, loss of teeth, hypertension, sweating, insomnia, irritability, and apathy. Mercury exposure can cause tremors, the so-called "Tremor Mercurialis." Tremor is a very typical symptom of acute and chronic mercury intoxication.

Note!

- Specimens, such as urine, blood, or hair, do not necessarily reflect the concentration of mercury at the main target organs, such as brain or kidney.[21]
- Mercury exposure can show delayed effects, months and years after the exposure, or get more severe, meaning that the time of exposure and the time of onset of effects can differ.[22]
- Mercury is excreted with a half-time of about 3 months. Effects can be persistent.
- There may be a lack of correlation between the symptoms and the level of exposure.[23,24,25]

References

1. Harada M. Minamata disease: methylmercury poisoning in Japan caused by environmental pollution. Crit Rev Toxicol. 1995; 25:1–24.

2. Akagi H, Grandjean P, Takizawa Y, Weihe P. Methylmercury dose estimation from umbilical cord concentrations in patients with Minamata disease. Environ Res. 1998; 77:98–103.

3. Grandjean P, Jorgensen PJ, Weihe P. Human milk as a source of methylmercury exposure in infants. Environ Health Perspect. 1994; 102:74–7.

4. Vimy MJ, Hooper DE, King WW, Lorscheider FL. Mercury from maternal "silver" tooth fillings in sheep and human breast milk. A source of neonatal exposure. Biol Trace Elem Res. 1997; 56:143–52.

5. Yoshida M, Satoh H, Kishimoto T, Yamamura Y. Exposure to mercury via breast milk in suckling offspring of maternal Guinea pigs exposed to mercury vapor after parturition. J Toxicol Environ Health. 1992; 35:135–9.

6. Sandborgh-Englund G, Elinder CG, Johanson G, Lind B, Skare I, Ekstrand J. The absorption, blood levels, and excretion of mercury after a single dose of mercury vapor in humans. Toxicol Appl Pharmacol. 1998; 150:146–53.

7. Henriksson J, Tjalve H. Uptake of inorganic mercury in the olfactory bulbs via olfactory pathways in rats. Environ Res. 1998; 77:130–40.

8. Fang SC. Comparative study of uptake and tissue distribution of methylmercury in female rats by inhalation and oral routes of administration. Bull Environ Contam Toxicol. 1980; 24:65–72.

9. Al-Saleh I, Al-Doush I. Mercury content in skin-lightening creams and potential hazards to the health of Saudi women. J Toxicol Environ Health. 1997; 51:123–30.

10. Palmer RB, Godwin DA, McKinney PE. Transdermal kinetics of a mercurous chloride beauty cream: an in vitro human skin analysis. J Toxicol Clin Toxicol. 2000; 38:701–7.

11. Deleu D, Hanssens Y, Al-Salmy HS, Hastie I. Peripheral polyneuropathy due to chronic use of topical ammoniated mercury. J Toxicol Clin Toxicol. 1998; 36:233–7.

12. Lucy Hannan. Companies still make hazardous cosmetics for Africa. Feature: Hazardous Cosmetics. *African Business* May 1988.

13. Lauwerys R, Bonnier CH, Evrard PH, Gennart PH, and Bernard A. Prenatal and early postnatal intoxication by inorganic mercury resulting from the maternal use of mercury containing soap. *Hum Toxicol* 1987; 6:253-6.
14. Grandjean P, Murata K, Budtz-Jorgensen E, Weihe P. Cardiac autonomic activity in methylmercury neurotoxicity: 14-year follow-up of a Faroese birth cohort. J Pediatr. 2004; 144:169–76.
15. Thurston SW, Bovet P, Myers GJ, Davidson PW, Georger LA, Shamlaye C, et al. Does prenatal methylmercury exposure from fish consumption affect blood pressure in childhood? Neurotoxicology. 2007; 28:924–30.
16. Drasch G, Bose-O'Reilly S, Beinhoff C, Roider G, Maydl S. The Mt. Diwata study on the Philippines, 1999—assessing mercury intoxication of the population by small scale gold mining. Sci Total Environ. 2001; 267:151–68.
17. von Mühlendahl KE. Feer's disease (acrodynia)—a strange disease. Umweltmed Forsch Prax. 2008; 13:73–9.
18. von Mühlendahl KE, Schulter-Wissermann H, Grips M, Feer M. Skin changes. Pädiatr Prax. 1995; 49:647–52.
19. Foulds DM, Copeland KC, Franks RC. Mercury poisoning and acrodynia. Am J Dis Child. 1987; 141:124–5.
20. Gattineni J, Weiser S, Becker AM, Baum M. Mercury intoxication: lack of correlation between symptoms and levels. Clin Pediatr. 2007; 46:844–6.
21. Drasch G, Schupp I, Hofl H, Reinke R, Roider G. Mercury burden of human fetal and infant tissues. Eur J Pediatr. 1994; 153:607–10.
22. Clarkson TW, Magos L. The toxicology of mercury and its chemical compounds. Crit Rev Toxicol. 2006; 36:609–62.
23. Clarkson TW, Magos L, Myers GJ. The toxicology of mercury—current exposures and clinical manifestations. N Engl J Med. 2003; 349:1731–7.
24. Counter SA, Buchanan LH. Mercury exposure in children: a review. Toxicol Appl Pharmacol. 2004; 198:209–30.
25. Bose-O'Reilly S, Lettmeier B, Gothe RM, Beinhoff C, Siebert U, Drasch G. Mercury as a serious health hazard for children in gold mining areas. Environ Res. 2008; 107:89–97.

Identification of mercury in skin-whitening creams.

The handheld XRP analyzer proved an excellent tool for screening mercury in skin creams, and could be particularly useful in developing countries because it is relatively inexpensive, requires no sample preparation or extraction, can be used by staff with little technical background, and can facilitate on-site education.

Reference

Murphy Thomas, Lim Sereyrath, Huong Srei Pisei, *et al.* Application of Handheld X-Ray Fluorescence Analyzers to Identify Mercury in Skin-Whitening Creams in Cambodia *Blacksmith Institute Journal of Health & Pollution.* June 2012; 2 (3): 21-31.

HYDROQUINONE

Introduction

Hydroquinone, also known as benzene-1, 4- diol or quinol, is an aromatic organic compound, that is a type of phenol, having the chemical formula C_6 H_4 $(OH)_2$.[1] It is a white granular solid. has aSubstituted derivatives of this parent compound are also referred to as hydroquinones. Hydroquinone (HQ) is a dihydric phenol with important derivatives viz. monobenzyl and monomethyl ether of hydroquinone. Hydroquinone variety of uses principally associated with its action as a reducing agent that is soluble in water. Hydroquinone was originally employed as an industrial chemical. It is a major component in most black and white photographic developers for film and paper where, with the compound Metol, it reduces silver halides to elemental silver. There are various other uses associated with its reducing power.[1]

Hydroquinone is a chemical agent whose melanin inhibiting properties were discovered quite by accident in 1938, when 17 black workers in a tannery plant in Waukegan, Illinois, complained of discolouration of the hands and arms. An internal investigation conducted by the plant authorities found out that the problem was caused by rubber gloves treated with monobenzyl ether of hydroquinone (HQ), a substance ironically designed to reinforce the gloves worn by the workers in order to prevent discolouration of the leather these workers were handling[2]. The incident found its way into the local media. As a result, by 1955, hydroquinone was being mass-produced in the United States for the purpose of skin-bleaching. By 1961, hydroquinone found a lucrative market in apartheid South Africa[3]. Hydroquinone came to the attention of the Western medical communities when in 1975 South African dermatologist G. H. Findlay and his colleagues published an article linking the use of hydroquinone-based skin-bleaching creams used by 35 South African black women to an irreversible skin condition called exogenous ochronosis[4]. Exogenous ochronosis from skin bleaching products was subsequently reported by other authors.[5,6] Exogenous ochronosis is a localized, blue-black hyperpigmentation in the epidermis, dermis and subcutaneous layers of the skin that can be induced by a number of different chemicals, including hydroquinone[7,8,9]. Dr Pick was the first physician who made the link between exposure of harmful chemical compounds similar to hydroquinone to humans and the damaging skin condition "exogenous ochronosis."[7] Exogenous ochronosis was also reported by Thomas and Ginsburg in 1961.[8]

Hydroquinone as a skin-bleaching agents[9-16]

The most common over-the-counter skin bleaching agent in the world, including North America and Europe, is hydroquinone. In human medicine, hydroquinone is used as a topical application in skin whitening to reduce the colour of the skin. This use is banned in some countries, including the member states of the European Union under Directive 76/768/ EEC: 1976[9,10] The ingredient has been banned due to numerous safety issues and serious toxicity concerns in Europe. Japan and several other countries. In the U.S.A however, the ingredient is still used in a wide variety of prescription and non-prescription skin bleaching products. Any product with a concentration of four percent or higher must be obtained via prescription only. However, it is 'easily prescribed by most dermatologists to women of color as well as women with lighter skin who are experiencing hyperpigmentation, brown or age spots and melasma.

Topical hydroquinone is used frequently throughout the world as a skin bleaching agent. Hydroquinone for cosmetic use is chemically synthesized. It may be found in concentrations up to 15% or more but a doctor's prescription is required by the FDA (United States) for preparations containing concentrations above 2%. The Cosmetic Ingredient review (CIR) Expert Panel states hydroquinone should not be used in "leave-on" cosmetic formulations. In spite of this, internet sites can easily be found that offer topical hydroquinone in concentrations over 2% and very commonly as high as 4% or more[11]

In the United States, topical treatments usually contain up to 2% in hydroquinone. Otherwise, higher concentrations (up to 4%) should be prescribed and used with caution. In 2006, the United States Food and Drug Administration revoked its previous approval of hydroquinone and proposed a ban on all over-the-counter preparations.[11] The FDA stated that hydroquinone cannot be ruled out as a potential carcinogen. This conclusion was reached based on the extent of absorption in humans and the incidence of neoplasms in rats in several studies where adult rats were found to have increased rates of tumors, including thyroid follicular cell hyperplasias, anisokaryosis, mononuclear cell leukemia, hepatocellular adenomas and renal tubule cell adenomas. The Campaign for safe Cosmetics has also highlighted concerns.[12-16]

Mechanism of action[17-19]

Hydroquinone is easily absorbed into the skin and its absorption increases dramatically when alcohols are present in a topical preparation. Hydroquinone reacts with the functional parts of individual cells and effects cellular metabolism. Hydroquinone is known to competitively inhibit melanin production by inhibiting sulfhydryl groups and acting as a substrate for tyrosinase. The melanosomes and ultimately the melanocytes are damaged by semiquinone free radicals released during the above reaction. Hydroquinone has cytotoxic (cell-killing or cell-damaging) activity on the pigment-producing cell of the skin, the melanocyte, as well as on many other cell types. The cell-toxic activity of hydroquinone is caused by a free-radical oxidation mechanism. Free radical development has the potential to damage the melanocyte on its own and may also damage neighboring cells or their physical structures.

Potential adverse effects[20-41]

Cases of intoxication have been reported after oral ingestion of hydroquinone alone or of photographic developing agents containing hydroquinone. The major signs of poisoning included dark urine, vomiting, abdominal pain, tachycardia, tremors, convulsions and coma. Deaths have been reported after ingestion of photographic developing agents containing hydroquinone.

Hydroquinone has been identified as both a potential clastogen and mutagen. A clastogen is a toxin that has the capability to cause breaks in chromosomes, cause sections of them to be destroyed, and to rearrange the sections and thus cause mutations which can lead to various types of cancer. A mutagen is a material that causes mutation and damage in DNA. When the DNA is altered, it can cause any number of chain reactions that can negatively impact the health, including cancerous growth of cells and cell division. In addition to its classification as a likely carcinogen, it has also been implicated as a disruptor or damaging presence to several other vital human functions and systems–one is the immune system. The chemical has shown immunity-weakening side effects in some of the animal testing that has been done. Animal testing has also shown an impact on the endocrine system, suggesting the material would also have an impact on the human endocrine system. Concerns that it is also a neurotoxin, which affects the nervous system and lungs have also surfaced. Hydroquinone can also cause a side effect that is worse than the very condition it is supposed to treat. This side effect becomes more likely with longer use of products containing the ingredient. The condition is called exogenous ochronosis which causes the skin to produce blue and black pigments which causes blotches of dark spots on the skin.

Combined exposure to hydroquinone and quinone airborne concentrations causes eye irritation, sensitivity to light, injury of the corneal epithelium, corneal ulcers and visual disturbances. There have been cases of appreciable loss of vision. Irritation has occurred at exposure levels of 2.25 mg/m^3 or more. Long-term exposure causes staining of the conjunctiva and cornea and also opacity. Slowly developing inflammation and discoloration of the cornea and conjunctiva have resulted after daily hydroquinone exposure for at least two years of 0.05-14.4 mg/m^3; serious cases have not occurred until after five or more years. One report described cases of corneal damage occurring several years after the exposure to hydroquinone had stopped.

It was once thought that concentrations of hydroquinone of 2% or less had negligible potential for adverse effects. It is now known that this is not true, as the medical literature reports problems occurring with lesser concentrations. There are case reports suggesting that skin lightening creams containing 2% hydroquinone have produced leucoderma, as well as ochronosis. Hydroquinone (1% aqueous solution or 5% cream) has caused irritation(erythema or staining). Allergic contact dermatitis due to hydroquinone has been diagnosed. The topical side effects after hydroquinone application are thought to be related to its mechanism of cytotoxicity. Another earlier myth was that only heavily pigmented skin suffered from adverse effects related to hydroquinone use. This also is untrue, as side effects in Asians, Hispanics, Caucasians and Blacks with less pigmentation have been reported in the medical literature.[31-36] Applying hydroquinone to skin and then exposing the skin to sunlight markedly increases potential toxicity. Additionally, hydroquinone is systemically absorbed through the skin with measurable amounts appearing in urine after topical application. Orally ingested hydroquinone is very rapidly absorbed by the gastrointestinal (GI) tract and is known to incite kidney and liver damage. In the presence of moisture and at room temperature, hydroquinone metabolizes to quinine which can cause serious issues such as eye irritation, leading to conjunctivitis (red eye) and erosions of the cornea (open sores over the central eye). The potential adverse effects involving inflammation (redness) and cell damage (related to free radical damage) potentially result in severe reactionary hyperpigmentation. The potential development of malignant cells is also of great concern.

Hydroquinone is readily absorbed through the skin and can be detected in urine as the intact parent substance (rather than a metabolite) after the 2% cream is applied. The evidence relating to kidney damage of orally ingested material raises concerns here, considering that hydroquinone applied to the skin must get through the blood stream and the rest of the body in order to be found in urine. This raises other questions about the cancer-causing (malignant) potential and other cell-damaging (cytotoxic) properties of hydroquinone that could occur with systemic absorption (passage through the skin to the remainder of the body). Blood cell toxicity and leukemia have been associated with hydroquinone absorbed throughout the body. In addition to these toxicity concerns, there is a secondary skin cancer risk. The chemical works to "bleach" the skin by inhibiting the production of melanin. This, in turn, prevents the skin from discoloring and helps to lighten already darkened areas on the skin such as liver spots, discoloration and melasma. The mechanism by which it inhibits melanin production also lets UV light penetrate the skin more deeply. This means it makes UV exposure more carcinogenic by increasing the depth at which the skin soaks up the DNA-damaging rays. This is why people who use hydroquinone products are always told to wear a sunscreen at all times, or preferably to use the product only before bed time when there is no risk of UV exposure.

Several adverse health effects have been reported as regards hydroquinone. Some of these are squamous cell carcinoma, irritant and allergic contact dermatitis (inflammation of the skin), dyschromia (abnormal patches of uneven skin-color), exogenous ochronosis which is a type of dyschromia. There are no adequate epidemiological data to assess the carcinogenicity of hydroquinone in humans. The majority of patients suffering from ochronosis have heavier genetic melanin production as it is especially frequent in African Blacks, who sometimes use as high as 27% concentration of hydroquinone in skin bleaching products. This disorder can also occurs in Asians, Hispanics and Caucasians with hydroquinone use.[31-36] Treatment is extremely frustrating because improvement occurs so slowly or not at all with this debilitating condition. Some other adverse effects are striae ("stretch marks"), fingernail yellow-brown discoloration,[37] and hydroquinone neuropathy[38]

The fallacy about the safety of "2 percent" hydroquinone[26-30]

In 1975, the first medical report linking hydroquinone-based skin bleaching chemical to irreversible skin damage, exogenous ochronosis, was published by G.H. Findlay *et al* in the British Journal of Dermatology.[4] By using Findlay's published medical report, members of the South African medical community, as well as lay people, put pressure on the pharmaceutical companies who were manufacturing and distributing hydroquinone. However, the apartheid regime refused to ban hydroquinone based skin bleaching chemicals being sold and manufactured in South Africa, instead, it agreed to "better regulate" its manufacture and sales.[40]

As a result of regulation, by 1980 the concentration of hydroquinone in skin-bleaching creams, soaps and ointments sold and or manufactured in South Africa had been reduced from an 8 percent to a 2 percent upper limit, though there was no medical evidence to indicate that 2 percent hydroquinone in over-the-counter hydroquinone skin-bleaching preparations was safe. On the basis of the arbitrary decision made by one of the most racist regimes of the modem era, today you can buy 2 percent hydroquinone based skin-bleaching creams, soaps and ointments in almost all drug stores and "beauty" shops, globally.

Six years after the concentration in over-the-counter hydroquinone skin-bleaching chemical agents was reduced to 2 percent, another South African dermatologist, N. Hardwick, conducted a survey in two Pretoria research hospitals by randomly selecting 194 outpatient subjects who came to these research facilities for reasons other than skin problems; 53 males and 141 females were selected[2]. The result of this research was that 68 patients (35 percent of the total 195 patients) had exogenous ochronosis. Of the 68 patients with exogenous ochronosis, 12 patients who started using hydroquinone-based bleaching preparations after 1983 had the condition. In their analysis, Hardwick *et al*[3] had chosen 1983 as a cut-off-period to give the old hydroquinone-based skin-bleaching preparations containing 8 percent concentration sufficient time to be off the market. However, this new finding, which contradicted the claim that 2 percent hydroquinone is a "safe" skin-bleaching chemical, did not change the legal status of skin-bleaching products in apartheid South Africa or in the West. Hardwick's findings suggest that even in 2 percent concentration, hydroquinone causes skin damage. In addition, Schulz *et al*[40] have argued that skin damage resulting from hydroquinone poisoning depends on the amount of hydroquinone absorbed by the skin which, in turn, depends on the frequency and duration of application and not on the concentration in hydroquinone.

The reasons for resisting a ban on these poisonous chemicals in the West and in South Africa are many and complex. One of the reasons why medical communities in the West, as well as in the Southern hemisphere nations, are reluctant to ban skin-bleaching chemical poisons like hydroquinone is that hydroquinone and its derivatives have entered, in the broadest sense, the cosmetics and dermatology industries. Some dermatologists have started using hydroquinone in their practices to treat women with skin "blemishes," "freckles," and "age spots" who are willing to pay the cost of "safe," "customized" hydroquinone preparations which meet their needs.[41]

Hydroquinone and other cutaneous depigmenting agents are widely used by dermatologists to treat pigmentary disorders. On 29 August 2006, the US Food and Drug Administration (FDA) published a monograph in the US Federal Register proposing to ban all hydroquinone products that have not been approved via a New Drug application process.[14] This proposal arose following the failure of manufacturers to comply to a request by the FDA for safety studies on hydroquinone. In addition, the FDA has cited many safety concerns about this product, including the occurrence of hydroquinone-induced ochronosis. Nonetheless, hydroquinone remains a popular agent for the treatment of pigmentary disorders in people with skin phototypes IV to VI.[41] Thus, the proposal to ban this agent has prompted many within the dermatological community to publish articles that address the concerns of FDA.[14,15,16,42] However, a review of the English-language scientific literature reveals that most of the reported cases of hydroquinone-induced exogenous ochronosis occur in Africa, where culture practice of skin bleaching is highly prevalent.[38-40] In Japan, the European Union, and Australia, hydroquinone has been removed from over-the-counter skin products and substituted with other chemicals due to concerns about health risks. In the U.S., over-the-counter creams containing up to 2 percent hydroquinone are recognized as safe and effective by the U.S. Food and Drug Administration. A proposed ban by the FDA in 2006 fizzled.

Currently, one can walk in to any American or Canadian drug store, or "beauty" salon serving blacks and other people of colour, and pay for skin-bleaching creams, ointments and soaps with names such as Ambi fade Crème, Esoterica, Parcelana, Vantex, and Venus de Milo. Most over-the-counter skin-bleaching chemicals available in the United States, Canada and Europe contain hydroquinone. In the United States, in 1990, $44 million of over-the-counter skin-bleaching products were purchased.[2] This figure does not reflect the use of hydroquinone-containing chemical agents sold as prescription drugs or in cosmetics which contain hydroquinone but which do not list it. In South Africa, in 1979, 25 million Rands worth of hydroquinone–based skin-bleaching products were purchased. In 1986, in South Africa, that figure jumped to 94 million Rands, or about $30 US million.[3] Most over-the-counter hydroquinone-based skin-bleaching preparations available in the United States, Canada and Europe following the 1983 South African 2 percent upper limit guideline; and some American dermatologists have vigorously advocated for the use of hydroquinone as a drug to treat various skin conditions such as acne and melasma[24]

The world Health Organization states: "It is recommended that over-the-counter sales of creams containing hydroquinone be restricted. Health education programs should be developed to discourage the use of hydroquinone-containing creams".[25]

References

1.Hydroquinone. *http://en.wikipedia.org/wiki/Hydroquinone.*

2. Russell Kathy, Wilson Midge, and Hall Ronald. The Color Complex: The politics of skin color among African Americans. *(New York, London, Toronto, Sydney, Auckland: Anchor Books,* 1992, p51

3. Hardwick N, Van Gelder LW, Van der Merwe CA and Van DerMerwe. Exogenous Ochronosis: An epidemiological study. *British Journal of Dermatology.* 1989; 120: 229-38

4. Findlay GH, Morrison JGL and Simson IW. Exogenous ochronosis and pigmented colloid millium from hydroquinone bleaching creams. *British Journal of Dermatology.* 1975; 93:613.

5. Horshaw Richard, Zimmerman Kent G and Menter Alan. Ochronosis like pigmentation from hydroquinone bleaching creams in American Blacks. *Arch Dermatol* Jan 1985; 121: 105-8

6. Lang Pearson G. Probable coexisting exogenous ochronosis and mercurial pigmentation managed by dermabrasion. *J American Academy Dermatol* 1988; 19 (5): 942-6.
7. Pick L. Uber Die Ochronosis. *Klin Wochenschrift* 1906; 43: 478.
8. Thomas AE, Ginsburg MA. Exogenous ochronosis and myxoedema from resorcinol. *British J. Dermatol* 1961; 73:378-81.
9. 76/768/EEC:1976 Council Directive 76/768/EEC of 27 July 1976 on the approximation of the laws of the Member States relating to cosmetic products. http:eur-lex.europa.eu/LexUriServ
10. Example of a product recall in Ireland (http://www.consumerconnet.ie/eng/News_+_Research/Product_Recalls/Clear_N_Smooth_cream_withdrawn.html)
11. United States Food and Drug Administration (2006). Skin Bleaching Drug Products for Over-the-Counter Product Use; Proposed Rule (http://www.fda.gov/OHRMS/DOCKETS/98fr/78n-0065-npr0003.pdf) Report) 1978 N – 0065
12. Campaign For Safe Cosmetics – Hydroquinone (http://www.safecosmetics.org/article/php?id=289
13. Danna Norek. Why hydroquinone, the skin bleaching chemical, is highly toxic. *Natural News* Saturday, March 23, 2013
14. U.S. Department of Health and Human Services, Food and Drug Administration. Skin bleaching drug products for over-the-counter human use; proposed rule. *Federal Register* 2006; 71: 51146-51155 (codified at 21 CFR Part 310).
15. Nordlund JJ, Grimes PE, Ortonne JP. The safety of hydroquinone. *J Eur Acad Dermatol Venereol* 2006; 20:781-7
16. Levitt J. The safety of hydroquinone: a dermatologist's response to the 2006 Federal Register. *J Am Acad Dermatol* 2007; 57:854-72
17. Lerner AB, Fitzpatrick TB. Inhibition of melanin formation by chemical agents. *J Invest Dermatol* 1952; 18:119-35.
18. Jimbow K, Obata H, Pathak MA et al. Mechanism of Depigmentation by Hydroquinone . *J Invest Dermatol* 1974; 62:436
19. De Haven Charlene. Hydroquinone. *www.innovativeskincare.com. http://www.isclinical.com/whitepapers/Whitepaper_Hydroquinone_July2014.pdf*
20. Snider Rebecca and Brace H Their. Exogenous Ochronosis. *Journal of the American Academy of Dermatology*. 1993; 28(4): 662-6.
21. Davis EC, Callende VD. Post inflammatory hyperpigmentation: a review of the epidemiology, clinical features, and treatment options in skin of colour. *J Clin Aesthet Dermatol.* Jul 2010; 3(7): 20-31.
22. Policarpio B, Lui H. Skin lightening and depigmenting agents. *eMedicine*/WebMD, Oct 26 2009.
23. Spencer MC. Topical Use of hydroquinone for depigmentation. *JAMA*. 1965; 194 (9): 114-6.
24. Engasser Patricia G and Howard I Maiback. Cosmetics and dermatology: Bleaching creams. *Journal of the American Academy of Dermatology* 1981; 5(2): 143-7
25. "Hydroquinone". WHO working group. Environmental Health Criteria. 1994; vi(157): 178

26. Amin RP, Witz G. DNA-protein crosslink and DNA strand break formation in HL-60 cells treated with Trans, Trans-muconaldehyde, hydroquinone and their mixture. *Int J Toxicol.* Mar-Apr 2001; 20(2): 69-80.
27. Ly F, Kane A, Deme A, Ngom NF, Niang SO, Bello R, Rethers L, Dangou JM, Dieng MT, Diousse P, Ndiaye B. First cases of squamous cell carcinoma associated with cosmetic use of bleaching compounds. *Ann Dermatol Venereol.* Feb 2010; 137(2): 128-31.

28. Topping DC, Bernard LG, O'Dnoghue JL, English JC. Hydroquinone: acute and subchronic toxicity studies with emphasis on neurobehavioral and neurotoxic effects. *Food Chem Toxicol.* Jan 2007; 45(1): 70-8 .
29. Olumide Yetunde M, Akinkughe Ayesha O, *et al.* Complications of chronic use of skin lightening cosmetics. *International Journal of Dermatology* 2008; 47: 344-53
30. Olumide Yetunde M. Use of skin Lightening creams. Lack of recognition and regulation is having serious medical consequences. *BMJ* 2010; 341: c6102 doi: 10.1136/bmj.c6102.
31. Howard KL, Furner BB. Exogenous Ochronosis in a Mexican-American Woman. *Cutis.* Mar 1990; 45 (3): 180-2.
32. Wen Chun Liu, Hong Liang Tey, Joyce Siong See Lee and Boon Kee Goh. Exogenous Ochronosis in a Chinese patient: use of dermoscopy aids early diagnosis and selection of biopsy site. *Singapore Med J.* 2014 Jan; 55(1): e1-e3.
33. Tan SK. Exogenous ochronosis in ethnic Chinese Asians: clinicopathological study, diagnosis and treatment. *J Eur Acad Dermatol Venereol.* 2011; 25: 842-50
34. Tan SK, Sim CS, Goh CL. Hydroquinone-induced exogenous ochronosis in Chinese%two case reports and a review. *Int J Dermatol.* 2013; 52: 413-7
35. Jonas Ribas, Antonio Pedro Mendes Schettini, Melissa de Sousa Melo Cavalcante. Exogenous ochronosis hydroquinone induced: a report of four cases. *An Bras Dermatol* Sept./Oct.2010; 88 (5). *http://dx.doi.org/10.1590/S0365-05962010000500017.*
36. Swati Sharma, Raghavendra Rao. Exogenous ochronosis masquerading refractory melasma. *Our Dermatol Online.* 2014; 5(4): 398-400.
37. Ozluer SM, Muir J. Nail staining from hydroquinone cream. *Australas J Dermatol.* Nov 2000; 41 (4): 255-6.
38. Karamagi C, Owino E, Katabira ET. Hydroquinone neuropathy following use of skin bleaching creams: case report. *East Afr Med J.* Apr 2001; 78(4): 223-4.
39. Levin CY, Maibach H. Exogenous Ochronosis. An update on clinical features, causative agents and treatment options. *Am J Clin Dermatol.* 2001; 2(4): 213-7.
40. Schulz EJ and Sher MA. Rescinding of legislation to ban hydroquinone-containing creams. *South African Medical Journal.* 1990; 77: 372. Reprinted in *the British Medical Journal* 1992; 305: 903-4.
41. Amina Mire. Skin-Bleaching: Poison, Beauty, Power, and the Politics of the Colour Line. *Resources for Feminist Research.* 2001; 28(3-4): 13.
42. Toombs EL. Hydroquinone–what is it's future? *Dermatol Ther* 2007; 20: 149-56.
43. Williams Hywel. Skin lightening creams containing hydroquinone: The Case for a temporary ban. *British Medical Journal* 1992; 305: 903-4.

Hydroquinone induced Exogenous Ochronosis

The term 'ochronosis' was first coined by Virchow in 1866 to refer to brownish-yellow accumulations of pigment found in the connective tissue of patients with endogenous ochronosis.[1] **Endogenous** ochronosis, also known as alkaptonuria, is a rare (1:250,000) autosomal recessive disease caused by the congenital absence of homogentisic acid oxidase, leading to the accumulation of homogentisic acid within various tissues of the body.[2] Cutaneous features of endogenous ochronosis include blue-black hyperpigmentation on the pinnae, nasal tip, cheeks, sclerae and axilla. Systemic deposition of homogentisic acid results in ochronotic arthropathy (mainly involving large joints and the vertebral column), deafness, genitourinary obstruction and cardiovascular complications (e.g. aortic valve calcification and stenosis). Diagnosis is usually made clinically or with urine tests using sodium hydroxide.

Exogenous ochronosis was first described by Pick in 1906.[3] This condition is often reported in the black population of South Africa as a result of the use of bleaching agents, particularly hydroquinone.[4] Other agents implicated include antimalarials, and products containing resorcinol, phenol, mercury or picric acid.[5] Classical features of exogenous ochronosis are asymptomatic blue-black macules with textural coarsening and sooty tipped papulations on the malar area, temples, inferior cheeks and neck. In 1979, Dogliotti et al[6] classified exogenous ochronosis into three clinical stages: (a) erythema and mild hyperpigmentation; (b) hyper-pigmentation, pigmented colloid milium (i.e. caviar-like lesions) and scanty atrophy; and (c) papulonodular lesions

References

1. Virchow R. Eii Fall von allegemeiner ochronose der knorpel and knorpelahnlichen theile. Virchows Arch (Pathol Anat) 1866; 37:212–9. German.

2. Srsen S. Alkaptouria. Johns Hopkins Med J. 1979; 145:217–26.

3. Pick L. Uber die Ochronose. Klin Wochenschr. 1906; 43:478–80. German.

4. Levin CY, Maibach H. Exogenous ochronosis. An update on clinical features, causative agents and treatment options. Am J Clin Dermatol. 2001; 2:213–7.

5. Hull PR, Proctor PR. The melanocyte: an essential link in hydroquinone-induced ochronosis. J Am Acad Dermatol. 1990; 22:529–31.

6. Dogliotti M, Leibowitz M. Granulomatous ochronosis – a cosmetic-induced skin disorder in Blacks. S Afr Med J. 1979; 56:757–60.

Pathogenesis

Exogenous ochronosis is a diffuse pigmentation of the face; and blue black macular patches on the face and external ears and sun-exposed arears of the upper chest, upper back and extensor surfaces of the extremities following prolonged application of hydroquinone. With prolonged application and stimulation, the depigmented melanocytes recover from the effect of hydroquinone and drops into the papillary dermis; they become taken up by fibroblasts, leading to altered elastic fibre production, excretion of abnormal material into new fibre bundles and degenerative changes in the collagen bundles. With prolonged application and sun stimulation, the melanocytes recover from the damaging effect of the hydroquinone which passes down into the papillary dermis of the skin. Hence they are actively taken up by fibroblasts and lead to altered elastic fibre production and excretion of abnormal material into new fibre bundles. Furthermore, benzoquinone acetic acid formed during the oxidative processes in which hydroquinone is involved, binds and cross link collagen fibres leading to degenerative changes due to altered physico-chemical bonds.[1,2]

Histology[3-6]

Histologic examination of exogenous ochronotic lesions reveals yellow-brown banana-shaped fibers in the papillary dermis. Homogenization and swelling of the collagen bundles is noted and a moderate histiocytic infiltrate may be present. Sarcoid-like granulomas with multinucleated giant cells engulfing ochronotic particles have been noted. Transfollicular elimination of ochronotic fibers has also been described. Fibers stain black with Fontana stain and blue-black with methylene blue stain. Ultrastructural examination reveals homogenous electron-dense, irregular structures embedded in an amorphous granular material infiltrating adjacent collagen fibril bundles. The source of these ochronotic fibers is not clear. Topical hydroquinones may inhibit homogentisic acid oxidase in the skin, resulting in the local accumulation of homogentisic acid that then polymerizes to form ochronotic pigment. Pigmented particles may be elastic or collagen fibers. Melanocytes may be involved; most cases involve sun-exposed sites and one case is reported of ochronosis that avoided areas of vitiligo. The changes in the collagen bundles may be responsible for the loss of elasticity and poor wound healing. Clinical features and some histologic features of exogenous ochronosis are similar to features of photoageing. Association of exogenous ochronosis with chronic sun exposure, presentation in sun exposed areas, and clinical and histologic similarity with photoageing may qualify it to be listed as feature of photodamage in the dark skinned.

Clinical manifestations of adverse effects of chronic application of hydroquinone on the skin

Complications of hydroquinone use that have been reported are dermatitis, exogenous ochronosis, cataract, pigmented colloid milia, scleral and nail pigmentation and patchy depigmentation[7]. The pigmented exogenous ochronotic lesions are most marked on sun-exposed areas of the body viz, face, upper chest and upper back. Dogliotte,[6] described 3 stages of this condition: (1) Erythema and mild pigmentation; (2) hyperpigmentation, black colloid milia and scanty atrophy; and (3) papulonodules with or without surrounding inflammation. Figures 13.1-20 show exogenous ochronosis. Since most commercial sex workers use these skin lightening creams, some of them are HIV positive; and in an attempt to bleach away the pruritic papular eruption (PPE) commonly seen in HIV/AIDS patients, the skin of the extremities appear scruffy with the excoriated papules on a background of ochronotic pigmentation on bleached skin as shown in Figures 13.19 and 20. A patient developed squamous cell carcinoma on the site of chronic exogenous ochronosis (Fig. 13.21). It is not clear if this is a chance finding or an expected sequelae of hydroquinone induced exogenous ochronosis with superimposed chronic sun damage on the vulnerable skin. Coalescence of multiple colloid milia may give rise to big nodular lesions particularly on the upper back.

Other complications of hydroquinone use include atrophy of the skin, pigmented colloid milia, sclera and nail pigmentation. The fawn colored pigmentation of all the twenty nails(Fig 13.6) may mimic the yellow nail syndrome—hence the authors call the phenomenon "*pseudo* yellow-nail syndrome." Abnormal repigmentation of depigmented skin has also been reported on discontinuing therapy. This abnormal repigmentation has been attributed to the Meirowsky effect of long wavelengths of ultraviolet light darkening melanin already present in the skin and leading to a skin color darker than that prior to bleaching. Because of this repigmentation, users find it compelling to continue to use the bleaching creams to maintain the newly acquired light colored skin. Hence, the inevitable complications from prolonged use. A more serious complication is loss of elasticity of the skin and impaired wound healing. When cutting through the skin, either for incisional biopsy or other surgical procedures, it is as if one was cutting through the skin of a cadaver. There is difficulty in apposing the edges of the wounds when stitching, hence the skin often tears through the suture material. Furthermore, there is often delayed wound healing. After major abdominal surgeries like Caesarian section, myomectomy, hysterectomy etc, there may be catastrophic wound dehiscence, burst abdomen, and death from overwhelming infection.

Legends of all the pictures are on Page 592

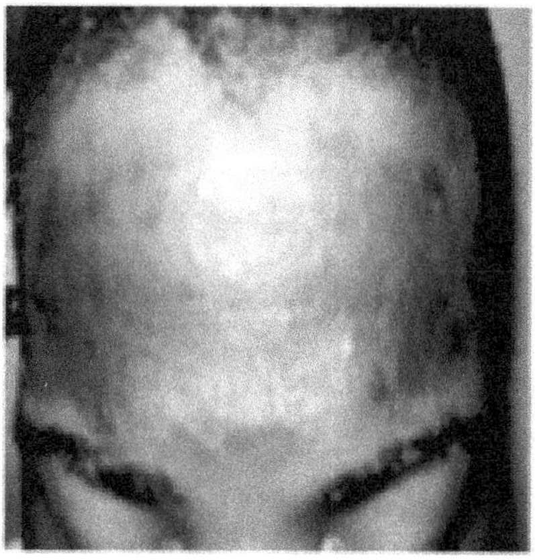

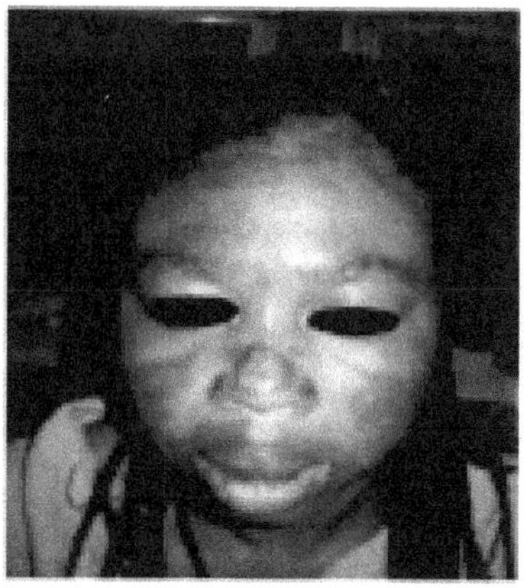

Fig 13.1 Fig 13.2

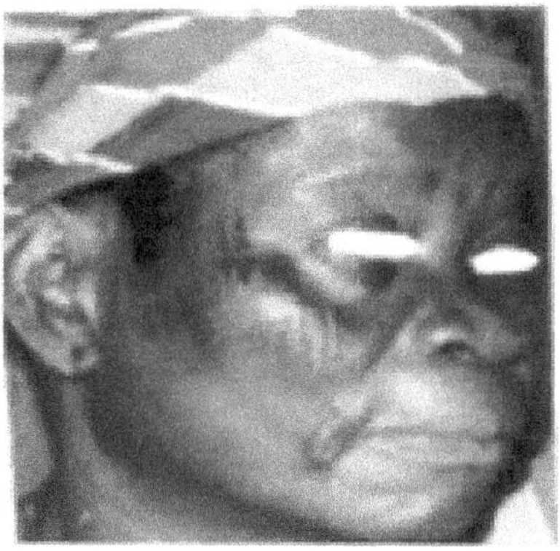

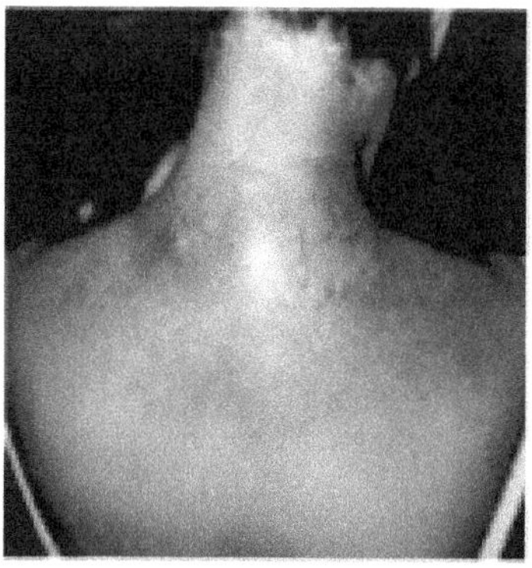

Fig 13.3 Fig 13.4

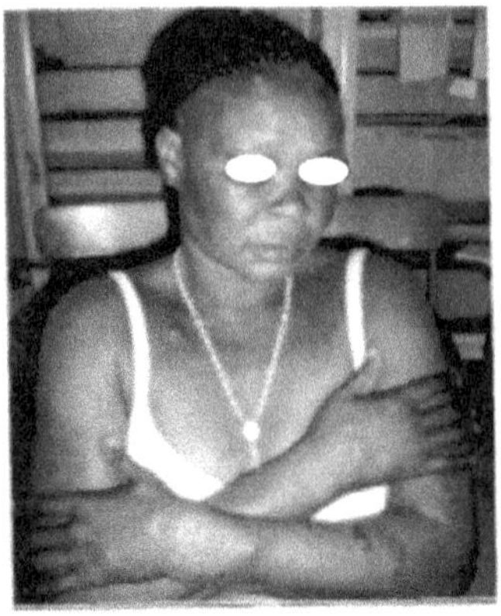

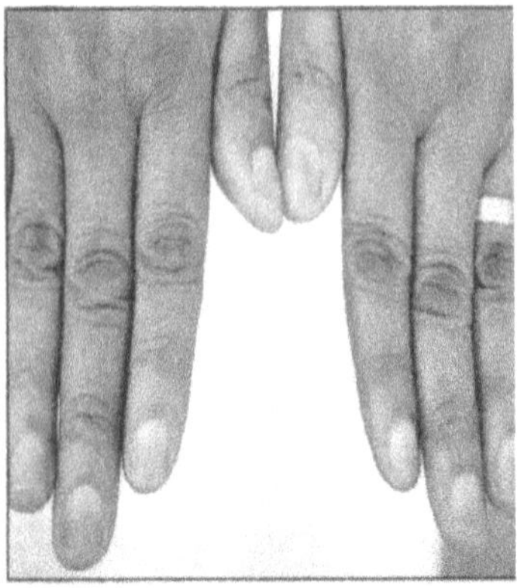

Fig 13.5 Fig 13.6

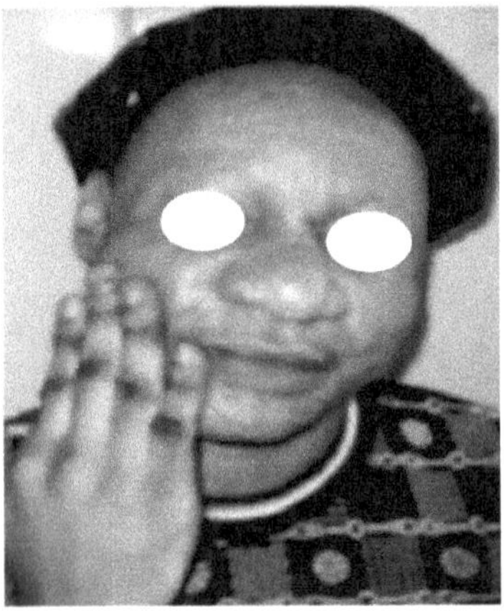

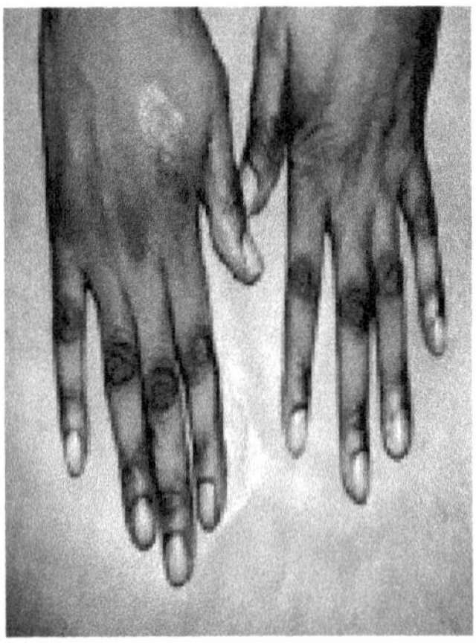

Fig 13.7 Fig 13.8

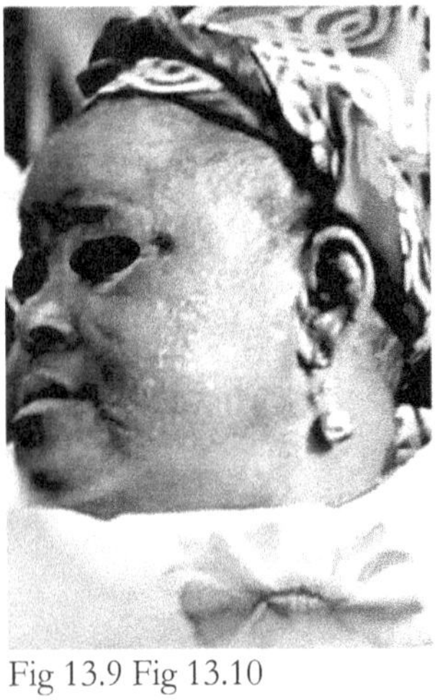

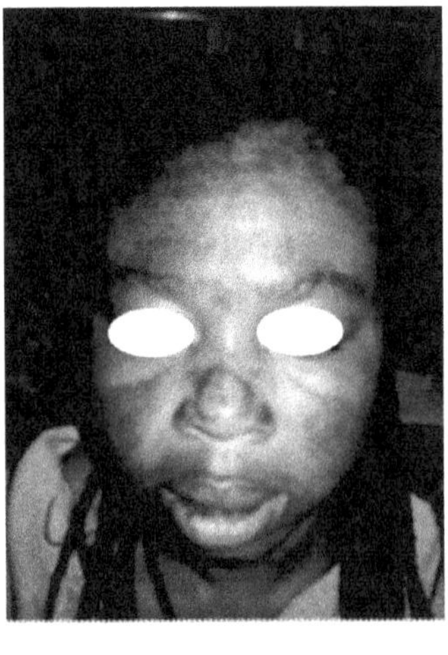

Fig 13.9 Fig 13.10

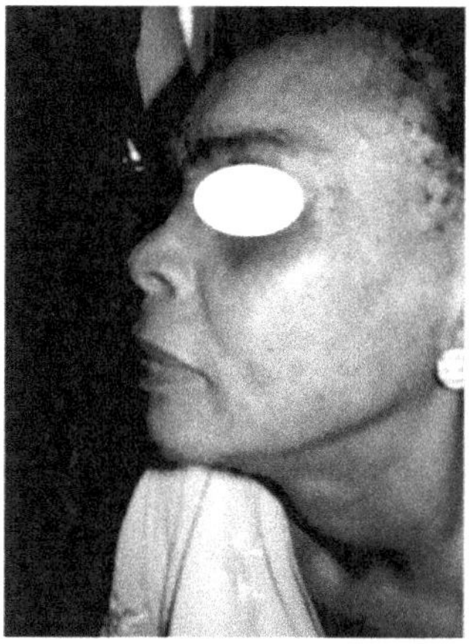
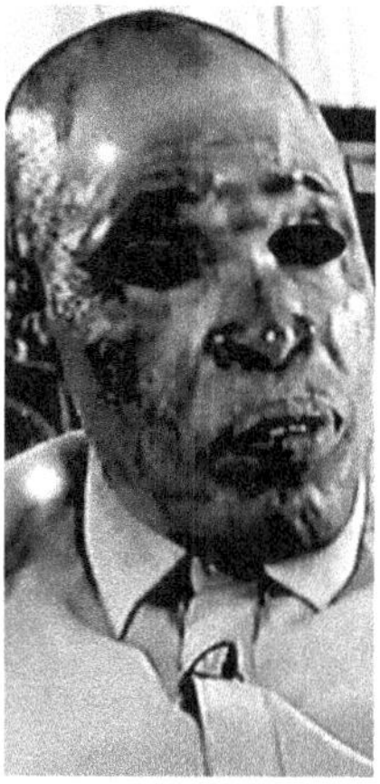

Fig 13.11 Fig 13.12

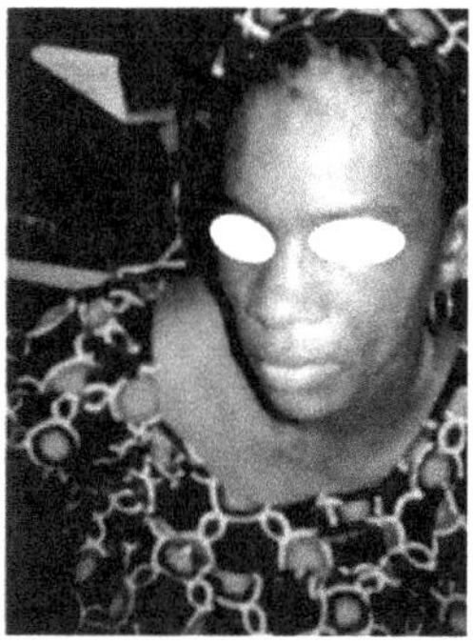
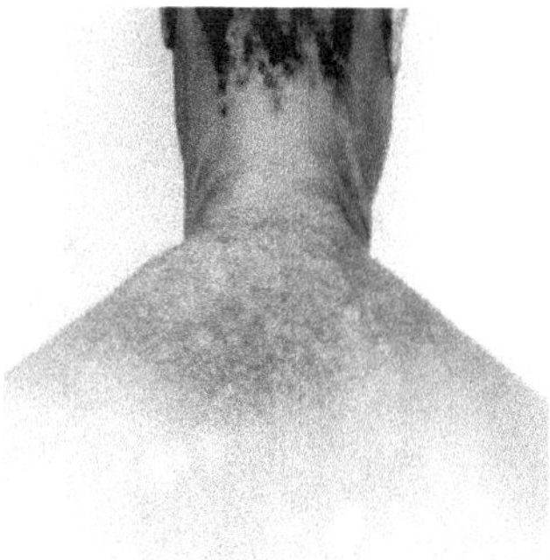

Fig 13.13 Fig 13.14

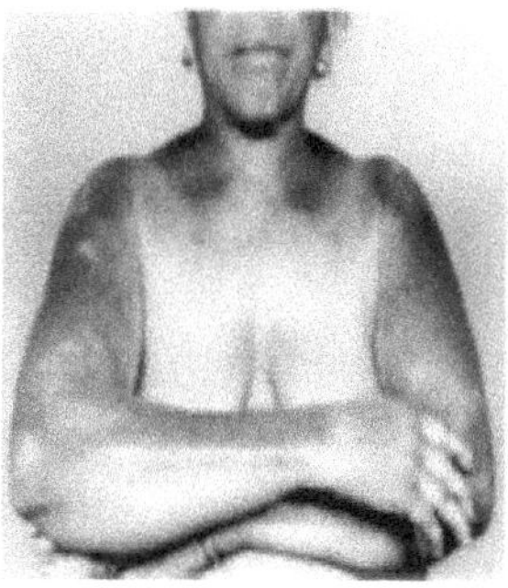
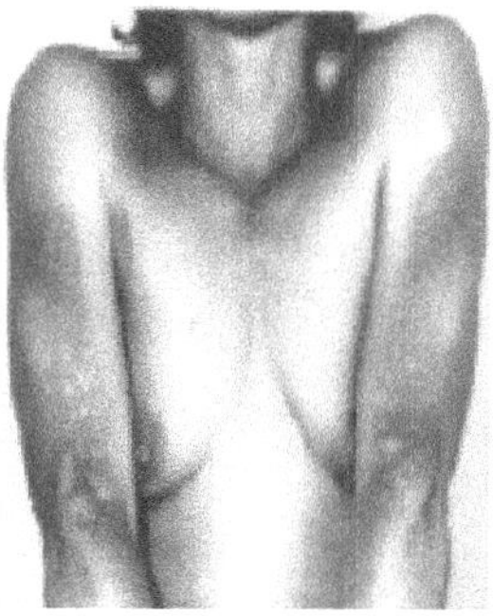

Fig 13.15 Fig 13.16

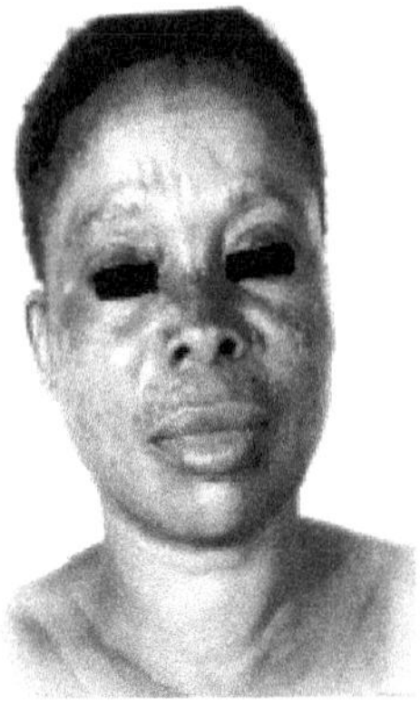
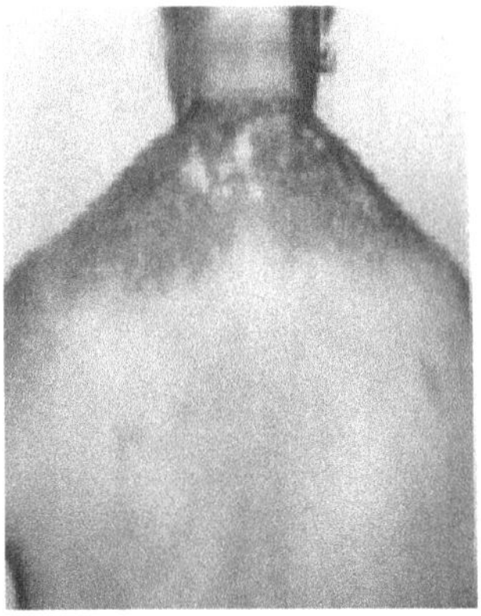

Fig 13.17 Fig 13.18

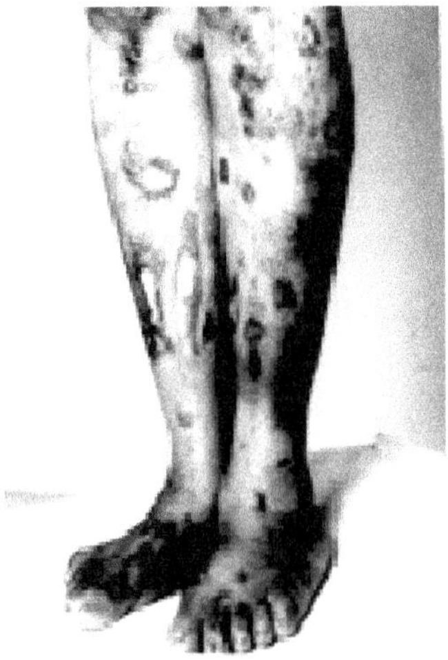
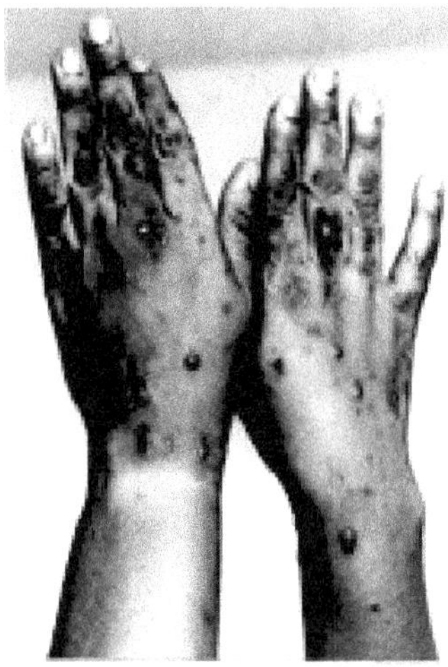

Fig 13.19 Fig 13.20

Figures 13.1-18 Hydroquinone-induced Exogenous Ochronotic Pigmentation
Note pigmented knuckles and yellow nails in figures 13.6, 7, 8
Note Fig 13.12 is a male patient
Figures 13.19, 20. Exogenous ochronosis superimposed on pruritic popular eruption in HIV/AIDS patient

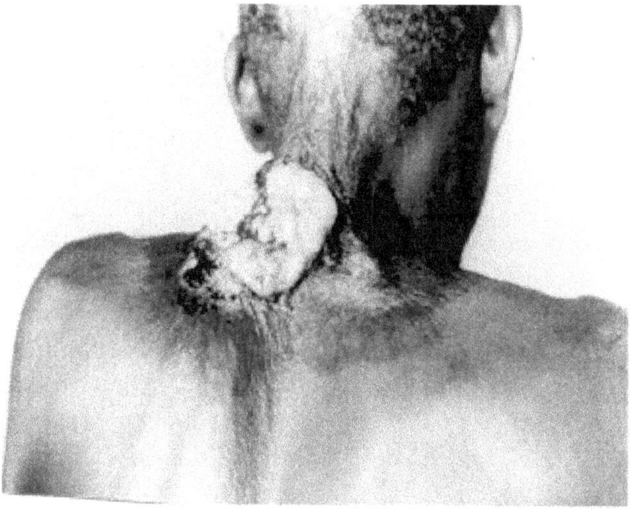

Fig 13.21 Squamous cell carcinoma on ochronotic pigmentation from hydroquinone

Hydroquinone also causes hyperchromia, presence of red cells with abnormally increased cell hemoglobin count; hypochromia, presence of cells with abnormally low cell hemoglobin content, neuropathy and diseases of the nervous system.

The fish odor syndrome

The chronic bleachers also exude an offensive fish odour in the sweat like the 'fish odour syndrome.'[8] The 'fish odour syndrome,' also known as trimethylaminuria, is characterised by body odour of rotten fish. This is due to excretion of a chemical, trimethylamine in the breath, urine, sweat, saliva, and vaginal secretions.

Trimethylamine (TMA) is produced in the gut mainly by bacterial degradation of choline and lecithin-rich foods, such as salt water fish, eggs, offals (such as intestines, liver, and kidney), and leguminous vegetables such as soya beans. Normally, this compound is converted by TMA oxidase into a stable non-odorous trimethylamine N-oxide (TMA-oxide) that is then excreted in the urine. In the presence of a defective TMA oxidase activity, the accumulated TMA is eliminated as a volatile product in the urine, sweat, and breath, giving the affected individual the characteristic fishy smell.

The TMA oxidase activity may be defective because of a congenital, inherited impairment of N-oxidation (*primary trimethylaminuria*) or for other acquired reasons that interfere with the action of the enzyme (*secondary trimethylaminurias*). Some of these causes are: (1) overload with TMA precursors, such as choline and lecithin, leading to the formation of an increased burden of TMA through enterobacterial degradation; (2) intake of inhibitors of TMA oxidase, both dietary (e.g., Brussels sprouts) and pharmacologic (e.g. thiourea), and (3) liver and kidney diseases. In all these cases, the causative agent may act rather as an inducing, precipitating factor in predisposed subjects, who are carriers of the potential defect as heterozygotes. Other causes of fish odour are bacterial vaginosis, and pemphigus vulgaris or foliaceus due to muco-cutaneous bacterial degradation of body fluids. Hydroquinone is an antioxidant, it may cause the fish odour by reducing the ability to oxidise trimethylamine in chronic bleachers, or hydroquinone may act rather as an inducing, precipitating factor in predisposed subjects, who are carriers of the potential defect as heterozygotes.

Treatment of exogenous ochronosis has been disappointing. Tretinoin gel, cryotherapy, and trichloroacetic acid have been tried without benefit. Cases of exogenous ochronosis successfully treated with dermabrasion and CO2 laser and Q-switched ruby laser have been reported.[9]

Clinical stigmatas of chronic bleachers. How to recognize the bleached skin when they deny.

The face in normal people is always darker than the other parts of the body that are covered by clothing because the face is permanently exposed to the tanning effect of the sun. However, in skin bleachers the face may be shades lighter than the arms, legs and the thighs if these parts are not bleached. The cheeks may be violetious, as if the skin is peeling. The knuckles, back of the elbows, front of the knees are dark, darker than the skin on the arm and face, which is quite fair. Skin bleachers may be so fair-skinned that the bluish green veins on the neck, arms and the backs of the legs are visible due to thinning (atrophy) of the skin from corticosteroid creams. Atimes the skin of the upper lip may be darker and hairy—the "moustache effect." The darker skin is often a sign of exogenous ochronosis from hydroquinone or the grayish pigmentation from ammoniated mercury; whilst the hairiness is a feature of steroid induced hypertrichosis (excessive hairiness). The nails also may be yellowish due to chronic use of hydroquinone; although this is often masked by the nail polish, though chronic use of nail polish may also result in yellowish tinge of the nails. Chronic bleachers also exude offensive body odor—'the fish odor syndrome.' Those who have been bleaching with steroid containing products may develop recalcitrant acne on the face, a

bloated face of cushionoid features and extensive bizarre shapes of tinea corporis—superficial fungal infections—'tinea incognito.' (See the clinical pictures on complications of bleaching products).
However, those who now bleach with high-end products such as pills, injectables and laser surgical depigmentation techniques may not have the above cutaneous stigmatas of bleaching. Nevertheless, when chronic bleachers cease to use the skin bleaching products, the face progressively repigments to a colour which is different from the pre-bleaching state—as the face acquires a sallow and, atimes, a cadaveric type of pigmentation.

The need for highly sensitive, simple, fast and economic test for hydroquinone

Manufacturers globally are aware of the ban on hydroquinone in cosmetics in most African countries, hence most packages for skin lightening products have boldly written "HYDROQUINONE FREE". Since it has been observed that this is not always true, there is need for a highly sensitive, simple and fast method to test the products Uddin *et al*[10] have established a method which is claimed to meet such requirements. The spectrophotometric method is based on using ammonium meta-vanadate as an oxidizing catalyst for conversion of hydroquinone to p-benzoquinone (BQ) in the presence of oxygen. As a result of higher absorption of UV light by BQ than by HQ, its signal has been utilized for determining HQ at the trace level.

The researchers claimed that the newly developed method has been successfully applied to diluted samples of various skin lightening creams for free HQ determination at the trace level. Comparing the results obtained by the proposed method with those by a previously reported method proved its validity.

A dip-stick method of testing for hydroquinone and mercury is necessary for use by consumers who may wish to verify the contents of a cosmetic product before use. As have been observed by Sylvia Arthur in Ghana,[11] it is becoming increasingly difficult to get safe non bleaching cosmetics and toiletries even for babies.

Other names for Hydroquinone

It is critical to note that, because the use of Hydroquinone in cosmetics has been banned in several countries, other names are often used on the ingredient labeling to camouflage the identity of the ingredient. Hence, other names for hydroquinone like Quinol, Tequinol, Benzene-1,4-diol, Idrochinone, 1-4 dihydroxy benzene, 1,4 hydroxy benzene, 1,4-Benzenediol, p-Diphenol, Hydrochinone, p-hydroxylphenol, Hydrochinonium, and Hydroquinol may be used.

References

1. Jackyk WK. Annular granulomatous lesions in exogenous ochronosis are manifestations of sarcoidosis. *Am J Dermatopathol* 1995:17:18-22.

2. Zannoni VG, Lomtevas N, Goldfinger S, *et al.* Oxidation of homogentisic and to ochronotic pigment in connective tissue. *Biochem Biophys Acta* 1979; 177:94.

3. Olumide YM, Elesha SO. Hydroquinone induced exogenous ochronosis *Nig Med Pract* 1986; 11: 103-6

4. Tidman MJ, Horton JJ, Macdonald DM *et al* Hydroquinone-induced ochronosis: Light and electron-microscopic features. *Clin Exp Dermatol* 1986:11:224.

5. Tidman MJ, Horton JJ, MacDonald DM. Hydroquinone-induced ochronosis—light and electron-microscopic features. *Clin Exp Dermatol* 1986;11:224-8.

6. Dogliotte M, Liebowitz M. Granulomatous ochronosis – a cosmetic-induced skin disorder in blacks. *S Afr Med J* 1979; 56:757-60

7. Olumide YM, Akinkugbe AO *et al.* Complications of chronic use of skin lightening cosmetics. *Int J Dermatol* 2008; 47:344-

8. Ruocco V, Florio M. Fish-odor syndrome: an olfactory diagnosis. *Int J Dermatol* 1995; 34:92-3.

9. Diven DG, Smith EB, Pupo RA, Lee M. Hydroquinone-induced localized exogenous ochronosis treated with dermabrasion and CO2 laser. *J Dermatol Surg Oncol* 1990;16:1018-22.

10. Uddin S, Rauf A, Kazi TG, Afridi TG, Afridi HI, Lutfullah G: Highly sensitive spectrometric method for determination of hydroquinone in skin lightening creams: application in cosmetics. Int J Cosmetic Sci, 2011 Apr; 33(2); 132-7.

11. Sylvia Arthur. The New Skin Bleaching Phenomenon. http://www.ghanaweb.com/GhanaHomePage/NewsArchive/artikel.php?ID=22240

CORTICOSTEROIDS

Topical corticosteroids TCs are subdivided according to strength (Class I–VII), with class I (i.e. clobetasol) being the most potent and class VII (i.e. hydrocortisone) the least potent.[1] The strength of TCs is determined by the vasoconstriction assay, in which potency is associated with the degree of blood vessel blanching in the upper dermis.[1,2] TCs have long been used for their skin lightening properties and are often the most commonly used skin lighteners in Africa.[3,4] TCs are believed to bleach the skin through inhibiting pro-opiomelanocortin (POMC), the precursor protein for α-melanocyte-stimulating hormone (α-MSH), which is produced in the intermediate lobe of the pituitary to stimulate epidermal melanin production.[5]

References

1. Levin C, and Maibach HI. Topical corticosteroid-induced adrenocortical insufficiency: clinical implications. *Am J Clin Dermatol.* 2002; 3: 141–7

2. McKenzie AW, and Stoughton RB. Method for comparing percutaneous absorption of steroids. *Arch Dermatol.* 1962; 86: 608–10

3. Wone I, Tal-Dia A, Diallo OF. et al. Prevalence of the use of skin bleaching cosmetics in two areas in Dakar (Senegal). *Dakar Med.* 2000; 45: 154–7 ([in French])

4. Mahe A, Ly F, Aymard G. et al. Skin diseases associated with the cosmetic use of bleaching products in women from Dakar, Senegal. *Br J Dermatol.* 2003; 148: 493–500

5. Olumide YM., Akinkugbe AO, Altraide D. et al. Complications of chronic use of skin lightening cosmetics. *Int J Dermatol.* 2008; 47: 344–53

Corticosteroids as a skin bleaching agents

Corticosteroids are *de facto* drugs, not cosmetic products. Corticosteroids constitute an ideal treatment for various inflammatory and autoimmune disorders due to their anti-inflammatory and immunomodulatory actions. One of the side effects of topical corticosteroids is bleaching of the skin hence people began to use it as a skin-lightening agent when they discovered its skin-lightening effect. People are often initiated into the use of corticosteroids as bleaching agents when they use it to treat acne on the face. Because of its anti-inflammatory effect, the acne improves, but when an attempt is made to stop the use of the drug, there is a flare-up of the acne lesion – a rebound phenomenon. This rebound phenomenon can only be treated by the recommencement of the corticosteroids treatment. This eventually leads to chronic use of corticosteroid cream. Hence chronic use leads to local complications on the skin and since corticosteroids are absorbed through the skin, more serious systemic complications like hypertension, diabetes and the deadly suppression of the hypothalamic pituitary-adrenal (HPA) axis ensue.

Fluorinated corticoids e.g Fluocinonide (Topsyn gel), Betamethasone dipropionate (Diprosone), and Clobetasol propionate (Temovate) rate as some of the strongest topical corticoids, and are among the commonly used bleaching agents in Nigeria. They are readily available in the market place among the battery of bleaching creams. Fluorinated corticosteroids are highly potent drugs that are normally available only on prescription in Europe, US, Canada and other developed countries. However in Nigeria and most parts of Africa, they are readily available as over-the-counter drugs-induced 'cosmetics'. They are often sold as cosmetic products in nonmedical stores without warning about adverse effects or contraindications. Indeed several years ago when the major transnational companies manufactured them in Nigeria, market women and other traders were among their distributors. When used as cosmetics, they are applied over a large surface area for prolonged periods—several months to years. This factor, coupled with the occlusive effect of the tropical environmental heat and humidity, promote percutaneous absorption, and hence, complications.

Mode of action of corticosteroid as a skin bleaching agent

Corticosteroids bleach the skin. It is believed that they lighten the skin due to inhibition of endogenous steroid production and thus a decrease in precursor hormone levels. This precursor hormone, propiocortin is also the precursor for melanocyte stimulating hormone and thus, such negative feedback will lead to decreased amounts of the hormone. Topical steroids are also cytostatic to the epidermis. When used over a prolonged period, they decrease the rate of epidermal turnover, with fewer, abnormal, and less pigmented melanocytes on histology. The skin lightening properties of these preparations have been found to be directly proportional to their vasoconstrictor (blanching) effect.[1]

Complications of chronic corticosteroid use

Corticosteroids constitute an ideal treatment for various inflammatory and autoimmune disorders due to their anti-inflammatory and immune modulatory actions. However, corticosteroids have a considerable number of side effects, including hypertension, diabetes, lipid disorders, sleep apnea, osteoporosis, myopathy, and disorders of coagulation and fibrinolysis, which are components of Cushings syndrome(CS)[2,3]

Corticosteroid-induced side effects are dependent on the formulation, route, dose, and time of exposure. However, the underlying pathogenetic mechanisms have not been clearly defined. A large body of evidence supports the role of an imbalance between vasoconstriction and vasodilatation with possible links to nitric oxide, prostanoids, angiotensin II, arginine vasopressin, endothelins, catecholamines, neuropeptide Y, and atrial natriuretic peptide. Increased oxidative stress, rennin-angiotensin system activation, increased pressor response, metabolic syndrome, and sleep apnea appear to be pathogenetically involved as well.

Although TCs are frequently used as skin lightening agents,[1, 2] they are associated with multiple dermatologic and systemic side effects.[3,4,5,6,7] Common cutaneous complications associated with TC application include acne vulgaris,[2,5,7] allergic contact dermatitis,[2,8,9] skin atrophy,[10,11,12] perioral dermatitis,[12] hypertrichosis,[5,7] rosacea,[4,5] striae atrophica[2,5,7,11] and telangiectasias.[7,10] The skin on the neck seems particularly prone to atrophy, sometimes producing a rippled, "plucked chicken" appearance, otherwise known as *pseudo-pseudoxanthoma* elasticum.[4] Chronic periocular TC use can cause ophthalmologic complications, such as cataracts and glaucoma.[4] TC users are also particularly prone to developing infections such as cellulitis,[4] dermatophytosis,[2,5,7] erysipelas,[4,5] folliculitis,[4] and scabies.[2,5] Dermatophyte infections are especially common[4] and include tinea incognito,[4] widespread tinea corporis[4] and tinea faciei, which can mimic roseacea[7] or lupus erythematosus.[14,15] Furthermore, chronic users are more likely to develop viral warts,[5] which tend to appear simultaneously on the neck and upper trunk, a finding that Olumide and colleagues[4] nicknamed the "*pseudo Leser-Trélat* sign."

TC use is also associated with various systemic complications such as hypothalamic-pituitary-adrenal (HPA) axis suppression, Cushing syndrome,[5,16,17] diabetes mellitus,[7] and hypertension.[18] The most worrisome of these complications is HPA dysfunction causing adrenal insufficiency,[19,16,20,21] which can be life-threatening. Adrenal suppression has long been regarded as a complication of high-dose TCs (i.e. >50 g/wk of clobetasol propionate), but patients taking low doses (i.e. 7.5 g/wk) have also experienced adrenal suppression.[22] In 2001, Perret and colleagues[23] assessed the functionality of the HPA axis among decade-long TC users in Sénégal and reported significantly lower plasma cortisol levels in response to cosyntropin stimulation compared with controls.

Another potential adverse effect from chronic daily use of a potent TC is "steroid addiction syndrome," which is characterized by intense burning and potentially permanent erythema due to withdrawal vasodilatation.[4] The irreversible form of pronounced erythema, often referred to as *homme rouge*, occurs more commonly in male users.[4]

Other less-common reactions reported with TC use include avascular necrosis of the femoral head[24] and squamous cell carcinoma.[25,26] Additionally, chronic use of TCs may mask other pathologic conditions, as was observed in a patient with leprosy.[27] The risk of these adverse reactions is potentiated when high-potency formulations are used on sites with fragile, thin skin (i.e. face, armpit, groin) for prolonged periods or under occlusion, which promotes penetration.[19,4] Individuals particularly at risk for developing adrenal suppression include infants and patients with damaged skin barriers.[19] A list of the complications is in Table 13.1

Clinical manifestations

Local complications of corticosteroids that manifest on the skin

The local cutaneous manifestations of the complications of chronic steroid use are steroid folliculitis, severe acneiform eruption, striae steroid addiction syndrome, predisposition to infections – fungal, bacterial, and viral, and allergic contact dermatitis.

Table 13.3 Complications of topical corticosteroids

Cutaneous

Atrophy of the skin (thinning and fine wrinkling)
Telangiectasia, purpura, persistent erythema
Skin fragility
Hypertrichosis
Perioral dermatitis
Pustular acneiform eruption (face)—steroid rosacea
Folliculitis
Striae
Hypopigmentation
Steroid addiction syndrome
Predisposition and masking of cutaneous infection
(e.g. Tinea incognito, multiple filiform warts)
Allergic contact dermatitis

Ophthalmologic

Glaucoma
Cataracts

Endocrinologic

Cushingoid syndrome with moon facies, buffalo
humps, supraclavicular fat pads
Hyperglycaemia and diabetes mellitus
Suppression of hypothalamic-pituitary-adrenal axis
Suppression of growth in children
Menstrual irregularities
Oedema
Electrolyte imbalance
Hypertension
Pseudotumor cerebri

Others

Aseptic necrosis of the head of femur
Predisposition to infection
Protein catabolism with negative nitrogen balance
Weakness, vertigo
Thrombophlebitis
Osteoporosis

Figures 13.22-48 show some of the complications of long-term use of topical corticosteroids as skin lightening cosmetics. The lower part of the axilla is a favored site for steroid folliculitis (Fig. 13.22) and both sides are usually symmetrically affected. Figures 13.23, 24 show steroid induced folliculitis and Figures 13.25-28 show steroid-induced acne on a background of bleached skin. Steroid-induced striae (stretch marks) (Figures 13.30, 34-36) are often erythematous and wide-gaping. Striae often accompany Cushing's syndrome. Overt features of Cushing's syndrome — 'mooning' of the face and truncal obesity (Figures13.29, 31, 34 & 36) are frequently seen. Some of them, at the time of presentation, have already developed systemic manifestations like glucose intolerance and hypertension.

Legends of all the pictures are on page 605.

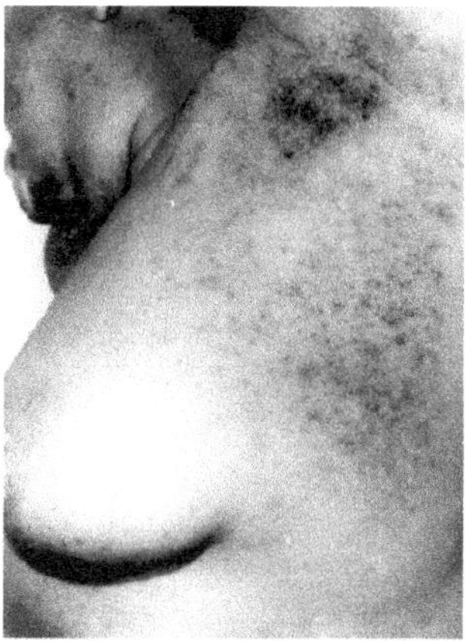

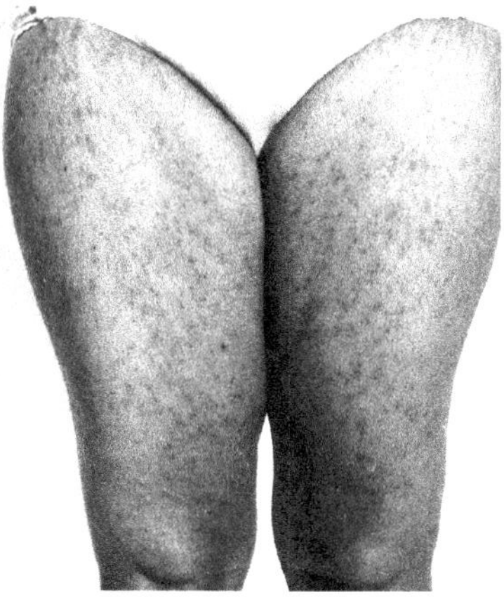

Fig 13.22 Fig 13.23

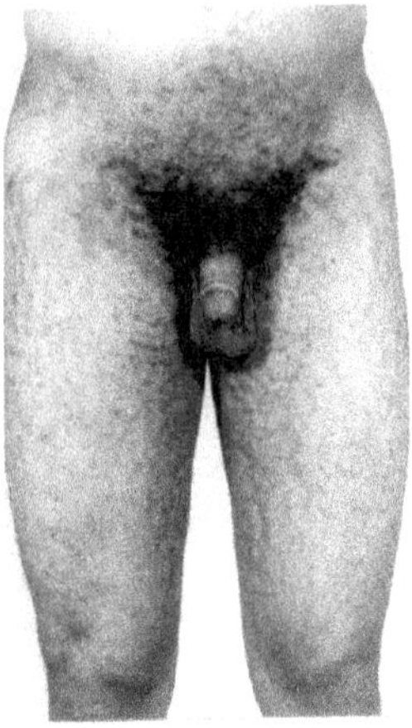
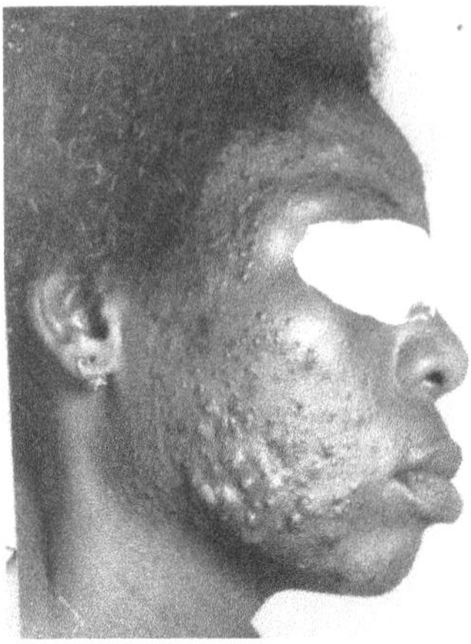

Fig 13.24 Fig 13.25

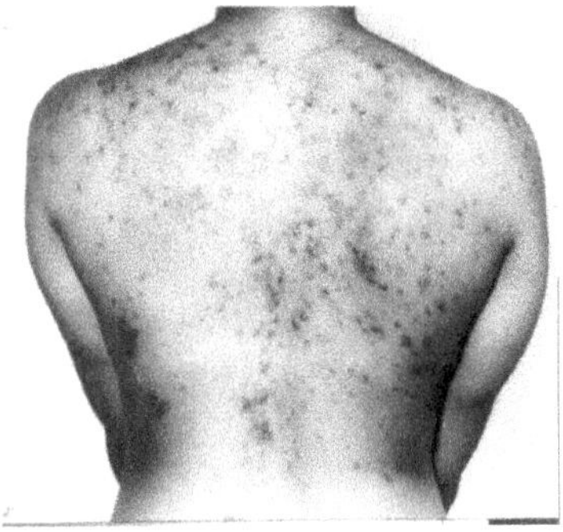
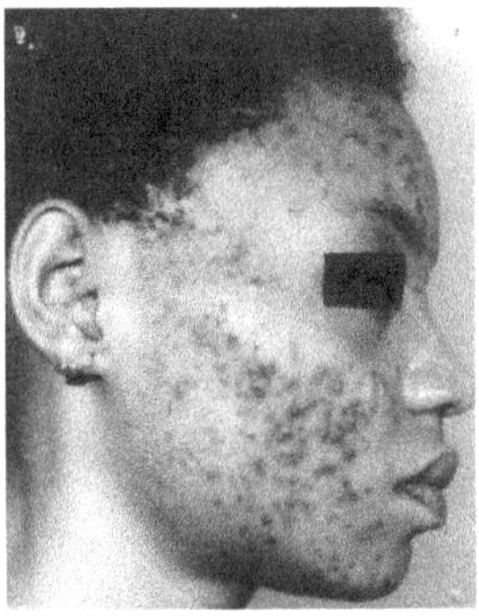

Fig 13.26 Fig 13.27

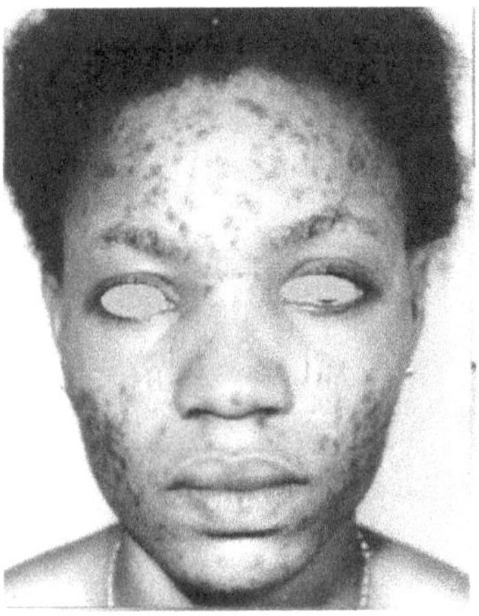
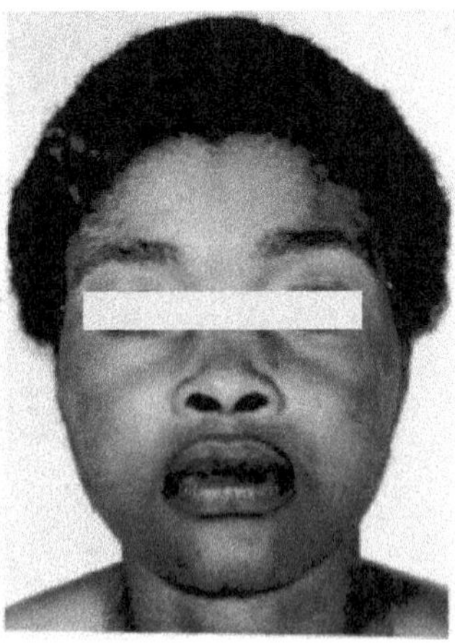

Fig 13.28 Fig 13.29

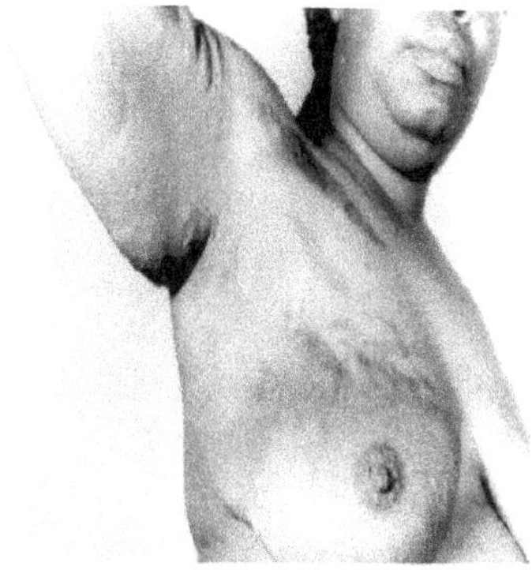
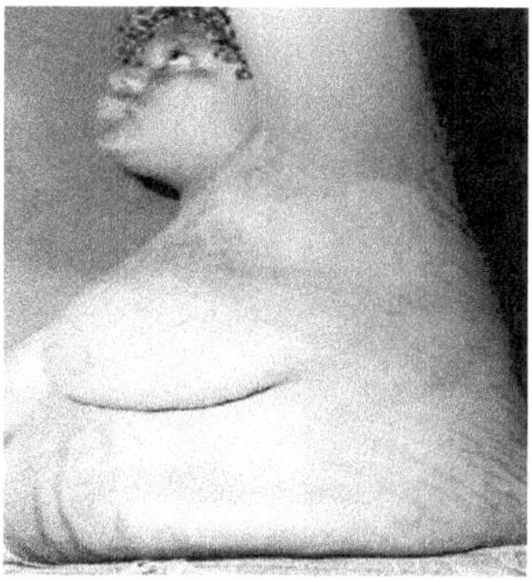

Fig 13.30 Fig 13.31

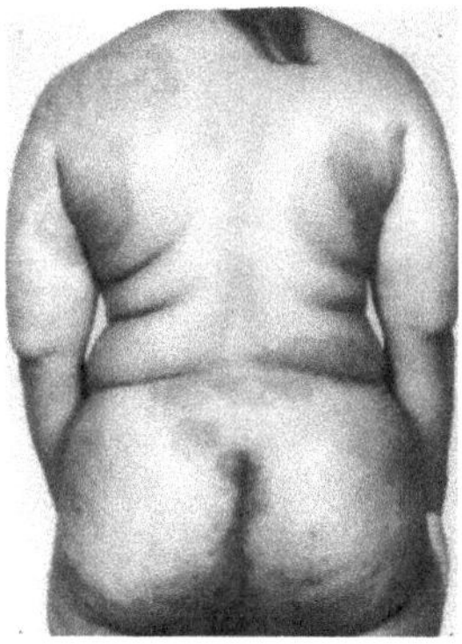
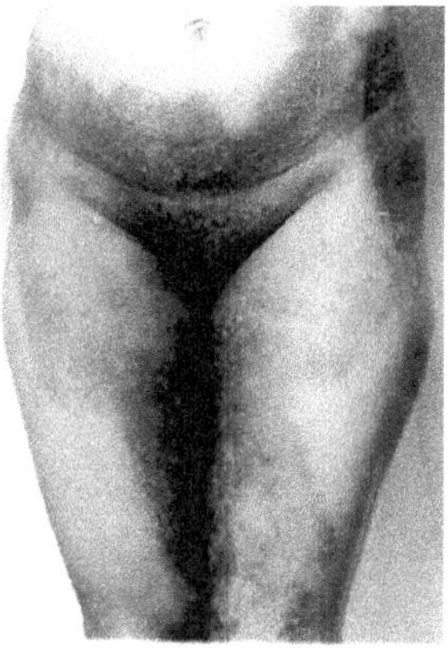

Fig 13.32 Fig 13.33

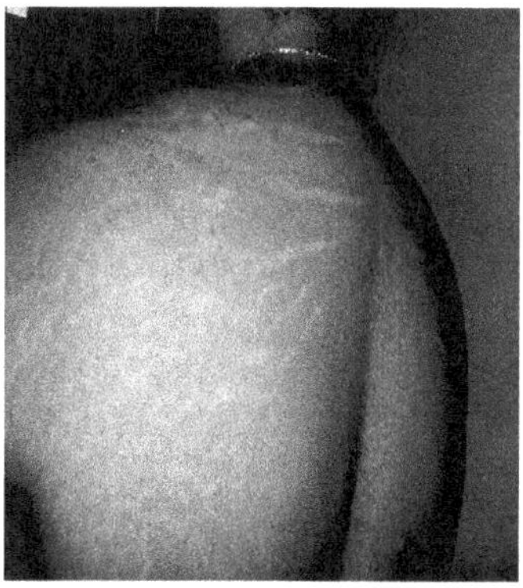
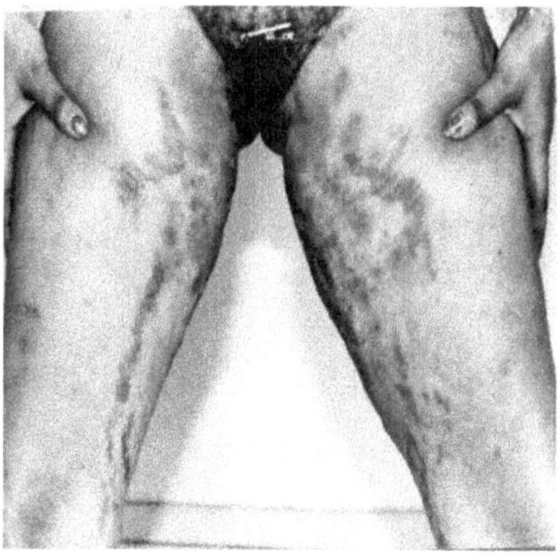

Fig 13.34 Fig 13.35

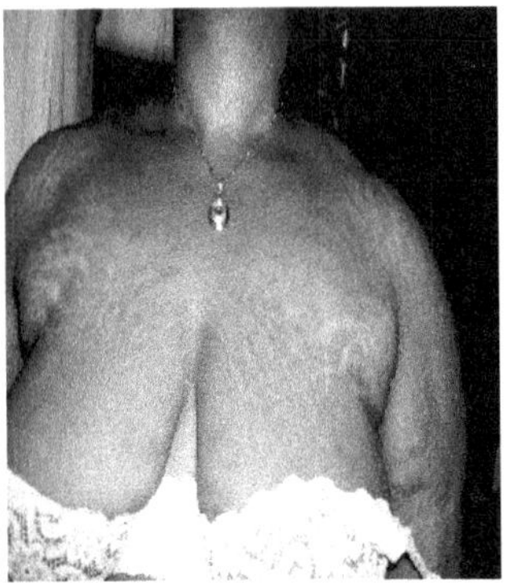
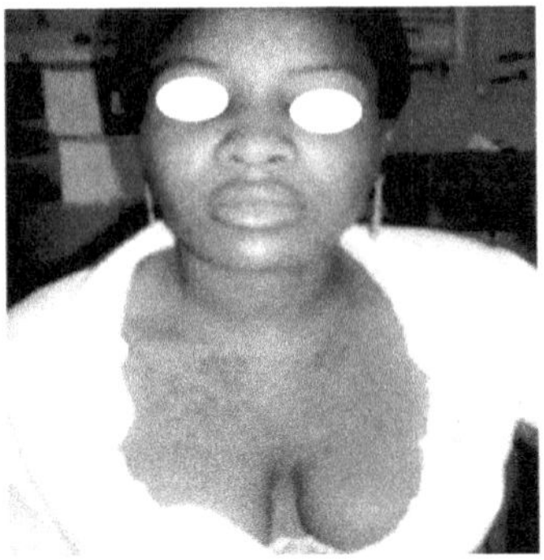

Fig 13.36 Fig 13.37

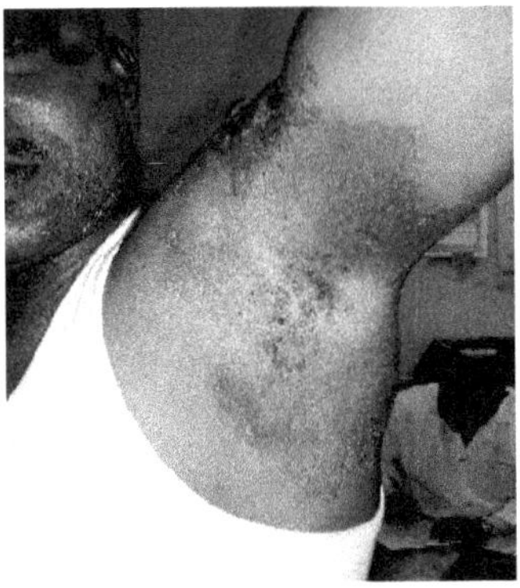
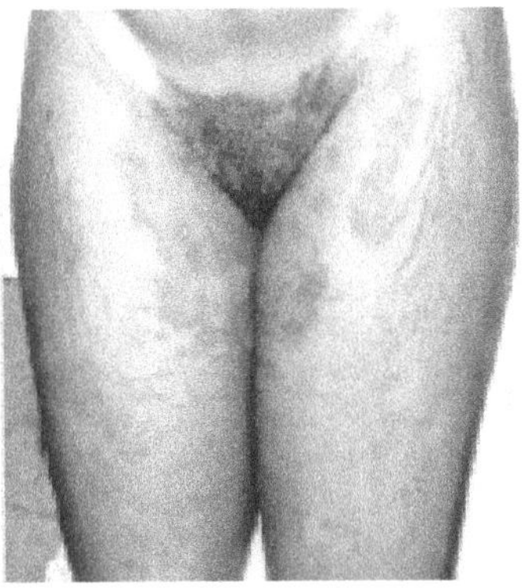

Fig 13.38 Fig 13.39

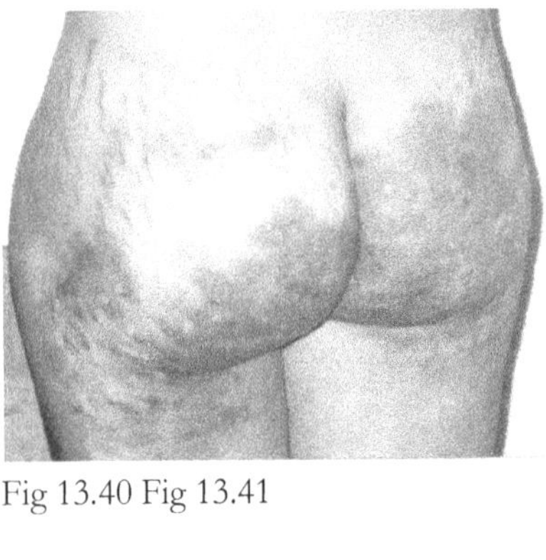
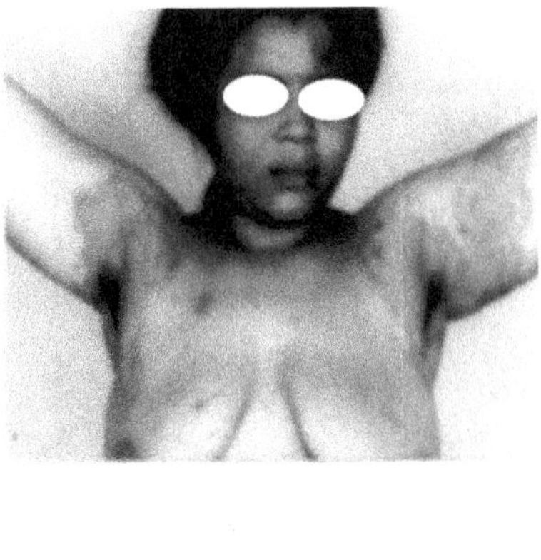

Fig 13.40 Fig 13.41

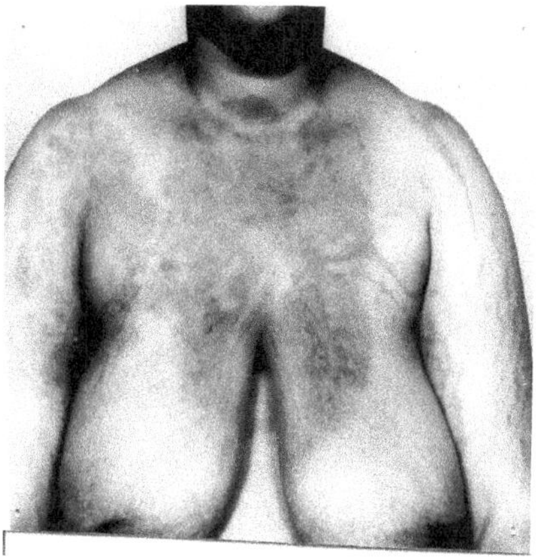
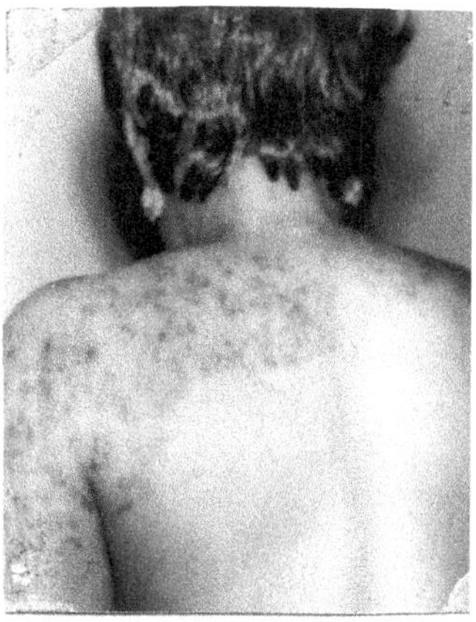

Fig 13.42 Fig 13.43

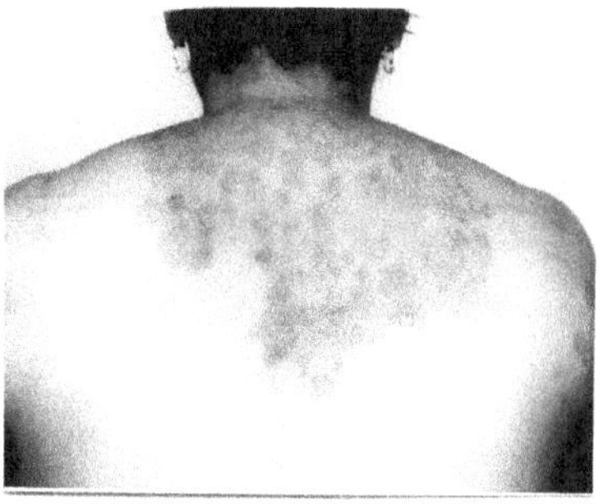
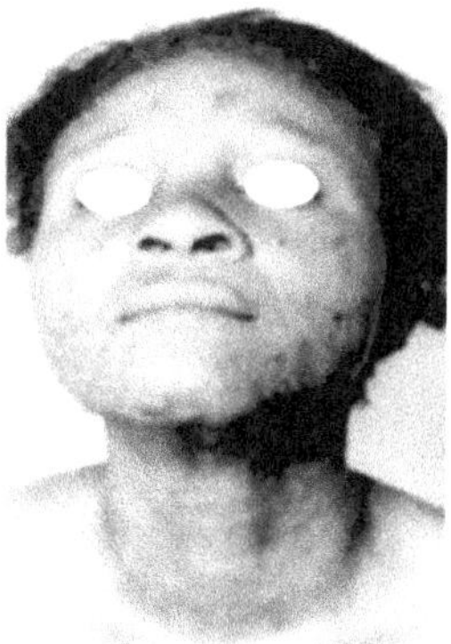

Fig 13.44 Fig 13.45

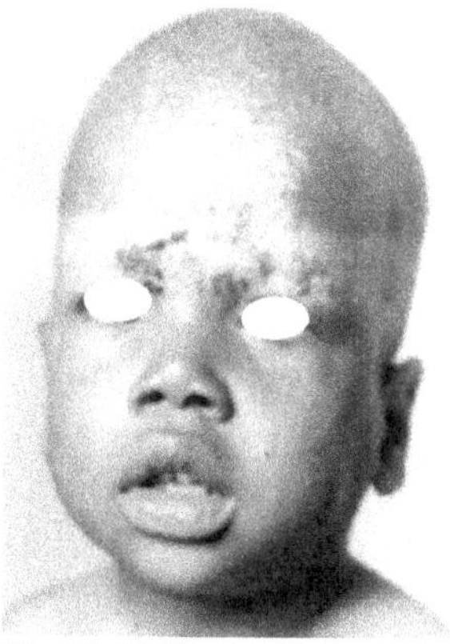
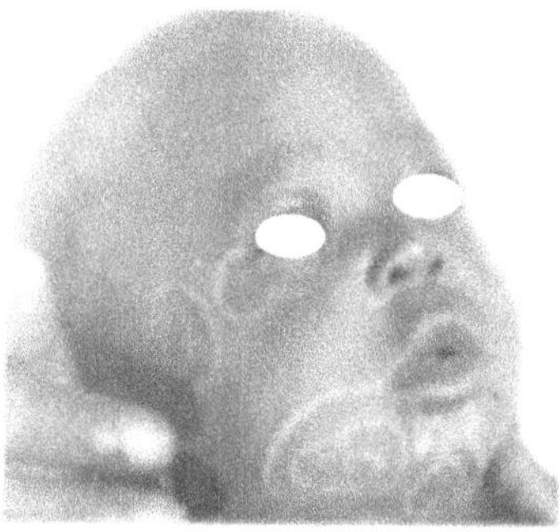

Fig 13.46 Fig 13.47

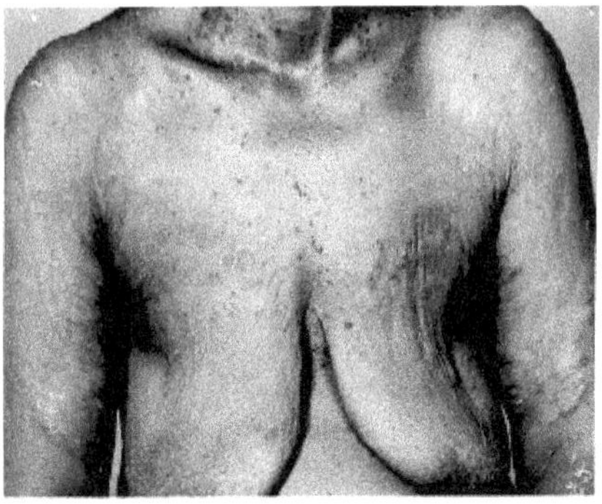

Figs 13.22-24, 37 Corticosteroid-induced folliculitis
Figs 13.25-28, Corticosteroid-induced Acne
Figs 13.29-31, Corticosteroid-induced Cushinoid features and striae
Figs 13.32, 33, 38-44 Corticosteroid-induced Tinea incognito
Figs 13.34,35,36 Corticosteroid-induced Striae
Fig 13.45 Corticosteroid-induced Tinea facies and "*Pseudo*-pseudo xanthoma elasticum" on the neck
Figure 13.46 & 47 Corticosteroid-induced fungal infections on babies acquired from the skin of mothers while breast-feeding
Fig 13.48 Corticosteroid-induced striae and eruptive filiform warts ("*Pseudo* Lesser Trélat sign")

Steroid addiction syndrome

The steroid addiction syndrome is the result of chronic daily application for greater than a month or more period of the application of a potent or moderately potent glucocorticosteroid preparation to the facial skin, neck, scrotum or vulva. These tissues become "addicted" to the topical steroid, so that withdrawing the topical steroid results in severe burning which is only relieved by further steroid applications. As application continues, the patient experiences a rebound vasodilatation. Permanent redness of the facial skin eventuates, with thinning and fine wrinkling of the skin. Indeed the redness is so striking that in our clinic we call the phenomenon "L'homme rouge." For unexplainable reason, this permanent redness is more pronounced on male bleachers. Furthermore, the thinning and wrinkling of the skin on the neck gives a rippling pattern like the neck of a plucked chicken, rather reminiscent of pseudoxanthoma elasticum—hence, in our clinic we call this complication of steroid "*pseudo*-pseudoxanthoma elasticum."(Figure 13.45). Some bleachers claim that they developed the habit of chronic steroid use while trying to treat acne. They experienced good response initially due to the anti-inflammatory effect of the steroids. Abruptly stopping the topical steroids preparation will result in increased numbers of papules and pustules over the subsequent days—a "rebound phenomenon." The patient soon finds it difficult to stop the steroid and the facial skin then develops persistent redness, and acneiform papules and pustules located on the nose, chin, cheeks, and lower eyelids—acne rosacea. Steroid induced acne usually occurs on a background of bleached skin or associated with hypertrichosis (Fig 13.29) or Cushing's syndrome (Fig 13.31).

Predisposition to infections

A very common observed complication of steroid on chronic bleachers is dermatophyte infection. Tinea faciei (Fig. 13.45) is common in these patients and may mimic cutaneous lupus erythematosus or rosacea. Very bizarre and extensive Tinea corposis and cruris (Figures 13.32, 33, 38-47) are often seen, which are readily transmitted to the spouse and baby. Hence, it is common to find the trio of wife, husband and baby with Tinea incognito. Older children are not part of this phenomenon. The wife often transmits the fungal infection to husband and baby because of close body contact. Figures 13.46 & 47 show children with Tinea incognito on the face, acquired from the infected skin of the mother while feeding on her breast. Steroid induced fungal infections are often extensive, involve unusual sites with bizarre configurations and atypical, hence they are called Tinea incognito because the diagnosis may be missed due to the atypical nature of the lesions. The patients with Tinea incognito usually have additional striae. Tinea versicolor could also be very extensive, and is usually pigmented with dirty brown scales.

Also, multiple histologically proven viral warts are frequently found on these chronic bleachers. They often appear in an eruptive manner—rather reminiscent of eruptive seborrheic keratosis (*Leser-Trélat sign*). Hence in our clinic we call this complication "*pseudo*-Leser-Trelat sign." They are multiple tiny filiform warts, common on the neck and upper trunk (Fig. 13.48).[4] Observations have also been documented on camouflaging of cases of leprosy due to skin bleaching[27]

Paradoxically, topical corticosteroid preparations may induce allergic contact dermatitis.[9] This complication should be considered in any patient with an eczematous dermatitis who becomes worse or is refractory to topical steroid treatment.[8]

Endocrinopathies complicating corticosteroids in topical bleaching agents[16-23]

Case studies

i. A Senegalese cohort study of 147 women showed a statistically significant increase in the risk of hypertension and diabetes linked to the use of skin-lightening agent[23]

ii. A middle-aged Nigerian lady was brought home to die a few years ago from a Western European country because she developed an uncontrollable diabetes mellitus and evidence of hypothalamic-pituitary-adrenal axis suppression.[4] On clinical examination, the lady had dense stigmatas of chronic use of skin lightening creams, which was confirmed through history. She died in the emergency room before detailed laboratory investigations could be done. Majority of medical practitioners outside Sub-Saharan Africa may not be familiar with this habit of bleaching the skin nor the cutaneous and extra-cutaneous complications of this widespread cosmetic habit of black Africans. Furthermore, these cosmetics and toiletries are not sold in the regular departmental stores nor pharmacy shops in Europe and North America. They are either manufactured purely for export to Africa or are exported from Africa to Europe and N. America so that they are sold only in local shops in ghettoes patronized by the black Africans. The paper sets out to give a brief review of this problem so that practitioners worldwide would be aware of these complications which may atimes be fatal.

iii. Endocrinopathy consistent with adrenal insufficiency in the setting of Cushing's syndrome secondary to corticosteroids used as bleaching agent was also reported in an African immigrant in Canada·[28] Systemic absorption of a noncortisol steroid would suppress the hypothalamic adrenal axis, resulting in low corticotrophin and cortisol levels.

The 46-year-old African immigrant woman who had been living in Canada for only 1 year presented to the emergency department with a several-day history of weakness, polyuria, polydipsia, and new-onset hyperglycemia (blood glucose level of 41.1 mmol/L. Her past medical history includes a 6-year positive HIV status, and she was receiving highly active antiretroviral treatment at the time of admission. Other past medical history included pulmonary tuberculosis, hepatitis C, pancreatitis secondary to isoniazid therapy, and ovarian abscess. There was no family history of diabetes mellitus or other endocrinologic disorders.

The patient reported a 5-kg weight loss in recent weeks and complained of fatigue, generalized weakness, and blurred vision without diplopia. She had a difficulty climbing stairs and standing from a seated position for month to years (symptoms of proximal muscle weakness—steroid myopathy). Further questioning elicited a history of easy bruising and oligomenorrhea. The patient denied observing a darkening of her skin tone; rather she said that her skin had become lighter secondary to a bleaching creams she had been using for several years. Upon arriving in Canada she had changed brands of bleaching product. She showed pictures taken at the time of her arrival in Canada in which her skin colour was considerably lighter than at presentation.

On examination, the patient was obese, with supraclavicular and dorsal-cervical fat fullness. Her blood pressure was 100/75mm Hg. and her pulse rate was 86 beats/min. She had all relevant endocrinologic laboratory tests including dynamic testing with 250μg of cosyntropin. The results reflected adrenal gland reduced cortisol reserve.

The diagnosis of exogenous Cushing syndrome was made. She discontinued the bleaching cream and was started on a tapering dose of hydrocortisone, as well as insulin for management of hyperglycemia. Imaging was undertaken to rule out an adrenal tumour, which had negative findings.

Follow-up blood tests completed 2 months after discontinuation of the bleaching cream demonstrated normalized corticotropin and cortisol levels. She was able to use half the original dose of Insulin to control the hyperglycemia. Later follow-up blood tests, however, showed cyclical low corticotrophin and morning cortisol levels, which is postulated to be due to the patient's difficulty in discontinuing use of bleaching products for physiologic (steroid addiction syndrome) as well as psychosocial reasons.

The findings of HIV seropostivity and tuberculosis in this patient is noteworthy. This has also been the observation of Olumide *et al* [4] because bleaching of the skin is highly prevalent among commercial sex workers (see chapter 4 on NIGERIA); and tuberculosis is a very common opportunistic' infection in HIV/AIDS patients. The occupation of the patient is not stated; she may have branded herself "a fashion designer"— as commercial sex workers usually code themselves in Nigeria.

One of the key points in this study as stated by the authors is:
"Most medical practitioners outside of Africa are unaware of the widespread use of skin-bleaching products. Physicians need to be aware that patients of African descent might be using these treatments to lighten their skin tone".

Olumide *et al*[4] also state:

"This paper sets out to give a brief review of this problem so that practitioners worldwide would be aware of these complications which may at times be fatal"

iv. Another case of endocrinopathy in an immigrant was reported in the UK. Read the case report of Gina in the relevant section titled "Toxic creams for sales as thousands seek whiter skin" by Antony Barnett and Zoe Smith. (See chapter 15 on UK).

References

1. Wone I, Tal-Dia A, Diallo OF. et al. Prevalence of the use of skin bleaching cosmetics in two areas in Dakar (Senegal). *Dakar Med.* 2000; 45: 154–157 ([in French])
2. Mahe A, Ly F, Aymard G. et al. Skin diseases associated with the cosmetic use of bleaching products in women from Dakar, Senegal. *Br J Dermatol.* 2003; 148: 493–50
3. Dadzie OE and Petit A. Skin bleaching: highlighting the misuse of cutaneous depigmenting agents. *J Eur Acad Dermatol Venereol.* 2009; 23: 741–750
4. Olumide YM, Akinkugbe AO, Altraide D. et al. Complications of chronic use of skin lightening cosmetics. *Int J Dermatol.* 2008; 47: 344–353
5. Ajose FOA. Consequences of skin bleaching in Nigerian men and women. Int J Dermatol 2005; 44: 41-3
6. Ly F. Skin diseases associated with the use of skin-bleaching products in Africa. *Ann Dermatol Venereol.* 2006; 133: 899–906 ([in French])
7. Nnoruka E and Okoye O. Topical steroid abuse: its use as a depigmenting agent. *J Natl Med Assoc.* 2006; 98: 934–939
8. Boyle J and Peachey RD. Allergic contact dermatitis to Dermovate and Eumovate. *Contact Dermatitis.* 1984; 11: 50–51
9. Lutz ME and el-Azhary RA. Allergic contact dermatitis due to topical application of corticosteroids: review and clinical implications. *Mayo Clin Proc.* 1997; 72: 1141–1144
10. Keane FM., Munn SE, Taylor NF. et al. Unregulated use of clobetasol propionate. *Br J Dermatol.* 2001; 144: 1095–1096
11. Ly F, Soko AS, Dione DA. et al. Aesthetic problems associated with the cosmetic use of bleaching products. *Int J Dermatol.* 2007; 46: 15–17

12. Otley CC and Sober A. Over-the-counter clobetasol propionate. *Arch Dermatol.* 1994; 130: 121

13. Lee SJ, Choi HJ, and Hann SK, Rosacea-like tinea faciei. *Int J Dermatol.* 1999; 38: 479–480

14. Meymandi S, Wiseman MC, and Crawford RI. Tinea faciei mimicking cutaneous lupus erythematosus: a histopathologic case report. *J Am Acad Dermatol.* 2003; 48: S7–8

15. Singh R., Bharu K, Ghazali W. et al. Tinea faciei mimicking lupus erythematosus. Cutis. 1994; 53: 297–298

16. Staughton RC and August PJ. Cushing's syndrome and pituitary-adrenal suppression due to clobetasol propionate. *Br Med J.* 1975; 2: 419–421

17. May P, Stein EJ, Ryter RJ. et al. Cushing syndrome from percutaneous absorption of triamcinolone cream. *Arch Intern Med.* 1976; 136: 612–613

18. Bwomda P, Sermijn E, Lacor P. et al. Glucocorticoid hypertension due to the use of bleaching skin cream, a case report. *Acta Clin Belg.* 2005; 60: 146–149

19. Levin, C. and Maibach, H.I. Topical corticosteroid-induced adrenocortical insufficiency: clinical implications. *Am J Clin Dermatol.* 2002; 3: 141–147

20. Tobin AM., Barragry J, Kirby B. et al. Adrenal suppression following topical use of clobetasol propionate illegally supplied as a bleaching agent. *Ir Med J.* 2005; 98: 118

21. Gilbertson EO, Spellman MC, Piacquadio DJ. et al. Super potent topical corticosteroid use associated with adrenal suppression: clinical considerations. *J Am Acad Dermatol.* 1998; 38: 318–321

22. Ohman EM., Rogers S, Meenan FO. et al. Adrenal suppression following low-dose topical clobetasol propionate. *J R Soc Med.* 1987; 80: 422–424

23. Perret JL, Sane M., Gning S. et al. Hypothalamo-hypophyseal-adrenal hypofunction caused by the use of bleaching cosmetics in Senegal. *Bull Soc Pathol Exot.* 2001; 94: 249–252 ([in French])

24. Hogan DJ, Sibley JT, and Lane PR. Avascular necrosis of the hips following longterm use of clobetasol propionate. *J Am Acad Dermatol.* 1986; 14: 515–517

25. Addo H. Squamous cell carcinoma associated with prolonged bleaching. *Ghana Med J.* 2000; 34: 3

26. Ly F, Kane A, Deme A. et al. First cases of squamous cell carcinoma associated with cosmetic use of bleaching compounds. *Ann Dermatol Venereol.* 2010; 137: 128–131 ([in French])

27. Mahe A, Ly F, Badiane C. et al. Irrational use of skin-bleaching products can delay the diagnosis of leprosy. *Int J Lepr Other Mycobact Dis.* 2002; 70: 119–121

28.Jamie Nathan Rosen, Elman Alseddeeqi, Juan Rivera. Cosmetic agents causing endocrinopathy in an African immigrant. *Canadian Family Physicians.* Febuary 2012; 58(2) 169-71.

Intimate Area Whitening (Private parts bleaching)

Prostitution is another significant factor which could be responsible for skin bleaching practice. The concept of the body, especially the female body, as a commodity may also be traced to prostitution. For example, in Kenya, the more successful prostitutes are invariably light complexioned.[1]

Private parts bleaching involves the bleaching of sexually sensitive parts of the body in order to become lighter. The private parts, which may be involved, include the breasts, penis, the vagina, the buttocks and the thighs. The purpose of private parts bleaching could be for sexual attraction of the opposite gender, which is popular among commercial sex workers. Indeed, in the skin clinic, commercial sex workers brand themselves as "fashion designers" to hide the identity of their trade. Midas care Pharmaceuticals in 2012 began selling its clean and Dry intimate wash that promises women a fair look for their vaginas.

Intimate cosmetic treatment like anal bleaching, genital bleaching, vaginal bleaching, and nipple bleaching, started as "Hollywood" trends, and were only offered in a few salons and spas in California and New York.[2] Since debut, these treatments have become very popular and many people are now searching for easier, practical alternatives for applications at home. Most individuals may prefer not to expose their private intimate areas to salon echnicians, let alone discuss this sensitive topic with others.

There are various bleaching products that contain strong ingredients that can be irritating to the skin. For example, skin bleaching products that contain the ingredient hydroquinone should be avoided due to the potential of side effects. Hydroquinone has been banned in countries such as France and the UK. "Ingredients that are potentially less harmful like, Alpha Arbutin" are recommended for such parts.

Anal bleaching is "frankly some sort of torture technique. An acid is applied to the client's freshly waxed anus and rubbed in". Most spas offer the initial application for about $100-150, then sell a set of bleaching lotion or gel to use at home. The whole in-spa process takes about 20 minutes. Depending on how dark the skin is, a client may need to reapply a number of times to see results and about twice a week for up to eight weeks. Customers could also opt for a package that includes both anal bleaching and vulva lightening, in which the bleach is applied to the opening of the vagina. Anal bleaching is heavily searched for online.

Gynecologists and dermatologists agree that anal bleaching is a risky procedure, no matter how nice and clean the place looks. There have been reports of burning, irritation, and even scarring from the practice. A New York dermatologist Doris Day, MD, said that anal bleaching can do more harm than good. The potential problems include strictures, which make the opening smaller and bowel movements difficult, and tears in the anal canal. "And if the spa isn't clean, there is the risk of acquiring herpes in the area or bacterial infection." Further, in addition to the risk of burns or scarring, the bleaching does not always give the desired result— "The darker pigmentation always comes back so the bleaching is not permanent. There is also a chance of total depigmentation [ie. totally white, rather than matching the skin colour], or in some cases, because of how one's skin reacts to the bleach, a paradoxical increased darkening of the area may occur.

References

1. McVicar KG. *Twilight of an East African Slum.* Ann Arbor, University Microfilms (UCLA Dissertation) 1968.
2.Intimate whitening. *http://intimatewhitening.com/anal-bleaching/*

Tooth bleaching

Dental bleaching, also known as **tooth whitening**, is a common procedure in cosmetic dentistry. According to the FDA, *whitening* restores natural tooth color and *bleaching* whitens beyond the natural color. There are many methods available, such as brushing, bleaching strips, bleaching pen, bleaching gel, and laser bleaching. Teeth whitening has become the most requested procedure in cosmetic dentistry today. More than 100 million Americans whiten their teeth one way or another; spending an estimated $15 billion in 2010.[1]

Bleaching methods use carbamide peroxide which reacts with water to form hydrogen peroxide. Carbamide peroxide has about a third of the strength of hydrogen peroxide. This means that a 15% solution of carbamide peroxide is the rough equivalent of a 5% solution of hydrogen peroxide. The peroxide oxidizing agent penetrates the porosities in the rod-like crystal structure of enamel and breaks down stain deposits in the dentin. Power bleaching uses light to accelerate the process of bleaching in a dental office. Another bleaching agent is 6-phthalimido peroxy hexanoic acid (PAP).

Tooth bleaching is not a modern invention. Ancient Romans, for example, used urine and goat milk in an attempt to make and keep their teeth whiter.[2]

References

1. Tooth bleaching. *Wikipedia,* the free encyclopedia https://en.wikipedia.org/wiki/Tooth_bleaching
2. "The History of Teeth Whitening¯Smiles Through the Miles" http://www.thehistoryof.net/the-histroy-of-teeth-whitening-html.09-11-2008.

SYSTEMIC SKIN WHITENING AGENTS

Glutathione as a skin lightening agents

Glutathione (GHS)

The most commonly used systemic skin whitening agent is GSH used alone or in various combinations, both as oral and intravenous formulations. Glutathione (GSH) is the most abundant low-molecular weight intracellular thiol in mammals.[1,2] It is a tripeptide composed of the amino acids L-cysteine (L-Cys), glutamate, and glycine. Glutathione is one of the five network antioxidants and has been recognized as a master antioxidant. It is involved in many important biological processes such as DNA and protein synthesis and the protection of cells through the metabolism of xenobiotics and carcinogens. It also functions to detoxify electrophilic compounds and acts as a reductant in the detoxification of peroxides, protecting cells from intracellular free radicals and reactive oxygen species (ROS).[1,2] Glutathione also serves as a reservoir for the amino acid cysteine.[3]

GSH is also available naturally in watermelon, avocado, broccoli, spinach and tomatoes. GSH exists in cells mostly in the reduced form (GSH) which is constantly oxidized forming oxidized GSH and its supply is replenished by the action of GSH reductase. GSH is involved in various biochemical processes especially those involving scavenging of free radicals and detoxification of toxic compounds, it acts as coenzyme and helps in the transport of amino acids across the cell membranes.[4,5] Lower GSH levels are implicated in many diseases and GSH has been tried in the management of Alzheimer's disease, Parkinson's disease, multiple sclerosis, alcoholic hepatitis, atherosclerosis, acquired immunodeficiency syndrome, and chronic fatigue syndrome. It has been commonly used to combat the neuro- and nephrotoxicity associated with cisplatin chemotherapy[6] and this is the only Food and Drug Administration (FDA) approved indication for the intravenous form of GSH. The role of GSH as a skin whitening agent was an accidental discovery when skin whitening was noticed as a side effect of large doses of GSH. This led to extensive studies establishing its role in melanogenesis and the recent use of GSH as systemic skin whitening agent.

How glutathione works to lighten the skin

GSH exerts its action as skin whitening agent at various levels of melanogenesis which include the following:[4-8]

- Interference with cellular transport of tyrosinase
- Direct inactivation of the enzyme tyrosinase by binding with the copper-containing active site of the enzyme
- Mediating the switch mechanism from eumelanin to phaeomelanin production as GSH is the major physiologic reservoir of cysteine and increase in cysteine levels results in switching of eumelanogenesis to pheomelanogenesis
- Quenching of free radicals and peroxides that contribute to tyrosinase activation and melanin formation.

Modulation of depigmenting abilities of melanocytotoxic agents.

The products

GSH for skin whitening is available in both tablet and injectable form. Parenteral administration of gluthathione, specifically through the intravenous (IV) route, is believed to provide faster and better results because it avoids the first-pass metabolism seen with the oral route. Intravenously administered GSH is not directly utilized by cells but is cleaved into its component amino acids and is resynthesized, to GSH intracellularly after transmembrane transport. After IV administration, most GSH is immediately oxidized and disappeared from the circulation with a half-life of 10 minutes, and the rest is broken down into its three component amino acids. However, safety of intravenous route continues to be a concern as there have been reports of adverse reactions. These range from mild, transient headaches and skin eruptions to severe drug reactions that have required hospitalization.

Conflicting reports exist about the bioavailability of oral intake of GSH. It was previously believed that GSH molecule could not pass through the intestinal lining of the gastrointestinal tract and had to be broken down into its components amino acids before absorption. When taken orally, GSH is hydrolyzed by intestinal and hepatic gamma-glutamyl transferase resulting in reduced bioavailability. Even when large oral doses were administered, it was found that most of the absorbed GSH remains within the gut luminal cells and only small and transient increases of GSH could be detected in the general circulation.[8] Thus, the effectiveness of exogenously administered GSH is hindered by its instability when crossing cell membranes and its rapid hydrolysis in the circulation by gamma-glutamyltranspeptidase found on the extracellular surfaces of cells.[9] On the contrary, intravenous GSH delivers very high doses directly into the systemic circulation, overloading the renal circulation.

Animal studies have shown that the intact GSH molecules can be absorbed through the small intestine. Plasma GSH levels increased three-fold 90 minutes after administration and remained elevated for 2-3 hours thereafter.[3,6,10] Other animal studies, have demonstrated that enteral intake of GSH precursors, specifically glutamine and cysteine (in the form of N-acetyl-L-Cys), increase intracellular GSH levels.[1] Reservations about oral ingestion of GSH capsules include the possibility that the capsule will not be digested, and thus GSH will not be made available for absorption in the small intestine. At the other end of the spectrum is the potential for the capsule to be digested too early in the stomach, preventing the glutathione from reaching the small intestine. Oral ingestion of GSH has been reported to produce variable results in terms of skin lightening, although most information is based on anecdotal evidence and testimonials. Large volume of pill load is required for oral GSH to have any measurable impact on skin lightening.

Oral GSH is in the "generally regarded as safe" category of FDA and is usually marketed as a food or dietary supplement and hence it does not certainly need to be FDA approved. There are no provisions in the law for FDA to approve dietary supplements for effectiveness before they reach the consumer. However, FDA has banned the use of intravenous form of GSH for skin whitening in view of commonly reported side effects like skin rashes, Stevens Johnson syndrome, toxic epidermal necrolysis, derangement in thyroid and renal function and severe abdominal pain.[11,12]

The promoters of GSH promote it at a dose of 20 and 40 mg/kg/body weight/day which is divided into two doses with a maintenance dose of 500 mg/day.[13] They claim that gradual systemic effect will be seen 1-3 months in medium brown skin, in 3-6 months in dark brown skin, in 6-12 months in very dark skin and in 2 years or more in black skin. Injectable GSH is given at a dose of 900 mg weekly by intravenous or intramuscular method and the sessions can be repeated 2-3 times a week. They claim skin whitening to occur as early as 2-3 weeks.[13-15]

Glutathione capsules come in strengths of 100 mg and 500 mg which lightens skin tone by two shades when taken once a day for three months. Even more dangerous is the off-label use of the drug in injectable doses of 1,200 mg, usually prescribed for 10 consecutive weeks after which people are asked to switch to the capsules to retain their newfound lighter complexion.[14]

GSH is also combined with many other agents like vitamin C to increase its absorption, N-acetyl cysteine to boost its level, alpha lipoic acid and other antioxidants like vitamin E and grape seed extract. Some oral preparations have dangerous combinations like monobenzone which causes irreversible depigmentation and hydroquinone which is banned by FDA as a carcinogen.[16]
In order to maximize absorption of the GSH molecule, the buccal mucosa may be a useful route of administration. Substances that are absorbed through the buccal route go directly into the systemic circulation. A novel preparation of glutathione, with absorption using the oral mucosal route, has been formulated to facilitate optimum absorption into the bloodstream without the side effects of IV administration and it bypasses the gastrointestinal (GIT) tract. Hence a novel preparation of GSH Lozenge has been formulated. Preliminary trials suggest that complications of sublingual and buccal medications are rare but can include inflammation of the mucous membrane including the gums[17]

L-cysteine peptide

Another agent promoted for skin whitening is L-cysteine peptide, which is claimed to be 3-5 times more potent than GSH.[18] Natural sources of L-cysteine include poultry, yogurt, egg yolks, red peppers, garlic, onions, broccoli, Brussel sprouts, oats, and wheat germ. L-cysteine along with L-glutamic acid and glycine is the rate-limiting precursor in the synthesis of GSH peroxidase and has been found that high concentrations of L-cysteine reduced the tyrosinase activity and produced more pheomelanin by way of cysteinyl dihydroxyphenylalanine DOPA, the building block of pheomelanin. The cysteinyl DOPAs can be formed in two ways-directly by nucleophilic addition of cysteine to DOPA quinone or indirectly from GSH DOPA by action of gamma-glutamyl transferase and peptidase.[19,20] Hence L-cysteine peptide is promoted as skin whitening agent but without much scientific evidence to support its use for this indication.

Tranexemic acid

Tranexemic acid (trans-4-aminomethyl cyclohexane carboxylic acid), a plasmin inhibitor, commonly used as a haemostatic agent owing to its antifibrolytic action is also promoted as a systemic skin whitening agent especially as oral or intradermal injections for melasma. The skin whitening effects of tranexamic acid was incidentally found when it was used in the treatment of aneurysmal subarachnoid hemorrhage. It is a synthetic derivative of lysine and its therapeutic role in melasma was first studied by Nijor as early as in 1979[21], but only limited data exist in the literature regarding its use in melasma. Plasmin, is a protease that enhances the intracellular release of arachidonic acid, a precursor of prostanoid, and also elevates alpha-melanocyte stimulating hormone (α-MSH) processed from pro-opio-melanocortin. Both arachidonic acid and α-MSH can activate melanin synthesis by melanocytes. Tranexemic acid by way of its antiplasmin activity depletes the keratinocyte pool of arachidonic acid involved in ultraviolet (UV) induced melanogenesis[21-26].

It has been used at a low dose of 250 mg twice a day for at least 3 months for the treatment of melasma and found to be effective.[24] But, it is not safe to use it for a long duration in view of its anti-hemorrhagic property resulting in side effects like venous thromboembolism, myocardial infarction, cerebrovascular accidents and pulmonary embolism. It is contraindicated in patients with acquired defective color vision, an active intravascular clotting condition, and hypersensitivity to tranexemic acid.[24] However, there is no scientific data available demonstrating the role of tranexemic acid as an overall skin whitening/lightening agent. It is even being promoted as intravenous injection for skin whitening at a dose of 500 mg every week for 1 or 2 months and 500 mg every month for maintenance.[27] Tranexamic acid has been found to produce good synergistic effect when combined with ascorbic acid or its derivatives and L-cysteine.[26]

Miscellaneous agents.[27-31]

Apart from these, large doses of vitamin C, hyaluronic acid, epidermal growth factor and combinations of multiple natural extracts (natural collagen extracts, bearberry extract, Glycyrrhiza glabra extract, Lycopene, Kelp, olive leaf extract, hawthorn, jujube, sea buckthorn, starch, coix seed, pearl extracts, etc.,) are also promoted for skin whitening in the form of food or dietary supplements with no scientific evidence.

Nevertheless, there are few animal studies and *in vitro* studies demonstrating the role of natural extracts like irradiated green tea polyphenol,[26] proanthocyanidin-rich extract from grape seeds,[27] ellagic acid-rich pomegranate extract,[28] and coumarin extracts from the plant *Angelica dahurica*,[29] in inhibiting melanogenesis resulting in skin whitening thereby recommending these agents as oral preparations for skin whitening. Procyanidins (pycnogenol, grape seed extracts) and *Polypodium leucotomos* have been found to be effective and safe in the treatment of melasma and to prevent UV A induced pigmentary changes respectively.[30] But there are no trials demonstrating their efficacy in the treatment of post inflammatory pigmentation or in improving the general skin color.

References

1.Exner R, Wessner B, Manhart N, *et al.* Therapeutic potential of glutathione. *Wien Klin Wochenschr* 2000; 112: 610-6.

2.Hagen TM, Jones DP. Transepithelial transport of glutathione in vascularly perfused small intestine of rat. *Am J Physiol* 1987; 252: G607-G613

3.Hagen TM, Wierzbicka GT, Sillau AH, *et al.* Bioavailability of dietary glutathione: effect on plasma concentration. *Am J Physiol* 1990; 259: G524-G529.

4.Villarama CD, Maibach HI. Glutathione as a depigmenting agent: An overview. *Int J Cosmet Sci* 2005; 27:147-53.

5. Malathi M, Thappa DM. Systemic skin whitening/lightening agents: What is the evidence? *Indian J Indian Dermatol Venereol Leprol* 2013; 79:842-6.2.

6. Hospers GA, Eisenhauer EA, de Vries EG. The sulfhydryl containing compounds WR-2721 and glutathione as radio- and chemoprotective agents. A review, indications for use and prospects. *Br J Cancer* 1999; 80:629-38.

7. Arjinpathana N, Asawanonda P. Glutathione as an oral whitening agent: A randomized, double-blind, placebo-controlled study. *J Dermatolog Treat* 2012;23:97-102.

8.Ebanks JP, Wickett RR, Boissy RE. Mechanisms regulating skin pigmentation; the rise and fall of complexion coloration. *Int J Mol Sci* 2009; 10: 4066-87

9.Hong SY, Gil HW, Yang JO, Lee EY, Kim HK, Kim SH, *et al.* Pharmacokinetics of glutathione and its metabolites in normal subjects. *J Korean Med Sci* 2005;20:721-

10. Hunjan MK, Evered DE. Absorption of glutathione from the gastro-intestinal tract. *Biochim Biophys Acta* 1985; 815: 184-8

11. Witschi A, Reddy S, Stofer B, Lauterburg BH. The systemic availability of oral glutathione. *Eur J Clin Pharmacol* 1992;43:667-9.

12. Injectable glutha not FDA-approved. Available from: *http://www.journal.com.ph/index.php/news/national/44605-injectable-glutha-not-fda-approved.* [Last accessed on 2013 Apr 2].

13. Skin whitening pills. Available from: *http://www.magicproducts.in.* [Last accessed on 2013 Apr 2].

14. Sanchita Sharma, India's fair skin obsession takes risky pharma turn. *Hindustan Times*, New Delhi *http://www.hindustantimes.com/wellness/india-s-fair-skin-obession...* Updated: Apr 05, 2015 09:27 IST.

15. Perfect white skin whitening and anti-aging tablets. Available from: *http://www.perfectwhiteaim.blogspot.in.* [Last accessed on 2013 Apr 2].

16. Levitt J. The safety of hydroquinone: A dermatologist2 s response to the 2006 Federal Register. *J Am Acad Dermatol* 2007;57:854-72.

17. Evangeline B. Handog, Maria Suzanne L Datuin, and Ivan A Singzon. An open-label, single-arm trial of the safety and efficacy of a novel preparation of glutathione as a skin-lightening agent in Filipino women. *Int Journal Dermatol* 2016; 55:153-7

18. Smit NP, Van der Meulen H, Koerten HK, Kolb RM, Mommaas AM, Lentjes EG, *et al.* Melanogenesis in cultured melanocytes can be substantially influenced by L-tyrosine and L-cysteine. *J Invest Dermatol* 1997; 109:796-800.

19. del Marmol V, Ito S, Bouchard B, Libert A, Wakamatsu K, Ghanem G, *et al.* Cysteine deprivation promotes eumelanogenesis in human melanoma cells. *J Invest Dermatol* 1996; 107:698-702.

20. Agrup G, Hansson C, Rorsman H, Rosengren E. The effect of cysteine on oxidation of tyrosine, DOPA, and cysteinyldopas. Arch Dermatol Res 1982; 272:103-15.

21. Nijor T. Treatment of melasma with tranexamic acid. *Clin Res.* 1979; 13:3129-31.

22. Ando H, Matsui MS, Ichihashi M. Quasi-drugs developed in Japan for the prevention or treatment of hyperpigmentary disorders. *Int J Mol Sci* 2010; 11:2566-75.

23. Tse TW, Hui E. Tranexamic acid: An important adjuvant in the treatment of melasma. *J Cosmet Dermatol* 2013; 12:57-66.

24. Karn D, S KC, Amatya A, Razouria EA, Timalsina M. Oral tranexamic acid for the treatment of melasma. *Kathmandu Univ Med J* (KUMJ) 2012; 10:40-3.

25. Wu S, Shi H, Wu H, Yan S, Guo J, Sun Y, *et al.* Treatment of melasma with oral administration of tranexamic acid. *Aesthetic Plast Surg* 2012; 36:964-70.

26. Tranexemic acid. Available from: *http://www.mcbiotec.com/products/?type=detail & id=33.* [Last accessed on 2013 Jun 17].

27. Beauty injections. Available from: *http://www.beautyinjections.com/products/Tranexamic-Acid.html.* [Last accessed on 2013 Jun 17].

28. An BJ, Kwak JH, Son JH, Park JM, Lee JY, Park TS, *et al.* Physiological activity of irradiated green tea polyphenol on the human skin. *Am J Chin Med* 2005; 33:535-46.

29. Yamakoshi J, Otsuka F, Sano A, Tokutake S, Saito M, Kikuchi M, *et al.* Lightening effect on ultraviolet-induced pigmentation of guinea pig skin by oral administration of a proanthocyanidin-rich extract from grape seeds. *Pigment Cell Res* 2003; 16:629-38.

30. Yoshimura M, Watanabe Y, Kasai K, Yamakoshi J, Koga T. Inhibitory effect of an ellagic acid-rich pomegranate extract on tyrosinase activity and ultraviolet-induced pigmentation. *Biosci Biotechnol Biochem* 2005; 69:2368-73.

31. Cho YH, Kim JH, Park SM, Lee BC, Pyo HB, Park HD. New cosmetic agents for skin whitening from *Angelica dahurica.* J Cosmet Sci 2006; 57:11-21.

Skin lightening Pills Side Effects—Dangers and Risks

Just like skin whitening creams and lotions, pills also have side effects. These products are the best in producing faster results when it comes to lightening skin. This is the major reason as to why they are preferred over skin whitening home remedies and other natural skin lightening methods.

Studies have been conducted and it has been revealed that pills have side effects and among them include the following:

- Allergic reactions: This include skin swelling and rashes on the skin surface that follows taking of the skin whitening pills and supplements.
- There is internal physical stress that is associated with symptoms such as nausea, insomnia, headaches, vomiting and drowsiness especially after a prolonged intake of the pills.
- Risk of liver conditions due to pill popping. Some skin lightening pills must to consumed in large volumes for effectiveness and this is risky to liver functioning.
- Hormonal imbalances due to the disruption of the normal body production of melanin.
- Hydroquinone is a harmful ingredient available in most skin whitening products including some pills.
- Use of some bleaching agents can cause a dry skin on the face, lips and arms, mainly associated with element that contains heavy metals such as lead.

These agents are being advertised on the internet and currently there are no market data available on the use of these agents

As already mentioned above, these agents are not FDA approved for skin whitening and **no scientific evidence exists** for their use. In addition, the injectable formulations are counterfeited and given by untrained people illegally and hence associated with the risk of sepsis, air embolism, transmission of human immunodeficiency virus, Hepatitis B, and use of non-sterile preparations that can lead to serious infections. Another major question that remains unanswered as yet is that whether this would result in an increased incidence of skin cancers.

As a general rule, the promoters of the systemic skin whitening agents list lactation, heart disease and hypersensitivity as contraindications for all these agents. Since there are not much human or animal studies advocating the role of these agents in skin whitening, there is no data on the relative and absolute contraindications, the appropriate dosing schedule and the long term side effects.

Side effects of Glutathione Injections
Hair loss
White spots on the nails
Numbness of extremities
Shivers and shakes
Depression and anxiety

Complications of Glutathione Injections
Allergy or Anaphylaxis (manifested by difficulty in breathing,tightness of chest, rashes, hives,and swollen skin)
Systemic Infection
Stevens–Johnson Syndrome
Toxic Epidermal Necrolysis or Lyell's Syndrome
Kidney Failure
Thyroid Dysfunction
Severe abdominal pain

The major concern is this: For any drug to be approved by the FDA, it must have undergone series of relevant clinical trials which should include follow up time. The point of the follow up period is to see if any side effects occur and to deduce how efficacious the drug is. So, if there have been no clinical trials on skin whitening injections to date, it means that those Africans, and Nigerians who inject themselves with these agents are in fact using themselves as experimental animals. This means that in 12-15 years time, when the drug has accumulated in the system, the true effect will be realized. If the thought of using oneself as an uncontrolled scientific experiment isn't scary enough, then what is? We will just have to wait a few years to see what happens.

Reference
Ify Aniebo. Skin whitening injections in Africa. Dec 05, 2013. *http://africahealthmagazine.com/2013/12/05/skin-whitening-injections-in-africa/*

Problems with Systemic Skin Whitening Agents
According to the FDA, the US drug watchdog, side-effects of the injection range from skin rashes, disruption in thyroid function, kidney damage, Stevens-Johnson syndrome and toxic epidermal necrolysis. The last two life-threatening conditions cause fever, severe rash, blisters and skin peeling. Affected people have to be treated in the hyper-sterile burns wards of hospitals.

Another major question that remains unanswered as yet is that whether switching the normal machinery from eumelanin (which is protective against UV radiation) to pheomelanin (which photosensitizes UV-induced deoxyribonucleic acid damage as observed in cultured human melanocytes) by an external agent for long duration would result in an increased incidence of skin cancers.

Conclusion

The desire for white and fair skin is a global phenomenon and it is being highly capitalized by both the cosmetic and dermatologic industries. It is an essential role of the dermatologist to make the public aware that skin lightening agents may progressively revert back from the facultative color to the constitutive level and normally this color change will not go beyond the constitutive level. If such a change is claimed, it should be considered to be dangerous as such alterations can become non-reversible resulting in vitiligo and may also predispose to other complications like skin cancer as the normal biochemical processes are altered. Till date, systemic skin whitening agents do not have much scientific evidence regarding their use and strict laws should be enforced to ban the use of these agents until well conducted randomized controlled trials are available ensuring the safety and efficacy of these agents.

Reference

Best Skin Lightening Pills — for Whitening Black, Dark People, African American Reviews and Side Effect. http://www.beautyclue/skin-whitening/best-skin-lightening-pills...

Illegal mixture of mercury containing skin lightening cream and alpha hydroxyl acid used as injection.

Skin lightening creams used as injectables

A worrying skin-lightening practice has emerged in Kenya and possibly some other African countries. There is a booming black market where creams that are intended for topical use are used as injectables by the wealthy Nairobi women for quicker action to lighter the skin because Kenyan men like women with whiter skin. The $70 US treatment is so 'strong', it is said to be capable of turning a user into 'albinos.' The shots contain alpha hydroxy acids and mercury-containing creams.

Beauticians claim "the injections can make customers look six years younger and their skin a shocking ten shades lighter; and they are gaining particular popularity on Nairobi's River Road— a busy marked place notorious for its black market commerce and bribed law enforcement. Rose, a beautician, who does the injecting says "The injection lightens you from inside. It makes women clean." She says most of her clients are wealthy and some are national celebrities. Many are Somali or Indians. But, those ones never come to my shop. They send a driver with a photo of their skin color and I supply what they need:"

Reference

Annabel Fenwick Elliott. Kenyan men like women with whiter skin: The rise of wealthy Nairobi women illegally injecting themselves with skin-lightening creams. *http://www.dailymail.co.uk/femail/article-2650766/Kenyan-men-like-women-whiter-skin-The-rise-wealthy-Nairobi-women-illegally-INJECTING-skin-lightening-creams.html*

Alpha hydroxy acids (AHAs)

Alpha hydroxy acids (AHAs), are a group of carboxylic compounds. AHAs most commonly used in cosmetic applications are typically derived from food products including glycolic acid (from sugar cane), lactic acid (from sour milk), malic acid (from apples), citric acid (from citrus fruits) and tartaric acid (from grape wine)! Glycolic acid is the smallest α hydroxy acid.

Safety

AHAs are generally safe *when used on the skin* as a cosmetic agent using the *recommended* dosage. The most common side-effects are mild skin irritations, redness and flaking. The severity usually depends on the pH and the concentration of the acid used. Chemical peels tend to have more severe side-effects including blistering, burning and skin discoloration, although they are usually mild and go away a day or two after treatment.

The FDA has also warned consumers that care should be taken when using AHAs after an industry-sponsored study found that they can increase photosensitivity to the sun[7]. Other sources suggest that Glycolic acid, in particular, may confer a photoprotective effect[8].

References

1. Alpha hydroxy acids" Wikipedia, the free encyclopedia. *http://en.wikipedia.org/wiki/Alpha-hydroxy-acid.*

2. Kempers S; Katz HI, Wildnauer R, Green B. An evaluation of the effect of an alpha hydroxy acid-blend skin cream in the cosmetic improvement of symptoms of moderate to severe xerosis, epidermolytic hyperkeratosis, and ichthyosis. *Cutis* 1998; 61: (6):347-50

3. Alpha Hydroxy Acids for Skin Care *Cosmetic Dermatology, Supplement:* 1-6. October 1994.

4. Kalla G, Garg A, Kachhawa D. Chemica/ peeling— Glycolic acid versus trichloroacetic acid in melasma. *Indian Journal of Dermatology, Venereology and Leprology* 2001, 67 (2): 82-4.

5. Atzori L, Brundu MA, Orru A, Biggio P. Glycolic acid peeling in the treatment of acne. *European Academy of Dermatology and Venereology* 1999; 12 (2): 119-22.

6. Peter Pacik. What is Glycolic acid?" (http:/howtogetridofacneeasily.com/whatisglycolicacid/)
7. Kurtzweil Paula. Alpha Hydroxy Acids for Skin Care. *(http:www.cfsan.fda.gov/~dms/fdacaha.html).* FDA Consumer. Archived *(http://web.archive.org/web20060207090619/http://www.cfsan.fda.gov/%7Edms/fdacaha.html)* from the original on February 7, 2006.
8. Perricone Nicholas V, DiNardo Joseph C. photoprotective and anitiinflammatory Effects of topical Glycolic acid. *Dermatologic Surgery*. May 1996; 22 (5): 435-37.

SKIN LIGHTENING SURGERY AND OTHER TECHNIQUES

Skin whitening surgery is a cosmetic treatment that involves restructuring some skin tissues in an attempt to lighten the skin tone and provide a more even skin tone.[1-4]

Skin lightening surgery uses a variety of methods, and peeling is considered as the most popular method. Tretinoin is usually applied in order to make the skin mature faster. Once it's done, surgeons can easily peel the skin off.

Skin lightening surgery, or skin bleaching plastic surgery is a depigmentation process or system that whitens a dark skin. This is the method used by celebrities with a dark complexion who turn out to be white almost instantly and the result is permanent. Skin whitening surgery treatment is a procedure that reduces the concentration of melanin pigment in the skin. The procedure is performed at the dermatologist's or surgeon's clinic. Usually the doctor will make an appointment with the client, discuss everything that is of concern when the client wants to bleach the skin permanently. The procedure is used for:

- Imperfections caused by melanin
- Lightening dark spots on the skin that are stubborn and won't go away
- Permanent skin lightening procedure for scars
- Getting rid of birthmarks such as port wine stains
- Uneven skin tone and permanent discoloration or hyperpigmentation
- Getting rid of freckles and brown sports.
- Dark spots caused by photo-aging

The method uses laser beams to reduce the concentration of melanin in the skin. An alternative method of reducing Melanin pigment is through Cryosurgery. Cryosurgery using liquid nitrogen is usually used for sensitive areas of the skin such as the genitals. The method destroys melanin cells and allows the skin to regenerate a new epidermis with a lighter shade. However, it is important to note that the efficacy of this surgery will depend on the depth of the melanin pigment, meaning that different people could get different dark skin whitening results with the same surgical procedure. After the initial procedure, the client usually needs two or three further appointments which may involve corrections of evenness and aftercare procedures. Clients may feel a little bit uncomfortable during and after laser surgery to whiten dark skin. After the procedure, daily application of sun block is recommended. This will not only protect your skin from sunburn, it will also prevent your skin from getting darker. Choose a sunscreen that can be worn under your make up.

The cost of permanent skin whitening surgery is not comparable to the temporary solutions. The costs vary depending on the countries where it is done e.g United States, UK, India, Israel, South Africa and other places. For instance, the cost for laser skin lightening for eczema spots is about $2300 US. The cost of laser melanin surgery to get a light complexion depends on the clinic and the area you want to have lightened. The following areas may have different costs:

- Dark armpit lightening surgery
- Face freckle removal laser skin lightening
- Full body skin brightening
- Arms and legs plastic surgery for skin lightening

The cost of erbium laser cosmetic surgery starts from £1500 (one thousand, five hundred pounds sterling) for a 5cm radius area for treatments and upward depending on size and what the skin disorder is. Full body skin lightening costs nothing less than $3000.

Laser Skin Resurfacing

Often skin lightening surgery is combined with laser skin resurfacing procedures. Some people, in addition, go under the knife to reshape their bodies, often in ways that Anglicize their facial features and body types. Ethnic rhinoplasty or nose surgery has also evolved recently.

Laser skin resurfacing is a popular cosmetic procedure that can help rejuvenate the skin and reduce the effects of the sun, aging and some facial skin disorders. During the laser skin resurfacing procedure a laser is used to dissolve the molecular bonds of the damaged skin cells layer by layer until a smoother, more uniform skin appearance is achieved. The procedure may also be referred to as laser skin rejuvenation because of its anti-aging benefits, or laser peel because the damaged layers of skin are peeled away.

With a qualified cosmetic surgeon, laser skin resurfacing treatment are a safe and effective way to correct fine lines, wrinkles, and other forms of skin damage. With that in mind, it is important to remember that all procedures carry with them some risks. The procedure has the possibility of resulting in heat injury, activation of cold sores, lightening or darkening of the skin, and, rarely, scarring or infection. Reddening of the skin may last for several weeks.

References

1. Skin Lightening Surgery—Cost, Before and After, Permanent, Procedure. *http://www.etopical.com/skin-lightening-surgery-cost-before-after-p...*
2. Laser Skin Resurfacing—Cost, Types, Risks, Recovery & Results. *http://www.docshop.com/education/dermatology/facial/skin-resurfacing*
3. skin Lightening South Africa- Check Prices and Compare Reviews. *http://whatclinic.com/beauty-salons/south-africa/skin-lightening.*
4. Laser surgery skin bleaching complications—Google Search. *https://www.google.com.ng/serach?q=laser+surgery+skin+bleaching...*

Microdermabrasion

Microdermabrasion (MDA) is a non-chemical, non-invasive procedure that uses a spray of aluminum oxide crystals and a vacuum device to remove the outermost layer of dry, dead skin cells and reveal younger, healthier-looking skin. Microdermabrasion also encourages the production of a new underlying layer of skin cells with higher levels of collagen and elastin, which further improves the skin's appearance. Microdermabrasion is much gentler than dermabrasion. Dermabrasion is a more intensive procedure used to treat deeper facial lines, extreme sun damage, and scars.

During an MDA treatment, the clinician directs a stream of tiny ("micro") aluminum oxide crystals through a hand piece that is placed against the skin. These dermabrasion crystals exfoliate the skin, and the mild suction created by the MDA system removes the skin debris and crystals. Sessions are spaced just as mentioned for peels. Chemical peels can be combined with MDA for a deeper effect, but this is only done for advanced peels in patients who have been taking regular peels for many months.

MDA helps produce thicker, healthier skin layers; multiple treatments are vital because they encourage the production of a new layer of skin cells that contains higher levels of collagen and elastin. Both of these components are essential for vibrant, healthy skin, and they will further improve your complexion and the overall appearance of your skin. Approximately five to twelve treatments spaced two to three weeks apart are usually necessary to reap full microdermabrasion benefits. Convenient and virtually painless, the microdermabrasion procedure takes only 30 to 60 minutes and is commonly referred to as the "lunch hour facial."

MDA is a safe, non-surgical, "lunch hour" procedure that provides many benefits. MDA reduces or eliminates fine facial lines, wrinkles, and other signs of aging; it improves the appearance of acne scars and other light scarring; and it gives skin of all colors and types a fresh, healthy-looking glow. It does all this with virtually no side effects. And because MDA uses non-allergenic crystals to treat the skin, it is an excellent treatment for skin that is sensitive to chemicals. MDA does not present any serious risks when it is performed by a qualified provider. Some people may experience slight skin irritation after MDA. Since everyone's skin and health history differ to some degree, the risks and benefits of MDA must be considered on a case-by-case basis.

Microdermabrasion for Acne

Microdermabrasion can be used to treat acne and the scars that acne causes. MDA treatments can eliminate or greatly reduce the appearance of lighter scarring. However, for deep acne scars (known as "pock marks" or "ice-pick acne scars") microdermabrasion may not be able to provide desired results. Deeper scars can usually be effectively treated with dermabrasion or an acne chemical peel. Patients with active acne may also benefit from microdermabrasion treatments, which exfoliate the skin and clear clogged pores of oil and dirt. Because the polishing action of the crystal and the removal of skin cells can aggravate acne, however, a consultation with a dermatologist or cosmetic surgeon is advised to help determine whether a patient's acne or acne scars can be effectively treated with microdermabrasion.

Normal side effects associated with microdermabrasion are increased skin sensitivity and risk of sunburn. However, these side effects are usually mild and brief. Microdermabrasion risks are minimal, but problems such as infection can occur if the treatment is not properly performed. MDA recovery and results are among the most favorable of all the noninvasive facial treatments available today.

The cost of microdermabrasion depends on factors such as the amount of MDA a patient needs, the number of treatments, the fees of the treating physician, and the geographic region where the treatment is administered. The cost of microdermabrasion is less expensive than that of some other cosmetic options for facial rejuvenation, particularly surgical procedures such as a face lift. The price of microdermabrasion treatments depends upon several factors, including the experience and qualifications of the person performing the procedure and the location of the spa or clinic. On average, microdermabrasion cost ranges from $75 and $200.

Chemical Peels– these are fruit acids, alpha and beta hydroxy acids which are used in various combinations to peel away the superficial tanned layer of the skin. Peels may only have one component like glycolic acid or salicylic acid or multiple components like retinol, lactic acid, mandelic acid, pyruvic acid, phytic acid etc. Peels can be short contact or leave on peels. Short contact peels are applied on the skin for 5-10 minutes and then neutralized. Leave on peels are left on for 6-12 hours and then washed off. These work deeper and typically cause more peeling of the skin which can continue for 5-7 days after the session. Peel sessions are repeated 2-3 weekly for 6-8 sessions after which maintenance sessions can be given once in 6 weeks.

Mesotherapy - this is a technique popular in Europe (particularly France) and involves injecting vitamins into the skin. This can be done superficially (called the 'nappage technique') or deep ('point to point' technique). Various vitamins can be used in isolation or as vitamin cocktails (e.g vitamin C, glutathione).

LED light devices - these contain blue, red and yellow light. Of these red and yellow stimulate the skin to make new collagen and this improves skin texture and gives it a glow. There is no effect on skin color though.

Fraxel laser treatment – this can be done for rejuvenating the skin (Fraxel Re:store) or for actually removing the superficial layers of the skin (Fraxel Re:pair). The latter laser can improve skin color and uniformity in patients with fair to light brown skin, not so much in Asian, brown or black skin.

References

1.http://www.docshop.com/education/dermatology/facial/mocrodermabrasion

2. Atlanta Blackstar. 15 Black Celebs Caught Whitening their skin *http://www.atlantablackstar.com/2013/08/19/15-black-celebs-caught-white…*

3.Dr Nair. How do celebrities lighten their skin tone? *http://www.justanswer.com/dermatology/77tvb-celebrities-lighten-skin..*

LIST OF APPENDICES

1. List of some publications by Nigerian Scientists on the skin bleaching culture.

2. Federal Republic of Nigeria-Official Gazette
   Lagos- 26th February, 1993 No3, Vol 80

3. Administrative Order completely banning Hydroquinone
Copy of Letter from the Federal Ministry of Health 24/4/91.

4. Federal Republic of Nigeria-Official Gazette
   Lagos 29th December, 1995 No 31c Vol 82

5. Feature Article on Hazardous Cosmetics by LUCY HANNAN.
   African Business May 1988.

6. Newspaper cuttings reacting to the **BANDUNG TV** Programme

7a & b Advert for *Venus de Milo* cosmetic bleaching cream in the Programme of 1st National Awareness Seminar of the Toiletries and Cosmetics Manufacturers Group of the Manufacturers Association of Nigeria. Wednesday 23rd November, 1988.

8 List of some feature articles in the Nigerian Press on the skin bleaching culture in Nigeria.

9 The Marriage Laws in Nigeria

10 Polygamy in Sub-Saharan Society

11 Bigamy in Nigeria

12 List of banned skin bleaching products in Kenya

13 Diagnosis of mercury intoxication; Environmental Monitoring; WHO Recommendations

14 How to naturally whiten skin at home

15 Some Literature Review on skin bleaching

Appendix 1

List of some publications by Nigerian Scientists on the skin bleaching culture

1. Olumide YM. (1985): Cosmetic Hazards and Legislative needs in Nigeria. *Nig. Med. Pract.* 9:7-12
2. Olumide YM, and Elesha SO. (1986): Hydroquinone Induced Exogenous Ochronosis. *Nig. Med. Pract.* 11:103-106
3. Olumide YM. (1986): Abuse of Topical corticoids in Nigeria. *Nig. Med. Pract.* 11:7-13.
4. Olumide YM. (1987): Photodermatoses in Lagos. *Int. J. Dermatol.* 26:295-299.
5. BLEACHING OF THE SKIN (What everyone should know) Publisher: Medical Women's Association of Nigeria 1988; 37 pages.
6. Olumide YM. (1989): Contact Leucoderma. *Nig. Quart. J Hosp. Med.* 4:53-62.
7. Olumide YM, Odunowo BD, and Odiase AO (1990): Depigmentation in Black African Patients. *Int J. Dermatol.* 29:3; 166-174.
8. Olumide YM. Toiletries and Cosmetics to Healthy Life (The Nigerian Perspectives) Proceedings of the Toiletries and Cosmetics Manufacturers Seminar 1997. pp20-24, 28.
9. Adebajo SB. An epidemiologic survey of the use of skin lightening cosmetics among traders in Lagos, Nigeria. *West Afr J Med* 2002; 21:51-5.
10. Ofondu EO. Cosmetic use of bleaching cream in Enugu. [*Nigerian FMCP dissertation*] National Postgraduate Medical College, Nigeria, 2003.
11. Ajose FOA. Consequences of skin bleaching in Nigerian men and women. *Int J Dermatol* 2005; 44(Suppl 1) 41-43
12. Nnorom IC, Igwe, JC, Oji-Nnorom CG. Trace metal contents of facial (make-up) cosmetics commonly used in Nigeria. *Afr. J Biotechnol* 2005; 4(10): 1133-8
13. Ofili AN. Eze EU, Onunu AN, Prevalence of use of Skin Lightening Agents Amongst University of Benin Undergraduates in Benin City, Nigeria. *Nigerian Medical Practitioner.* 2006; 49:24-7
14. Nnoruka E, Okoye O J Topical Steroid Abuse: its use as a depigmenting agent. *J. Natl Med Assoc* 2006; 98(6) 934-9

15. Olumide YM, Akinkugbe AO, Altraide Dan, Mohammed T, Ahamefule N, Ayanlowo S, Onyekonwu C, Essen N. Complications of chronic use of skin lightening cosmetics. *Int J Dermatol* 2008:47; 344-353.
16. Ayenomo JG, Yusuf AM, Adekunle AS, Makinde OW. Heavy metal exposure from Personal Care Products. *Bull Environ Contam Toxicol* 2009; 84(1): 8-14.
17. Olumide YM Editorial: Use of skin lightening creams. *British Medical Journal (BMJ)* 2010;341:c6102 (Published 23 November 2010)
18. Onwordi CT, Orizu CO, Wusu AD, Ogunwande 1A. Potentially toxic metals exposure from body creams sold in Lagos, Nigeria. *Researcher*, 2011; 3(1) http://www.sciencepub.net/researcher
19. Iyanda AA, Anetor John and Adeniyi FAA. Altered Copper lead and renal dysfunction in Nigeria women using skin-whitening agents. Jan 21, 2011 www.ncbi.nim.nih.gov/pubmed/21253890
20. Ayanlowo OO, Olumide YM, Akinkugbe AO, Ahamneze N. Photodamage on the background of chronic use of skin lightening cosmetics *Household and Personal Care Today* Health Issues-Skin Lightening (Peer reviewed article) n2/2012. pp22-24.
21. CNN documentary on Skin Lightening Cosmetics. http://edition.cnn.com/video/?/video/world/2013/10/09/pkg-duthiers-skinwhitening.cnn&on.cnn=1 Wednesday 9th Oct 2013. Interviewed by Vladimir Duthiers. Correspondent CNN.
22. Ekpunobi UE, Okonkwo EO, Udeh, CV, Ogbuagu AS, Duru CB, Determination of hydroquinone and mercury concentrations in some skin lightening lotions and creams sold in Southeastern Nigeria. *International Journal of Biotechnology Research* March 2014; 2(1) 011-16

Appendix 2

Federal Republic of Nigeria-Official Gazette. No 3, Vol 80

Extraordinary Reprint

Federal Republic of Nigeria Official Gazette

No. 3 Lagos-26th February, 1993 Vol. 80

Government Notice No. 3

The following is published as Supplement to this *Gazette* :-

Decree No.	*Short Title*	*Page*
1 5	National Agency for Food and Drug Administration Control Decree 1993	[illegible]
1 9	Drugs and Related Products (Registration, etc) Decree 1993	[illegible]

Printed and Published by The Federal Government Press, Lagos, Nigeria.

FGP 13/196/1,000

Annual Subscription from 1st January, 1991 is Local : ₦400.00 Overseas : ₦450.00 (Surface Mail) ₦600.00 (Second Class Air Mail). Present issue (Including Supplement) ₦50.00 per copy. Subscribers who wish to obtain *Gazette* after 1st January should apply to the Director, Federal Government Press, Lagos for amended Subscription.

Appendix 3
Administrative order completely banning Hydroquinone.

24/4/91

Dear Prof. Olumide

Compliments of the season!

Your request refers.

1. Hydroquinone: The position now is that the Fed. Min. of Health has banned the use of hydroquinone in all cosmetics (so-called bleaching creams). Previously 2% was permitted, but now it is completely banned. This is by the Administrative Order of the Hon. Min. The legal document is not yet out.

2. Tobacco products: The Decree on Tobacco & Smoking was promulgated last year. I have not yet got the document from the Ministry, and therefore, the details.

3. IRGASAN (= Proprietary name)
Generic Name = Triclosan

It is a bacteriostatic skin disinfectant used in soaps, creams, deodorants (etc cosmetic products) in concentrations of 0.5 – 2%.

There are no regulations governing its manuf, importation & sale in Nigeria, that I am aware of.

Dr. E.C. Chidomere

24/4/91

Appendix 4

Federal Republic of Nigeria-Official Gazette. No. 31c, Vol 82

Cosmetic Products Prohibition Regulation

Extraordinary

Federal Republic of Nigeria
Official Gazette

No. 31c	Lagos-29th December, 1995	Vol. 82

Government Notice No. 54c

The following is published as Supplement to this *Gazette* :

Printed and Published by The Federal Government Press, Lagos, Nigeria.
FGP 316 (95)/ 896 / 1,500 (OL 111)

Annual Subscription from 1st January, 1996 is Local ; ₦5,200.00 Overseas: ₦8,200 [Surface Mail] ₦10,200.00 [Second Class Air Mail]. Present issue ₦100.00 per copy. Subscribers who wish to obtain Gazette after 1st January should apply to the Federal Government Printer, Lagos for amended Subscription.

S. I. 20 of 1995

NATIONAL AGENCY FOR FOOD AND DRUG ADMINISTRATION AND CONTROL DECREE, 1993
(1993 No. 15)

COSMETIC PRODUCT (PROHIBITION OF BLEACHING AGENTS, ETC.) REGULATIONS, 1995

Commencement : 11th August, 1995

In exercise of the powers conferred on it by sections 5 and 29 of the National Agency for Food and Drug Administration and Control Decree 1993 and of all other powers enabling it in that behalf, the Governing Council of the National Agency for Food and Drug Administration, with the approval of the Minister of Health and Social Services, hereby makes the following Regulations -

Sale of adultrated cosmetics products.

1.-(1) No person shall sell or offer for sale any cosmetic product which is adulterated or which contains any substance which when used according to the directions on the label accompanying the cosmetic product is likely to cause injury to the health of the user.

(2) No person shall manufacture, sell, offer for sale, distribute or cause to be distributed any cosmetic product which contains any of the skin bleaching agents listed in the Schedule to these Regulations.

(3) A person who contravenes the provisions of paragraph (1) or (2) of this regulation is guilty of an offence and liable on conviction to a fine of ₦5,000 naira or imprisonment for a term of 6 months or to both such fine and imprisonment.

Meaning of adultrated cosmetic product.

2. A cosmetic product shall be regarded as adulterated if it -

(a) contains more than a trace of mercury or any mercury salt which under normal condition of manufacturing practice is unavoidable; or

(b) contains more than a trace of mercury or any mercury salt calculated as the metal or preservative; or

(c) contains hydroquinone; or

(d) bears or contains any poisonous or deleterious substance as to render it injurious to a user under the conditions prescribed in its labelling or under such conditions of use as are customary or usual for the cosmetic product; or

(e) has been prepared, packed or held under insanitary conditions thereby rendering it likely to be injurious to health; or

(f) the container in which it is packed is composed in whole or part of poisonous or deleterious substance which may render the contents injurious to health; or

(g) contains more than the permissible limit of an ingredient.

Citation. 3. These Regulations may be cited as the Cosmetic Products (Prohibition of Bleaching Agents, Etc.) Regulations, 1995.

SCHEDULE *Paragraph 1(2)*

SKIN BLEACHING AGENTS

1. Hydroquinone.
2. Corticosteroids
3. Mercury and Mercury Compounds.

MADE at Lagos the 16th day of August, 1995.

PROFESSOR G. E. OSUIDE,
Director-General
National Agency for Food and Drug Administration and Control

EXPLANATORY NOTE

(This note does not form part of the above Regulations but is intended to explain its effect)

The Regulations, among other things, prohibit the inclusion of skin bleaching agents in cosmetic products manufactured, sold or distributed in the Nigerian market and further specify the penalty for any person who contravenes any of the provisions.

Appendix 5

Feature Article on Hazardous Cosmetics by LUCY HANNAN. African Business May 1988

Feature: Hazardous cosmetics

Companies still make hazardous cosmetics for Africa

European safeguards have now outlawed the sale of certain hazardous cosmetics such as mercury soap and skin lighteners in European markets. But *AB* investigations have discovered that a number of European companies continue to manufacture these harmful products specifically for sale to African markets. *AB*'s LUCY HANNAN carried out on-the-spot inspections to see what is still on offer in the African marketplace and where it comes from.

Mercury-based soaps were banned in the EEC in 1976 because it had been discovered that absorption of mercuric iodine through the skin could cause renal deficiencies, miscarriages and skin damage.

Originally manufactured as an antiseptic product, mercury soaps have more recently found a new purpose: they are boiled down to make a cream which, if applied up to three or four times a day, has been adopted as a skin-lightening agent. The product is sold predominantly in West Africa and Zaire.

European manufacturers have managed to capitalise on the pigment-destroying ability of mercury and to transform the trade from a redundant medicated one to an extremely profitable cosmetic one.

It is a classic case of "dumping", with a particularly cynical twist in its tail. Manufacturers within the EEC are legitimately able to continue producing for export purposes only.

The notion of "lighter is better" in Africa is a complex one. In the late 1980s, a growing number of sophisticated young African men and women are abandoning this old idea, which has its roots in Africa's colonial past. But a still significant number of Africans continue to cling to the concept, so much so that they constitute an important market for these products.

The colonial association of lighter shades of skin with a high social and economic status is perpetuated through the effects of Western influence and through advertising which seeks to change perceptions of physical beauty and acceptability.

Apart from causing harm to consumers, foreign-manufactured mercury soaps also damage the domestic markets of the West African countries they plague. In a survey carried out in January in the Lagos markets, *AB* found that at least 90% of the total trade in skin lighteners were British-made.

Nigeria, in contrast to most other West African countries, has taken comparatively severe measures against the skin-lightening trade. All mercuric products were banned in 1982, and the level of hydroquinone (the legitimate pigment-destroying agent used in creams) was limited to 2%.

Nevertheless, most of the imported products found during a two-week survey broke the law, either in strength or in content – and vendors reported that they were in far greater demand than the legal products because their relative "effectiveness" is perceived as greater than that of the safe, domestically manufactured, government-regulated products.

It is a classic case of "dumping", with a cynical twist in its tail.

Preventing these illegal soaps from coming into the country has proved impossible for Nigeria over the last six years. Many of the brands find their way in through cross-border smuggling, which cannot be curbed without massive resources to mount a counter-policing operation and which some British distributors openly exploit to sell their products.

Philip Winner & Co of London, which distributes a 3% mercuric soap called Sukisa Bango, were delighted to hear that their soap had found its way into Nigeria and, in response to an enquiry about supplies to Lagos, proposed a regular transaction through the Republic of Benin.

During the January survey, the petty traders of Lagos were evidently unaware that their goods are illegal, and they unreservedly showed receipts that identified the suppliers. The source proved to be Balogun West, a major market on Lagos island, where whole streets are devoted to an exclusive stock of all available brands of mercury soaps and skin-lightening creams.

While *AB* was unable to determine who the actual importers are, the thriving success of the trade at Balogun West was evident. It was also evident that the operation is not on a small scale, as new stock constantly arrived in vans carrying "Government Licensed Imports" labels – suggesting that the smuggling and trading involves corruption at a high level.

A market flooded by foreign goods in this way encourages a consumer preference for imported products and has the additional effect of undermining the nascent domestic industries. Some entrepreneurs circumvent consumer demand by producing "Made in England" fakes, but the end result is a severely disadvantaged domestic market.

For all these reasons, many African government officials contend that the EEC must recognise the necessity of stopping *production* of any dangerous products at source, rather than leaving it to the importing countries to attempt to clear their markets through legislation.

British manufacturers prefer to maintain the position that it is "paternalistic" to take decisions on behalf of their foreign markets and that it must be up to the African governments to take any necessary measures to prevent importation of goods they believe are harmful.

When the Irish Development Authority (IDA) provided a £750,000 sterling ($1.4m) grant to expand **W & E Products'** mercury-soap operation in County Wicklow, it defended the decision by claiming that the

X

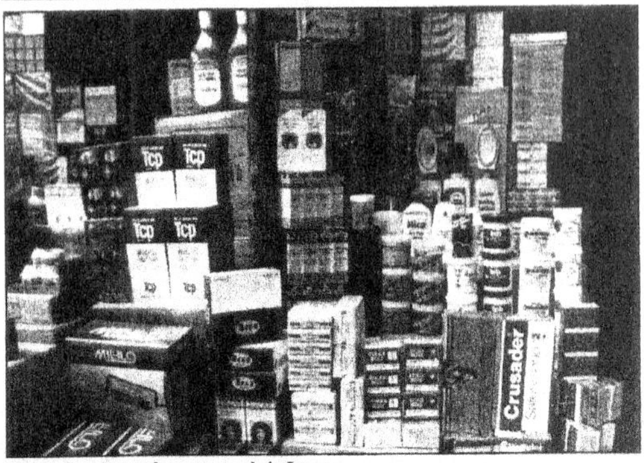

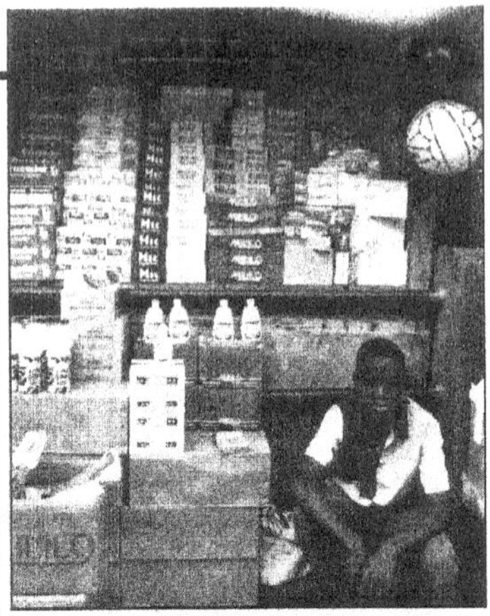

Skin lighteners and soaps on sale in Lagos.

IDA is "not in the business of making moral decisions for other countries".

Michael Tattersall, Financial Director of the main British factory of W & E Products, has, moreover, continued to insist, despite a public and parliamentary campaign to stop the trade, that the soaps are actually completely harmless – whether used according to the instructions on the packet (which carry a mandatory "poison" warning) or as a skin-lightener. According to Tattersall, mercuric soaps have been available in Africa for over 50 years, and "if there were any problems with it, they would have come to light by now."

UK Euro MP Michael Hindley, in whose constituency W & E Products operates, dismisses any excuse from the manufacturers for a trade which he says is evidently dangerous. Hindley claims, "Given the number of countries that have found it necessary to ban the soap, there is *ipso facto* enough evidence; even South Africa bans skin-lighteners, and South Africa is hardly known for protecting the interests of its black citizens."

Hindley has run a two-year campaign to stop production of the soap within the EEC and maintains that continued production is based on the notion that it is "perfectly acceptable to exploit other countries with dangerous products for as long as there is a market".

He points out that the economic and political situation in many of the African markets facilitates sales despite any appropriate legislation – and he has, in fact, produced samples of the soap found in British and Belgian markets. Their presence challenges the effectiveness of the EEC's own internal ban. Responding to Tattersall's remarks, Hindley contends that it is unrealistic to expect any consumer complaints to reach the factories when consumer-complaint facilities in Africa are so notoriously poor.

Yetunde Olumide, a dermatologist from the Lagos University Teaching Hospital, who has been researching the effects of mercuric soaps and skin-lighteners for the government, also dismisses Tattersall's claims. She charges that manufacturers are simply sheltering behind the difficulties all developing countries face when it comes to producing corroborative statistical and laboratory evidence.

Olumide describes herself as being "propelled into research . . . by the number of people who flood the clinic with hopelessly damaged and blistering skin". It is only the tip of the iceberg, she adds, as many people do not come to the clinic until the symptoms are far advanced.

> ***"Even South Africa bans skin-lighteners, and it is hardly known for protecting its black citizens."***

Different people, she explains, absorb different quantities of mercury when they use the soaps, but the permanent danger is that it accumulates in the body and eventually concentrates in the liver and kidneys.

In an interview in January, the doctor pointed to the economic strength of manufacturers which are able to continue to make profits in Nigeria even when their products have been banned, and she asserted that the trade realistically can be stopped only when it is destroyed at the root. "Banning the importation is not the panacea," she notes. "Stopping the production from the source is manifestly the solution."

The UK Department of Trade & Industry (DTI), which has justified its policy of *laissez-faire* as being "based on the principle that all countries are responsible for the health and safety of their own consumers", responded to pressure last year by asking the manufacturers to substantiate their defence that the product is completely harmless.

Although the DTI acknowledges that it has been receiving many complaints from African governments, the main political leverage against the factories appears to be domestic pressure concerning the effects of mercuric poisoning on the workforce.

A female worker who gave birth to a baby suffering from muscular spasms, stiffness and high muscle tone – all symptoms of heavy mercuric poisoning – has taken legal action which is now pending. The baby was found to have 10 times more mercury in his body than the amount tolerable for an adult.

Another woman working at W & E Products in the UK gave birth to a baby with no kidneys, who died at three months.

Both the BBC and *The Observer* of London drew attention to the controversy growing around mercury-soap production, which, along with the pressure from Hindley, forced the DTI to reconsider its position.

Then in February, as a result of the January survey in Lagos, Nigerian Health Minister Olikoye Ransome-Kuti announced a ban of 34 brands of British-manufactured mercuric soaps and skin lighteners and called on the exporting countries to "inform their industries that it is an offence to import into Nigeria any cosmetic products that contain mercury".

On 18 February the DTI wrote to the factories and told them to "stop exporting or supplying the products for exporting, or a prohibition notice will be served". ▶

The DTI explained that the move was made because of its "impatience" with manufacturers for their failure to produce any convincing evidence that their products are harmless.

The DTI cannot stop actual production, but under the Consumer Safety Act it has the power to prohibit supply for export as well as the home market "if evidence were to emerge that the soap containing mercury was causing problems in the importing countries". A spokesman from the DTI's Nigeria desk did suggest that it is "pretty irresponsible really to continue exporting a product that has been banned as dangerous in the EEC". In looking into the situation regarding W & E Products, the DTI discovered two other UK manufacturers. They are **International Generics** of Hove in Sussex, which stopped production in March, and **Shakespeare Soaps** of Manchester, which at the time of going to press had not responded. The DTI told *AB* it will serve a prohibition order on Shakespeare Soaps to halt production of the mercury-based soaps if the company does not comply with their instruction voluntarily.

It is, of course, by no means the end of the trade. W & E Products are simply moving production to their Irish branch in County Wicklow – and will in all probability profit from the closure of the other British factories.

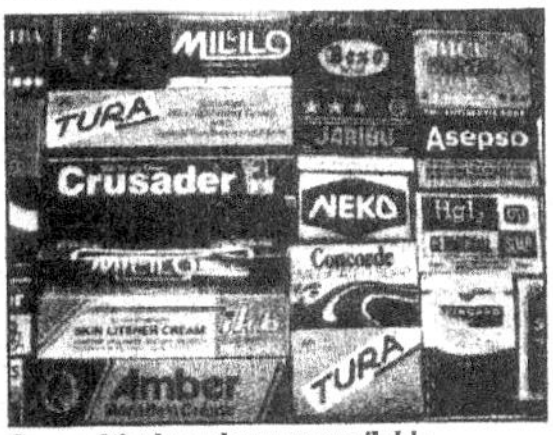

Some of the brand names available.

According to Tattersall, over 20 other factories within the EEC are producing mercuric soaps, and plenty of other countries are eager to get a share of a profitable market – estimated by those familiar with it to be worth £20m ($37m) a year for the Nigerian trade alone. He claimed that many of the brands are produced in the Far East and named Korea as one country that is eager to join the market.

In Lagos, the effect of the Health Minister's new crackdown has, ironically, been a dramatic upward surge in demand. Vendors of the banned products are reportedly buying up stock in the markets to sell later at inflated prices, and some have removed them from the shelves to make profitable under-the-counter deals.

One of the British manufacturers included in the ban, however, told *AB* that Minister Ransome-Kuti indeed "has their blessing".

Martal Cosmetics of London, which produces a range of skin-lightening creams called Symba, has been on the market for over 16 years and sells in the EEC as well as in Africa. Its content of hydroquinone is legitimate, at only 2%.

Their packaging clearly states: "This product complies with the Federal Government of Nigeria Health Directives 1987."

Many legitimate manufacturers and distributors have pointed out that the illegal 5% preparations on the market have been seriously undermining sales of products bearing the correct percentage.

Martal is now re-packaging its product according to the new requirements. The company recognises that ultimately it can only be good business to comply with government regulations – especially where health hazards are concerned.

Over the last decade, the legitimate manufacturers have seen a plethora of new and dangerous preparations introduced into Africa, and they state emphatically that they welcome any necessary measures African governments may take to clear a flooded, not to mention hazardous, market ■

Appendix 6

Newspaper cuttings reacting to the London BANDUNG TV programme

Soaps danger exposed

British firms sell banned skin cosmetics in Africa

COSMETIC products, banned in Europe, are causing skin cancer, death and aborted foetuses in Africa.

by RONNIE SMITH

Well-known British companies like Reckitt and Colman, makers of Robinson's Barley Water, are accused of exporting dangerous skin-lightening creams and medicated soaps in Channel 4's Bandung File, to be shown next Tuesday.

The programme, A Whiter Shade of Black, investigates the devastating results of the sale — both legal and illegal — of dangerous skin-lightening cosmetics to black people.

Sale of these products, which contain mercury and hydroquinone, is banned in Europe although their manufacture for export is not, despite evidence to suggest that workers making them can suffer miscarriages and their children suffer kidney failures.

Dr Yetunde Olumide, from the University Teaching Hospital in Nigeria, accuses the Common Market of "immorality" in allowing the manufacture of products which can cause irreversible skin damage.

The programme shows that the EC is itself funding their production.

Britain's biggest manufacturer, W & E Products, recently moved operation from Lancashire to Ireland — after complaints from the Nigerian government — and received funds from the Irish Development Authority, an EC-backed body.

Current EC rules on the amounts of both mercury and hydro-quinone are too high say contributors to the programme.

In strong sunlight the creams accelerate the destruction of pigment cells causing irreversible skin damage and increasing the risk of cancer.

In parts of Africa use of these creams and medicated soaps, whose mercury content can cause brain damage especially if the skin is broken, is reaching epidemic proportions.

Dr Olumide says that 90 per cent of the patients in her Lagos skin clinic suffer from the effects of mercury soaps.

Some of these products are openly on sale in Britain where the black population is being sucked into the US and South African mentality of thinking "lighter is better."

Some African countries have taken steps to ban these products but are unable to prevent them from being smuggled into their countries.

TELEVISION PREVIEWS

MAKING IT

Sunday 10.30-11.15 LWT

Mark Sanderson

She needs to lose a ton of weight and her Samantha Fox hair-do. Poor old Lorraine wants to be a dancer so much that to finance her career she works in the holidays as a greencoat on the Isle of Wight. But with 'wobbly thighs at 18' and *sequins* on her costume, Arlene Phillips, founder of Hot Gossip and one of the judges of the 1987 Cosmo/C&A Dance Award, doesn't reckon her chances. Milton Astley (20) from Rotherham drives a fork-lift truck during the day before slinking into a leotard at night. Another subsidises her art by working in MacDonalds; the lucky ones have a daddy who does lots and lots of overtime to pay his darling daughter's exorbitant training fees. Filmed at Sadler's Wells, this two-part documentary follows the fortunes of 47 aspiring hoofers. This week it's the turn of the contemporary crew; next week it's the turn of the ballet brigade and the final result. Because the interest is in who gets through and who doesn't it could just as well feature prospective members of the Groucho Club but you do pick up a few tips about fancy footwork. You can join in the talent-spotting too but most of the enjoyment comes from the comments of the judges (who include an unusually quiet Michael Clark): 'Look at that smile, she's got lockjaw'.

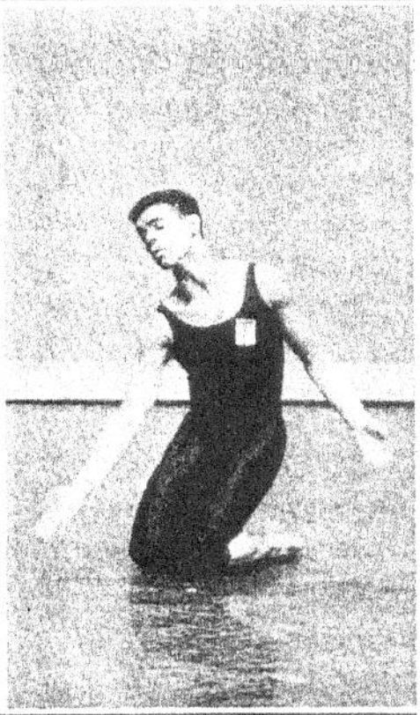

BANDUNG FILE

Tuesday 9.00-10.00 C4

Alkarim Jivani

Several decades after blacks declared themselves beautiful, there is a nagging feeling that beige is better. The most horrifying aspect is that it is blacks themselves who feel this and whites, surprise surprise, are more than willing to exploit that feeling. It is a sobering thought that although we can intellectually dismiss all the shit about whiter being nicer, emotionally some of us still want lighter skins. This thought-provoking report looks at the market in skin lightening soaps and creams — 16 different brands can be bought in Brixton alone. In one year the Nigerians got through £20m worth of the stuff and that's not counting the dozens of other African countries where it is sold. The cost is not paid in cash alone. Nor is it restricted to the silent shame that at some subliminal level we too feel that white skin is superior. The penalty is paid physically as well as in moral and financial terms. According to the medicos interviewed, the products cause your skin to become very dry, causing it to crack which allows the chemicals to enter the bloodstream where they cause untold damage. And that's not to mention the risk of skin cancer. The chief manufacturers of the products are British, some of whom are indirectly given grants by the EEC which, in another bitter irony, won't permit the sale of the same products in Europe. As one Nigerian doctor says in the programme: 'The preservation of human health is the collective responsibility of all nations. If the manufacturers in Britain cannot do anything to better the health of people in Africa at least they should not do anything to worsen the plight of Africans. It is totally immoral, totally unjustifiable to export these chemicals which have been banned in your countries to my people.' Quite.

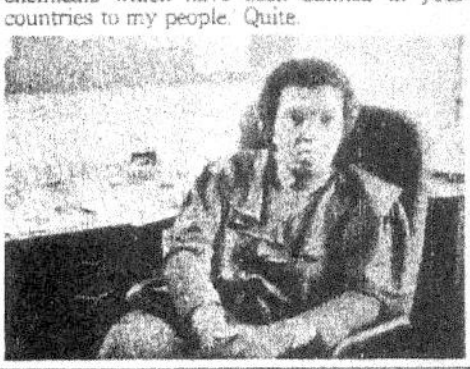

SCANNERS

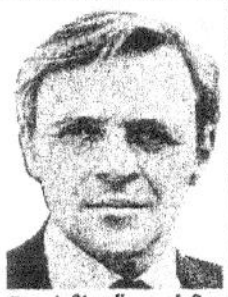

Great Storylines of Our Time. Aunty's daffodil division — BBC Wales — is making great play about the fact that Anthony Hopkins is returning to the valleys to do a great play. We-e-e-ll, as great a play as can be made out of a 'story of one man's conflict with the EEC agricultural policy'. No doubt a heroic tale full of wheat and beet signifying subsidy. Wait before you mock, though. After all would you have stuck a cigar in Sam's breastpocket if he'd come to you with a manuscript which involved two tramps waiting on stage for nothing to happen. This could be the best thing since 'How Green Was My Valley'. But we're not holding our breaths. Or indeed anything else.

Incontrovertible evidence that there is life after 'Brookside'. Simon O'Brien, aka Damian, fresh from braving crocs, bonds dealers and smashing his nose up on a desert island off the coast of Sri Lanka, is about to take on a job fraught with far more risks — as a compere on a kiddies' series for Aunty. Not quite the RSC, we know, but better than disappearing into a black hole somewhere in the vicinity of the Mersey Tunnel like all too many other escapees from the Close — not least the much missed Karen. Meanwhile if Terry was making a bid for a breakout with a bit part in 'Chelmsford 123' it clearly hasn't worked. Never mind Tel, we hear that they're auditioning moustaches for a remake of 'Viva Zapata'.

TELEVISIO

The Refug

Wednesday 11.00-

Don Perrett

The Refus

You could have knocked me do
verbial plume when I found ou
ity was being recommissioned.
was *so* bad, far worse in fact t
C4 sitcoms which got only one c
ing consigned to the great arc
that one was relieved by the th
volved would be spared any fur
ment. But no. Witness a secor
marks no improvement whatsc
decessor, a factor which damns
The shame of it is that in essen
is a great idea and sounds like t
C4 should be airing, a series ab
populated almost exclusively by
kind of right-on context that
make fun of without underm
premise. Something like 'The (
fact. Instead what we have is an
paper thin stereotypes, pop-up
who charge around delivering t
lines best reserved for a Brown

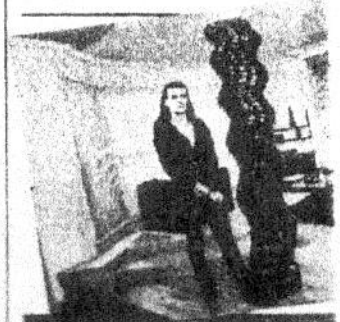

TELEVISION

Room For Cha

Thursday 7.30-8.00

Alkarim Jivani

Design Fo Living

Anyone who cannot go by a li
without glancing in for a quick
ghastliness within or, alternati
with envy, will find this c
watchable. The producer, Anne C

RADIO

RADIO RESEARCH

John Marshall

Is More Less?

The dearth of good research about radio has always hampered discussion of the medium. The lack of clear understanding about why and how audiences listen has created a general background to debate which relies on assertion and special-interest pleading rather than convincing analysis. A recent report from the Broadcasting Research Unit, commissioned by the Home Office, is therefore welcome not just because of its findings but because it indicates, at last, a desire to treat radio seriously.

The study — 'The Listener Speaks' by Steven Barnett and David Morrison — was an attempt to examine how radio is used at a time when the de-regulation and expansion of the radio system is being planned. Many of its findings confirm generally held views about the importance of radio: it concludes, for example, that 'Radio is an integral and highly valued part of people's lives, which frequently structures patterns of daily behaviour'. It also, predictably, found that people talk of radio in terms of it being 'genuine, typical, intimate and real'. This apparently contrasts with attitudes to television, with one interviewee stating, for example, that since his move from radio to TV, Terry Wogan had 'lost contact with the audience and the ordinary people'. While listening to radio was usually a 'secondary activity', the study found that many people structured their lives in order to catch favourite programmes and there were tales of factories interrupting production for Simon Bates' Our Tune and drivers sitting in their cars after arriving at a destination in order to listen to The Archers.

If forced to give up one of them, more people overall would miss television than radio. This is most true of listeners to Radio 1 (28 per cent for radio, 63 per cent for television) but is almost balanced in the case of Radio 4 (47 per cent for radio, 48 per cent for television). It was also found that station loyalty is not so entrenched as conventional wisdom suggests and that over the course of a week, a majority will listen to more than one station. This finding, the report suggests, 'means that the opportunities for new stations to detach listeners from their customary resting places may be more enhanced.'

Given that one aim of the study was to examine the background to de-regulation and the demand for new stations, it set out to find whether audiences actually wanted greater choice. Here it found that there was demand for new services as long as they didn't imply tinkering with the known and loved. In particular there was evidence of demand for more specialist music, especially big band, jazz and country.

The general problem with asking folk whether they want more and different radio is the need to compare the known and liked with the unknown. Satisfaction with radio is very high, much greater than for television, and so a fear of the unknown might be expected to show itself. As the report states, 'listening habits tend to be fairly entrenched and . . . four out of five listeners will listen to no more than two radio stations a week. The objects of their affection, which serves them well, are therefore jealously guarded.'

Much of the study's research deals with opinion across the board but in the two specialist groups it dealt with — ethnic minorities and Londoners — it found greater demand for new services than the average. If factories are

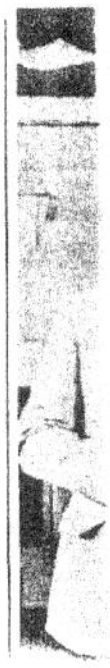

TV Mail

Dark side of a love affair

PETER PATERSON'S TELEVISION REVIEW

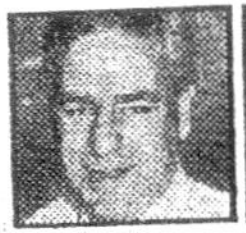

IN DEFIANCE of modern convention, and just as one was speculating that no-one nowadays could write The Hunchback of Notre Dame, or even Snow White and the Seven Dwarfs, without stirring protests, director Phil Young focused last night's play, **Crystal Clear** (BBC 1) firmly on a selfish, ruthless and disagreeable individual who happened to be visually handicapped or, as we used to say, blind.

Art dealer Richard (Anthony Allen) started the play with the sight of one eye intact, which made him king in his relationship with blind-from-birth Thomasina (Philomena McDonagh) — something pointed up when he deliberately echoed the title of Radio 4's programme for the handicapped by asking her: 'Do you take sugar?' He was, however, diabetic, and careless of the precautions he was required to take, so he crossed over from the world of the sighted to blindness.

Richard was not only negligent towards his health. He also treated his women with contempt, carrying on with Thomasina without disclosing that he was already heavily involved with (fully sighted) Jane (Vivienne Ritchie). Much of the action of the play showed his attempts to make a final break with Jane, and the change that came over his new affair with the loss of his sight.

Nothing in this uncomfortable drama was designed to provoke pity for Richard, a sarcastic, emotionally crippled and arrogant man, but his attempts to cope with complete blindness — scalding himself making the coffee, crawling around the floor of his room searching for things, his wretched cries of 'Oh God! Oh God!' — nevertheless had that effect.

The greatest tragedy was the discovery that far from her lifetime of blindness allowing her to cope with his affliction, Thomasina's strength and will seemed to evaporate as she struggled to end the relationship. And in the darkest scene in the play she explained the compounded misery of two blind people living together, neither able to help the other, finally bursting out: 'The only way for a blind girl is to be with someone sighted.'

If you managed to stay the whole distance with this melancholy morality play, with its defensible use of four-letter words and bleak view of human nature, you will have appreciated the emotionally battering performances of Allen, McDonagh and Ritchie. Director Young, having brought it to TV from the stage, made all the adjustments necessary without losing an ounce of its main ingredient, despair.

□ NOT the least of the ironies of the modern world is that while millions of white people lie out under the sun to make their skins darker, large numbers of dark-skinned people smother themselves in preparations they believe will make them lighter. Last night's **Bandung File** (C4) investigated these special soaps and skin lighteners, which provide lucrative, and sometimes illegal, export opportunities for British companies, some of them household — or household soap — names.

Horrific film from Nigeria showed the disfiguring rashes caused by chemicals in the skin lightening creams and compounds, while the mercury in the soaps can cause kidney failure, miscarriages and brain damage. Much closer to home, the Bandung team discovered that despite a ban on such preparations by the Common Market, 16 different brands can be bought in Brixton market.

TELEVISION

Misdirected passion

IT MAKES one feel an awful louse to be unmoved by a play in which a diabetic man falls in love with a blind girl and then goes blind himself. There was much despair in **Crystal Clear** (BBC-1), a play which, being created by improvisation under the direction of Phil Young, makes a good case for the usefulness of writers.

Being created by actors, it is full of acting, by which I mean there is a great deal of strong, showy emotion: hysterics, rage, bitterness, sobbing. "Sod the futon," gasps a harrowed actress at one stage, trying and failing to lug her boyfriend's bed across the floor. It was hard to tell whether it was meant to be funny or not. A little lower emotional pitch, and a higher awareness of character development and structure, might have made the play more genuinely affecting and would certainly have left fewer question marks at the end.

The play began with a first sexual encounter between diabetic Richard (Anthony Allen) and blind Thomasina (Philomena McDonagh). This scene should have been moving, but coming so early in the play, it was faintly embarrassing. One hadn't yet been properly introduced. Next came a girlfriend clearly on the way out who staged a big scene about the direction of the "relationship". Richard was evasive and passive, and there was the play's greatest flaw. It was hard to care about him.

The climax was another grand row in which Richard forced Thomasina into the shocking admission that she would like to see. I found this wholly unsurprising. I imagine all blind people would like to see. The rest of Thomasina's message I found less acceptable. It was that life was intolerable for the blind unless they lived with sighted people who could tell them whether their clothes matched or not. This is nonsense. Many blind people live happily alone. Some blind people are happily married to other blind people. Some have children. The aftertaste of "Crystal Clear" was not insight or compassion, but self-pity, negativism and a great deal of artistic self-indulgence.

After this, it was a pleasure to see a piece of television which had a clear direction, professional discipline and a strong point to make. **The Bandung File** (C4) looked at the cynical way in which British companies illegally exploit the absence of consumer protection in Africa by selling toxic skin lighteners which can cause permanent, irreversible skin damage and which, in the case of soaps containing mercury, are linked with foetal malformation, abortion and kidney damage. Nor is the trade confined to Africa. In Brixton the team found 16 different kinds of illegal soaps on sale.

The tragedy here is less the vast profits being made by the companies concerned, more the discontent and inferiority felt by millions of black women and men who long to have lighter skin. Colour prejudice is felt among blacks as well as between blacks and whites. Black magazines go for lighter skinned models. Blacks with lighter skins find it easier to get jobs. Here were uncomfortable issues well aired, and an excellent justification for minority programming.

Lesley Garner

D.T.

Watching Brief

Sandy Smithies

Bandung File (Channel 4, **9.0**). An insidious and profitable spin-off from racist attitudes is the huge market for skin-lightening products for black people. For many who use them, particularly in South Africa, skin-lighteners are used for pragmatic, not cosmetic reasons. The market raises moral issues — but on top of that there is an alarming medical aspect. Tonight's report presents evidence that skin-lightening soaps and creams are causing irreversible skin damage to thousands, increasing susceptibility to cancers; that they are responsible for kidney failure, brain damage and miscarriages, and that 40 per cent of black South African women are suffering from their effects. Many of these products, although banned by the EEC for sale in Europe, are being made in Britain for export to Africa — by companies which are household names here.

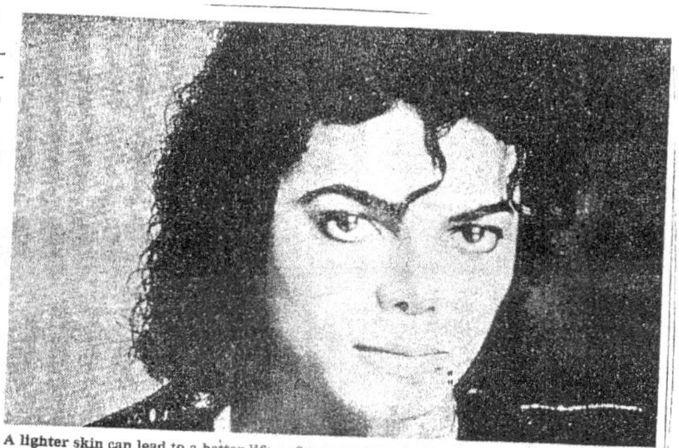

A lighter skin can lead to a better life — for some. But at what risk to health?

TUESDAY

Crystal Clear* (9.30-10.50pm, BBC1). Phil Young's improvised stage piece successfully transfers to television. The play is about a diabetic man (Anthony Allen) who loses the sight of one eye as well as his hard-bitten girlfriend. An affair with a blind woman (Philomena McDonagh) also appears to be for the chop as he becomes increasingly bitter about his plight and she perceives the harsh realities of a future life together, in which the blind will be leading the blind. Allen's manic-depressive performance is quite stunning, and McDonagh's portrayal of a sightless person entirely convincing.

Bandung File (9.00-10.00pm, C4). C4's magazine programme, aimed at ethnic groups, often boasts some of the most professional and comprehensive journalism on television. Tonight's programme contains a report on the horrifying effects of the skin-lightening creams and soaps which are used by those people who don't have the bank balance of Michael Jackson.

Appendix 7a

Toiletries and Cosmetics Manufacturers Group

OF THE MANUFACTURERS ASSOCIATION OF NIGERIA

1st National Awareness Seminar

THEME:

NIGERIA'S HEALTH & BODY-CARE UNDER SIEGE

At

Lagos Sheraton Hotel, Ikeja

On

Wednesday 23rd November, 1988

7b

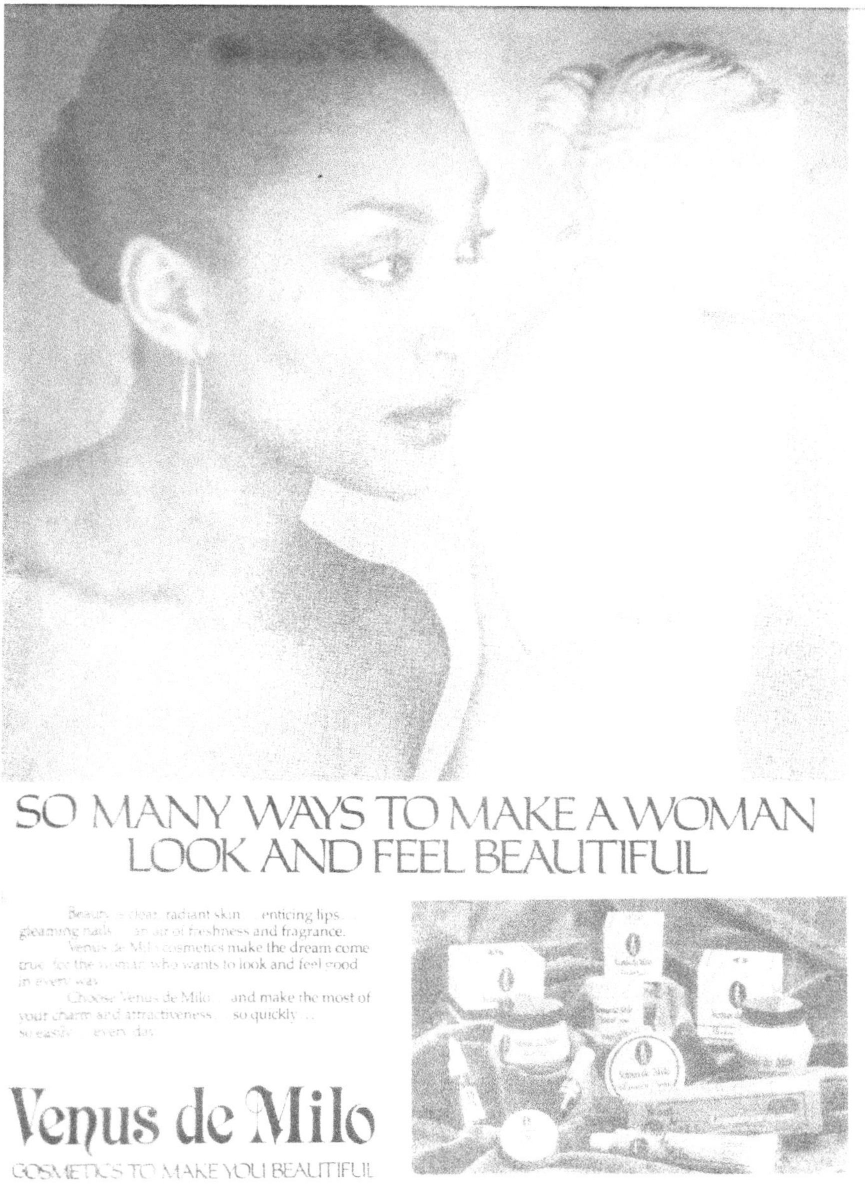
SO MANY WAYS TO MAKE A WOMAN LOOK AND FEEL BEAUTIFUL
Beauty is clear, radiant skin ... enticing lips ... gleaming nails ... an air of freshness and fragrance.
Venus de Milo cosmetics make the dream come true for the woman who wants to look and feel good in every way.
Choose Venus de Milo ... and make the most of your charm and attractiveness ... so quickly ... so easily ... every day.
Venus de Milo
COSMETICS TO MAKE YOU BEAUTIFUL

Appendix 8

List of some feature articles in the Nigeria Press on the skin bleaching culture in Nigeria

1. Tunde Alao. Staff Reporter. Lagosians and the bleaching scourge. THE GUARDIAN. Thursday, February 6, 2003 p 13.
2. Bleach perfect: Nigeria No. 1 for skin-bleaching products. June 22, 2012 ynaija.com/bleach-perfect-nigeria-no-1-for-skin-bleaching-products-says… 1 for skin-bleaching products says World Health Organisation. Doyin Jaiyesimi. The Punch.
3. Help! Nigerian women are killing themselves / National Mirror Nationalmirroronline.net/…/help-nigerian-women-are-killing-themselves/ Jun 27, 2012 – An array of bleaching cream in Nigerian market… Amid classification by the World Health Organization recently that Nigerian women are…
4. 9jatravel – Nigerian Women Lead the World in Skin Bleaching http://www.facebook.com/9jatravel/posts/422175034556421
5. Nigerian women lead in skin bleaching – WHO – Vanguard… www.vanguardngr.com/.../nigeria-women-lead-in-skin-bleaching-who/ June 3, 2013
6. Nigerian women Lead in Skin Bleaching – WHO – Fashion… www.nairaland.com/1312406/nigerian-women-lead-skin-bleaching/8 June 4, 2013
7. Interview by Aljazeera http://www.aljazeera.com/indepth/features/2013/04/201345148459
8. Lara Adejoro. What would make an older woman bleach? http://www.dailytimes.com.ng/article/what-would-make-older-wom..... Daily Times NG. Article May 10, 2014
9. Britni Danielle. Jan 20, 2014. Nigerian Singer Releases 'Whitenicious' Skin Lightening Cream and its sold out. http://www.xojane.com/issues
10. Kingsley "Rukus" Okafor. In: Britni Danielle. Jan 20, 2014. Nigerian Singer Releases 'Whitenicious' Skin Lightening Cream and its sold out. http://www.xojane.com/issues http://www.xojane.com/issues/nigerian-singer-releases-whitenicious
11. Jide Ojo. Nigeria as the world capital for skin bleaching http://www.punching.com/opinion/nigeria-as-the-world-capital-of-sk... March 26, 2014.
12. Danielle Kwateng. Nigerian Singer pushes Bleaching Products/Style Blazer http://styleblazer.com.ng/21109/denia-skin-bleaching/Jan 16,2014.
13. Gbenga Adebambo. Stop Bleaching Away Your Destiny I, II, III #Say No To Bleaching. *YOUTHMAGAZINE. THE GUARDIAN*. May 7, 14, 21. 2016.
14. Reuben Abati. The bleaching, chameleon crowd. The Guardian 29 July, 2016
15.

Appendix 9
The Marriage Laws in Nigeria

In Nigeria, there are basically three types of marriage recognized by the law. These are **statutory** marriage, **customary** marriage and **Islamic** marriage. Under civil law, Nigeria does not recognize polygamous unions. However, 12 out of the 36 Nigerian states recognize polygamous marriage as equivalent to monogamous marriage, as all twelve are governed by Sharia law. Polygamous unions are recognized by customary law in Nigeria, providing a handful of benefits for those in polygamous unions ranging from inheritance rights to child custody.[1]

The present Nigerian criminal justice system is part of Nigeria's inheritance from colonial Britain. Bigamy is a statutory offence under the statutory marriage. "Bigamy" is an act described as a crime under the Criminal Code Act in Nigeria. It is the act of contracting or entering into any other form of marriage with another person while a valid statutory marriage (marriage under the law) subsists. Surprisingly, bigamy in most laws in Africa is an act of criminal offence.

The law of Bigamy States:

"Any person who having a husband or wife living, marries in any case in which such marriage is void by reason of its taking place during the life time of such husband or wife, is guilty of a felony and is liable to imprisonment for seven years."

As of 2009, there has yet to be any debate of introducing a measure that would allow for civil polygamous marriages to be recognized within the entire country of Nigeria, letting the legislation play out on a state-by-state basis rather than introducing a nationwide measure.

There are no requirements based on religion in the North, therefore Christians are legally allowed to form polygamous unions just as Muslims may do. Christian church leaders such as Archbishop Peter Akinola of the Anglican Church of Nigeria have condemmed the practice of polygamy by Christians, with Akinola going on to write "The observation [of polygamy] will destroy our witness if not firmly addressed. We cannot claim to be a bible-believing church and yet be selective in our obedience.[2] Reports of Nigerian Mormons practicing polygamy have also surfaced.[3]

Lagos State, which has Nigeria's most populous city, Lagos, has silently amended the Lagos State Criminal Code and expunged bigamy from its statutes.[4] The state Attorney General and Commissioner for Justice, Mr Adeola Ipaye, confirmed the development, saying the old law was no longer useful. He said "bigamy was expunged from the amended criminal code. It was necessitated by the need to decriminalize it. What this means is that it is no longer a criminal offence when a man or woman who is legally married to contract another marriage. Instead, the marriage remains null and void. The argument for the expulsion of bigamy was premised on the fact no single person has been convicted in respect of the crime in decades.

The old Criminal Code of Lagos state Cap C17, section 370 stated: "Any person who having a husband or a wife living, marries in any case in which such marriage is void by reason of its taking place during the life of such husband or wife is guilty of a felony and is liable to imprisonment for seven years."

Decriminalizing bigamy means that a person charged with bigamy in Lagos State may escape conviction, if he or she is able to prove that the first marriage has been dissolved or that the first spouse has died or that the first spouse has not been seen for a space of seven years.
Some Reactions to the decriminalization of bigamy in Lagos State.

- "The regulation of monogamous marriages is governed by the Marriage Act, a **Federal law** and it is still an offence under Section 39 of the marriage Act. And, the law still applies to Lagos".
- "This is the most stupid law making I have ever seen. If one man is allowed more than one wife at the same time, are women allowed to legally marry and sleep with 2 or 3 men at the same time?

- "Lagos State Govt. lacked the power to grant a criminal of a **federal** offence a waiver. Therefore, this so-called amendment is an exercise in futility"

Furthermore, there are clear well defined Legal requirements of marriage under Nigeria's marriage Act.[5] Once the parties satisfy the Registrar that there is no impediment to their marriage, the Registrar will issue them with the certificate to marry. On receipt of the certificate, the parties can celebrate their marriage in a church **duly licensed** for the celebration of statutory marriages or in a marriage registry. Section 22 of the marriage Act forbids a minister of religion to celebrate any marriage until the parties have delivered to him the Registrar's certificate or a special license from the governor under section 13. Section 43 imposes a maximum penalty of five years imprisonment for performing a marriage in defiance of the Act.

The sanctity of marriage is crucial to the moral fabric of every society. The Nigerian Marriage Act has clearly attempted to provide very solid benchmarks and requirements that would ensure that the very essence and sanctity of marriage is not violated or trampled upon. In doing this, the marriage Act is invariable protecting the moral sanctity of the Nigerian society.

References

1. "Nigeria" Genderindex.org. Retrieved 21 November 2014. https://en.wikipedia.org/wiki/Polygamy_in_Nigeria
2. Liberty Sugar. "Polygamy makes a Mocker of Christians." *POPSUGAR love & Sex*. Retrieved 21 November 2014.
3. "How Nigerian marmons started practicing Polygamy in Nigeria." *Yeyeolade. Wordpress.com*. Retrieved 21 November 2014.
4. The legal Requirements of marriage under Nigeria's marriage Act.

http://thelawyerschronicle.com/the-legal-requirements-of-marriage-under-nigerias-marriage-act/

5. Davidson Iriekpen and Jaiyeola Andrews. In Lagos, Bigamy is No Longer a Crime. http://www.thisdaylive.com/articles/in-lagos-bigamy-is-no-longer-a-crime/105094/
6. Ferdinard Olufemi. Decriminalisation of Bigamy in Lagos State And Its Legal Implications. http://topeadebayollp.wordpress.com/2012/02/15/decriminalisation-of-bigamy-in-lagos-state-and-its-legal-implications/

Appendix 10

Polygamy in Sub-Saharan societies

Sub-Saharan societies are highly polygamous, with over 40% of wives living in polygamous unions[1]. Polygamy creates a situation where many women are competing for the attention and favour of one man in the home.

"We are all competing for mates, and we do whatever we can to give ourselves an advantage over the next person." (Lewis et al –Tanzania)

"In predominantly Muslim Senegal, where polygamy is prevalent, rival wives lighten their skin to compete for their husbands favour". (Dr Pierre–Andre Aka).

Increasingly, single motherhood is becoming the norm as Nigerian women are content to just having a child for a married man. Africa is entering a new social environment. African men seek self-reliant women who can raise children largely on their own. Increasingly, African women are supporting themselves and their children through work in service economy–with its emphasis on charm and visual presentation. The circumstances of life are now promoting rather than hindering the aesthetic preference for lighter-skinned women.

The prevalence for polygamous union in Africa may even be higher because

1. We are told the muslim culture permits polygamous unions.
2. Marriage contracted through customary law does not forbid polygamy.
3. The Law on "Bigamy" has been rendered irrelevant in the African society.

Although the Christian faith permits only marriage between one man and one woman; and the Civil law permits only marriage between one man and one woman, African men have found a way to circumvent this restriction. Church goers (not necessarily, Christians) who want to cover themselves with a veneer of "western" civilization or Christianity, marry one wife in the church and/or through the Civil Law (Statutory marriage), but keep many women as concubines or undocumented wives outside the matrimonial home.

However, the legal wife remains powerless except she is ready to divorce the bigamous man. This she can only do if she is adequately empowered to take care of herself and her children. Furthermore, while acts of adultery in a man in some Western countries may be serious enough to pull down a government, in Africa, the shameless man may even show off his numerous wives and concubines as a sign of 'virility' even in his old age! Also, in Africa, the culture puts a **burden** on the women to marry and to bear children. This is a major contributory factor that leads the women to dehumanizing body modification practices like skin bleaching to make them competitive in the marriage market. (See the sections on THE MARRIAGE PRESSURE)

Reference

1. Frost P. Polygamy and sex ratios. *Encyclopedia of Birth Control*, ed by V.L. Bullough, Santa Babara (Cal): ABC – CLIO, pp. 218-23.
2. Lewis KM, Harris S, Camp C, KALala W et al, the historical and cultural influences of skin bleaching in Tanzania. In: The Melanin Millennium: Skin color as 21st Century International Discourse. Publisher Spinger Netherlands 2013pp 19-38.
3. Aka Pierre-Andre. In: Penangnini Toure. Skin bleaching on rise in Africa. *The Toronto Star.* 10 March, 1997. *http://www.biyokulule.com/view_content.php?articleid=5534*

Appendix 11
Bigamy in Nigeria

Bigamy in Africa (generally) is a reality and not just a myth. Many a times we found out that most people in marriage advertently or inadvertently contracted a bigamous marriage. Surprisingly, bigamy in most laws in Africa is an act of criminal offence. In Nigeria in particular, various national Laws made it a criminal offence punishable with various jail terms. Yet the practice persists, in that majority of those in the so-called polygamous marriages have committed the crime of bigamy but, the long arm of the law never catches up with them.

The act of bigamy has been variously defined, but it means the act of legally marrying more than one wife at a time or the act of legally marrying more than one husband at a time. (See the section on MARRIAGE LAWS OF NIGERIA). Therefore, basically it is an offence that can be committed by both spouses to a marriage. However, this act of bigamy in Nigeria and indeed other parts of Africa is committed exclusively by men. There have been no cases recorded and unrecorded of incidents of bigamy involving women as culprits. The act of committing bigamy in Africa has been solely an all-male affair.

There are various reasons why the law on bigamy has remained largely ineffective. The position of our national laws will also be looked into and remedies will be proffered on how to make this law effective and absolutely functional.

Our world (Africa) has been derogatively called a *third world* because of some of the things that obtain in our society and the rampant occurrence of bigamy can be identified as one of the practices that hurls a pail of disgust on us. Making our societies more conducive would entail the complete eradication of some of our traditional practices that are harmful and unjust to a section or a group of our society. This will definitely make our society more civil and amenable to the needs of individual members of each society. The problem besetting us right here in Africa is indeed multi-facet and grappling with each of these problems often results to volatile issues being touched off. This rampant occurrence of the offence of bigamy comes with a religious and cultural undertone, this account for its state of inertia and it has turned it into a moribund law.

Now we have to make a distinction between bigamy and polygamy. We must acknowledge here that due to cultural and religious leaning, polygamy has become an everyday affair in Africa; people now view it as our normal way of life without blinking an eyelid. This has been carried over to bigamy because people do not know where polygamy stops and where bigamy starts and as a result all is muddled up.

Polygamy is divided into two, namely polygyny and polyandry. Unlike bigamy which involves the practice of both human sexes, polygyny is an act whereby a man marries simultaneously more than one wife. Polyandry in the same vein is an act whereby a woman marries simultaneously more than one husband. Unlike in Statutory Law, in Islamic and Cultural Laws, polygyny is permissible and the practice thrives in those spheres. Polyandry is not allowed by these laws and like bigamy to civil law, it is abominable in the sight of these laws. From the above short definition of polygamy, it is quite evident that the type of polygamy allowed by Islamic and Cultural Laws is the one that is favourable to men and unjust to women. The aspect of polygamy that is favourable to women and unjust to men is decreed an abomination and is thrown into the gutter.

Chambers Dictionary also defines polygamy as "the state or custom of having more than one wife or husband at the same time". Going by this definition of Chambers Dictionary, there is no difference between polygamy and bigamy, it is all an act of marrying more than one wife or husband simultaneously. In Britain and most Western world, a marriage contracted by two consenting adults without any impediment as to affinity or other impediments to a valid marriage, is deemed legally binding. But in Nigeria, the case is not the same; there are three types of marriages obtainable, the Islamic marriage, cultural marriage and statutory marriage. All these marriages are legally binding to whoever contracts it.

However, Islamic law and customary law allow polygamy while statutory law prohibits polygamy and sanctioned it with the offence of bigamy. **Therefore, for one to commit the offence of bigamy in Nigeria, such a person must have married twice simultaneously under statutory law or must have married simultaneously once under Islamic and Customary law and once under Statutory law.** This is where the issue of **legality** comes in, in any definition of bigamy. A man can marry as many as four wives under Islamic law and has not committed any act of bigamy. Four wives is the limit placed by Islamic laws on the number of wives a man can marry. However, there is no sanction that awaits anybody who violates this limit and marries as many as twenty or more. It is a religious law whose sanction awaits any violator in the life after death. Also, in Customary law, there is no limit placed on the number of wives a man can have, so under Customary law, a man can marry as many as forty wives without having committed any crime known as bigamy. Therefore, the need arises to distinguish such Customary and Islamic marriages by adding the word *legal* in the definition of bigamy. **Besides, customary and Islamic marriages are not registered, therefore, there is no written or documented evidence to show that such marriages ever occurred.**

There is no doubt that such chaotic state of our marriage laws has contributed immensely towards the ineffectiveness of the law of bigamy in Nigeria.

Reference

Bigamy in Nigeria.
http://www.okeyeni.com/2012/08/law-journal-003-bigamy-in-nigeria-part-1.html

Appendix 12

List of banned products in Kenya

Some Corticosteroid creams and other bleaching products containing harmful substances (2009 Whiter Skin.com)

Corticosteroid creams misused as skin-lightening products

BETNOVATE
MEDIVEN
DIPROSONE
NERISONE
DERMOVATE
HYDROCORTISONE

Creams containing Benzoyl peroxide usually used to treat acne (pimples) but skin lightening products

OXY 5 AND OXY 10

Skin Lightening Creams Containing Hydroquinone:

JARIBU CREAM
MEKAKO CREAM
AMIRA CREAM
TURA SKIN TONING CREAM
YESAKO MEDICATED BEAUTY CREAM
RICO COMPLEXION CREAM
MADONNA MEDICATED CREAM
MREMBO MEDICATED BEAUTY CREAM
SHIRLEY CREAM
KISS -MEDICATED BEAUTY CREAM
UNO21 CREAM
PRINCESS PATRA LUXURY COMPLEXION CREAM
ZARINA MEDICATED SKIN LIGHTENER CREAM
ENVI SKIN TONER
VIVA SUPER LEMON
AMBI SPECIAL COMPLEXION CREAM
LOLANE CREAM
NADINOLA CREAM
GLOTONE COMPLEXION CREAM
NINDOLA CREAM
CLAIRE CREME MIC SKIN LIGHTENER CREAM
TONIGHT NIGHT BEAUTY CREAM
FULANI CREME ECLAIRCISSANTE
CLERE LEMON CREAM
CLERE EXTRA CREAM
BINTI JAMBO CREAM
BUTONE CREAM
MALAIKA MEDICATED BEAUTY CREAM
DEAR HEART WITH HYDROQUINONE CREAM
MIKI BEAUTY CREAM
CRUSADER SKIN TONING CREAM
NISH MEDICATED CREAM
ISLAND BEAUTY SKIN FADE CREAM
MALIBU MEDICATED CREAM
PALMER'S SKIN SUCCESS FADE CREAM
CARE PLUS FAIRNESS CREAM
TOPICLEAR CREAM
CAREKAKO MEDICATED CREAM
BODY CLEAR CREAM
A3 SKIN LIGHTENING CREAM
AMBI AMERICAN FORMULA
DREAM SUCCESSFUL
SYMBA CREME SKIN LITE 'N' SMOOTH
Ikb MEDICATED CREAM
CLEARTONE SKIN TONING CREAM
CLEAR ESSENCE MEDICATED FADE CREAM
AMBI EXTRA COMPLEXION CREAM FOR MEN
CLEARTONE EXTRA SKIN TONING CREAM
O'NYIA SKIN CRÈME
A3 TRIPPLE ACTION CREAM PEARL LIGHT
ELEGANCE SKIN LIGHTENING CREAM
MR. CLERE CREAM
FAIRLADY SKIN LIGHTENING CREAM
FADE OUT CREAM
TOP LEMON PLUS CREAM
CLEAR TOUCH CREAM
CRUSADER ULTRA BRAND CREAM
ULTIME SKIN LIGHTENING CREAM
RICO SKIN TONE CRÈME
BARAKA SKIN LIGHTENING CREAM
PEAU CLAIRE CRÈME ECLAIRCISSANTE
PRINCESS MEDICATED BEAUTY CREAM
IMMEDIAT CLAIRE LIGHTENING BODY CREAM
SOFT AND BEAUTIFUL CREAM00
LEMONVATE CREAM
SECRET GEL
TCB GEL PLUS
UNIC CLEAR SUPER CREAM
TOPIFRAM CREAM
SKIN BALANCE LEMON CREAM
PEAU CLAIRE GEL PLUS
DARK & LOVELY GEL
DERMO -GEL PLUS
PEAU CLAIRE CREAM

FASHION FAIR GEL PLUS
HOT PROSONE GEL
SKIN BALANCE CREAM WRINKLE REMOVER
DARK & LOVELY CREAM
VISIBLE DIFFERENCE GEL
SIVOCLAIR CREAM
ACTION DEMOVATE CREAM
REGGE LEMON GEL
ULTIMATE LADY GEL
TOPIFRAM GEL PLUS
AGE RENEWAL CREAM
FAIR & WHITE GEL PLUS
PEAU CLAIR GEL PLUS
FASHION FAIR CREAM
FIRST CLASS LADY CREAM
SKIN SUCCESS CREAM
NEU CLEAR CREAM PLUS
JARIBU BETA - β CREAM
BODY TREAT CREAM SPOT REMOVER
CLAIR & LOVELY GEL
PEAU CLAIR CREAM
SOFT & BEAUTIFUL GEL
ACTION DEMOVATE GEL PLUS
PROSONE GEL
SKIN BALANCE GEL WRINKLE REMOVER
ULTRA-GEL PLUS
PRO-ONE GEL MCA
BETALEMON CREAM

Skin Lightening Body Oils Containing Hydroquinone:

PEAU CLAIRE LIGHTENING BODY OIL
SOAPS CONTAINING HYDROQUINONE
M.G.C. EXTRA CLEAR
TOPICLEAR BEAUTY COMPLEXION SOAP
LADY CLAIRE
BLACKSTAR
AMIRA
ULTRA CLEAR
BODY CLEAR MEDICATED ANTISEPTIC SOAP
IMMEDIATE CLAIRE LIGHTENING BEAUTY SOAP
CHERIE CLAIRE BODY BEAUTY LIGHTENING & TREATING SOAP

Soaps Containing Mercury and its Compounds:

MOVATE
MEKAKO
JARIBU
TURA
ACURA
RICO
FAIR LADY
ELEGANCE
MIKI
JAMBO

Skin Lightening Lotions Containing Hydroquinone:

JARIBU SKIN LIGHTENING LOTION
AMIRA SKIN LIGHTENING LOTION
A3 CLEARTOUCH COMPLEXION LOTION
A3 LEMON SKIN LIGHTENING LOTION
KISS LOTION
RICO SKIN LIGHTENING LOTION
PRINCESS LOTION
PEAU CLAIRE BEAUTY BODY LOTION
CLEAR TOUCH LOTION
FAIR & WHITE BODY CLEARING MILK
SIVOCLAIR LIGHTENING BODY LOTION
EXTRA CLAIR LIGHTENING BODY LOTION
PRECIEUX TREATMENT BEAUTY LOTION
CLEAR ESSENCE SKIN BEAUTYFYING MILK

Skin Lightening Gels Containing Hydroquinone:

ULTRA CLEAR
TOPICLEAR
BODY CLEAR

Skin Lightening Creams Containing Mercury and its Compounds:

PIMPLEX MEDICATED CREAM
NEW SHIRLEY MEDICATED CREAM

Cream Preparations Containing Hydrogen Peroxide (H_2O_2):

JOLEN CREAM

Skin Preparations Containing Steroids:

MOVATE CREAM
SKIN SUCCESS GEL
HOT MOVATE GEL
AMIRA -C
NEU CLEAR GEL
TENOVATE
BODY CLEAR CREAM SPOT REMOVER
TOP GEL PLUS

Appendix 13

Diagnosis of Mercury Intoxication

A medical history, including an environmental history, a complete physical examination, plus results of mercury measurement in human tissue can exclude or substantiate the diagnosis of mercury intoxication. It is important to handle the collection and analysis of urine and blood mercury tests carefully.[1]

Urine levels reflect the acute exposure situation better than blood and much better than hair levels.

Organic Mercury Methylmercury should be measured in blood or hair. In the general population usually the mercury level in hair is 1 part per million or less.[1]

Clinical Signs and Symptoms—Acute Intoxication

Acute intoxication causes symptoms, depending on the exposure pathway, such as bronchitis, pneumonia, gastroenteritis with blood in the feces, leading to disorders of kidney function. If the history including the environmental history, clinical picture, and mercury levels in urine are concordant, the diagnosis of acute mercury intoxication can be made.[2]

The symptoms of chronic mercury intoxication in childhood are as follows:

- **Cerebellar and psychological, vegetative signs:** Muscular hypotonia followed by refusing to walk, stand, or sit, disturbed, negative behavior, apathy, loss of appetite, weight loss, nightly sleeping disorders, sleepiness during the day, tremor, ataxia, coordination problems, excessive salivation, metallic taste, increased sweating, severe itchiness, increased blood pressure, tachycardia, light sensitivity, slowly increasing process over weeks.
- **Skin symptoms:** Symmetrical erythema of the nose, hand, and feet, mainly distal, volar and plantar (acrodynia), in cold surroundings more cyanotic and wet, transient, urticaria-like, morbiliform or rubeoliform exanthema, urticaria rubra (scarlatiniform, little pustules), lamellar desquamation of hands and feet.
- **More neurological symptoms of teenagers:** Tremor, dysarthria, paresthesia, ataxia, change of personality, erethism, loss of memory,

depression, loss of ability to see colors, concentric narrowing of visual field, unspecific symptoms, such as lack of energy, tiredness, loss of appetite, weight loss, dizziness, headache, concentration problems, sleep disorders.

Measurement of Mercury in Other Body Fluids
Under specific circumstances, it may be important to collect samples other than urine, blood, or hair.

Breast Milk Methylmercury and inorganic mercury are present in human breast milk

Feces are rarely used to establish the diagnosis of pediatric mercury exposures.[3,4,5,6,7] Methylmercury is mainly excreted in feces and therefore this measurement reflects the burden of methylmercury.

Nails In most epidemiologic and exposure studies, mercury exposure is assessed by analysis of hair, blood, or urine. However, nail analyses have been extensively used to assess body burdens of metals, often in the context of nutritional epidemiology

Environmental Monitoring
Monitoring the environment for mercury indicates the extent of external mercury exposure for children. Media used for environmental monitoring include the following[8,9,10]

- **Air:** Mercury can be analyzed in air, either with personal mercury vapor samplers, which are analyzed latterly using atomic absorption spectrometry, or with passive diffuse samplers. Mobile analyzers, such as, eg, the Lumex, can measure elemental mercury in air continuously.
- **Food:** Mercury can be analyzed in food and other biota. The analysis of mercury in fish is common. Speciation is essential to determine the amount of methylmercury.
- **Soil and sediments:** Mercury can be monitored in soil and sediments. It is important to ensure a proper sampling protocol. Total mercury and methylmercury can be determined.
- **Water:** Mercury can be monitored in water. It is important that the sample is representative and that sample containers are free of mercury contamination.

Environmental Guidelines

Guidelines for water, air, and soil have been set nationally and internationally. International guidelines for air, water, soil and food are as follows:

Air

The World Health Organization guideline value for inorganic mercury vapor is 1 $\mu g/m^3$ as an annual average.[11] A tolerable concentration is 0.2 $\mu g/m^3$ for long-term inhalation exposure to elemental mercury vapor, and a tolerable intake of total mercury is 2 $\mu g/kg$ body weight per day.[12]

Fish

Food and Agriculture Organization/World Health Organization Codex Alimentarius—Commission guideline levels for methylmercury in fish 0.5 mg/kg for predatory fish (such as shark, swordfish, tuna, pike and others) is 1 mg/kg.[13]

Food

For methylmercury, the Joint Food and Agriculture Organization/World Health Organization Expert Committee on Food Additives (JECFA) set in 2004 a tolerable weekly intake of 1.6 $\mu g/kg$ body weight per week to protect the developing fetus from neurotoxic effects.[14] JEFCA[15] confirmed this provisional tolerable weekly intake level, taking into account that adults might not be as sensitive as the developing fetus, in 2003 (JECFA/61/SC http://www.who.int/ipcs/food/jecfa/summaries/en/summary_61.pdf) and 2006 (JECFA/67/SC http://www.who.int/ipcs/food/jecfa/summaries/summary67.pdf).[16,17]

Soil

United Nations Environment Programme Global Mercury Assessment quotes for soil, preliminary critical limits to prevent ecological effects due to mercury in organic soils with 0.07-0.3 mg/kg for the total mercury content in soil.[8]

Water

The WHO guideline value is 1 $\mu g/L$ for total mercury.[18]

Preventing Mercury-Related Human Health Effects
Because mercury is hazardous to children's health, attention needs to be drawn to prevention.

Preventing Mercury Exposure
Food Advisory Children ingest mercury mainly due to the consumption of methylmercury in carnivorous fish.

Hygiene and Behaviors Children should not live close to mercury emissions, such as gold mining areas. Separation of housing and mining is essential. Children should not work as miners or in any other way with immediate contact to mercury. Children should not play with liquid mercury.

Cultural Practices Children should not use skin lightening creams because they contain mercury. Traditional medicine, such as Ayuvedic medicine, that contains mercury and other toxic metals should not be given to children.

In the Medical Domain Mercury should be removed from medical devices if possible. Because electronic thermometers may be available and are easier and safer to use, the unnecessary risk of mercury-containing thermometers should be avoided. In dentistry, non-mercury-containing composite is preferable.

Broken Bulbs There are some suggested ways to prevent exposure to mercury through broken bulbs. The US Environmental Protection Agency web site lists actions to reduce exposure when a compact fluorescent light bulb breaks,

World Health Organization Recommendations National, regional, and global actions, both immediate and long term, are needed to reduce or eliminate releases of mercury and its compounds to the environment. The WHO has committed to work with the health sector and national, regional, and global health partners in these efforts.[19]

World Health Organization Recommendations to Reduce Mercury Exposure

Reduce mercury exposure

—Eliminate the use of mercury wherever possible

—Promote the development of alternatives to the use of mercury

Elimination of mercury-related diseases requires strategic action to

—Conduct national assessments of mercury usage and disposal and implement educational activities for the health, environment, and other sectors.

—Promote the use of mercury-free alternatives, eg, for manometers and thermometers, and ensure that mercury-containing devices are taken back by the manufacturer or properly disposed of.

—Develop mercury cleanup and waste-handling, storage, and safe-handling procedures; promote environmentally sound management of health-related waste-containing mercury (as set out in the UN, Basel convention on the control of trans-boundary movements of hazardous wastes and their disposal).

—Encourage countries to develop and implement policies and legislation on mercury; highlight the role of the health sector in dealing with mercury-containing material, health-care waste, and emission reduction; and promote effective ways to control mercury emissions from cremation.

—Encourage international agencies to work with manufacturers, wholesalers, and retailers to develop and make widely available inexpensive mercury-free products and facilitate their procurement.

—Assist countries in preparing advice for pregnant and lactating women and children, about the risks and benefits of fish consumption, indicating the type of fish that may be eaten and how often. WHO strongly recommends breastfeeding because the presence of methylmercury in breast milk is not sufficient to outweigh its benefits.

—Identify traditional practices, folk medicines, and cosmetics involving mercury and disseminate information on mercury hazards, exposure prevention, and how to clean up spillages.

—Promote long-term monitoring (including biological measurements of exposure) and programs to reduce occupational exposure.

Education The protection of children's health depends on members of the family and community, as well as on local, regional, national, and international bodies. Childhood exposure to elemental mercury often accrues due to inappropriate handling and cleanup. Health education and policy initiatives are needed as primary prevention.[20] The WHO has provided good examples of how to protect children.[21]

References

1. LR, Shannon MW. Committee on Environmental Health, American Academy of Pediatrics. Technical report: mercury in the environment: implications for pediatricians. *Pediatrics.* 2001; 108:197–205.
2. Von Muhlendahl KE. [cited 2010 12th of May];Paediatric guideline mercury. 2004 Available at:
http://www.gpaev.de/typo/fileadmin/user_upload/GPA/dateien_indiziert/Leitlinien/umw_Leitlinie_Quecksilber.pdf.
3. Pichichero ME, Gentile A, Giglio N, Umido V, Clarkson T, Cernichiari E, et al. Mercury levels in newborns and infants after receipt of thimerosal-containing vaccines. *Pediatrics.* 2008; 121:e208–14.
4. U.S. Environmental Protection Agency Mercury Study. *Report to Congress.* 1997; Volume IV: An Assessment of Exposure to Mercury in the United States
5. Bjorkman L, Sandborgh-Englund G, Ekstrand J. Mercury in saliva and feces after removal of amalgam fillings. *Toxicol Appl Pharmacol.* 1997; 144:156–62.
6. Engqvist A, Colmsjo A, Skare I. Speciation of mercury excreted in feces from individuals with amalgam fillings. *Arch Environ Health.* 1998; 53:205–13.
7. Ishihara N. Excretion of methyl mercury in human feces. *Arch Environ Health.* 2000; 55:44–7.
8. Drasch G, Horvat M, Stoeppler M. Mercury. In: Merian E, Anke M, Ihnat M, Stoeppler M, editors. Elements and their compounds in the environment. *Wiley-VHC Verlag; Weinheim, Germany:* 2004. pp. 931–1005.
9. United Nations Environment Programme-Chemicals. Global Mercury Assessment. Geneva: 2002. Available at: http://www.unep.org/gc/gc22/Document/UNEP-GC22-INF3.pdf.
10. United Nations Environment Programme - Chemicals. Toolkit for Identification and Quantification of Mercury Releases. Geneva: 2005. pp. 1–275.
11. World Health Organization. Air Quality Guidelines, global update 2005. *WHO; Copenhagen:* 2006.
12. Risher JF. The Concise International Chemical Assessment Document Series. World Health Organization; Geneva: 2003. Elemental Mercury and inorganic compounds: human health aspects. Available at: http://www.who.int/ipcs/publications/cicad/en/cicad50.pdf.
13. General C. Standard for contaminants and toxins in foods—CODEX STAN 1993-1995. FAO; 2007. Rev 3-2007.
14. Joint FAO/WHO Expert Committee on Food Additives. In: Evaluation of certain food additives and contaminants. World Health Organization, editor. WHO; Geneva: 2004. (Technical Report Series).
15. Joint FAO/WHO Expert Committee on Food Additives. Evaluation of certain food additives and contaminants. Geneva: 2007. (Technical Report Series). http://whqlibdoc.who.int/trs/
16. Joint FAO/WHO Expert Committee on food additives. In: Summary and conclusions. Jecfa, editor. FAO/WHO; 2006.
17. Joint FAO/WHO Expert Committee on food additives. In: Summary and conclusions. Jecfa, editor. FAO/WHO; 2003.
18. World Health Organization . In: Guidelines for Drinking-water Quality. 3rd ed. World Health Organization, editor. WHO; Geneva: 2004. pp. 1–515. p. 1-515.
19. World Health Organization. Exposure to mercury: A major public health concern. WHO, Public Health and Environment; Geneva: [cited 2010 July]. 2007. Available at: http://www.who.int/phe/news/Mercury-flyer.pdf.

20. Lee R, Middleton D, Caldwell K, Dearwent S, Jones S, Lewis B, et al. A review of events that expose children to elemental mercury in the United States. *Environ Health Perspect.* 2009; 117:871–8.

21. Boese-O'Reilly S, Shimkin MKE. Taking action to protect children from environmental hazards. In: Pronczuk-Garbino J, editor. Children's health and the environment - a global perspective. WHO press; Geneva: 2005. pp. 253–72.

Appendix 14

How to Naturally Whiten Skin at Home

How to Lighten Skin Tone in A Cost Effective Way

Skin lightening or whitening is probably the most searched term on the internet when we talk about beauty. People from all walks of life, from Asia to America, men and women, all want to know how they can significantly whiten their skin without burning holes in their pockets. Indeed, tons of so-called best skin whitening products are out on the market, all of which promise a fairer more radiant skin tone. However, not all of these products claiming to whiten your skin can really lighten and improve the color of your skin. Most of them are also priced incredibly expensive but there are some priced affordable; you only need to be patient as whitening with the help of these products takes time.

If you want to even out your skin tone, make it lighter in color as well as more radiantly glowing, remove marks brought about by acne and other skin conditions, all at a price you could truly afford, there are some skin whitening products you can make at home at a price you could truly afford. If you are tired of using those skin lightening serums or gels that whiten your skin but burdens your pocket at the same time, try these simple home skin whitening tips without burning holes in your pockets. These tips are also applicable for consumers with limited budget on hand who cannot afford to purchase some of the best skin lightening products known to mankind.

Homemade Best Skin Lightening Products

You don't actually need to go to your favorite drugstore and buy couple of solutions to mimic artificial skin whiteners. All listed below are natural skin whiteners known to effectively lighten the skin with very little to no side effects at all depending on your skin type and sensitivity to the ingredients. The ingredients you will see here can all be found in your kitchen, refrigerator or grocery items. To achieve best results, it is advised to apply these natural skin lightening mask concoctions and body washes regularly with three to four days interval. If you can include them as a part of your everyday routine, the better it is. You can likewise apply these whitening masks once or twice a day depending on your needs as well as desires.

How to Naturally Whiten Skin at Home

Three Methods: Using Natural Lighteners; Changing Habits for Brighter Skin; Knowing What to Avoid

If you'd like your skin to be paler, using natural items can lighten it a few shades without the harsh side effects that come with chemical whitening products. The simple practice of staying out of the sun will also keep your skin from getting darker. There's no magic potion that will lighten your skin more than a shade or two, so keep your expectations realistic — and most importantly, remember that dark skin is beautiful too.

Method 1:

Apply a lemon juice solution. Lemon juice has been used for thousands of years as a natural skin lightener. It contains acids that lightly bleach the skin and exfoliate the top layer of darker skin cells. Since pure lemon juice can be irritating to skin, make a lemon juice solution by mixing one part lemon juice to one part water. Take a cotton ball and spread the solution on your skin. Let it sit for 15 minutes, then wash it off with warm water.

- Limit your application of lemon juice solution to just two to three times per week. Applying it more often could lead to skin irritation. Apply a moisturizer after rinsing off the lemon juice because the juice can dry out your skin.
- You should begin to see results after three to four weeks of using the solution several times per week. While lemon juice doesn't provide instant lightening effects, it's the most effective natural solution available.
- Use caution if you ever attempt to put any kind of citrus juice on your face. Phytophotodermatitis can be caused by a reaction photosynthesizing chemicals found in citrus fruits.[1] While it's fine to

use lemon juice on your skin, you need to wash it off thoroughly before going out in the sun[2]

Try a lemon milk soak. For a soothing full-body lightening treatment, start by drawing a bath of warm water. Pour in a cup of full-fat milk and squeeze the juice of an entire lemon into the tub. Swirl the mixture around so that the milk and lemon are evenly distributed in the tub. Soak in the bath for 20 minutes, then rinse yourself off with clean water.

- The milk in this soak has enzymes that gently lighten the skin. It also moisturizes the skin, offsetting the drying properties of the lemon juice.
- Try a milk soak once a week, and you should see results after a month or so

Make a yogurt honey mask. Like milk, yogurt contains enzymes that can gently lighten skin. Honey has moisturizing and antibacterial properties. Together, the two ingredients make a nourishing mask. Mix one part honey and one part yogurt, then spread the mixture on your face and body. Allow it to sit for 15 minutes, then rinse it away with warm water.

- Be sure to use plain, unsweetened yogurt. Sugary or flavored yogurt will get too sticky.
- In place of honey, try mashing up an avocado or using aloe instead. Both ingredients have a wonderful moisturizing effect.

Try a lightening paste. For more concentrated benefits, try making a thick paste using natural ingredients that help lighten the skin. Spread a paste on your freshly washed face, leave it in place for 15 minutes, then rinse it away with warm water. Here are two recipes for natural lightening pastes:

- Gram flour paste. Pour ¼ cup of gram flour into a bowl. Add enough lemon juice or milk to make a thick paste.
- Turmeric paste. Pour 1 tablespoon of turmeric into a bowl. Add enough lemon juice or milk to make a thick paste.

Milky Honey and Almond Face Mask

- 1 teaspoon milk powder of your choice
- 1 teaspoon of natural honey
- 1 teaspoon of fresh lemon juice
- 1 teaspoon of almond oil

Method 2: Changing Habits for Brighter Skin

Exfoliate your skin. The buildup of dead skin cells on the surface of your skin can make the skin appear a little dull. To brighten your skin, it's important to exfoliate regularly. One excellent way to exfoliate the skin is to use a body scrub composed of sugar or salt. In the bath or shower, wet your skin and rub the scrub in a gentle circular motion over your entire body. In this way you can "polish" your skin until it has a healthy gleam.

- To exfoliate your face, use a gentler facial scrub. Ground up oatmeal or almonds have good exfoliating properties that won't damage your fragile facial skin.
- Using a dry brush to brush the dead skin cells from your body is another good exfoliating method Find a brush made from natural fibers, and brush your body before you get into the bath or shower.

Keep it moisturized. Keeping your skin moisturized will prevent dead skin cells from building up and sloughing off so quickly. For brighter skin, use a daily moisturizer after you get out of the bath or shower. Choose a creamy moisturizer that doesn't contain alcohol, since alcohol can actually dry out your skin.

- Coconut oil is another great moisturizer that keeps skin looking glowing and youthful. Spread coconut oil on your arms and legs after getting out of the shower. Wait ten minutes for it to absorb into your skin before you put your clothes on.
- Jojoba oil also has moisturizing properties and is great for the skin. Olive oil or almond oil can also work wonders.

Limit your sun exposure. It's hard to stay out of the sun every day, but exposure to the sun darkens your skin. You don't have to stay cooped up inside, though — just spend some time preparing your skin for sun exposure before you go out for the day. To keep your skin from getting too tanned, take the following measures:

- Use sunscreen with a high SPF. 30 SPF or higher is best, since lower SPF sunscreen still allows the sun's rays to tan your skin. Reapply it throughout the day as necessary.
- Wear a wide-brimmed hat. This will keep the sun out of your face and off of your neck and shoulders.
- Wear long-sleeved shirts and long pants. During the summer, choose cool, swishy fabrics so you won't get too hot.

- Be careful not to stay out of the sun completely. Your body depends on some sun exposure to produce vitamin D, which is essential to bone health and other vital functions.

Method 3: Knowing What to Avoid

Never use bleach or other dangerous chemicals on your skin. There are a few dangerous myths going around regarding using bleach, ammonia, and other household cleaning products on your skin to try to lighten it. These chemicals are extremely harmful to skin, and they can do long-term damage. Damaged skin actually looks darker, so using these chemicals will end up doing the opposite of what you want. Avoid them.

Don't buy into false beauty standards. No matter what your skin color might be, it's beautiful just the way it is. It's fine to use safe items like lemon juice to lighten your skin a little, but don't seek to completely change your skin color from its natural state. Instead of trying to have a different skin color, accept yourself for who you are. If you were born with dark skin, embrace your beauty, and don't let anyone tell you to change.

- Many women across the world hold themselves to beauty standards that prize light skin over darker skin. Many other women go to great lengths to get darker skin, paying for tanning beds and risking skin cancer to get a few shades darker. Doesn't make a lot of sense, does it?
- When it comes to having beautiful skin, the most important thing you can do is keep your skin healthy. It's your body's largest organ, and it deserves a high level of care. Eat well, stay hydrated, and exfoliate and moisturize your skin to keep it looking vibrant and healthy.

Tips

- You can also apply tomato puree on your face and leave it for 20 minutes.

- Do not avoid the sun completely. Sunlight has harmful ultraviolet waves, but it also helps the body make Vitamin D.
- Applying this mixture every alternate night can dramatically lighten your skin tone. Do not forget to completely protect your skin from

direct sun exposure during the day to prevent further darkening of skin.
- Drink lots of water! Wear sun block.
- Apply a paste of apple cider vinegar and wheat flour twice a week. It will surely help to lighten your skin

Warnings

- Individuals with sensitive skin should be careful not to use too much lemon juice, as it can be drying.

References

http://shikenan.tumblr.com/post/21789635149/how-to-lighten-skin-to...
http://www.wikihow.com/Naturally-Whiten-Skin-at-Home...

Some natural skin care remedies to maintain natural skin tone

We live in under harsh environmental conditions with adverse effects on our skin. Consequently, the need to care for skin in order to reduce these effects will always be there. Below are some natural skin care remedies you can adopt to maintain your natural skin tone without necessarily resorting to bleaching which leaves you with permanent damages.

- **Use Yoghurt**: A by-product of milk containing lactic acids, yoghurt has essential ingredients with less bleaching properties suitable for all skin types. Tip 1: To apply it, gently rub plain yogurt onto your skin, wait for a few minutes and wash it off with lukewarm water.
- **Try Honey**: Having antibacterial properties, honey helps to fade age spots and acne scars. It also acts as a moisturizing agent. Tip 1: Once every day, you can apply pure honey to your face, leave it on for a few minutes and then wash it off with lukewarm water. This will help remove dead skin cells, and make your skin appear brighter and fresher than before.
- Tip 2: A second option is to mix a half-tablespoon of the honey with a tablespoon of fresh yogurt and apply the mixture on your face and neck. Leave it for 10 to 15 minutes and wash. Doing this daily to improve your skin tone and complexion. Tip 3: Alternatively, you can make a with it by combining one teaspoon each of honey and lemon juice, one tablespoon of powdered milk, and one-half teaspoon of almond oil. Then apply the mixture gently on the skin.

Leave it on for 10 to15 minutes and then wash it off with cold water. Do this every other day.

- **Lemons**: High in vitamin C, lemons encourage the regrowth of cells and have natural bleaching agents due to the acidic properties, as well as antioxidants in them which is good for evening out skin tone. Note that due to its acidic content, lemons can cause pain in open wounds. Tip 1: Add a bit of lemon juice and some oatmeal to yogurt to make a thick paste, and apply it as a face mask to keep your skin supple and moisturised. Tip 2: You can simply squeeze the lemon juice on a cotton ball and apply directly to your face too.
- Cut the lemon and apply the juice directly to your face. Leave it on for at least an hour and wash with water. If you do this daily, you will do away with and prevent scars on your face. Tip 3: Mix three teaspoons of lemon juice and one teaspoon of turmeric powder or tomato juice to make a paste. The paste can also be applied on the skin and left for half an hour before washing with water. Do this once daily. Tip 4: Alternatively, you can mix together one teaspoon each of lemon juice, powdered milk and honey and apply it on your skin. Wash after 15 to 20 minutes and rinse. Do this daily or every other day for better results.
- **Aloe Vera** is also good: It alleviates hyperpigmentation, which is the main cause of uneven skin tone, and restores the skin's original color. The cooling effect of aloe vera also helps to regenerate new cells and rebuild damaged tissue, which is important for healthy skin. This simple remedy using aloe vera gel can lighten dark spots and improve your overall skin complexion.
- Tip1: Cut the outer layers of an aloe vera leaf and Squeeze out the thick, jelly-like substance. Apply the gel thoroughly on your skin. Leave it on for about 30 minutes, and then wash it off with water. Do this at least twice daily for two weeks. Tip 2: Make a paste by combining two tablespoons of orange juice and a pinch of powdered turmeric. Apply the paste on your face and neck before going to bed. You can also apply it on your hands and legs. Wash it off the next morning.
- **Take Oranges**: The most important ingredient in skin care is vitamin C, which you can get in abundance from oranges. It has been found that regular consumption of fresh orange juice can greatly improve the overall texture of your skin as well as its suppleness.

Tip1: Make a paste by combining two tablespoons of orange juice and a pinch of powdered turmeric. Apply the paste on your face and neck before going to bed. You can also apply it on your hands and legs. Wash it off the next morning. Do this daily. Tip2: Grind dried orange peels into powder. Mix one tablespoon of the powdered peels with one tablespoon of plain yogurt to make a paste.

- **And Garam Flour**: It is one of the best ingredients for people who wish to lighten their skin complexion. It contains various nutrients that help keep your skin very healthy. Using the remedy below every other day will help remove excess oil from your skin while retaining your skin's natural moisture. Tip1: Mix some garam flour with a small amount of water or rose water to make a thick paste. Apply it on your face, hands, and legs. Leave it on until the paste dries. Then wash it off with water.

http://www.top10homeremedies.com/how-to/lighten-skin-naturally.html

http://www.top10homeremedies.com/kitchen-ingredients/honey-benefits.html

http://www.top10homeremedies.com/home-remedies-for-black-spots-on-face.html

Appendix 15

SOME LITERATURE REVIEW

SKIN BLEACHING IN AFRICA: AN OVERVIEW

Although several studies surrounding its dangers have surfaced in the past couple decades, skin bleaching is still very prevalent in the Western and Central region of Africa. Existing studies on the topic discuss the usage rates, side effects, and motives for bleaching in the regions. Using a chronological approach, the following literature review comprises a sample of works on topics dealing with the practice of skin bleaching.

In **Tenderheaded: A Comb-Bending Collection of Hair Stories,**[1] Pamela Johnson recalls during a trip to Africa how skin bleaching products are sold heavily in the black market in nations where they are prohibited. Johnson uses the term of "aesthetic assimilation" to describe the need for Africans to bleach to be more acceptable to former colonizers.

A. Mahé[2] did a study using a randomly selected sample of 368 Senegalese women and 452 other Senegalese women who actually practice skin bleaching. In the random sample, it was found that 52% of the women bleached their skin, and 92% of the women in the 425 person sample applied products to their entire body every day for a median period of four years. He also collected statistical data concerning the chemicals in the bleaching products and physical side effects.

Robert Baran's **Textbook of Cosmetic Dermatology**[3] discusses exogenous ochronosis, which is a difficult to treat thickening of the skin. Baran suggests that it is more prevalent among those who use products containing hydroquinone, which is a chemical found in many inexpensive skin bleaching products. **An Imperfect Fit: Advanced Democracy and Human Nature**[4] by Vít Klemeš introduces the skin bleaching culture of Senegal, in which skin bleaching is commonly known as "xessal." Klemeš also states that skin bleaching is a "nightmare" for African dermatologists, as the products make the skin extremely susceptible to damage.

Lynnea Stephen states the approximated percentage of women skin bleaching in the Central African nation of Mali and the rest of the region in **The black tax: Skin tone and social stratification in the United States.**[5] Stephen also discusses the side effects of skin bleaching products, particularly cheaper products (which are the types most people in the region use).

Sylvia Arthur's "Dying to Be White"[6] is an article which gives an in-depth look at the skin bleaching craze in the nation of Ghana. Arthur notes the huge profits companies make in selling the products, which are usually banned in Europe, to Africans desperately in need of lighter skin. Also mentioned is the time and dedication many Africans put into bleaching their skin, some taking up to many hours a day.

Racism in the 21st Century: An Empirical Analysis of Skin Color[7] by Ronald E. Hall discusses how the tone of one's skin color has developed to be the new discriminating factor as opposed to race in the 21st Century. Specifically, Hall discusses talks he had with women in African nations who have bleached themselves or know of others who bleach. Additionally, Hall discusses steps some African nations have taken to limit the popularity of its use.

Melanie Miyanji de Souza, MD[8] writes an article that gives a very comprehensive look at skin bleaching in Africa. Souza discusses plausible reasons for why some Africans feel lighter skin is more desirable, the rapid growth of skin bleaching amongst the population, the side effects, and the desired response from the international medical community.

In **A Princess Found: An American Family, an African Chiefdom, and the Daughter Who Connected Them All**,[9] Sarah Culberson details the viability of skin bleaching products. Culberson discovers that in Sierra Leone, many request skin bleaching products shipped from abroad as gifts. Culberson also talks about side effects she witnessed in skin bleachers such as puffiness and excessive blemishes. Hugh L.J. Makin's Steroid Analysis[10] examines the dangers of corticosteroid usage. This is relevant to the topic of skin bleaching because corticosteroids such as hydrocortisone are paired with agents like hydroquinone to create inexpensive bleaching products. Makin states that women in Sub-Saharan Africa who use skin bleaching products containing corticosteroids risk harm not only to themselves but their unborn children.

The review shows that there have been many thorough and informative studies on the background, popularity, and dangers of skin bleaching in Central and Western Africa. However, with the exception of Souza's 2008 article, there are not enough tangible solutions provided to reduce the percentage of people using these dangerous products. This study not only provides a critical analysis, it also aims to present more feasible suggestions in efforts to end the epidemic of skin bleaching in the regions.

References

1. Johnson Pamela. *Tenderheaded: a Comb-bending Collection of Hair Stories*. New York: Pocket. 2001.
2. Mahé A. "Skin Diseases Associated with the Cosmetic Use of Bleaching Products in Women from Dakar, Senegal." *US National Library of Medicine. National Institutes of Health*. Retrieved 2003, on 06 October 2011 fromhttp://www.ncbi.nlm.nih.gov/pubmed/12653741.
3. Baran Robert *Textbook of Cosmetic Dermatology*. London: Martin Dunitz. 1998.
4. Klemes Vít. *An Imperfect Fit: Advanced Democracy and Human Nature*. Victoria B.C: Trafford. 2004.
5. Stephen, Lynnéa Yuvella. *The Black Tax: Skin Tone and Social Stratification in the United States*. Berkeley, CA: University of California - Berkeley. 2007.

6. Arthur, Sylvia (2008). "Dying to Be White." *Clutch Magazine*. Sutton New Media LLC. Retrieved on 05 October 2011 from http://www.clutchmagonline.com/2008/01/dying-to-be-white/
7. Hall, Ronald E. *Racism in the 21st Century: An Empirical Analysis of Skin Color*. New York: Springer. 2008.
8. De Souza, Melanie M. "The Concept of Skin Bleaching in Africa and Its Devastating Health Implications." *US National Library of Medicine*. National Institutes of Health. Retrieved on 2008 11 October 2011 from http://www.ncbi.nlm.nih.gov/pubmed/18280901.
9. Culberson, Sarah. *A Princess Found: an American Family, an African Chiefdom, and the Daughter Who Connected Them All*. New York: St. Martin's.2010.
10. Makin H LJ. *Steroid Analysis*. Dordrecht: Springer. 2010.

INDEX

I

J

K

L

S

STORY HIGHLIGHTS

Chapter 2
The Invention of Racism

Biblical Christianity debunking the ideology of racial superiority

www.ingramcontent.com/pod-product-compliance
Lightning Source LLC
LaVergne TN
LVHW052011200926
848481LV00005B/1465
* 9 7 8 9 9 5 6 7 6 3 5 6 6 *